Winter Sports Medicine

CONTEMPORARY EXERCISE AND SPORTS MEDICINE SERIES
ALLAN J. RYAN, M.D., Editor-in-Chief

Winter Sports Medicine

MURRAY JOSEPH CASEY, M.D., M.S., M.B.A.
Editor-in-Chief

CARL FOSTER, M.Ed., Ph.D.
Associate Editor
(Skating; Basic and Applied Sports Science)

EDWARD G. HIXSON, M.D.
Associate Editor
(Skiing; Sliding; Climbing, Trekking, and Winter Camping)

CONTEMPORARY EXERCISE AND SPORTS MEDICINE SERIES
ALLAN J. RYAN, M.D., Editor-in-Chief

 F. A. DAVIS COMPANY • Philadelphia

Last digit indicates print number: 10 9 8 7 6 5 4 3 2 1

NOTE: As new scientific information becomes available through basic and clinical research, recommended treatments and drug therapies undergo changes. The author(s) and publisher have done everything possible to make this book accurate, up-to-date, and in accord with accepted standards at the time of publication. However, the reader is advised always to check product information (package inserts) for changes and new information regarding dose and contraindications before administering any drug. Caution is especially urged when using new or infrequently ordered drugs.

Library of Congress Cataloging-in-Publication Data

Winter sports medicine.

    (Contemporary exercise and sports medicine series)
    Includes bibliographies and index.
    1. Winter sports—Physiological aspects. 2. Winter sports—Accidents and injuries. 3. Sports medicine. I. Casey, Murray Joseph. II. Foster, Carl. III. Hixson, edward G. IV. Series. [DNLM: 1. Cold Climate. 2. Sports Medicine. QT 260 W787]
RC1220.W55W56 1990   617.1′027   89-11682
ISBN 0-8036-1683-X

The editors of this book, dedicate their work

To our families

And to our students and the participants in winter sports, the staffs
and researchers who make this book worthwhile.

Preface

The uneasy relationship between the so-called winter sports and other sports dates back to the fact that in the first quarter of the 20th century the snow sports were practically confined to the Scandinavian countries. The Nordic Games, which included Nordic skiing, ski jumping, and bandy (a variety of ice hockey), were held every 4 years from 1901 to 1917 and in 1922 and 1926. The annual Holmenkollen Week in Norway began in the 19th century. Ice skating had a long history as a recreational sport in Holland and Scotland, where the first skating club was founded in Edinburgh in 1642.

Figure skating was the first sport to hold European and world championships. Fancy skating, as it was called, became possible only after 1850, when steel blades were introduced by Bushnell, an American inventor. Then ballet master Jackson Haines, also an American, went to Vienna in 1864 and began to teach ballet classes on ice. This was the foundation of modern figure skating. His Canadian pupil, Louis Rubinstein, became the first world champion at St. Petersburg, Russia, in 1890.

Although Baron Pierre de Coubertin opposed the introduction of winter sports when he revived the Olympic Games in 1896 as "too divisive," figure skating was introduced to the London Games just 12 years later in 1908, and competitions in ice hockey were introduced at the Antwerp Games of 1920. The Chamonix International Winter Sports Week of 1924 was recognized retrospectively in 1926 as the first Olympic Winter Games. It was specified in the charter, however, that although the Olympic Winter Games "are subject to all rules of the Olympic protocol, the prizes, medals and diplomas must be different from those of the Olympic Summer Games, and the term Olympiad shall not be used in this connection."

The Second Olympic Winter Games marked the beginning of a new field of medicine. Thirty-three physicians meeting in St. Moritz during the 1928 games initiated the formation of the Association Internationale Medico-Sportive. This group subsequently became the Federation International Medico-Sportive, which now consists of worldwide membership from 70 national associations. Meetings such as the Annual Lake Placid Sports Medicine Conference and the knowledge and expertise displayed in the chapters assembled in this book owe much to these beginnings.

As this volume demonstrates, sports medicine today is a multidisciplinary field. Although physicians continue to be leaders of the therapeutic team, it is the work of coaches, exercise physiologists, nutritionists, psychologists, experts in kinesiology and biomechanics, equipment manufacturers, and the athletes themselves, collaborating in the field and laboratory research, that brings greater safety and higher levels of performance to winter sports. The importance of these efforts is great for competitive athletes but even greater in terms of numbers and needs for the many thousands who participate in recreational winter sports.

ALLAN J. RYAN, M.D.

Acknowledgments

We acknowledge the help of Anne Marie Borenstein, staff assistant, Department of Family Practice, Albany Medical College; Mary Margaret Newsome, head, Department of Education, US Olympic Committee; and Barbara Keator, executive secretary for Medical Services Lake Placid Olympic Organizing Committee and now for the Olympic Regional Development Authority; and we thank them. We thank our staffs—Joan Glans, Lynnette Liebelt, Jayne Vanderwerker, and most particularly Carol Budny and Jeni Williams—for their dedicated technical assistance.

We acknowledge our colleagues of the Lake Placid Sports Medicine Society and the board of directors and staff of that organization which was founded for the advancement of winter sports through good science, high-quality medical practice, and education.

Contents

Contributors

JAMES D. ANHOLM, M.D.
Assistant Professor of Medicine
Loma Linda School of Medicine
Loma Linda, California

Dr. Anholm, a Fellow of the American College of Sports Medicine, is a member of the Pulmonary Section of the Jerry L. Pettis Memorial Veterans Hospital and the Pulmonary and Intensive Care Section of the Department of Medicine, Loma Linda University School of Medicine. He has carried out research and published extensively on cardiopulmonary physiology, as well as studying many aspects of physiology and adjustment to high altitudes. Dr. Anholm has worked specifically with elite speed skaters, rope skippers, cross-country skiers, weight lifters and endurance athletes.

RODNEY S. W. BASLER, M.D.
Assistant Professor of Internal Medicine
Division of Dermatology
University of Nebraska Medical Center
Consultant in Dermatology
University of Nebraska-Lincoln
Lincoln, Nebraska

Dr. Basler is a widely published dermatologist with special interest in skin problems associated with sports and exercise. He is Director of the Forum on Sports Medicine, American Academy of Dermatology. He is also a member of the Society for the Review of Dermatologic Advancements and the Society for Investigative Dermatology.

JOHN H. BLAND, M.D.
Professor of Medicine—Rheumatology
University of Vermont College of Medicine
Burlington, Vermont

Dr. Bland has a long-standing interest in fitness and health maintenance, exemplified by his personal athletic participation and his research and many publications, which range broadly across the fields of clinical medicine and basic medical sciencies. Dr. Bland has written extensively on problems of the joints and musculoskeletal system, cardiovascular disease, metabolism, and aging and endurance. A frequent participant in cross-country ski marathons, he competes regularly in the American Birkebeiner 50-kilometer ski race at Cable, Wisconsin. Dr. Bland has been a member of the U.S. Masters Nordic Cross-Country Ski Team since 1983. Among many national and international skiing honors, Dr. Bland won a bronze medal in the World Masters Cross-Country Championship at Hirschau, Germany, in 1985, and in 1986 he took home both bronze and silver medals from the World Masters Cross-Country Championships at Lake Placid. Dr. Bland is a member of the U.S. Nordic Ski Team Medical Supervisory Team, and he served as Chief Medical Officer for the Nordic Division at the XIII Olympic Winter Games in Lake Placid. He is a consultant to the National Institute on Aging, and he was recently honored as a Master Physician in the American College of Rheumatology.

DAVID BRADLEY, M.D.

Policy Studies Program
Amos Tuck School of Business Administration
Dartmouth College
Hanover, New Hampshire

Dr. Bradley was raised in Madison, Wisconsin, where he first became acquainted with ski jumping. As an undergraduate student, Bradley captained the Dartmouth College Ski Team. In 1938 he was U.S. cross-country and Nordic combined champion, in 1939 he was the European collegiate four-event champion, and in 1940 he was a member of the U.S. Olympic Ski Team. After graduating from Harvard Medical School, Dr. Bradley served in the U.S. Army Medical Corps, working with the Bikini A-bomb tests—an experience that led to his best-selling book, No Place to Hide. Dr. Bradley is also the author of Lion Among Roses—A Memoir of Finland, Robert Frost: A Tribute to the Source, and many publications on outdoor life, skiing, and ski jumping. He was Manager of the U.S. Nordic Ski Team in 1960, and served as Chief of First Aid at the ski-jumping venue during the XIII Winter Olympic Games at Lake Placid in 1980. In 1984 he was named to the U.S. Ski Hall of Fame. Dr. Bradley was a member of the New Hampshire State Legislature for 10 years, serving on the Education, Ways and Means, and Environment and Agriculture Committees.

KEVIN R. CAMPBELL, Ph.D.

Department of Musculoskeletal Research
The Cleveland Clinic Foundation
Cleveland, Ohio

Dr. Campbell joined the Cleveland Clinic Foundation in 1986 as a member of the Section of Biomechanics in the Department of Musculoskeletal Research. From 1982 until 1986, Dr. Campbell was on the faculty of the University of Massachusetts, Amherst, Department of Exercise Science. Since 1980 he has been a consultant to the U.S. Ski-Jumping Team.

MURRAY JOSEPH CASEY, M.D., M.S., M.B.A.

Professor and Chairman
Department of Obstetrics and Gynecology
Creighton University School of Medicine
Omaha, Nebraska

Dr. Casey is past President of the Lake Placid Sports Medicine Society, 1984-1986. During the XIII Winter Olympic Games, Dr. Casey was a member of Medical Services, Lake Placid Olympic Organizing Committee and served as a medical officer and gynecologic consultant at the Olympic Village Polyclinic. He has been a member of the U.S. Nordic Ski Team Medical Supervisory Team, and from 1983 through 1988, Dr. Casey was engaged in clinical care, research, and follow-up of the women's U.S. Speed Skating Team in the Human Performance Laboratory of Mount Sinai Medical Center in Milwaukee while he was a professor at the University of Wisconsin Medical School. Dr. Casey served as a medical officer during the Women's World Speed Skating Championships in 1987 and the World Sprint Speed Skating Championship in 1988 as well as other national and international skating events held in West Allis, Wisconsin. Previously, Dr. Casey was a Research Staff Associate in the Laboratory of Infectious Diseases, National Institute of Allergy and Infectious Diseases of the National Institutes of Health, Bethesda, Maryland, during testing phases of respiratory virus vaccines. There he conducted research in viral oncogenesis and the definition of virus-induced tumor antigens. From 1971 until 1980, Dr. Casey was Director of Gynecologic Oncology at the University of Connecticut Health Center, and from 1980 until 1989 he was Head of Gynecologic Oncology at the University of Wisconsin Milwaukee Clinical Campus.

LESTER M. CRAMER, D.M.D., M.D.

Vice Chairman
Sports Medicine Committee
U.S. Figure Skating Association
Colorado Springs, Colorado

Dr. Cramer has been Chairman of the Sports Medicine Committee of the American Society of Plastic and Reconstructive Surgery since 1982. Following his training in plastic surgery in 1959, Dr. Cramer joined the faculty of the University of Rochester, where he remained until 1966. From 1966 until 1977, Dr. Cramer was Professor and Chairman of the Department of Plastic and Hand Surgery at Temple University. Dr. Cramer is a past Chairman of the Plastic Surgery Research Council, and past President of the American Society of Maxillofacial Surgeons and the Plastic Surgery Educational Foundation. He served as a Director of the American Board of Plastic Surgery from 1976 to 1981 and was Examination Chairman for the Board from 1977 to 1981. He has been a medical consultant to the U.S. Figure Skating Association since 1983, and he now serves as Coordinator of the U.S. Figure Skating Association's Sports Science Program at the U.S. Olympic Training Center in Colorado Springs and is Director of the Association's Sports Medicine and Science Elite Program. He was physician for the U.S. Junior World Figure Skating Team in 1984 and physician for the U.S. World Figure Skating Team in 1985 and 1988.

MICHAEL CROWE, B.S.
National Team Coach
U.S. Speed Skating Team
Butte, Montana

Mr. Crowe has been U.S. Speed Skating National Team Coach since 1985, and he coached the U.S. Speed Skating Team of the XV Winter Olympic Games in Calgary during 1988. Since becoming National Team Coach, Mr. Crowe has been actively involved with researchers of the University of Wisconsin, evaluating and developing speed skating athletes through their program at the Human Performance Laboratory of Mount Sinai Medical Center in Milwaukee. Mr. Crowe previously worked in the Exercise Physiology Laboratory of Washington University in St. Louis. As a member of the U.S. Speed Skating Team, he personally competed in a number of international events.

JACK DANIELS, Ph.D.
Assistant Professor
Department of Physical Education and Athletics
State University of New York
Cortland, New York

Dr. Daniels is the Head Track and Cross-Country Coach of the State University of New York, Cortland. Dr. Daniels was a member of the 1956 and 1960 U.S. Olympic Teams and is an Olympic medal holder in Modern Pentathlon. He is an internationally recognized authority on altitude training, having served extensively as a consultant to U.S. national swimming and athletic teams.

JAMES O. DAVIS, Ph.D.
Professor of Psychology
Southwest Missouri State University
Associate Director, Sleep Disorder Center
Cox Medical Centers
Springfield, Missouri

Dr. Davis is a member of the U.S. Olympic Committee Sport Psychology Registry and Director of Sports Science and Medicine for the U.S. Olympic Yachting Committee. From 1985 to 1986, Dr. Davis was a resident psychologist with the U.S. Olympic Committee's Sports Science Program. He also has served on the U.S. Judo Sports Medicine Committee and the Sports Medicine Committee of the U.S. National Swim Team.

ELLIOT C. DICK, M.S., Ph.D.
Professor of Preventive Medicine
Chief, Respiratory Virus Research Laboratory
University of Wisconsin Medical School
Madison, Wisconsin

Dr. Dick has been extensively involved in research on the natural transmission of infectious diseases, particularly those of the respiratory tract. He also has worked in the testing phases of antiviral drugs and vaccine development. His investigation of respiratory infections at McMurdo Station gained Dr. Dick the Antarctic Medal of the United States. Dr. Dick is a Fellow of the Explorers Club and a member of the

American Academy of Microbiology and the Infectious Disease Society. He is a founding member of the American Society of Virology.

MICHAEL EASTERBROOK, M.D., F.R.C.S.(C)
Associate Professor
Department of Ophthalmology
University of Toronto
Toronto, Ontario
Canada

Dr. Easterbrook is Consultant Eye Surgeon to the Toronto Maple Leaf National Hockey League team and serves as an eye consultant to both the Canadian and American Squash and Racquetball Associations. Dr. Easterbrook is the author of many publications on eye injuries, and now with the great reduction in ocular injuries from ice hockey, his attention has turned to accomplishing the same reduction of ocular injuries resulting from the indoor racquet sports. Currently Dr. Easterbrook is Chairman of the Canadian Standards Association's Task Force for Eye Protection in Racquet Sports and a member of the Sports Medicine Committee of the Canadian Ophthalmological Society.

CARL FOSTER, M.Ed., Ph.D.
Associate Professor of Medicine
University of Wisconsin Medical School
Milwaukee Clinical Campus
Director, Human Performance Laboratory
Mount Sinai Medical Center
Milwaukee, Wisconsin

Dr. Foster is Chairman of the Sports Medicine Committee of the U.S. International Speed Skating Association. He is Director of Cardiac Rehabilitation and Exercise Testing at the Mount Sinai Medical Center, Milwaukee, where he and his group have followed and helped prepare the U.S. Speed Skating Team since 1979, through ten seasons of international competition and three Winter Olympic Games. Dr. Foster is a Fellow of the American College of Sports Medicine, and he served that organization as Vice-President, Basic and Applied Science, from 1985 until 1987. A rehabilitation and sports physiologist, he has studied both basic and practical aspects of nutrition, metabolism, and gastrointestinal function in soccer players and elite speed skaters.

NANCY L. GREER, M.S., Ph.D.
Assistant Professor
School of Physical Education and Recreation
University of Minnesota
Minneapolis, Minnesota

Dr. Greer is a biomechanist on the faculty of Physical Education at the University of Minnesota. Prior to that, she conducted biomechanical research in the Department of Exercise Science at the University of Massachusetts, Amherst, and served as a research assistant in the Biomechanics Laboratory at the U.S. Olympic Training Center in Colorado Springs. She has been a research associate in ice hockey in the Sport Science Program of the U.S. Olympic Committee and is currently a member of the Sport Science Committee for USA Hockey. From 1979 until 1981, Greer served as varsity coach for men's and women's tennis and women's field hockey at the University of Wisconsin, River Falls.

GENE R. HAGERMAN, M.A., Ph.D.
Coordinator, Sports Medicine Program
U.S. Alpine Ski Team
Sports Performance Orthopedic Research Training, Inc.
South Lake Tahoe, California

Dr. Hagerman codirected the Sports Physiology Laboratory at the U.S. Olympic Training Center, Olympic Valley, California, from 1977 until 1980 and was Head of the Sports Physiology Laboratory of the U.S. Olympic Training Center, Colorado Springs, from 1980 until 1982. Dr. Hagerman's work with rowers, swimmers, track and field athletes, wrestlers, and basketball players has led to numerous publications and presentations in his field of sports physiology. Dr. Hagerman has been a member of the sports medicine committees of the U.S. Rowing Association, the U.S. Biathlon Team, and the U.S. Alpine Ski Team.

MURRAY P. HAMLET, D.V.M.
Director, Cold Research Division
U.S. Army Research Institute of Environmental Medicine
Natick, Massachusetts

Dr. Hamlet has been Director of the Cold Research Division of the U.S. Army Research Institute of Environmental Medicine since 1972. Prior to that, Dr. Hamlet was an investigator in the U.S. Army Veterinary Laboratory at Fort Wainwright, Alaska. Dr. Hamlet is widely published on many aspects of experimental hypothermia and cold injury on the clinical management of cold injury, frostbite, and hypothermia. He is a member of the Polar Research Board of the National Research Council.

WALTER R. HAMPTON, M.D.
Clinical Associate Professor of Medicine
University of Connecticut
School of Medicine
Farmington, Connecticut

Dr. Hampton is a faculty member of Mountain Medicine, Inc., and has been the Medical Director of Mountain Medicine Trek/Seminars to Mount Everest and Kathmandu, Nepal, in 1981, 1983, 1984, and 1987. Dr. Hampton was a physician with the Nordic Ski Patrol during the XIII Winter Olympic Games in Lake Placid, 1980. He now serves as Secretary-Treasurer of the Lake Placid Sports Medicine Society.

KENNETH J. HARKINS, M.S.
Director, Cardiovascular Rehabilitation
St. Mary's Medical Center
Duluth, Minnesota

Mr. Harkins is a past member of the U.S. Ski Team, participating as a ski jumper from 1967 until 1973 and from 1975 until 1978. He has conducted research projects in physiology with the U.S. Nordic Ski Team, the U.S. Speed Skating Team, and the University of Wisconsin hockey team.

JACK HARVEY, M.A., M.D.
Clinical Assistant Professor of Pediatrics
University of Colorado Medical School
Director of Sports Medicine
Orthopedic Center of the Rockies
Fort Collins, Colorado

Dr. Harvey is an Affiliate Professor of Physical Education at Colorado State University, a Clinical Assistant Professor of Pediatrics at the University of Colorado Medical School, and Medical Director of the Human Performance Laboratory at the University of Colorado-Boulder. He serves as a team physician to the U.S. Nordic Ski Team, the U.S. Swimming Team, the U.S. Biathlon Team, and he is the Chief Physician for the U.S. Wrestling Team. Dr. Harvey is also a member of the U.S. Biathlon Sports Medicine Council and has worked for Medical Services of a number of national and international competitions. He is widely published on topics relating to the participation of children and youth in sports.

JEFF HASTINGS, B.S.
Ski Jump Coach
U.S. Ski Team
Hanover, New Hampshire

Mr. Hastings is the Head Jumping Coach for the U.S. Nordic Combined Ski Team. He was graduated from Williams College and was a member of the 1984 U.S. Olympic Ski Jumping Team.

DAVID R. HILL, M.D.
Assistant Professor of Medicine
Director, International Traveler's Medical Service
University of Connecticut School of Medicine
Farmington, Connecticut

Dr. Hill has a special interest in the infections of the alimentary tract that are most likely to afflict athletes, travelers, and their support staffs. His personal research and publications have included work with *Escherichia coli, Salmonella, Giardia lamblia,* and prevention of illness during travel. He has been honored with the Young Investigator Award of the Infectious Diseases Society of America for his studies on the immune response to giardiasis.

EDWARD G. HIXSON, M.D.
Chief Medical Officer
Olympic Regional Development Authority
Chief Physician-in-Residence
U.S. Olympic Training Center
Lake Placid, New York

Dr. Hixson, a member of the Adirondack Surgical Group in Saranac Lake, New York, has been a central figure in the development of sports medicine in and around the Lake Placid region. Dr. Hixson was Vice-Chairman of Medical Services for the Lake Placid Olympic Organizing Committee during the XIII Winter Olympic Games, 1980, and served as President of the Lake Placid Sports Medicine Society from 1986 to 1988. He is a Fellow of the American College of Sports Medicine.

As Chief Medical Officer for the Olympic Regional Development Authority, Dr. Hixson is often consulted regarding issues of equipment safety and design. He now serves as Chairman of the Medical Supervisory Team for the U.S. Nordic Ski Team and is team physician for the National Guard Biathlon Team. He is a past editor of the feature "Nordic M.D." in *Nordic Skiing* magazine.

Dr. Hixson, an experienced climber, was a member of the 1982 China-Everest Expedition, the 1983 German-American Everest Expedition, and the 1984 China Expedition. He has personally climbed the highest peaks of North America, and has reached several of the high Himalayan summits, including ascents to more than 28,000 feet. Also an enthusiastic kayaker, Dr. Hixson participated in the 1981 American Bhutan Himalayan Kayak Descent.

STEPHEN J. INCAVO, M.D.
Clinical Assistant Professor
Department of Orthopedic Surgery
University of Vermont College of Medicine
Burlington, Vermont

Dr. Incavo, a practicing orthopedic surgeon, joined the clinical faculty of the University of Vermont in 1988. During the course of his postgraduate training, Dr. Incavo worked extensively with Dr. Robert Johnson in the study of skiing accidents, injuries and equipment. He has written on intermedullary nailing techniques for fractures of the femur, lateral ankle ligament strain, and Achilles tendon rupture.

ROBERT J. JOHNSON, M.D.
Professor of Orthopedic Surgery
Head, Division of Sports Medicine
University of Vermont College of Medicine
Burlington, Vermont

Dr. Johnson has researched and written extensively on the topics of skiing injuries and their relationship to technique, biomechanics, and equipment. He has served on the Board of Directors and as Vice President of the International Society for Skiing Safety. He is a member of the editorial boards of several sports medicine journals.

JOHN M. KELLY, M.S., D.P.E.
  Professor of Physical Education
  Director, Human Performance Laboratory
  St. Cloud State University
  St. Cloud, Minnesota

Dr. Kelly directs the Human Performance Laboratroy and the Adult Fitness Program at St. Cloud State University, where he has taught and conducted research in human physiology for nearly 20 years. He is a Fellow of the American College of Sports Medicine and has served as President of the Northland Chapter of that organization.

JULIE ANN LICKTEIG, M.S., R.D.
  Associate Professor
  Department of Dietetics
  Cardinal Stritch College
  Milwaukee, Wisconsin

Ms. Lickteig is Director of the Dietetics and Food Management Program at Cardinal Stritch College. She has extensive experience in dietary administration and the preparation of menus for sports venues and trekking expeditions to the highest ranges of five continents. Participation in numerous trekking adventures to the Bolivian and Peruvian Andes, Mount Kilimanjaro in Africa, Mount McKinley in the Alaskan Range, and the Nepalese and Tibetan Himalayas has given Ms. Lickteig firsthand experience in menu development and food packaging for mountain expeditions in foreign lands. She is an active member of the American Dietetic Association and a founding member of Sports and Cardiovascular Nutritionists (SCAN).

JOHN G. McMURTRY, M.A.
  Director of Athletic Development
  U.S. Ski Team
  Sports Performance Orthopedic Research Training, Inc.
  South Lake Tahoe, California

As an undergraduate at the University of Denver, Mr. McMurtry was a member of the National Collegiate Athletic Association Champion Ski Team. From 1980 until 1984, Mr. McMurtry was Head Slalom and Giant Slalom Coach for the U.S. Ski Team, and he was Head Slalom and Giant Slalom Coach of the Women's Olympic Ski Team for the XIV Winter Olympic Games, Sarajevo, 1984. Coach McMurtry's 1981–1982 U.S. Women's Ski Team won the overall Nations Cup Trophy—the first ever Nations Cup for a U.S. ski team. From 1987 to 1988, John McMurtry was Director of Athlete Development for the U.S. Ski Team, and he has been Alpine Program Director for the U.S. Ski Team since 1988.

CRAIG H. McQUEEN, M.D.
  Associate Clinical Professor of Orthopedic Surgery
  University of Utah School of Medicine
  Member, Sports Medicine Committee
  U.S. Figure Skating Association
  Salt Lake City, Utah

Dr. McQueen is in the private practice of orthopedic surgery and President of Utah Orthopedic Associates. In addition to his activities with the U.S. Figure Skating Association, Dr. McQueen is a consultant to Ballet West and a member of the Board of Trustees of the School of Ballet West. Dr. McQueen also is team physician for the Utah Trappers professional baseball team.

JAMES B. McQUILLEN, M.D.
  Attending Neurologist
  Mansfield General Hospital
  Mansfield, Ohio

Dr. McQuillen is a practicing neurologist and a neuropathologist. As a consulting neuropathologist to the Office of the Chief Medical Examiner, State of Vermont, Dr. McQuillen had the opportunity to study fatalities resulting from skiing accidents and to relate these to clinical neurology. Dr. McQuillen is now an attending neurologist on the staff of the Mansfield General Hospital, Mansfield, Ohio. He was previously a member of the faculty of the University of Vermont College of Medicine, where he was an Associate Professor of Neurology and Pathology (Neuropathology) and Chief of the Electromyography Laboratory from 1976 until 1986.

JAMES V. MOGAN, M.D.
Clinical Assistant Professor
Department of Orthopedic Surgery
University of Vermont, College of Medicine
Burlington, Vermont

Dr. Mogan, a practicing orthopedic surgeon in Burlington, Vermont, has extensive training and experience in sports medicine and special interest and expertise in surgery of the hand. Dr. Mogan has published and presented many papers on sports injuries, particularly regarding those involving the hand.

DAVID H. MOORE, M.S.
Chief of First Aid and Director
National Ski Patrol
Intervale MacKenzie Olympic Ski Jump
Lake Placid, New York

Mr. Moore has over 25 years of experience with the National Ski Patrol. Mr. Moore is certified in emergency medical technology and cardiopulmonary resuscitation. He is an instructor for both these disciplines as well as a mountaineering instructor for the National Ski Patrol. Presently, Mr. Moore is a member of the Mount Van Hoevenberg Nordic Patrol and First Aid Chief and Director of the National Ski Patrol at the Intervale MacKenzie Olympic Ski Jump. Previously, Mr. Moore was Section Chief of the North Adirondack National Ski Patrol. He is Superintendent of the Bushton-Moira Central School in the Adirondack area of New York State.

WILLIAM J. MULLALLY, M. Med. SCI., M.D.
Sports Medicine Council
U.S. Luge Association
Headache and Neurologic Associates
Princeton, New Jersey

Dr. Mullally is a member of the Sports Medicine Council of the U.S. Luge Association. As a neurologist with special interest in headaches, he has paid particular attention to this ubiquitous problem in sledders. Dr. Mullally is a Clinical Instructor in Neurology at the Robert Wood Johnson Medical School of the University of Medicine and Dentistry of New Jersey.

WILLIAM EDWARD PETERSON, B.S.
President, Peterson Laboratories
Lake Placid, New York

Mr. Peterson, educated as an engineer, is a designer, fitter and manufacturer of orthotic devices. He has consulted and provided prescription footwear for the United States and Canadian national ski teams, the United States Biathlon Team, the United States Disabled Ski Team and the Professional Ski Instructors of America.

WILLIAM E. PIERSON, M.D.
Clinical Professor of Pediatrics and Environmental Health
University of Washington School of Medicine
Seattle, Washington

Dr. Pierson is Chairman of the organizing committee of Asthmatic Athletes of America and has served as a member of the U.S. Olympic Committee's Drugs and Performance Committee. Dr. Pierson has been a member of the Board of Directors of the American Board of Allergy and Immunology. He was Chairman of the Section on Allergy and Immunology of the American Academy of Pediatrics and served as

Chairman of the Academy's Liaison Committee with the National Institute of Allergy and Infectious Diseases. He also has been a member of the Board of Directors and President of the Joint Council of Allergy and Immunology. Dr. Pierson was on the Pulmonary Allergy Drugs Advisory Committee of the U.S. Food and Drug Administration. He is presently Chairman of the Sports Medicine Committee of the American Academy of Allergy and Immunology.

JAY J. RAND, B.A.
Director, Intervale Ski-Jump Complex
Olympic Regional Development Authority
Lake Placid, New York

Mr. Rand has managed the Intervale Ski-Jump Complex since 1978. He is a graduate of the University of Colorado, where as a member of the ski-jumping team he was NCAA Champion in 1970. Mr. Rand was a member of the U.S. Ski Team from 1966 through 1976 and participated in the 1968 Olympics, the 1970 World University Games, and the 1974 World Championships. He has coached soccer, skiing, and lacrosse at the Cardigan Mountain School, Canaan, New Hampshire, and ski jumping at the University of Vermont.

HUBERT F. RIEGLER, M.D.
Clinical Assistant Professor
Department of Orthopedics
University of Rochester School of Medicine
Rochester, New York

Dr. Riegler is a member of the medical staff of both the University of Rochester-Strong Memorial Hospital and the Highland Hospital, Rochester, New York, where he is Director of the Athletic Injury Treatment Center. Dr. Riegler is a consultant in orthopedics and Team Physician at Rochester Institute of Technology, Nazareth College, and the State University of New York-Brockport, where he is also an Adjunct Professor of Physical Education. Dr. Riegler has served as a physician at numerous national and international sporting events, including World Cup competitions. He has published on an extensive number of subjects concerning sports medicine and injuries.

ALLAN J. RYAN, M.D.
Director, Sports Medicine Enterprise
Editor-in-Chief, Fitness in Business
Minneapolis, Minnesota

Dr. Allan J. Ryan, founding editor of *The Physician and Sportsmedicine*, is one of the world's best-known and most respected experts in sports medicine and fitness. Trained as a surgeon, Dr. Ryan joined the faculty of the University of Wisconsin Medical School in 1965, following an early career in private practice. After 11 years as a member of the Department of Rehabilitation Medicine at the University of Wisconsin, Dr. Ryan left to devote his professional energies totally to research and writing. Dr. Ryan has published extensively and authoritatively. His bibliography ranges from infectious diseases to many aspects of surgical management and technique to cancer detection and care, and, of course, to sports and fitness. Besides his long tenure as Editor-in-Chief of *The Physician and Sportsmedicine*, Dr. Ryan has been Editor-in-Chief of *Postgraduate Medicine*, and he is currently Editor-in-Chief of *Fitness in Business*. Dr. Ryan has been the President and Trustee of the American College of Sports Medicine, and he served as Secretary General of the International Federation of Sports Medicine. He now is a member of the Advisory Board of the Instructional Center for Sports Science and Medicine.

JOANN SCHONNING, M.S., A.T.C.
Sports Medicine Coordinator
Fort Collins Orthopedic Associates
Fort Collins, Colorado

Ms. Schonning holds her master's degree in physical education. She has served as an athletic trainer at many important centers and events, including the U.S. Olympic Training Centers in Colorado Springs; Lake Placid; and Marquette, Michigan. She served at the World Cross-Country Championships in 1984 and was Medical Coordinator for U.S. athletes during the Winter World University Games at Cortina,

Italy, in 1985. Most recently Ms. Schonning was the U.S. Luge Team trainer during the 1987 World Cup Circuit.

ARNOLD SHERMAN, O.D.
Associate Clinical Professor of Optometry
State College of Optometry
State University of New York
New York, New York

Dr. Sherman is in the private practice of optometry in Merrick, L.I., New York and is president of the Sports Vision Enhancement Institute, Ltd. From 1982 to 1984, Dr. Sherman was the Director of Vision Programs in the U.S. Olympic Committee program for Elite Athletes and consultant to the U.S. National Teams in archery, fencing, and handball and to the junior development program in tennis. He has also served as a consultant to St. John's University Athletic Department, the New York Jets National Football League team, the New York Knicks National Basketball Association team, and the New York Rangers National Hockey League team.
Dr. Sherman was a founder and past chairman of the Sports Vision Section, American Optometric Association. He is a Diplomate in Binocular Vision and Perception, a Fellow of the American Academy of Optometry, and a Fellow of the College of Optometrists in Vision Development.

HOWARD M. SILBY, M.D.
Assistant Clinical Professor of Neurology
George Washington University
School of Medicine
Chairman, Sports Medicine Committee
U.S. Figure Skating Association
Chevy Chase, Maryland

Dr. Silby has served as a U.S. Figure Skating Association World Team Physician since 1982. He was Assistant Team Leader for the 1988 Olympic Figure Skating Team. Dr. Silby currently is Chairman of the U.S. Figure Skating Association Sports Medicine Committee. In 1981, he was Assistant Chief for Doping Control during the World Figure Skating Championships. Dr. Silby practices neurology in Chevy Chase, Maryland.

JAMES STRAY-GUNDERSEN, M.D.
Assistant Professor of Surgery and Physiology
University of Texas Southwestern Medical Center
Director of the St. Paul-University of Texas Southwestern Medical Center
Human Performance Center
Dallas, Texas

Dr. Stray-Gundersen is a general surgeon and a clinical physiologist who directs the Human Performance Center at St. Paul-University of Texas Southwestern Medical Center in Dallas. He currently serves as Sports Medicine Coordinator for the U.S. Nordic Ski Team.

GLENN M. STREET, Ph.D.
Assistant Professor of Physical Education and Director of Research
Human Performance Laboratory
St. Cloud State University
St. Cloud, Minnesota

Dr. Street is a multifaceted researcher who pursued investigations in the Biomechanics Laboratory of the Pennsylvania State University before joining the faculty of St. Cloud State University in 1988. Prior to that, he worked as an exercise physiologist in the Sports Medicine Department of the Cleveland Clinic. From 1981 until 1984, Dr. Street served as a physiology consultant to the U.S. Cross-Country Ski Team. Dr. Street's research and publications range broadly from cardiovascular physiology to human kinetics, and from body composition to sports biomechanics with special emphasis on cross-country skiing and skiing equipment.

WILLIAM N. TAYLOR, M.D.
Physician Crew Chief
U.S. Olympic Committee Drug Control Program
Student Health Services
Washington State University
Pullman, Washington

Dr. Taylor has been one of the most outspoken voices calling attention to the harmful effects of anabolic steroids in sports. He has written extensively on this topic and is frequently called to testify before major legislative and regulatory bodies. Dr. Taylor has been a member of the U.S. Powerlifting Sports Medicine Committee since 1983 and has served as Crew Chief of the U.S. Olympic Committee Drug Control Program since 1986. Dr. Taylor is a Fellow of the American College of Sports Medicine and a member of the Board of Governors of the American Academy of Sports Medicine. He is now in the private practice of sports medicine in Gulf Breeze, Florida.

NANCY N. THOMPSON, M.S.
Chief Technologist
Human Performance Laboratory
Mount Sinai Medical Center
Milwaukee, Wisconsin

Ms. Thompson received her bachelor's degree in physical education at Iowa State University and her master's degree in adult fitness and cardiac rehabilitation at the University of Wisconsin-LaCrosse. She joined the research team in the Human Performance Laboratroy of Mount Sinai Medical Center, Milwaukee, in 1984, where she has been engaged in both physiological and nutritional investigations.

ROBERT O. VOY, M.D.
Director of Sports Medicine and Science
U.S. Olympic Committee
Colorado Springs, Colorado

As Chief Medical Officer and Director of Sports Medicine and Science for the U.S. Olympic Committee, Dr. Voy supervises all of the Committee's official research efforts. He is also responsible for recruitment, assignment, and evaluation of volunteer health professionals. Dr. Voy has been active in developing numerous educational programs in the medical sciences for athletes, coaches, and health professionals. He takes a keen personal interest in developing team and sports physicians for participants at all age levels, recognizing that the elite athletes of tomorrow and their health care givers will come from these ranks. Dr. Voy, a pharmacist and family physician by background, has been instrumental in the development of the U.S. Olympic Committee's Drug Control Program and Hotline.

DAVID W. WEBB, M.D.
Associate Director
Center for Sports Medicine
St. Francis Hospital
San Francisco, California

Dr. Webb, a specialist in emergency medicine, has a long-standing interest in sports traumatology and applied exercise physiology. In 1986, Dr. Webb served as Chief Race Physician for the World Banked-track Speed Skating Championships. Since 1985, Dr. Webb has served as a race physician for the Coors International Bicycle Classic, and since 1987 has been Chief Race Physician for that event. Dr. Webb was previously a troupe physician for the San Francisco ballet and a team physician at the City College of San Francisco. He is a Fellow of the American College of Sports Medicine.

ROBERT G. WESTPHAL, M.D.
Clinical Professor of Medicine
University of Vermont College of Medicine
Medical Director
Vermont-New Hampshire Region
American Red Cross Blood Services
Burlington, Vermont

Dr. Westphal has studied and written extensively on problems of anemia and transfusion, including the predeposition of blood for later autotransfusion. He has been a member of the University of Vermont faculty and has served as a director of the Vermont-New Hampshire regional Red Cross Blood Services for over 15 years.

MICHAEL P. WOODS, M.D.
Assistant Professor of Anesthesiology
Medical College of Wisconsin
Milwaukee, Wisconsin

Dr. Woods was a member of the U.S. International Speed Skating team from 1973 through 1980 and from 1983 through 1984. He was a member of three U.S. Olympic Teams—1976, 1980, and 1984. Dr. Woods placed first in the 10,000-meter race of the 1980 World Speed Skating Championships, and second in this same race at the 1984 World Championships. Dr. Woods was the U.S. Olympic Team Captain during the XIII Winter Olympic Games in Lake Placid, 1980, and he placed fourth in the 10,000-meter and seventh in the 5,000-meter speed skating events in those games. At the 1984 Winter Olympic Games in Sarajevo, Dr. Woods placed seventh in the 10,000-meter race and 12th in the 5,000-meter event. He currently serves as Vice President, Executive Board Member, and Sports Medicine Committee Secretary of the U.S. International Speed Skating Association, and he is Vice President of the Wisconsin Olympic Ice Rink Foundation. Dr. Woods also is active as a track, cycling, and speed skating coach.

JAMES R. WRIGHT, JR., M.D.
Department of Pathology
Isaak Walton Killam Hospital for Children
Dalhousie University Faculty of Medicine
Halifax, Nova Scotia
Canada

Dr. Wright, a pediatric pathologist, holds a Master's degree in the History of Medicine. In 1985, Dr. Wright became the first recipient of the Lake Placid Sports Medicine Society's Young Investigator Award for his work on ski-jumping injuries. He is a member of the National Ski Patrol and the Canadian Ski Patrol Service. Dr. Wright has worked as a physician during competitions at the Intervale Olympic Ski-Jump Complex and the Whiteface Mountain Alpine Ski Area in Lake Placid.

CHAPTER 1

Winter Sports Medicine: Introduction and Overview

MURRAY JOSEPH CASEY, M.D.

In his preface to this book, Dr. Allan J. Ryan dates the beginnings of sports medicine to 1928, with the establishment of Association Internationale Medico-Sportive during the Second Olympic Games in St. Moritz. When medical historians in years to come look for the beginnings of winter sports medicine, they will find them rooted in the 1980 Winter Olympic Games and the subsequent founding of the Sports Medicine Society in Lake Placid.

Winter sports medicine is not a confined, specific discipline. It is a topic of professional education dealing with the development, training, and care of participants—competitive and recreational—who engage in winter sports. This body of knowledge is interdisciplinary. Many skills and many specialties are represented. It is the whole of this knowledge—the amalgamation of this science and the application of this practice—that is embodied in winter sports medicine.

Winter sports medicine draws heavily on the expertise of professionals who work specifically with participants in the individual sports. Each sport has its own particulars regarding preparation, skills, strengths, stresses, and injuries, and these are discussed in their respective sections of this book. There are also common problems that are encountered in the care of all participants in winter sports, their supporting staffs, and even the spectators. The winter wind and cold and the higher altitudes at which winter sports are often performed place special de-

mands on nutrition and physiology. Trekking, skiing, camping, and mountaineering under these extreme conditions can test the very boundaries of human endurance. Competitive athletes pressing their limits at great speeds and often great risk are liable to injuries among the most severe known in sport. The confines of travel and close living quarters, contact with contagion, extremes of temperature, physical and emotional exhaustion, and sojourns to backwoods and exotic lands render the participants in winter sports susceptible to illnesses that might not affect their countrymen who are not thus engaged.

Winter sports medicine is involved not only with the techniques and preparation of athletes for their individual sports but also with the prevention of injuries and illnesses to which winter athletes are subject. Through investigation and study of physiology, biomechanics, and psychology; through research in the design and promotion of safe equipment and safe facilities; through efficient scientific planning and administration of training programs and competitive events; and through the promulgation of this knowledge by education those involved with winter sports medicine seek to assist elite and developing athletes in their quests for individual best performances while protecting them from avoidable accidents and illnesses. Inherent in all of this is the necessity of providing services not only to the athletes but also to their supporting staffs and spectators (Table 1–1) and the need to assure the avail-

1

Table 1–1. PATIENTS BY CATEGORY: MEDICAL SERVICES LAKE PLACID OLYMPIC ORGANIZING COMMITTEE, XIII WINTER OLYMPIC GAMES, LAKE PLACID, 1980

Athletes and team officials	542
Staff and security	330
Support personnel	379
Spectators and accredited personnel	1,286
	2,537

Compiled from Hart.[2]

ability and safe, efficient function of evacuation techniques and methods of conveyance for persons ill or injured in the often remote localities where winter sports are performed.[1,2]

In the United States, more than two million persons engage in recreational skiing and sledding, and there are nearly one and a half million recreational ice skaters.[3] A great deal of what has been learned through the

Table 1–2. DIGEST OF DIAGNOSTIC CATEGORIES: MEDICAL SERVICES LAKE PLACID OLYMPIC ORGANIZING COMMITTEE, XIII WINTER OLYMPIC GAMES, LAKE PLACID, 1980

Infection	
Acute upper-respiratory tract	787
Bronchitis/pneumonia	11/5
Gastroenteritis	39
Trauma	
Fractures	61
Sprains	166
Dislocations	12
Head	7
Open wounds	107
Cold Injury	
Frostbite	24
Hypothermia	12
Miscellaneous	
Dermatitis/skin infection	34/2
Back pain	24
Headache	20
Chest pain	11
Malaise and fatigue	10
Nausea and vomiting	10
Cough	6

Compiled by ICD-9 Diagnostic Code from Hart.[2]

testing, preparation, and care of elite performers in these sports is now available for application to improve the efficiency, safety, and enjoyment of recreational participants. Moreover, what can be learned in the production of sports extravaganzas—such as World Cup competitions and the Olympic Games—is applicable in our management of future contests at all levels. And knowledge gained through staging major climbing and trekking expeditions is useful to the winter hiker, snowshoer, and camper.

This book covers virtually every aspect of winter sports medicine. The experiences of our individual authors and the excellent records available through the Lake Placid Olympic Organizing Committee and the Olympic Regional Development Authority[1,2] allow identification of the frequency of reported illnesses and injuries among elite, developing, and recreational athletes, staffs, and spectators during training, recreational participation, and championship events. This experience and the compilations of these data (see Tables 1–2 to 1–9) have aided us in focusing on the most common questions and most frequent and important problems confronting athletes, coaches, and administrative staffs as they prepare for winter sports.

Though complete in its intent, it is impossible for a volume of this size to treat comprehensively every issue that its chapters raise. We believe that a greater service is done by disseminating the unique insights of the authors while providing selected references for those who wish to delve more deeply. Though introductory, the references are sufficiently extensive to provide direction without belaboring the reader with a tedious preliminary search. It must be recognized, however, that much of the information contained in this book has little precedent and therefore depends heavily upon the observations and authority of the writers and the editors.

The first section of this book, General Topics, addresses from the standpoint of winter sports several topics that are often covered in general textbooks on sports medicine. The next two sections discuss the most frequently encountered medical problems common to participation in winter sports. The final three sections are devoted to specific medical and scientific aspects of the skating, skiing, and

Table 1-3. ANATOMIC SITES OF TRAUMA: MEDICAL SERVICES LAKE PLACID OLYMPIC ORGANIZING COMMITTEE, XIII WINTER OLYMPIC GAMES, LAKE PLACID, 1980

	Upper Extremity	Lower Extremity	Neck/Back	Head/Face	Clavicle and Ribs
Fractures	15	30	10	2	4
Sprains	29	125	12	—	—
Dislocations	6	6	—	—	—
Lacerations	65	—	—	46	—

Compiled by ICD-9 Diagnostic Code from Hart.[2]

Table 1-4. CATALOG OF INJURIES BY VENUE: OLYMPIC REGIONAL DEVELOPMENT AUTHORITY, LAKE PLACID, 1983-1984

Venue	Fractures	Sprains	Dislocations	Lacerations	Contusions	Strains	Frostbite
Ski jump	4	5	2	1	14	1	0
Bobsled and luge	27	12	5	54	126	5	0
Cross-country ski	3	2	2	0	5	2	6
Skating arena	2	7	1	42	33	1	0
Alpine ski	73	114	16	51	96	6	2

Compiled from Dick, Hornet, and Pazienza.[1]

Table 1-5. FRACTURES BY VENUE: OLYMPIC REGIONAL DEVELOPMENT AUTHORITY, LAKE PLACID, 1983-1985

Venue	Upper Extremity	Lower Extremity	Neck and Back	Head and Face
Ski jump	2	1	0	0
Bobsled and luge	8	11	2	2
Cross-country ski	3	2	1	0
Skating arena	3	0	0	0
Alpine ski	88	43	1	0

Compiled from Dick, Hornet, and Pazienza.[1]

Table 1-6. SPRAINS BY VENUE: OLYMPIC REGIONAL DEVELOPMENT AUTHORITY, LAKE PLACID, 1983-1985

Venue	Upper Extremity	Lower Extremity	Neck and Back
Ski jump	0	5	0
Bobsled and luge	3	8	1
Cross-country ski	0	2	0
Skating arena	2	5	0
Alpine ski	6	109	9

Compiled from Dick, Hornet, and Pazienza.[1]

Table 1–7. CONTUSIONS BY VENUE: OLYMPIC REGIONAL DEVELOPMENT
AUTHORITY, LAKE PLACID, 1983–1985

Venue	Upper Extremity	Lower Extremity	Trunk	Head and Face
Ski jump	2	4	6	2
Bobsled and luge	40	48	25	16
Cross-country ski	0	1	2	2
Skating arena	8	3	9	5
Alpine ski	6	29	27	34

Compiled from Dick, Hornet, and Pazienza.[1]

Table 1–8. LACERATIONS BY VENUE: OLYMPIC REGIONAL DEVELOPMENT
AUTHORITY, LAKE PLACID, 1983–1984

Venue	Upper Extremity	Lower Extremity	Trunk	Scalp and Face
Ski jump	0	0	0	1
Bobsled and luge	15	13	1	25
Cross-country ski	0	0	0	0
Skating arena	5	6	1	29
Alpine ski	4	2	2	42

Compiled from Dick, Hornet, and Pazienza.[1]

Table 1–9. HEAD AND VERTEBRAL
INJURIES: MEDICAL SERVICES LAKE
PLACID OLYMPIC ORGANIZING
COMMITTEE, XIII WINTER OLYMPIC
GAMES, LAKE PLACID, 1980

Skull fracture (base)	1
Vertebral column fracture	6
Concussion	3
Intracranial, unspecified	3

Compiled by ICD-9 Diagnostic Code from Hart.[2]

sliding sports and the mountain sports of
climbing, trekking, and winter camping. To
each of the chapters in these sections, the
several authors bring their considerable experience as participants and as researchers
and care providers working with winter athletes and staffs. We believe that sport, science, and medicine are advanced by this
collection.

REFERENCES

1. Dick, B, Hornet, J, and Pazienza, J: Sports injuries at
Lake Placid: 1983–1985, A descriptive study. Department of Family Practice, Albany Medical College, Albany, NY, 1986.
2. Hart, GG: Final report, frequency of visits by ICD-9
diagnostic code. Medical Report of the XIII Winter
Olympic Games. Lake Placid Olympic Organizing
Committee Medical Services, Lake Placid, NY, 1980.
3. Statistical Abstract of the United States 1986, ed 106.
US Department of Commerce, Bureau of the Census,
Washington, DC, 1986.

PART I

General Topics

CHAPTER 2

Year-round Preparation of the Winter Sports Athlete

MICHAEL CROWE, B.S.

Winter sports athletes face several problems unique to the medium upon which they perform. One of the foremost of these problems is the lack of venue availability during the summer months. As of the summer of 1988, there were still no 400-meter speed skating rinks available for the summer training of North American skaters. Unless travel to southern hemisphere locations or to a few glaciers is undertaken, there is no place to practice for skiers of the northern hemisphere. Even the availability of indoor ice facilities for figure skating, hockey, and short-track speed skating is limited. In many ways this would be comparable to the closing of swimming pools, running courses, and cycling venues during the winter preceding summer competitive sports. For the winter sports athlete the problem is increased by the considerable importance of maintaining highly developed skills for performance at optimal levels. Speed skating and Nordic skiing—the winter equivalents of track and cross-country running—depend as much on the effectiveness of delivering power to the ice or snow as they do on the physiologic capacities of the competing athletes (Fig. 2–1). Thus, much of the coaching of winter sports athletes is concerned with trying to maintain their skills in the absence of suitable facilities during the off-season.

Other problems for the coach of winter sports athletes are less unique, yet still substantial. These include balancing of the training program while providing motivation and

DETERMINANTS OF PERFORMANCE

$$\text{VELOCITY} = \frac{\underset{\substack{\text{VO}_2\text{max} + \text{An P} \\ \text{Pre Extension Knee Angle} \\ \text{Strength}}}{\text{POWER OUTPUT}} \times \underset{\text{Skill}}{\text{EFFECTIVENESS}}}{\underset{\substack{(\text{Frontal Area} + \text{Ice Friction}) \\ \text{Pre Extension Knee Angle} \\ \text{Hip Angle} \\ \text{Body Size}}}{\text{RESISTANCE}}}$$

Figure 2–1. Conceptual model of the factors related to average velocity, which is the primary determinant of performance in energy-demand sports, such as speed skating. For many winter sports athletes the *effectiveness* of the delivery of power to the propulsive medium (snow/ice) is very much more important than that for summer sports athletes.

managing a variety of other factors that might have impact upon athletic performance. This chapter reviews several approaches to these problems which have been undertaken with the United States Speed Skating Team. Although our problems and solutions are somewhat unique to the sport of speed skating, they suggest some common avenues which may be pursued by coaches, sports scientists, and health care providers involved with other winter sports.

YEARLY PROGRAM

Our program is broken down into three phases: transition, preparation, and competition.

Transition Phase

The transition period is a time of nontraining and is intended to give the athlete some needed "R and R"—rest and relaxation—after the conclusion of the competitive season. During this period, we encourage active participation in sports other than skating.

Traditionally, this period has been March and April. However, the development of the World Cup series and the availability of indoor 400-meter rinks in the Netherlands, the German Democratic Republic, and Canada have extended the competitive speed skating season until well into March. Also, the short

track World Championship usually takes place in late March or early April. These events act to extend the season significantly for many athletes. With the development of short-track skating as a demonstration sport in the 1988 Olympic Winter Games and as a full part of the Olympic program in 1992, the trend toward longer competitive seasons is likely to continue. Thus, the duration of the transition phase of training is likely to suffer.

Preparation Phase

The preparation phase is the longest phase of training. For American speed skaters it includes five 40-day periods from mid or late April to late October or early November. During the preparation phase, the athlete is *acquiring* the physiologic, technical, and mental aspects necessary for good performance. The preparation phase of training is used to develop the athletes progressively from general conditioning to more specific technical aspects which we hope to transfer onto the ice. Throughout the early phases of preparation there is considerable emphasis on general conditioning, with cycling, running, and weight training as primary modes of activity. We accept as a first principle that a good base of endurance conditioning is important because it allows the athletes to accomplish more skating-specific training later in the preparatory and the competitive phases. Because of the common requirement for great strength and endurance of the hip and knee extensors, speed skaters often make good cyclists, and cycling is very good training for speed skating. We encourage competition in cycling events during this phase of training because competition often engenders enthusiasm. However, at the elite level of skating we remind our athletes that cycle racing should be viewed as a means to an end and should not interfere with their training for skating. In our view, excessive time spent resting before cycling races and missing skating-specific training are not fair trade-offs for speed skaters who wish to achieve maximum success in their primary sport. Also, we remind our skaters that although there have been several skaters who became outstanding cyclists after their competitive skating days were over (Sheila Young, Connie Pariskevin, Connie Carpen-

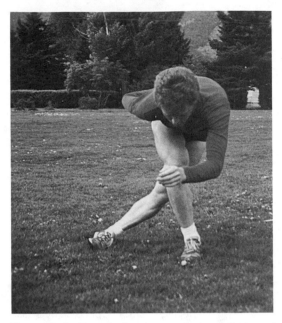

Figure 2–2. Dry skating is a technique designed to mimic the muscular requirements of speed skating without the necessity of using ice during the summer months.

ter, Beth and Eric Heiden), there is yet to be a cyclist who became a great skater. The techniques required for speed skating are just too difficult to learn later in life. Similarly, we do not object to other low-level competitive sporting activities during the preparation phase, as long as they are viewed as means to an end.

Later in the preparatory phase, the focus of training shifts to include more skating-specific activities such as dry skating (standing on the ground in August and pretending to be skating 50 km per hr around an oval in bitter cold January weather—Fig. 2–2), slideboarding (pretending that a formica-covered plank is a patch of ice and using sock-covered tennis shoes as skates to simulate the speed skating motion and form—Fig. 2–3), and more or less specialized weight-training activities (doing one-legged squats while carrying a sandbag on the back—Fig. 2–4). In recent years we have begun doing some on-ice drills in hockey rinks to teach skate-edge control and balance. We also do some skating for conditioning using short-track skates. These workouts might be compared to ski

jumping on plastic or using roller skis. Although not quite the same, such activities provide some similarities to the primary sports. Finally, toward the end of the preparatory phase, many athletes travel considerable distances for the opportunity to get early season ice time. Thus, many American athletes are off to Europe in late September to finish their preparation. It is hoped that the availability of the new 400-meter indoor rink in Calgary and the new high-altitude rink in Butte, Montana, will at least minimize the travel requirements for North American speed skaters.

Competition Phase

During the competitive phase, the athlete is *stabilizing* the same factors that are acquired during the preparation phase and

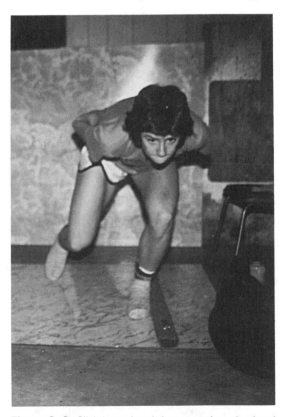

Figure 2–3. Slideboard training, another dry-land technique, is designed to mimic the muscular requirements of speed skating.

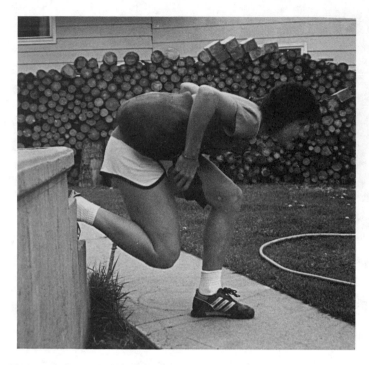

Figure 2–4. Weight training using sandbags to provide resistance and to allow exercise in a more skating-specific position. Speed skaters also do large amounts of traditional weight training.

working toward a peak performance. In the competitive phase of the speed skating year, the training emphasis shifts to specific on-ice drills designed to allow the athletes to use their skating strengths and skills. Competitive-phase training generally follows a pattern of relatively hard workouts with little rest prior to early season competitions. Then relatively easy training with plenty of rest is the norm prior to late season competitions. However, even during periods of very hard training, we continue to reinforce the necessity of rest to allow the athletes to skate correctly. It has been our experience that athletes who are overly tired make technical mistakes that may be just as detrimental to their performances as true overtraining. During this phase of the year we typically maintain a reduced schedule of dryland training that is intended only to minimize the loss of physiologic gains made earlier in the year.

OTHER TRAINING PROBLEMS

Athletes are individuals. Regardless of how well an overall scheme of preparation for competition is planned, no two athletes are going to respond in the same way. Even in a sport like speed skating, in which all-around competition is greatly emphasized, there are substantial differences in the events with which athletes feel comfortable and in the manner in which they respond to subtle differences of training. Individualization of training schedules is essentially a ceaseless job that is complicated by injuries, travel, and so forth (see Chapter 11). Just as the management of a particular patient with a chronic disease many times takes a physician months or years, so the individualized preparation of athletes requires considerable time.

Athletes are highly motivated individuals. In the winter sports, particularly, in which travel requirements and equipment costs may be substantial, an intrinsically motivated athlete is essential. Nevertheless, even the most highly motivated athlete will need short-term goals, and will require supportive and critical counseling to remain focused on the problem of preparing adequately. In many winter sports, notably speed skating, the travel and economic requirements of top-level competition select for young athletes who are very often still supported by their parents. There are few skaters who remain competitive into their mid-20s, and even the few older skaters who do remain competitive are often isolated from many of the job, education, and social aspects of "normal life." Thus, part of the motivation problem revolves around the coach's role as surrogate parent and counselor. Simply being available to provide a consistent set of rules or a sympathetic ear is often as important as the details of the next week's training schedule.

SPORTS MEDICINE AND SPORTS SCIENCE

In recent years media attention to the development of sports medicine and sports science as clear-cut academic disciplines has served to create a view that these technologies may pave the way for monumental leaps in performance. The failure of this to happen has often been cause for grave disappointment, particularly on the part of coaches. Based on our experience in speed skating, we believe that at least part of the problem is structural, and this may be amenable to a structural solution.

Traditionally, the primary source of support for athletes has been their coaches. The coach has provided virtually everything from advice on training to diet to injury prevention and treatment. Given the fact that coaches are also human, their knowledge and expertise concerning many important issues is superficial at best. In years past, American medicine has been traditionally reactive, giving care only after an illness or injury. Even when excellent medical care was available, there was often a lack of understanding by medical professionals regarding the specific problems of individual sports. This often limited the effectiveness of physicians in dealing with athletes (see Chapters 11 and 28). For example, when a speed skater says, "I can't sit down properly," he or she more likely has something wrong with the knee than with the posterior. Moreover, the scientific community has rarely understood the practical realities of sports. Strapped for funding and sometimes not seeing beyond their next abstract, they often did not give athletes and their coaches the type of long-term attention that was needed.

More by serendipity than by design, we have been fortunate to develop a sports med-

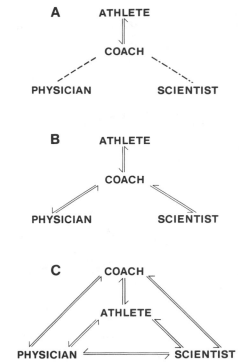

Figure 2–5. Structural models of the support structure for athletes. (A) The traditional model, with limited involvement of sports medicine/sports science; (B) the coach-centered model, with little direct interaction with the athlete from sports medicine/sports science; (C) the triangular model, featuring multiple lines of communication. In our experience, the triangular model has proven to be very effective.

icine/sports science structure that has proven to be utilitarian (Fig. 2–5). Thanks to the economic support of the Sports Science Division of the United States Olympic Committee and of Ross Laboratories, we have had the financial capacity to develop a program at Mount Sinai Medical Center in Milwaukee that works for us. Over the last decade, the physicians, physical therapists, trainers, and sports scientists in this group have come to understand the medical problems of speed skaters. Moreover, they have developed an appreciation of the time restrictions and special lifestyle and financial problems faced by many speed skaters. Today this group provides an additional dimension to the preparation of our athletes and the prevention of injuries. When they

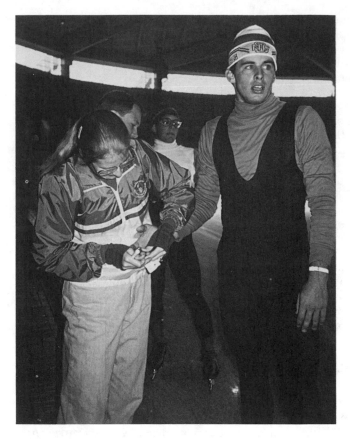

Figure 2–6. Field studies of blood lactate metabolism at the Olympic Oval in Calgary. Application of this technology by sports scientists who are conversant with the coaches' and athletes' needs provides a useful tool for fine tuning the preparation of our athletes.

join us at competitions they often function more as assistant coaches than as "docs." The application of their technology thus becomes a practical tool for the coach, rather than a scientific exercise (Fig. 2–6). This has required considerable goodwill and patience on the part of many coaches as well as the willingness of the sports science group to take a longer view of their work. Today for American speed skaters, the support structure can be thought of as a triangular platform upon which the athletes stand in the quest of their goals, rather than merely balancing on the shoulders of their coaches. At the points of the triangle are the coaching staff, the sports medicine staff, and the sports science staff. Communication among all three points of the triangle, as well as from each of the points of the triangle to the athlete, provides support not heretofore attainable in this country. This structure allows the coach to concentrate on more purely coaching-oriented functions while providing a dependable resource for medical or scientific

information. Our model is not perfect. None of the sports medicine/sports science people are skaters themselves, and many subtleties of our sport still escape them. Furthermore, they are very dependent upon competitive funding sources and continued goodwill of the medical center at a time when hospitals are having to reevaluate many programs on economic grounds. It remains, however, an important part of our overall program.

SUMMARY

Winter sports athletes are limited primarily by venue availability. In events that have a large technical component, it is difficult at best, and often impossible, to provide for adequate skill training during much of the training year. Many coaching issues are centered around ways to do effective "dry land" training during the summer months. Other primary concerns regard the individualization and balancing of training and competition. In speed skating, we have been fortunate to develop a sports medicine and science program in which the clinical and scientific staffs understand many of the basic problems unique to our sport and so can often function more as assistant coaches than as doctors or professors. This structural relationship with the coach and the athletes has enhanced strictly clinical and scientific functions. Building this structure has not been easy. It has required considerable luck, as well as patience, on the part of the coaching staff, the sports medicine/sports science staff, and the athletes. It has also required a considerable institutional commitment and support from multiple funding sources. However, its presence and continued operation has allowed us to focus more effectively on our primary goal—helping our skating athletes achieve their competitive goals.

CHAPTER 3

Altitude Training

JACK DANIELS, Ph.D.

Historically, early concern relative to the effects of altitude on human work and performance was paramount in the minds of mountaineers, aviators, and laborers who were hired to perform heavy work at "high" altitudes (above 3000 meters). These early concerns over altitude were simply related to performing physical tasks, most of which were noncompetitive in nature.

Only in the last 30 years or so have we become sensitive to the effects of altitude on athletic performance and how a low-lander might approach training for competition at altitude. In the past 15 years, concern over this issue—preparing for competition at high altitude—has been placed on hold while athletes have become infatuated by the potential benefits that altitude training may hold for athletes who wish to reach new highs of performance at sea level.

The progression of interest—from the effects of altitude on work and performance of required duties, to preparing for competition at altitude, to using altitude training as a means for improving sea-level performance—has not been accompanied with defined research to answer the questions that have arisen. The use of altitude training to improve sea-level performance has become relatively widespread. However, well-controlled research supporting the hypothesis that altitude training improves sea-level performance over comparable training at sea level is practically nonexistent. This lack of evidence has fed the mystique that altitude training is capable of producing superhuman performances and has led to the development of a variety of devices and training methods that provide the user with the "benefits" of altitude training without having to go to a higher elevation. It should be clarified that although the effects of altitude increase exponentially with increasing elevation and decreasing barometric pressure, concerns over altitude training—whether for competition at altitude or at sea level—are normally limited to *moderate* altitude in the range of 1000 to 3000 meters (3281 to 9843 feet) above sea level.

THE EFFECTS OF ALTITUDE ON HUMAN PERFORMANCE

The effects of altitude on various types of human performance are depicted in Figure 3–1. Strength and flexibility are not affected at altitude. On the other hand, skill of performance may be either adversely or positively affected, depending upon whether or not the activity being performed has a high-endurance or high-speed component. For example, marksmanship, weight lifting, shot putting, and diving may not be affected at all; whereas wrestling, boxing, and fencing may be adversely affected; and triple jumping, which combines speed of movement with particular skills, can be expected to be performed better at altitude. Pure overground speed events, such as sprint running and cycling, are performed better at altitude because the body is being moved against a less dense atmosphere, and therefore the resistance to movement is decreased. When the medium is water, as with sprint swimming,

the body is not moving against lessened resistance and swim times will not be better at altitude. Among the winter sports, performance in the speed events—sprint skating, ski jumping, Alpine skiing, luge, and bobsled—would generally be improved at altitude because of lower atmospheric resistance to movement, whereas altitude may be expected to have an unfavorable influence on the winter events that require some level of endurance such as hockey, figure skating, Nordic skiing, biathlon, and the longer speed skating races.

Performance in pure endurance events suffers at altitude because the relatively low atmospheric oxygen tension results in lower blood oxygen content, and ultimately reduced amounts of oxygen are presented to the exercising muscles. In short, in anaerobic events, a decreased aerobic capacity will not affect the outcome of the effort, but as the duration of activity increases and aerobic capacity becomes more and more critical to performance, the relative hypoxia of altitude becomes a detrimental factor and performance suffers. It should be pointed out that in some land endurance events, in which velocities are higher than can be reached in running (e.g., speed skating and cycling), performance is actually enhanced, because the benefits of lowered air resistance outweigh the negative effects of a diminished maximum oxygen consumption ($\dot{V}O_{2max}$). In fact, it is common to see endurance cycling records broken at moderate altitude. Most of the current world records in speed skating were recorded at high altitude. Still, endurance athletes can expect to further improve

BETTER AT ALTITUDE

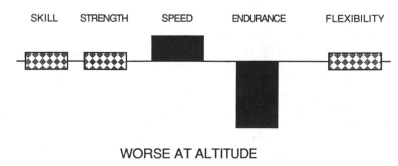

Figure 3–1. Summary of the effects of moderate altitude on various aspects of human performance (skill, strength, and flexibility are virtually unaffected).

WORSE AT ALTITUDE

their performances at altitude with appropriate altitude training.

TRAINING FOR A COMPETITIVE EFFORT AT ALTITUDE

Acclimatization to Altitude

Several facts became quite clear as a result of the considerable research conducted during the three or four years leading up to the 1968 Olympic Games, held at Mexico City's 2237-meter (7380-foot) altitude. First, as mentioned above, through an adverse effect on $\dot{V}O_{2max}$, altitude tends to hinder performance in many endurance events. Second, training at altitude (altitude acclimatization) improves this lowered altitude $\dot{V}O_{2max}$ to a level somewhere between the original sea-level value and the acute altitude exposure value.

Presently, there is little agreement among authorities as to how long it takes to become "fully acclimatized."[1-4] Notwithstanding, it has been generally accepted that many, if not all, physiologic adaptations are about as complete as they will ever be in a matter of a couple of months.[1-4] This is not to say that altitude acclimatization, as a whole, is complete in 6 to 8 weeks.

There are at least two, somewhat unrelated, aspects of acclimatization which must take place before optimum performance can be expected at altitude. One of these is physiologic in nature and includes an increase in red blood cell production and concentration and possibly an eventual increase in total blood volume. Acute exposure to altitude usually results in some dehydration and loss in plasma volume, which also results in higher red blood cell concentrations, and can be quite misleading when acclimatization is monitored through simple hemoglobin concentration and hematocrit tests. Another acute physiologic adjustment to altitude is an increase in pulmonary ventilation ($\dot{V}_E$) in an attempt to regain normal alveolar and arterial P_{O_2}. It is actually common to measure immediate increases in $\dot{V}_E$ upon acute exposure to altitude because the less dense air results in greater volumes being ventilated with the same ventilatory effort. Beyond this, however, further increases in maximum pulmonary ventilation (max $\dot{V}_E$) will occur over time.

"Competitive acclimatization" refers to learning to compete at altitude. Competitive acclimatization comes not only from training at altitude but also from competing at altitude. Merely subjecting the body to altitude initiates some degree of physiologic adaptation. Training at altitude increases both the rate of acclimatization and the degree to which the process proceeds. But some competitive experience at altitude is necessary for the athletes to become fully acclimatized for optimum performance at those heights. Learning to race at altitude takes time and requires a variety of attempts to learn the strategy that works best for the individual athlete at that particular height. An important observation in this regard is that competitors who learn how to pace their efforts and competitive tactics at particular altitudes tend to maintain their competitive acclimatization for months—if not years—after the initial period of exposure. Physiologic acclimatization, on the other hand, wanes relatively rapidly following return to sea level. Additionally, it has been the experience of numerous athletes that they may perform even better after they return to altitude following a week or two at sea level.

Training Strategies for Altitude Competition

Given the fact that the training needed for best performance in an altitude event is primarily designed to counteract the adverse effects altitude has on endurance, the training program must be specially designed for optimal results. In any endurance event, intensity of effort (often identified as speed or velocity of racing) is a function of the fraction of $\dot{V}O_{2max}$ at which the competitor can perform for the duration of the event. There is a given intensity of activity which is maintainable for any given duration of effort. When either economy of exercise or $\dot{V}O_{2max}$ is changed, this intensity becomes related to a different velocity of movement.

Figure 3–2 shows how the combined changes of economy of running and $\dot{V}O_{2max}$ result in a new speed of running being related to performance at the same relative intensity (same % $\dot{V}O_{2max}$). Figure 3–2 shows the typical economy curves for a distance runner at sea level and at altitude. With a better economy at altitude because of low-

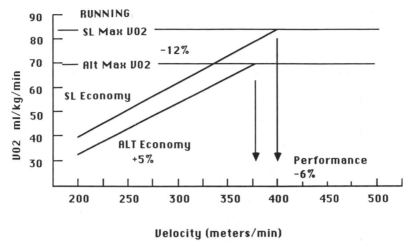

Figure 3–2. Typical effects of altitude on running economy and race pace at $\dot{V}O_{2max}$. Because of the similarity of competitive speeds, these results would be generally applicable to Nordic skiing.

ered air resistance, the typical 12 percent reduction in $\dot{V}O_{2max}$ expected at an altitude of about 2000 meters does not relate to an equal reduction in performance in a race run at 100 percent of the individual's $\dot{V}O_{2max}$ (a race lasting about 10 to 12 minutes). Naturally, in a longer race, the athlete could run at less than 100 percent of $\dot{V}O_{2max}$, but the resulting altitude decrement in performance would still be a combination of the drop in aerobic capacity and the improvement in economy. In speed skating the higher absolute velocity will tend to magnify the improved economy and for many distances will allow for im-

proved performances despite a lower $\dot{V}O_{2max}$ (Fig. 3–3). It is interesting to note that even though economy is not different for swimming at altitude and sea level, the 12 percent drop in $\dot{V}O_{2max}$ is associated with only about 6 percent reduction in performance, because of the configuration of the $\dot{V}O_2$/velocity relationship, which produces a much steeper slope in swimming (Fig. 3–4).

For running and skiing training, this implies that intervals that are typically performed at 95 to 100 percent of $\dot{V}O_{2max}$ will not necessarily have to be slowed by the same 12 percent that $\dot{V}O_{2max}$ is diminished at altitude.

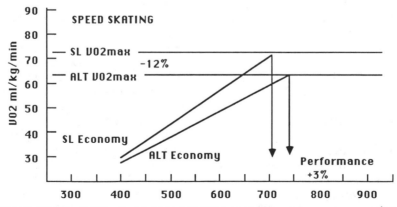

Figure 3–3. Typical effects of altitude on speed skating economy and race pace at $\dot{V}O_{2max}$. Because of the higher absolute speeds, the effects on economy are magnified when compared with those of running.

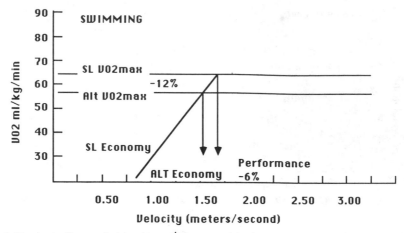

Figure 3–4. Typical effects of altitude on $\dot{V}O_{2max}$, swimming economy, and race pace at $\dot{V}O_{2max}$.

On the other hand, it is just as great a mistake to attempt to train at the same interval intensity at altitude as that used in sea level training, because this would result in a greater demand on anaerobic metabolism and a more rapid accumulation of blood lactate for the same amount of work performed. Conversely, for skating training the same relative intensity might be attained at a higher absolute velocity. Because the goal of training is to spend various amounts of time training at various relative intensities of effort, adjustments must be made at altitude to avoid "overtraining." For instance, a 2-hour run at 70 percent $\dot{V}O_{2max}$ or 70 percent of the maximum heart rate (HR_{max}) will be at a slower speed at altitude, even though the same speed may be possible by working at a higher percent of $\dot{V}O_{2max}$ at altitude.

The result of these intensity considerations is that when training at altitude for a race at altitude, usual relative training intensities—not usual speeds—should be employed, and these new training speeds will be appropriate for the new racing speed. With acclimatization, altitude $\dot{V}O_{2max}$ normally improves toward the sea level value, and the same relative intensities are associated with similar improvements in running velocity.

There has been no evidence that suggests that normal amounts of training need be curtailed upon exposure to moderate altitude, provided that consideration is given to maintenance of proper training intensities. However, it is recommended that unfit individuals should begin and increase their training load gradually, just as they should do when beginning a training program at sea level.

When preparing for a competitive endurance effort at altitude, the available time is an important consideration. If an individual has 5 days or fewer for acclimatization, it is advisable to arrive at the altitude site immediately prior to the competition. The usual reaction to acute exposure to altitude is to feel quite normal the first day. This is then followed by a decline in performance through days 3 to 5. By the end of the first week, most people are able to perform as well or a little better than they would the first day. Further improvements will come with several more weeks of altitude training. Thus, those who have the time would benefit from spending several weeks adjusting to altitude before an important competition. It has been found that alternating between periods of a couple of weeks at altitude and a week at sea level, with the altitude performance coming at the beginning of a reexposure, produces particularly good results. Athletes who must perform over a period of days cannot apply this procedure to each day's effort, but it is still satisfying to feel good on the first day, and subsequent competitive efforts do not drop off as they would during the first week of exposure. On the other hand, multiple-day competitors who do not have a week available prior to the first day of competition are in somewhat of a dilemma. They will often see their performances deteriorate over the course of the competition, and most likely it is the later days that are the more important ones. In this case, it would be advisable to time the most important competition day so that it comes after as many days as possible at altitude, with the understanding that performance during the middle days may be relatively disappointing.

Just as it is important to adjust training to match normal sea-level intensities, so must normal sea-level relative intensities be matched as closely as possible during competition at altitude. It is important to be particularly cautious at the beginning of an endurance event to avoid undue lactate accumulation, which will be carried, or even increased, throughout the event. Since different types of endurance events are affected differently, there is no general velocity or pace adjustment that applies to all sports. Therefore it is advisable to use some subjective evaluation of effort in order to judge proper pace. In most sports, a good means of controlling intensity is to be aware of breathing patterns. If the respiratory rate appears to be faster or the depth of breathing more labored than usual, chances are that the pace is too intense. With very little practice, ventilatory rate can be used to quite satisfactorily establish a reasonable competitive pace.

Special Training at Sea Level to Prepare for Altitude Competition

Probably the best approach to use when preparing at sea level for competition at altitude is to be informed of how altitude will affect performance. Endurance events will be slowed unless the speed of performance is particularly fast, as in cycling or speed skating. Altitude natives have an advantage, and evenly paced efforts will produce the best results for them. It should also be emphasized that a finishing "kick" at the end of a race may be as effective at altitude as it is at sea level if a prudent approach to the total performance is followed.

Since it is common for those unaccustomed to altitude to "go out" too fast at the start of a competition, thereby accumulating blood lactate at a faster-than-usual rate, there might be some subjective benefit to have athletes start practicing some sea level

workouts or races too fast. This could help increase their awareness to the consequences of a poorly paced effort. Use of special training devices or climate chambers which simulate altitude conditions may also aid in producing an adjustment to the feeling one will experience at altitude. Ventilatory muscles may be stressed somewhat harder. However, there may be a negative effect of artificially acclimatizing in climate chambers because the athlete may overestimate the benefits that can be derived and not compete as cautiously as might be the case without such preparation.

ALTITUDE TRAINING FOR A COMPETITIVE EFFORT AT SEA LEVEL

As suggested earlier, there has been a widely accepted use of altitude training as a means to improve performance at sea level—although research supporting this practice is lacking. There is no doubt that following a period of altitude training, an endurance athlete feels better competing at sea level. And in some cases sea-level performance actually is better. There are numerous testimonials to the benefits of altitude training presented by individuals who have moved to higher altitude "to become a better athlete." The very commitment to becoming better may produce better results.

Most studies designed to assess the effects of altitude training on performance at sea level take a group of sea-level natives to altitude for several weeks and administer pre-tests and post-tests. Usually, the results have actually been positive. However, such studies have typically been done at the start of summer with subjects who often leave stressful, warm, humid, polluted environments for the dry, cooler, cleaner, less stressful conditions of altitude. There are seldom any demands placed on the test subjects aside from training, eating, sleeping, and relaxing. The benefits of such a desirable overall environment are not measured; yet improvements in performance are invariably attributed to the effects of training at altitude.

Recent research, however, does suggest that altitude-trained athletes can perform better at sea level than do their equally trained sea-level counterparts.[5] Notwithstanding the relative lack of quantifiable data from better-controlled studies to support the benefits of training at altitude for improving sea level performance, many athletes and coaches will make this decision for subjective reasons.

There are some guidelines worthy of consideration when training at altitude for performance at sea level. The first, and probably foremost, is to plan the final 2 to 4 weeks of training to prepare for the specific conditions under which the important sea-level competition will occur. A good example of this applies to preparation for a marathon race. In this case, depletion of muscle glycogen, rise in body temperature, and dehydration are the main foes to be avoided or combated. Characteristically, locations at altitude are cool and dry, and if a sea-level marathon race is held in warm humid weather, the runner trained at altitude is at a real disadvantage. If altitude training is used in this case, it would be wise to spend the final 2 or 3 weeks training in the conditions that will be faced during the race. Any benefits that may have resulted from training at altitude will not be lost, provided that adequate time can be given to heat and humidity acclimatization.

In shorter endurance events, it is particularly important to prepare for the sea-level pace that is anticipated. As previously pointed out, the same relative intensity of effort is associated with a slower absolute pace at altitude for running and skiing; and when training for an altitude race, relative intensity is the important ingredient of training. Therefore, when a sea-level race is the goal, attention must be given to training at sea-level intensity. If training sessions include a particular amount of work repeated a defined number of times, at a particular intensity with a constant recovery period between individual bouts of work, primary emphasis should be on maintaining sea-level intensity. This is accomplished first by sacrificing recovery time between bouts of work. Then, if necessary, the duration of the individual bouts of work is shortened. In this way, the total amount and normal intensity of training can be maintained. For example, a typical sea-level interval running session involving eight repetitions of 800 meters at 2 minutes 20 seconds each with 2-minute recovery periods between each run might be changed to

8×800 meters at 2:20 with longer recovery periods, or more likely to 16×400 meters at 70 seconds each, with 1 to 2 minutes recovery after each run. In any case, the athlete at least must attempt to maintain the speed of training that would be required to accommodate the anticipated race pace at sea level. A simple rule to follow is that when a workout is designed to train a particular physiologic system, particular attention should be paid to *relative* intensity. When mechanics or speed is of primary importance, emphasis must be placed on *absolute* intensity.

Just as alternating between altitude and sea level training appears to work well in preparing for an altitude race, it seems to be a good method for preparing to race at sea level as well. Brief returns to sea level afford the opportunity to perform a few quality sea-level training sessions, assuring the athlete that performance at sea level has not deteriorated to the extent altitude training sessions might have suggested.

When considering altitude training as a means to performance enhancement, there are a few additional factors that warrant consideration: (1) The facilities must accommodate the sport for which the athlete is training; (2) the altitude should be kept between about 1525 and 2450 meters (5000 to 8000 feet); (3) general living conditions (e.g., housing, social activities, family consideration, weather) must be considered; and (4) finances must receive considerable attention, particularly if periodic returns to sea level are planned.

CONCLUSION

There is no doubt that altitude training will continue to be used by various athletes in a variety of sports; some will realize personal best performances, but some others will be very disappointed. Possibly the best way to look at altitude training is to treat it like any other type of training. It works better for some people than it does for others. How it is employed makes a considerable difference in the outcome. Until additional research provides us with a more definitive answer as to the possible benefits of training at altitude, these methods should continue to be considered as only *possible* means to performance enhancement.

REFERENCES

1. Astrand, PO and Rodahl, K: Textbook of Work Physiology, ed 3. McGraw-Hill, New York, 1986, pp 683–723.
2. Brooks, GA and Fahey, TD: Exercise Physiology: Human Bioenergetics and Its Applications. John Wiley & Sons, New York, 1984, pp 471–502.
3. Daniels, JT and Chosy, JJ: Epinephrine and norepinephrine exertion during running training at sea level and altitude. Medicine and Science in Sports 4:219–224, 1972.
4. Daniels, J and Oldridge, N: The effects of alternate exposure to altitude and sea level on world class middle distance runners. Medicine and Science in Sports 2:107–112, 1970.
5. Daniels, J, Troup, J, Telander, T, Miller, K, and Daniels, N: The effects of altitude training on sea-level swimming performance. In preparation.

CHAPTER 4

Nutrition for Winter Sports

JULIE ANN LICKTEIG, M.S., R.D.

CARL FOSTER, Ph.D.

Fluctuating environments and a wide variety of activities provide a range of nutritional problems for winter sports players, competitors, coaches, parents, health professionals, dietitians, and trainers. Lighted ski slopes and hockey rinks mean longer hours of activity, often late into the cold of the night. Competition continues despite snow, sleet, or chinook winds. Meals and snacks are scattered between occupations, schoolwork, practice sessions, and competition. Further disruption of living and eating patterns is caused by travel to sports activities occurring at higher altitudes and in different time zones.

A myriad of food products on the market tempt and often confuse the athlete. Some athletes believe that eating a special food will provide the margin of victory. However, a magic menu will not make up for lack of either talent or preparation. Nutritional supplements will not correct lifetime habits of incorrect eating. But, in the presence of adequate skill, practice, coaching, desire, and a healthy body, diet can make a difference.

Because of the individuality of winter sports and participants' needs, information in this chapter focuses on practical applications for the health care professional to implement rather than on a thorough review of the literature. Assessment of food patterns, activity levels, and body composition with techniques for collecting food-recall data will be presented. This is followed by an overview of protein, fat, carbohydrate, vitamin, mineral, energy, and fluid requirements.

DIETARY ASSESSMENT DATA

Complete nutritional assessment requires data from three areas:

1. *Clinical information:* a medical history, physical examination, anthropometric measurements, and dental and x-ray information. An ancillary role of the routine history and physical examination is to establish baseline parameters and rapport prior to the crisis precipitated by illness/injury. Anthropometric examination is often a useful guide to the gross nutritional needs of the participant.

2. *Dietary history:* a written questionnaire including eating patterns, food preferences and intolerances, food diaries, alterations in weight or appetite, supplements, digestive disorders, and possible nutrient-drug interactions.

3. *Biochemical data:* hemoglobin, hematocrit, cholesterol, serum sodium, serum potassium, serum albumin, serum protein, and other nutrient-related tests. Because of costs, the biochemical data are not always feasible. Furthermore, the value of these tests in the routine evaluation of clinically healthy individuals has not been established. In the absence of a serious deficiency apparent in the diet history or by clinical evidence, routine laboratory tests should be considered as research procedures.

Anthropometric Examination

It may be regarded almost as axiomatic that sports participants will be more successful as they get leaner and as they gain lean body mass. However, there are practical limits to the reduction of adiposity and, in gravity-resisting sports such as Nordic skiing and the various types of climbing, a high lean body mass may be counterproductive. Although hydrostatic weighing is the accepted gold standard for body composition studies, the time, expense, and inconvenience of this procedure limits its practical usefulness. We have found that the measurement of selected skinfold thickness, according to well-standardized methodology,[24] provides an accu-

rate assessment of percent fat in 5 minutes or less. Lean body weight may then be derived mathematically. For males younger than 30 years of age, we feel that 15 percent fat represents a practical upper limit of adiposity for even the recreational participant. For athletes, values in excess of 10 percent fat are thought to be excessive. On the other hand, percent fat values of less than 5 percent should be treated with caution, because this may signal an overall caloric deficiency. Athletes in this range should be monitored closely for signs of deteriorating performance. A similar pattern is recommended for female participants, although the absolute degree of adiposity is higher because of the secondary sex differences between males and females (see Chapter 6). We feel that for women less than 30 years of age, 23 percent fat represents a practical upper limit of adiposity. For serious competitors, values in excess of 17 percent fat are probably undesirable, and values less than 10 percent fat should be closely monitored as representing potential underfeeding. For all classes of participants, the recommended adiposity is increased about 1 percent fat for every 5 years after age 30 years. We cannot document that this is necessarily ideal but, in our experience, this weight gain seems to be inevitable. Because of the high prevalence of eating disorders in female athletes[26] and the association between *perceived* overweight and eating disorders, examiners should be very cautious when counseling. If in an attempt to achieve some "magic number" the athlete undereats or falls prey to an eating disorder, more may have been lost than gained. This may also be of importance for younger male athletes during periods of growth. Achieving ideal levels of body composition before completion of growth may limit adult stature and lean body mass. Accordingly, the need for strict control of body composition in this population is probably relatively low.

Diet History

The diet history is composed of (1) a food preference questionnaire and (2) a 24-hour food diary. On the food preference questionnaire appear questions related to the number of meals eaten away from home, amount of fast food, who does the cooking and shop-

Table 4–1. 24-HOUR FOOD DIARY

NAME: <u>Ann Sport</u> DATE: <u>March 2, 1986</u> SPORT: <u>Downhill Skiing</u>

TYPE DAY: <u>X</u> Training _____ Precompetition _____ Travel _____ Competition _____ Rest

TEMPERATURE RANGE DURING SPORTS ACTIVITY: <u>30°F</u> High <u>22°F</u> Low

DIRECTIONS:

1. Write down everything you ate or drank yesterday from the time you got up until you went to bed. It may help you remember by thinking about the time of day: breakfast, mid-morning, lunch, afternoon, dinner, and before bed.
2. Write down what time and where you ate or drank each food.
3. Describe each food fully. Tell whether it was raw or cooked. If cooked, tell how it was prepared (e.g., fried, boiled). Also, tell what it was served with (e.g., with cream sauce, with french dressing).
4. For casseroles or mixed dishes, list the major ingredients (e.g., hamburger casserole—hamburger, macaroni, tomatoes, onions).
5. Write down the amount of each food and beverage. Please give the amounts in exact measurements or units (e.g., 1 *slice* bread, 1 *medium* apple). (Do not give the amount as 1 bowl, 1 glass, etc.) If you are uncertain about the quantity, please discuss with registered dietitian; list water in addition to other beverages.
6. Describe emotions, level of anxiety, physical condition, and so forth.

EXAMPLE OF ONE MEAL:

Time	Place	Food Eaten	Amount
6:30 PM	Home	Toasted cheese sandwich made with	
		whole wheat bread	2 slices
		American processed cheese	1 slice
		margarine	1 tsp (5 gm)
		Cream of tomato soup (Campbell's)	1 8-oz bowl
		made with whole milk	250 ml
		Peanut butter cookies	3 (2″ size) (5 cm)
		Water	2 8-oz glasses (500 ml)

COMMENTS: Tired, worried   Weight: 136 lb

Adapted from Wisconsin Department of Health and Social Services,[34] p 82.

ping, some idea of income, number of meals eaten alone or with others, type of cooking facilities, food cravings, access to garden produce, use of special diets, supplements, drugs, alcohol, known allergies, gastrointestinal disturbances, cultural or religious features, and food fads.[1,16] Athletes keep *24-hour food diaries* for 3 to 5 days. Mason, Wenberg, and Welsh[21] cited numerous studies showing values in either 3- or 7-day food diaries. Averaging nutrient intake over 5 to 8 days is suggested by the National Research Council, which establishes the United States Recommended Dietary Allowances.[6] A particular nutrient, such as iron, may be better analyzed throughout a full week. However, cooperation by the client and the ability to record data accurately may be the overriding factors in choosing the appropriate length of

time for keeping the diary. Complete food diaries are kept for each 24-hour period; one meal is shown in Table 4–1.

Accurate reporting of serving sizes and the completeness of the diary are of utmost importance. Often food models, measuring cups, spoons, and scales need to be incorporated into the training of the recorder. Typical days should be chosen that represent the current eating pattern. For athletes going into a strict training routine, the menus of a 3-day basic cycle are compared with a 3-day training cycle. To emphasize the contribution of water to the total diet, the athlete should also be encouraged to record the total fluid consumption. Evaluating fluid and food replacement after heavy training or a competitive event is a valuable tool. Directly relative to the individual is the importance of capturing the day in total: Was it a competitive day, a regular training day, or a day of emotional peaks and valleys? A 24-hour activity diary form, presented later in this chapter (see Table 4–4), will complement the food recall. The athlete should enter the time spent in each activity level and multiply that time by the appropriate Kcal/min expenditure to yield the kilocalories for each category. These figures, added together, will provide the total energy expenditure for the 24-hour period.

Computer Application

Analysis of 24-hour diaries can be quickly accomplished by computer. It is our experience that nutritional software, which breaks down dietary recalls into subtotals for each meal and snack, is more helpful in counseling than dietary printouts showing only total consumption for the day. For endurance sports such as climbing and ski touring, meal and fluid subtotals graphically illustrate to an athlete the need to eat and to drink small amounts frequently. The database for nutritional analysis needs to be reliable and updated. Approved sources are United States Department of Agriculture (USDA) Handbooks No. 8,[30] 8-1 through 8-12,[29] USDA Handbook No. 456,[31] the USDA Home and Garden Bulletin No. 72,[32] Pennington and Church,[23] and University Nutritional Research Banks.[27] Programs should include analysis of fast foods and cultural foods of ethnic backgrounds.

ANALYZING THE FOOD DIARY

Recommended Dietary Allowances

Strict dietary analysis is judged against the average daily amounts of nutrients consumed by healthy populations over a certain period of time, known as the Recommended Dietary Allowances (RDA). Computer programs can illustrate by charts and graphs the percent of intake on a daily basis, providing the athlete with an individual learning tool. Dr. Sarah Short of Syracuse University[27] states that the RDAs are best used as a baseline for athletes, with modifications for weight, height, and activity. She refers to a cut-off of 66 percent of the published nutrient values[6] as the danger point for "low" or "poor" intakes. It is more difficult to judge overconsumption or "overly high" values, such as mineral intake of 200 percent of a given RDA.

Basic Four Food Groups

Professionals are more likely to use the RDAs, but the amateur finds the Basic Four Food Groups, shown in Table 4–2, an easier pattern to follow.

In the Milk Group, 250 ml (1 cup) of any form of milk equals one serving. Other equivalents are 240 gm (1 cup) yogurt, 200 gm (1½ cups) ice cream, 250 gm (1 cup) pudding with milk, 460 gm (2 cups) cottage cheese, 60 gm (2 oz) processed cheese food, and 40 gm (1⅓ oz) swiss or cheddar cheese.

Table 4–2. NUMBER OF SERVINGS PER FOOD GROUP IN THREE DIETARY PATTERNS RECOMMENDED FOR ADULTS PARTICIPATING IN WINTER SPORTS

	Basic*	Training†	Carbohydrate Loading‡
Milk products	2	2	2–3
Meats	2	2	2–3
Fruits and vegetables	4	8	8
Grains	4	8	12

*Recommended for recreational Alpine and cross-country skiers, hockey players, and ice skaters. Endurance athletes who are carbohydrate loading should follow this pattern during precompetition days 7, 6, 5, and 4.

†Recommended for short-distance speed skaters and Alpine and cross-country skiers as well as competitive hockey players. Athletes who work out daily for 2 hours or more should follow this pattern.

‡Recommended for endurance athletes (cross-country marathoners, long-distance speed skaters) or precompetition days 3, 2, and 1 of carbohydrate loading.

From Lickteig,[20] with permission.

In the Meat Group 60 to 90 gm (2 to 3 oz) of lean beef, veal, lamb, pork, poultry, fish or shellfish, 60 gm (2 oz) of seeds or nuts, 100 to 150 gm (½ to ¾ cup) cooked legumes, dry beans, peas, soybeans or lentils, 30 gm (2 tablespoons) peanut butter, or 2 eggs equal one serving.

The Vegetable and Fruit Group uses 120 gm (½ cup) cooked product as a serving, or a typical portion such as one orange, half a grapefruit, one medium potato, a bowl of salad, or half a cantaloupe. Use one good source of vitamin C daily, and frequently include deep yellow and dark green vegetables for vitamin A. Fiber found in this group is also a valuable component of the diet.

The Grain Group includes whole grain or enriched flour products. One serving may be

Table 4–3. MENUS FOR THREE DIETARY PATTERNS USING THE BASIC FOUR FOOD GROUPS

Basic	Training	Carbohydrate Load
Breakfast		
Orange juice (120 ml, ½ cup) Bran flakes with raisins (17 gm, ½ cup) Milk, skim (120 ml, ½ cup) Whole-wheat toast, 1 slice Coffee/tea	Orange juice (250 ml, 1 cup) Bran flakes with raisins (35 gm, 1 cup) Milk, skim (250 ml, 1 cup) Whole-wheat toast, 1 slice Jelly (10 gm, 2 tsp) Coffee/tea	Orange juice (250 ml, 1 cup) Bran flakes with raisins (52 gm, 1½ cups) Milk, skim (375 ml, 1½ cups) Whole-wheat toast, 2 slices Jelly (30 gm, 2 tbsp) Coffee/tea
Lunch		
Sandwich: ham (60 gm, 2 oz) Cheese, 1 slice (30 gm, 1 oz) Lettuce, tomato (½ medium) Enriched bread, 2 slices Apple (1 medium) Coffee/tea	Sandwich: ham (90 gm, 3 oz) Cheese, 1 slice (30 gm, 1 oz) Lettuce, tomato (½ medium) Whole-wheat bread 2 slices Salad dressing (10 gm, 2 tsp) Apple (1 medium) Coffee/tea	Sandwich: ham (90 gm, 3 oz) Cheese, 2 slices (60 gm, 2 oz) Lettuce, tomato (½ medium) Whole-wheat bread 2 slices Salad dressing (10 gm, 2 tsp) Apple (1 medium) Sugar cookies, 2 Coffee/tea
Dinner		
Beef roast (90 gm, 3 oz) Baked potato (1 medium) Broccoli (80 gm, ½ cup) Milk, skim (250 ml, 1 cup) Strawberries (150 gm, 1 cup)	Beef roast (120 gm, 4 oz) Baked potato (1 medium) Broccoli (80 gm, ½ cup) Whole-grain roll, 1 Margarine (5 gm, 1 tsp) Milk, skim (250 ml, 1 cup) Angelfood cake (1/16) with strawberries (75 gm, ½ cup)	Beef roast (120 gm, 4 oz) Baked potato (1 large) Broccoli (80 gm, ½ cup) Pasta salad (100 gm, ½ cup) Whole-grain roll, 1 Margarine (10 gm, 2 tsp) Milk, skim (250 ml, 1 cup) Angelfood cake (1/12) with strawberries (75 gm, ½ cup) and ice milk (40 gm, ⅓ cup)
Snacks		
Cucumber slices (1 small cucumber) Carrot sticks (3–4 strips) Cheese cube (30 gm, 1 oz)	Peach, fresh (1 medium) Fig cookies (6)	Peach, fresh (1 medium) Fruit-flavored yogurt (180 gm, ¾ cup) Banana, 1 medium (180 gm, 6 ounces)
1500 Kcal—50% CHO	2400 Kcal—50% CHO	3200 Kcal—58% CHO

1 slice of bread; 1 waffle; 1 pancake; 30 gm (1 oz) dry cereal; 120 gm (½ cup) cooked cereal, cornmeal, pasta; 18 gm (3 cups) popcorn; or 3 graham crackers.

A streamlined Basic Four, using skim milk and a low-calorie approach to food preparation, contains a variety of foods yielding the basic nutrients. However, it may produce only 1200 to 1500 calories—far below the needs of most active athletes. Thus the level of activity becomes a major consideration to be added to any basic nutrition program. Adaptions are shown in Table 4–2 for the training and higher carbohydrate patterns. Once the minimal pattern of the four groups is incorporated into the daily diet, the athlete can include additional calories. The extra calories may come from enlarged portions or the "others" category, including fats and sugars such as cake, pie, cookies, soft drinks, salad dressings, chocolates, and potato chips. By using the Basic Four plan as a guide, the athlete is consuming the 10 primary nutrients, which are protein, carbohydrate, fat, vitamin A, vitamin C, thiamin, riboflavin, niacin, calcium, and iron. The other 40 or so nutrients are most likely included in a mixed diet if adequate amounts are consumed. Single food sources are discouraged in favor of a diet with a wide variety of foods. Table 4–3 illustrates the translation of the Basic Four pattern into menus for basic, training, and carbohydrate-loading diets.

Professional Dietary Analysis

Dietary recalls of food and fluid intake can be compared with the Basic Four food guides for a rough estimation of nutrient value. Comprehensive analysis provides greater detail but needs interpretation by a professional. Additional time, equipment, and financial resources are needed to provide the type of expertise often desired. Even one session with the proper specialist in sports nutrition (usually a registered dietitian) may well be worth the dollars spent on vitamin and mineral supplements or self-help books written by nutritionists of self-appointed stature. One valuable specialist, a registered dietitian, may be located through Sports and Cardiovascular Nutritionists (SCAN), a practice group of the American Dietetic Association (ADA), 216 West Jackson Boulevard, Chicago, Illinois, 60606-6995.

ENERGY

Basic Daily Requirements

The RDAs are more uniformly established for minimal nutrient levels than for energy requirements. Daily energy needs depend on such variables as length of exercise, speed, body size, age, climate, altitude, and special needs for pregnancy and lactation. Excluding pregnancy and lactation, three categories encompass the basic energy requirements:[17] (1) *basal metabolic rate (BMR)*—a composite of chemical action which maintains a resting body, including heart, kidneys, liver, brain, gastrointestinal system, adipose tissue, and muscles; (2) *activity*—physical exercise and related muscular tension owing to increased arousal at competition; (3) *dietary thermogenesis (DT)*—involves all metabolic processes of digestion, absorption, and delivery of nutrients to the cells. DT adds about 10 percent to the total daily energy needs of the body. Protein is the nutrient requiring the most activity, especially in relation to oxygen, and it is the one that causes the greatest dietary thermogenesis—a factor to be noted especially when adjusting to performance at altitudes of over 2450 meters (8000 feet).

Our suggested approach to estimating daily energy needs is outlined below.

Calculations for Estimated Daily Energy Expenditures

1. To obtain a basal metabolic rate (BMR), determine the lean body weight in kilograms by the use of skinfold measures. Multiply this value by 28.9. For a 130-pound woman at 14 percent fat this becomes

$$\frac{130 - (130 \times 0.140)}{2.2} \times 28.9$$
$$= 1469 \text{ Kcal/day}$$

2. Activities of daily living for nonobese individuals require approximately 38 percent above the BMR.[25] Thus, for our female subject described above, the requirement for daily activities may be computed as

$$1469 \times 1.38 = 2027 \text{ Kcal/day}$$

3. For organized exercise, the energy requirements of various activities have been estimated[22] and are included in Table 4–4. Analysis of a typical week of training will give a reasonable estimate of energy needs.

Table 4—4. SAMPLE 24-HOUR ACTIVITY DIARY FORM—AVERAGE MALE-FEMALE

Activity Level	Time (Min)	Male—70 kg Kcal/min	Female—58 kg Kcal/min	Total Kcal
Sleep, reclining		1.0–1.2	0.9–1.1	
Very light		2.5	2.0	
Seated or standing activities, waiting for races, snowmobiling				
Light		2.5–4.9	2.0–3.9	
Level walking (2.5–3 mph), ice boating,* trapping, hunting				
Moderate		5.0–7.4	4.0–5.9	
Walking (3.5–4 mph), skiing (soft snow, leisure), ice skating, ski jumping,* bobsledding,* tobogganing*				
Heavy		7.5–12.0	6.0–10.0	
Climbing (alpine light), snowshoeing, ice hockey, speed skating, skiing (hard snow, alpine)				
Very heavy		12.1+	10.0+	
Skiing (uphill), racing cross country, dogsledding,* climbing (alpine heavy)				
			24-hour total:	

*Estimated

Adapted from Appendix D of McArdle, Katch, and Katch,[22] and from Committee on Dietary Allowance, Food and Nutrition Board,[6] p 24.

For our female subject, assuming her to be a speed skater training 2½ hours per day:

2027 + (9 Kcal/min × 150 min)
= 3377 Kcal/day

4. The DT from metabolism of food is estimated at 10 percent of the total Kcal:

10% × 3377 = 338 Kcal

5. Add the DT Kcal to the total in step 3:

3377 + 338 = 3715 Kcal/day

6. Comparison of the basic value for energy expenditure versus recorded intakes and weight history will allow for titration of individual needs.

Thermal Adjustments

Further adjustments to energy needs relative to winter sports include exposure to cold for extended time periods. Work at mean temperatures below 14°C (57.2°F) requires about 5 percent more energy than in warmer conditions.[6,33] Wearing heavier clothes, boots, and sporting gear may cause an additional 2 to 5 percent increase in energy expenditure. Thus, exercising under very cold conditions requiring heavier clothing may increase the requirement of exercising in the third calculation above by about 10 percent. Therefore, it is our recommendation that careful weight records should be maintained for winter sports participants to identify caloric deficits as early as possible. Recent reports have also remarked upon the surprisingly low energy intake in various groups of athletes.[3] A hypothesis of increased food efficiency in individuals with low levels of adiposity has been proposed. Although this hypothesis has not been adequately tested, it does serve to explain why computed energy requirements are often very different from recorded dietary intakes. Until this issue is resolved, the clinician should certainly be conservative when making energy intake recommendations to athletes.

BASIC NUTRIENTS

Protein

Approximately 11 to 12 percent of the daily caloric intake is in the form of protein. Contrary to past training-table practices, it is not the preferred energy source. Protein with only 4 Kcal/gm is an inefficient source of energy. Unfortunately, it is usually accompanied by fat in fairly large percentages and may jeopardize carbohydrate intake. At an RDA of 0.8 gm/kg of body weight per day, the 70 kg man is satisfied with 56 gm of protein and the 55 kg average woman with 44 gm per day. The Basic Four more than adequately covers this amount. For example, 1 slice of bread yields 3 gm, 180 gm (6 oz) beef yields 45 gm, and 1 glass (250 ml, 1 cup) of milk yields 9 gm. Beyond this contribution—namely, to supply nine essential amino acids for building and maintaining all body cells—the excess is used for energy. However, the average man is not an average athlete, or at least not an average Olympic hopeful. For athletes involved in heavy-resistance training programs, more research is needed to establish protein requirements. Although noting a lack of clearly supportive evidence, many authorities suggest that higher relative protein intakes may be desirable in athletes.[19] By eating 3000 Kcal per day with even 10 percent content, the 0.8 gm/kg can be met. However, many athletes consume less than 10 percent protein in an effort to replace protein with more complex carbohydrates for the endurance sports. If these athletes indeed need to consume between 1.3 and 1.5 gm of protein per kilogram body weight daily, a relative deficiency may occur. Athletes in activities requiring increased lean body weight may thus be at a disadvantage by following the RDA.

Normal protein foods, not special high-protein supplements, are still the best. Low-fat, high-protein suggestions include skim milk, yogurt, low-fat cheeses, broiled or baked poultry, legumes, fish, and eggs. Using the Basic Four, two to three servings each are listed from the meat and milk groups which will help to furnish protein needs. Remember that protein, although varying in quality, is available from all four food groups; for example, 8 gm in 30 gm (1 oz) of dried beans, 2 gm in 120 gm (½ cup) of vegetables, 2 gm in one serving of cereal, and 7 gm in 30 gm (1 oz) of cheese.[4] Vegetarian athletes should carefully match their proteins using one of the reliable current nutrition books, such as Cataldo and Whitney[4] or Hamilton, Whitney, and Sizer,[17] as a reliable source of information.

Fat

The training tables of yesteryear contained steak, potatoes with sour cream, and all the whole milk one could drink. But to reach the levels of carbohydrate needed for training and to maintain protein intake, the balance will need to come from decreasing fat intake. At 9 Kcal/gm of fat, even lowering a small amount of fat content in the diet frees up calories to be taken in the carbohydrate area. A decrease from the current daily consumption of 42 percent fat to 30 percent is encouraged.[17] The method of preparation is as important as the food; begin with lean meats, remove excess fatty skin and all visible fat. Minimize the use of eggs and organ meats, substituting leaner cuts, dry beans and peas, fish, and poultry. Cutting back on the sweet, syrupy desserts of cakes and sweet rolls makes room for complex carbohydrates and avoids further inclusion of fat in the diet. One of the easiest areas of minimizing fat intake involves evaluating fast foods. Substitute 250 ml (1 cup) skim milk for vanilla shakes, or baked chicken for fried chicken.

Carbohydrate

Endurance athletes will benefit by following Table 4–2, which illustrates a tripling of the grain group and fruit and vegetables. Carbohydrates yield 4 Kcal/gm. In the normal diet, carbohydrates are responsible for 46 percent of the calories. For athletes in training, the carbohydrate levels should be increased to 55 percent or more, especially coming from the complex sources such as potatoes, pastas, and whole grain products. Some high-carbohydrate, low-fat choices are given in Table 4–5.

Research studies from several laboratories have shown that severe training in athletes is associated with more or less chronic glycogen depletion.[7,13] This often leads them to cut back the intensity of their training which may reduce the value of the training efforts.

Table 4–5. HIGH-CARBOHYDRATE, LOW-FAT CHOICES IN THE FOUR FOOD GROUPS

Milk products	Low-fat yogurt and cheese, cottage cheese, skim milk, ice milk
Meats	Chicken, turkey, fish, eggs, lentils, dried peas, pork, and beans
Fruits and vegetables	Dried apricots, banana chips, grape juice, pear nectar, corn, fresh or frozen peas, potatoes, carrots
Grains	Crackers, bread, cornbread, noodles, rice, bran flakes, pancakes, bread dressing

From Lickteig,[20] p 203, with permission.

In certain sports, such as skiing, loss of technique may result and so may lead to an increased risk of injury.[13] High-carbohydrate diets have been shown to be effective in supporting muscle glycogen stores through several days of training.[10,14] However, it is equally well documented that athletes routinely fail to consume high-carbohydrate diets, despite the advice of the medical community.[2,12,18] In recent years the development of high-carbohydrate liquid nutritionals for the athlete has been shown to be a safe and effective method of enhancing carbohydrate intake and promoting muscle glycogen synthesis while also contributing to fluid replacement.[28] The development of liquid nutritionals based on polymerized forms of glucose allows administration of fairly high concentrations of carbohydrates (17 gm/100 ml) with minimal gastrointestinal upset.

Work that we have done with the United States Speed Skating Team has shown favorable alterations in the dietary pattern during weeks on and off the supplement (400 ml taken after each workout) (Table 4–6). Carbohydrate consumption increased both absolutely and as a percentage of total kilocalories. Both protein and fat intakes were depressed during this period, although total protein intake remained at 1.5 gm/kg/day. These dietary alterations were associated with favorable subjective responses during training and by enhanced performance during both submaximal and supramaximal exertion in the laboratory (Table 4–7). That these supplements can contribute to the twin goals of rehydration and carbohydrate consumption soon after exercise argues in favor of their use. Recent evidence that muscle glycogen synthesis is favored by feeding immediately following exercise suggests that they should be used in the training room. Our experience has been that a mild suppression of appetite occurs for 2 to 3 hours following consumption of 400 ml of these carbohydrate supplements. However, as long as the athlete is capable of adjusting mealtimes to ensure adequate intake of other nutrients, this appetite suppression is not critical.

Table 4–6. DIETARY RESPONSES DURING CONTROL AND SUPPLEMENT PERIODS FOR SPEED SKATERS DURING ONE WEEK OF TRAINING WITH OR WITHOUT A LIQUID CARBOHYDRATE SUPPLEMENT

Total Intake	Control	Supplement
Energy (Kcal/day)	3054 ± 750	3570 ± 590
Protein (gm/day)	120 ± 35	105 ± 30
Fat (gm/day)	125 ± 40	110 ± 31
Carbohydrate (gm/day)*	388 ± 95	538 ± 93
Percent of Kcal*	49 ± 9	64 ± 7

*p <0.05, control versus supplement

Table 4–7. METABOLIC AND PERFORMANCE
RESPONSES DURING SUBMAXIMAL AND
SUPERMAXIMAL EXERCISE IN SPEED SKATERS
AFTER ONE WEEK OF TRAINING WITH OR
WITHOUT A LIQUID CARBOHYDRATE
SUPPLEMENT

	Control	Supplement
Submaximal HR (beats/min)	149 ± 28	147 ± 30
Submaximal RPE* (Borg)	5.4 ± 1.0	4.7 ± 0.7
Time to fatigue* (min)	2.06 ± 1.05	2.33 ± 1.15
Max lactate* (mM)	8.5 ± 3.0	10.4 ± 2.9

*$p < 0.05$, control versus supplement

Vitamins and Minerals

Unless a known deficiency exists or an athlete is not able to consume the Basic Four, supplements are normally not given. Iron and calcium intake is a major concern for women. Daily intake of iron should exceed 18 mg, and although the RDA of calcium for women between 19 and 50 years of age is 1000 mg, calcium intake should exceed 1500 mg daily in women 50 years of age or beyond their menopause (see Chapter 6). It is often difficult to argue with the popular logic taken by supplement manufacturers that since we do not fully understand the difference between a nondeficiency state and "optimal health," supplements should be taken prophylactically. However, when one considers the real risk of hypervitaminosis states that are sometimes observed as the result of megadose supplementation and the dangers of iron storage in those with genetically determined enzymatic defects (see Chapter 13), it is possible to argue that these supplements may not be harmless. In the absence of documentable benefit, their use becomes difficult to justify. A reasonable compromise may be the use of a "one-a-day plus iron" type supplement. This certainly will cover any deficiencies attributable to an inadequate diet and is unlikely to be associated with deleterious side effects.

Fluid

It seems that the most important nutrient is the most neglected, as we do not need to go out and purchase water on a normal basis. Rarely is one aware of the amount consumed until such times as snow camping, when there is a conscious effort to melt snow for cooking and drinking. One half to three fourths of our body weight comes from water. Forty percent of this is inside the cells, and 15 percent is extracellular.[4]

Weighing before and after practice will convince the athlete of the need to replace the water pound for pound—a 0.91 kg (2 lb) loss equals 1 liter of fluid. Most hydration should occur prior to or following exercise, when gastric emptying is around the resting rate (20 ml/min). During heavy exercise, the rate of gastric emptying slows and may be only 5 ml/min,[9] thereby preventing adequate replacement of bodily losses. Plain water continues to be a good fluid replacement; when desiring fluid plus energy, choices revolve around some combination of a glucose/sucrose/fructose solution with approximately 5 to 7.5 gm sugar per 100 ml of water (about 1 to 1½ tsp per ½ cup). Gatorade is 6 percent carbohydrate and Exceed is 7.2 percent. By comparison, ordinary fruit juices range from 10 to 15 percent and Coca-Cola is 11 percent. Due to possible gastric complications and no known performance benefits, fructose should constitute no more than 2 percent of the total carbohydrate.[5]

Recent research shows that sodium as found in most sport drinks ranges from 10 to 12 mEq/8 oz glass. This is acceptable as plasma normally is 140 mEq/liter. Small amounts of sodium help to sustain blood volume during endurance exercise in a hot environment and to prevent the hyponatremia that is occasionally observed when athletes take our recommendations to drink water liberally too literally.

Glucose polymers are also an appropriate carbohydrate source, especially when 20 to 25 percent solutions are needed for replenishing muscle glycogen after long, heavy exercise. Examples are unflavored Carboplex and Polycose and flavored Gatorlode and Exceed.[5] Our experience has been that concentrated carbohydrate-containing beverages tend to produce osmotic diarrhea in many athletes. We feel that about 17 percent carbohydrate represents a practical upper limit for carbohydrate beverages.

It takes some planning and foresight to anticipate fluid needs before truly significant thirst alerts us to deprivation. Cold, wind, rain, and snow tend to make small, frequent water stops uncomfortable, but coaches, fellow athletes, and race directors have an obligation to provide ready access to fluids.

COMPETITION

One of the most difficult judgments for coaches and teams is when to eat before an event. Ideally, the athlete should consume food at least 3 hours before an event to allow the stomach to be relatively free of digestive activity. Excitement and emotional stress may account for a favorite food ritual. Since little is gained in performance by last-minute calorie stuffing, athletes should be free to choose a comfortable pre-event pattern. The meal should be small (500 to 1000 calories) and consistent with the concepts of high-carbohydrate, low-fat, moderate-protein, and low simple sugar contents. In no case should the athlete begin an event with plasma insulin still elevated in response to a previous meal. Hyperinsulinemia has been shown to increase the rate of glycogen utilization[8] and to influence performance negatively.[15] Because of the time course of plasma insulin responses following exercise, a minimum of 3 hours from the last meal to competition is often required.

In prolonged intermittent events—such as sprint skating, ski jumping or alpine racing, which may last all day—continued small intakes of fluids and foods will maintain blood sugar levels and water balance. Recent evidence suggests that sustained hyperglycemia

during prolonged exercise may allow continuation of high-intensity exercise even after depletion of muscle glycogen stores.[11] Thus, during very protracted exercise the need for more or less continuous feeding is evident.

SUMMARY

Nutrition for the winter sports participant is remarkably simple and follows the general guidelines for good nutrition. Observation of the Basic Four eating plan, with particular care to ensure adequate intake of water and carbohydrates, represents the "golden rule" of nutrition. Dietary requirements may be influenced by specific training or environmental circumstances but generally represent common-sense modifications of well-accepted principles.

ACKNOWLEDGMENT

We thank Judith Tharman, M.S., R.D., for reviewing the original manuscript.

REFERENCES

1. American Dietetic Association: Handbook of Clinical Dietetics. Yale University Press, New Haven, 1981.
2. Blair, SN, Ellsworth, NM, Haskell, WL, Stern, MP, Farquham, JR, and Wood, PD: Comparison of nutrient intake in middle-aged men and women runners and controls. Medicine and Science in Sports and Exercise 13:310–315, 1981.
3. Brownell, KD, Steen, SN, and Wilmore, JH: Weight regulation practices in athletes: Analysis of metabolic and health effects. Medicine and Science in Sports and Exercise 19:546–556, 1987.
4. Cataldo, CB and Whitney, EN: Nutrition and Diet Therapy: Principles and Practice. West Publishing, St Paul, 1986.
5. Coleman, E: Eating for Endurance, ed. 3. Bull Publishing, Palo Alto, Calif, 1988, pp 85–89.
6. Committee on Dietary Allowance, Food and Nutrition Board: Recommended Dietary Allowances, ed 9. National Academy of Sciences, National Academy Press, Washington, DC, 1980.
7. Costill, DL, Bowers, R, Branham, G, and Sparks, K: Muscle glycogen utilization during prolonged exercise on successive days. J Appl Physiol 31:834–838, 1971.
8. Costill, DL, Coyle, E, Dalsky, G, Evans, W, Fink, WJ, and Hoopes, D: Effects of elevated plasma FFA and insulin on muscle glycogen usage during exercise. J Appl Physiol 43:695–699, 1977.
9. Costill, DL and Saltin, B: Factors limiting gastric emptying during rest and exercise. J Appl Physiol 37:679–683, 1974.
10. Costill, DL, Sherman, WM, Fink, WJ, Maresh, C, Witte, M, and Miller, JM: The role of dietary carbo-

hydrates in muscle glycogen synthesis after strenuous running. Am J Clin Nutrition 34:1831–1836, 1981.

11. Coyle, EF, Hagberg, JM, Hinley, BF, Martin, WH, Ehsani, A, and Halloszy, JO: Carbohydrate feeding during prolonged strenuous exercise can delay fatigue. J Appl Physiol 55:230–235, 1983.

12. Ellsworth, NM, Hewitt, BF, and Haskell, WL: Nutrient intake of elite male and female nordic skiers. The Physician and Sportsmedicine 13(2):79–93, 1985.

13. Eriksson, E: Ski injuries in Sweden: A one year study. Orthopedic Clin North Am 7:3–9, 1976.

14. Eriksson, E, Nygaard, E, and Saltin, B: Physiological demands of downhill skiing. The Physician and Sportsmedicine 5(12):29–34, 1977.

15. Foster, C, Costill, DL, and Fink, WJ: Effects of preexercise feeding on endurance performance. Medicine and Science in Sports 11:1–5, 1979.

16. Grant, A: Nutritional Assessment Guidelines, ed 2. Seattle, WA, 1979.

17. Hamilton, EN, Whitney, EN, and Sizer, FS: Nutrition: Concepts and Controversies, ed 3. West Publishing, St Paul, 1985.

18. Jacobs, I, Westlin, N, Karlsson, J, Rasmusson, M, and Houghton, B: Muscle glycogen and diet in elite soccer players. Eur J Appl Physiol 48:297–302, 1982.

19. Lemon, PWR, Yarasheski, KE, and Dolny, AG: The importance of protein for athletes. Sports Medicine 1:474–484, 1984.

20. Lickteig, JA: Fueling Winter Sports. The Physician and Sportsmedicine 14(1):200–205, 1986.

21. Mason, M, Wenberg, BG, and Welsh, PK: The Dynamics of Clinical Dietetics, ed 2. John Wiley & Sons, New York, 1982.

22. McArdle, WD, Katch, FI, and Katch, VL: Exercise Physiology Energy, Nutrition and Human Performance, ed 2. Lea & Febiger, Philadelphia, 1986.

23. Pennington, JAT and Church, HN: Food Values of Portions Commonly Used, ed 14. Harper & Row, Philadelphia, 1985.

24. Pollock, ML, Schmidt, DH, and Jackson, AS: Measurement of cardiorespiratory fitness and body composition in the clinical setting. Comprehensive Therapy 6:12–27, 1980.

25. Ravussin, E, Lillioja, S, Abbott, W, and Bogurdus, C: Variability of 24 hour energy expenditure, resting metabolic rate and sleeping metabolic rate in man. Clinical Research 34:73A, 1986.

26. Rosen, LW, McKeag, DB, Hough, DO, and Durley, V: Pathogenic weight control behavior in female athletes. The Physician and Sportsmedicine 14(1):79–90, 1986.

27. Short, SH: Computerized sports nutrition. Sports-Nutrition News 3:1–5, 1984.

28. Snyder, AC, Lamb, DR, Baun, TS, and Prah, GL: Muscle glycogen loading with a carbohydrate drink. Physiologist 24:176A, 1981.

29. United States Department of Agriculture, Consumer Nutrition Center: Composition of Foods, Revised USDA Handbooks 8, 1–12, Washington, DC, 1976–1984.

30. United States Department of Agriculture, Consumer Nutrition Center: Composition of Foods–Raw, Processed, Prepared, Revised USDA Handbook 8, Washington, DC, 1963.

31. United States Department of Agriculture: Nutritive Value of American Foods in Common Units, USDA Handbook 456. Washington, DC, 1976.

32. United States Department of Agriculture: Nutritive Values of Foods, Home and Garden Bulletin No. 72, ed 7. Washington, DC, 1971.

33. Williams, SR: Nutrition and Diet Therapy, ed 5. Times Mirror/Mosby College Publishing, St Louis, 1985.

34. Wisconsin Department of Health and Social Services, Division of Health: Nutrition Screening and Assessment Manual. Madison, 1979.

CHAPTER 5

Winter Sports and the Young Athlete

JACK HARVEY, M.D.

JOANN SCHONNING, A.T.C.

Providing medical care for the young athlete participating in winter sports requires a knowledge of the sports medicine and training needs of the young athlete, as well as an understanding of the problems posed by exercise in a cold environment. The young athlete does differ from the adult counterpart in several physiologic aspects which dictate differences in training programs. The psychologic aspect of the child's participation in sport and competition is also an extremely important factor. Finally, the young athlete doesn't tolerate exercise in the cold as well as the adult athlete, and careful preparation and adult supervision are necessary for safe participation.

BASIC SPORTS SCIENCE

As has been often stated, children are not merely small adults, and their bodies do not respond to training stimuli in the same manner as adults' bodies. Research is just beginning to accrue about the trainability of enzymes, muscles, nerves, and organ systems of children. At the molecular level, the cell anatomy and enzyme systems for aerobic trainability are already in place in childhood. To what degree and how best to train them is the question. Recent papers have shown that prepubescent boys and girls can improve their aerobic capacity by endurance training and that capacity increases with age. In adolescent athletes, aerobic power correlates with lean body mass and maturity. In boys, $\dot{V}O_{2max}$ increases with age to 18 years, but does not increase in girls much beyond 14 years of age.[1,10]

Practical experience and research indicate that anaerobic potential can be developed in the adolescent athlete. Recent data also indicate that prepubescent children have limited potential for development of the anaerobic system.[6] The advisability of this type of training in the prepubescent child and the younger, less experienced adolescent athlete is questioned. In general, the longer-duration, higher-frequency, and higher-intensity training programs should be utilized for the more advanced teenage athlete. Intense training programs run the risk of physical and psychologic injury to the younger, less experienced athlete.

Strength training is often of interest to many youth sport coaches, parents, and athletes. It certainly has its place for the more experienced adolescent athlete, but again the practice must be questioned in the prepubescent athlete. It is well known that the presence of testosterone greatly enhances the effect of a strength program. Two groups of young athletes lack this hormone: prepubescent boys and all girls. This does not mean these groups of athletes cannot develop strength with a properly designed exercise program that enhances recruitment patterns of muscles. However, hypertrophy of muscle mass will not occur, because this aspect of body building requires the presence of testosterone.

In younger athletes, a strength-training program should be a very minor part of the overall training regimen. It should probably be pursued only in the few prepubescent children who enthusiastically want to participate in a weight program. Fun, proper technique, and perhaps some strength gains should be the focus of the closely supervised program for younger athletes.[9] Calisthenics, light free weights, or machines that can accommodate pediatric-size anatomy should be the tools. Higher repetitions (15 to 25 repetitions), low sets (1 to 2), and proper technique should be the emphasis. However, the adolescent athlete will perform better and perhaps be less prone to injury if a good pre-season strength program is combined with

an in-season strength-maintenance program as part of the sport. Recent trends indicate that this is important for the female athlete as well. This properly designed program will require increased frequency and sets (3 to 5) but fewer repetitions (6 to 10). Again, careful supervision with free weights and/or machines emphasizing good technique and intensity will give the best results.[15]

As previously mentioned, hypertrophy of muscle mass requires the presence of testosterone. Augmentation of this process by the use of anabolic steroids is condemned (see Chapter 12). These substances are not only unethical and illegal in competition and training but present several hazards to the performance and health of the athlete. Although steroids do produce profound strength increases, they do not enhance in any manner the endurance performance of the athlete. Psychologic changes, which include aggression and impatience, jeopardize athlete–coach and athlete–athlete relationships. The positive aspects of teamwork are often destroyed. Health consequences are many, with shortness of stature being unique to the growing athlete. Female athletes develop permanent masculine changes of voice, hirsutism, and other secondary sexual characteristics. Alteration of several body enzyme systems and reproduction function presents health concerns for the future. Of particular concern is also an increase in atherosclerotic deposits in the coronary arteries. This may well accelerate the development of coronary artery disease in steroid abusers.[3] By no stretch of the imagination do the benefits of steroid use justify the risks.

More important than a strength program for the younger or inexperienced athlete is learning and perfecting the basic skills of the sport. The athlete's performance and enjoyment of a sport will be more profoundly influenced by learning these skills than by participating in a strict conditioning program. Only after mastery of the skills of the sport should strength training and conditioning be emphasized in the young athlete's approach to a sport.

The psychologic aspects of the young athlete's participation in the sport must be monitored carefully. Young athletes need to have reached a maturational level that coincides with the demands of their sport. Readiness to compete in a sport also requires parental tolerance and the willingness of a coach to prepare the child for that sport.[7] Children can grasp the idea of competition around 6 to 8 years of age. However, undue emphasis on competition and winning will likely result in early burnout. Rigorous training and competition need to be delayed for later years.[13] As long as the competitive concept is used constructively in setting goals, motivation, and striving to do one's best, the psychologic effect will be positive. Coaches, parents, and team physicians need to understand the importance of fulfilling the psychologic needs of young athletes participating in sports. The positive attributes of fun, worthiness, teamwork, setting goals, and accomplishment should not be overshadowed by anxiety, fear of failure, and undue emphasis that the outcome of the competition must be winning.

Martens and colleagues[8] have developed a "Bill of Rights for Young Athletes" that coaches, parents, trainers, program directors, and physicians should keep foremost in mind.

BILL OF RIGHTS FOR YOUNG ATHLETES

Right to participate in sports
Right to participate at a level commensurate with each child's maturity and ability
Right to have qualified adult leadership
Right to play as a child and not as an adult
Right of children to share in the leadership and decision making of their sport participation
Right to participate in safe and healthy environments
Right to proper preparation for participation in sports
Right to an equal opportunity to strive for success
Right to be treated with dignity
Right to have fun in sports

THE YOUNG ATHLETE AND COLD ENVIRONMENT

Young athletes are especially susceptible to the effects of environment on their performance and health. First, compared with adults, they have a larger body surface area per weight; so extremes of temperature will have a more profound effect in terms of overheating or overcooling. Second, children do not have a good understanding of how they may monitor their body functions and make

appropriate adjustments regarding levels of exertion, clothing, nutrition, and hydration during exercise. When these factors are combined with the pressures of a demanding coach or parent, the young athlete may surpass his/her physiologic limits and become injured.

Cold environment per se does not affect the physiologic performance of a child. However, if there is a few degrees drop in the child's core body temperature, then aerobic capacity, strength, and agility, as well as performance, all decrease. Some studies seem to indicate that athletes with an increased level of fitness may have increased tolerance to low temperatures; however, in spite of this tolerance, performance levels tend not to improve in the cold.[5]

Although more is known about the detrimental effects of heat on the exercising young athlete than of cold, some studies on the effects of cold are beginning to appear. Unlike exercising in a hot environment, there is no adaptation to cold tolerance. Athletes exercised continually for several days in a cold environment did not tolerate that environment any better.[4] The young athlete's increased surface area allows for more rapid loss of body temperature while exercising in the cold. The young athlete is therefore at greater risk to hypothermia than the adult counterpart. The increased surface area is also augmented by the lack of body fat in some young endurance-trained athletes. These factors make proper clothing of the young athlete the most important aspect for prevention of hypothermia. Inadequate clothing or excess clothing (which will promote sweating and then rapid cooling) or the lack of a hat all may contribute to placing the young athlete at risk for hypothermia. Unfortunately, most young athletes are often dressed for training or competition by parents who do not understand these principles. Once the competition begins, the young athlete is also less likely to adjust clothing as conditions change. A charge for the coach should be to see that each athlete is properly clothed prior to the event, that the environment is safe, and that appropriate equipment adjustments are made during the training or competition as the temperature or other conditions change. In the event that the weather deteriorates, the health of the young athlete obviously must be of utmost concern to coaches and team physicians; and these considerations should take precedence in any decision about continuing competition during adverse climatic conditions.

ILLNESS

Overtraining, travel stresses, poor nutrition, and social intimacy among the team all increase the athlete's risk of illness. Experience has shown that it is more often the minor illnesses (see Chapter 14) than the catastrophic injury that thwarts the athlete from his or her final goal. It is not coincidental that this often happens at the most inopportune time—at the peak of training or during the competitive season, when stresses and overtraining are also at their peaks.

As with injury, the younger the athlete, the more conservative the physician/coach needs to be in decisions regarding allowing the ill athlete to practice or to play. The more advanced athlete in serious training or competition needs to weigh the possibility of prolonging the illness or of developing more serious complications by continuing while sick. The sick athlete does not perform well, and often acceptance of the illness and a rational course of medical consultation, rest, and good hydration and nutrition will produce a well athlete in the shortest period of time. Contraindications to training and competition should include

1. fever greater than 100°F (37.8°C)
2. diarrhea or vomiting with dehydration
3. respiratory illness with poor air exchange (coughing, wheezing, shortness of breath)
4. malaise or myalgia
5. early physical signs of serious illness (e.g., pneumonia, mononucleosis)

Commonly these illnesses are minor respiratory or gastrointestinal viral illnesses that are of short duration and self-limiting (see Chapters 15 and 16). Accurate diagnosis, careful medical observation, adequate rest, supportive treatment, and appropriately supervised use of medication are indicated. Many common over-the-counter medications used in the symptomatic treatment of these maladies have been banned by the United States Olympic Committee (USOC) and the International Olympic Committee for use by athletes training and competing

under their jurisdictions, and use of these drugs will make the athlete test positive in drug screens (see Chapter 12). When there is any doubt about a specific medication, the USOC Drug Control Hot Line (telephone 800-233-0393) should be consulted before using substances that could possibly disqualify an athlete.

Obviously, the key to the problem lies in prevention. Minimizing the various stressors (fatigue, poor nutrition, and crowding) and careful monitoring to prevent overtraining (see Chapter 9) are very important. The nutrition, hydration, and sleep of team members should be monitored by their coaching staff. Well athletes should be isolated from members of the team who are ill, and proper hygiene should be observed to avoid the use of common drinking containers, towels, toothbrushes, and so forth.

Overtraining is a prime factor in precipitation of illness. Training schedules have to allow for periods of rest, especially before and after competition or sessions of intense training. Monitoring the athlete's sleeping or early morning resting heart rate is often a good early indicator of overtraining, possible onset of illness, anxiety, or other stresses. A rise of 8 to 10 beats per minute in the resting heart rate should caution athlete and coach against intense training for a period of time. A less sensitive but otherwise reliable method is just for the athlete to "listen to his or her body." If the athlete is tired, unenthusiastic, and finds training a drudgery, then a period of rest is indicated—no matter what the prearranged training schedule dictates.

INJURIES

The chief objectives for children in sports are to teach fundamentals, to promote sportsmanship, and to provide the young athlete with an enjoyable experience. With these goals in mind, injuries can be kept to a minimum; however, even in the safest environment injuries do occur.

As with other athletes, injuries can be divided into two types. Acute traumatic injuries—such as contusions, strains, and sprains—occur because of the single application of a large amount of force. Overuse injuries, which are becoming much more common in many sports because of increased practice time, occur by repetitive application of small amounts of force. The guidelines for treatment of these two types of injuries do not differ appreciably from those used in their adult counterparts. As with illness, team physicians and coaches need to be conservative in allowing young athletes to return to competition after an injury.

First aid for acute traumatic injuries is rest, ice, compression, and elevation, which can be remembered by the mnemonic RICE (see Chapter 21). Contusions, sprains, strains, and even nondisplaced fractures can be initially managed this way. Rest starts at the time the injured athlete is seen on the practice field or competition arena. After careful evaluation to rule out spinal injury and unstable fractures, the injured athlete can be helped or carried by teammates or stretcher if appropriate. When assessment at the sideline reveals only mild to moderate soft-tissue injury, ice, compression, and elevation should be applied immediately. During the first 24 to 36 hours, ice should be applied for 20 to 30 minutes of each hour, whereas carefully observed compression should be used continuously. If there is any question of associated fractures, x-rays and possibly stress views to illustrate epiphyseal plate injuries must be obtained.

In case of overuse injuries, rest is the most important treatment factor. Complete inactivity or immobilization is usually not indicated; but intensity, frequency, and duration of workout should be markedly curtailed. Also, the use of alternative exercises that do not stress the injured extremity but allow conditioning of the rest of the body are extremely helpful. These alternative exercises may include swimming, running in the deep end of the pool, or use of a stationary bicycle. Gradual return to full activity is necessary to prevent a recurrence. Often a stretching and strengthening program will help in prevention; however, it is important to note that a vast majority of overuse injuries are caused by overtraining. The frequency, intensity, and duration of the training program need to be carefully analyzed by the coach.

Before returning a young charge to practice and competition, the young athlete must be fully prepared both physically and mentally. From a physical standpoint this means pain-free full range of motion. Strength, power, and endurance must be gradually rehabilitated to approach and to complement the uninjured contralateral extremity. Lastly, functional skills must be instituted to assure that the athlete has the proper agility, coordination, and balance necessary for execution of any complex skills that the sport requires.

Hockey

Hockey is one of the most popular winter sports for children. The Amateur Hockey Association of the United States (AHAUS) reports that there are 11,200 teams currently registered, with 200,000 young athletes competing in six AHAUS classifications. With the growth of Little League hockey, young athletes compete at an early age. Hockey sticks designed to shoot the puck harder and faster increase the intensity of play, and schedules have increased the number of games per season.

A major injury factor in youth hockey involves fatigue. Fatigue can set in as early as the first shift, due to the higher intensity of the game. Endurance tests show that within 25 to 30 seconds, players become less biomechanically efficient.[2] Skill development in young athletes will be hampered if learning is mixed with endurance training and the quality of play will be sacrificed for quantity.

Improper use of the stick and lack of enforcement of the high sticking rule have resulted in 41 percent of the injuries caused by the hockey stick.[11] In recent years, the use of mandatory protective equipment has produced a decrease in injuries. This is especially true of facial lacerations and eye injuries. Head injuries now occur predominantly in recreational hockey when the players are not wearing helmets. The youngster who has suffered concussion is very vulnerable to reinjury. Should a concussion be suspected as a result of head trauma, the young player should be removed from the game immediately and given an obligatory follow-up 3-week rest (see Chapter 22).

The most common injuries to the upper body in young hockey players include clavicle fractures, epiphyseal injuries to the proximal humerus, acromioclavicular sprains, and sternoclavicular separations at the epiphyseal plate. Shoulder dislocations seem to be rare in these young athletes. Injuries to the lower body commonly include knee ligament sprains. However, following any knee injury in a young athlete, epiphyseal fractures must be ruled out. Due to lack of conditioning, groin strains occur to goalies most commonly at summer camps and in early season. Thigh contusions are probably the most common hockey injuries. Proper care of the contusion is necessary to prevent myositis ossificans in the young athlete. This management usually entails a period of rest followed by a pain-free stretching and strengthening program.

Prevention of injuries in the young hockey player requires use of properly fitted protective equipment in practice and games (see Chapter 29). Enforcement of rules regarding stick use and limiting the number of games during each season will also help decrease injuries. Finally, it has been suggested that each player should have the opportunity to play and that all players should receive awards for their efforts, with scoring deemphasized until age 14.[11]

Figure Skating

The young recreational skater needs a properly fitted skate boot, rigid enough to support the ankle with blades sharp enough to hold a secure edge. Children should be dressed to provide warmth but to allow freedom of movement. Skill learning should begin with instructions on falling. Telling the novice to bend the knees and to sit down when feeling unstable is an effective injury prevention technique. As is true for all sports, proper progression of skill learning is necessary.

Injuries encountered in skating include a wide variety of overuse injuries which can be expected in the athlete who practices 4 to 6 hours a day 6 days a week. Twenty-one of 25 figure skaters seen at Boston Children's Hospital Medical Center in 1982 had extensor mechanism dysfunction.[14] These included patellar tendonitis, patellofemoral syndrome, and jumper's knee. Stress fractures of the tibia and metatarsals are often seen in adolescent girls who combine the stresses of increasing intensity of workouts while attempting to lose weight. Low-back problems are common in young skaters and are associated with repetitive hyperextension and frequent jumping and landing (see Chapter 28). The effect of repeated landings on growth plates is unknown.

Typically, the stretching program of the young competitive skater is inadequate, entailing warm-up times of less than 5 minutes before they begin to practice jumps and spins. Implementation of a stretching and concurrent strengthening program is needed for prevention of problems. This program should include stretching of the low back, hamstrings, and hip extensors and adductors with strengthening for muscle balance to include abdominal back and hip flexors.

Alpine Skiing

Skiing statistics show that young skiers are more frequently injured than their elders. Approximately 200,000 injuries occur yearly in North America to skiers under 16 years of age, with the highest injury rate in the 11- to 14-year-old group.[11] Children are at a greater risk because a large percentage of them are novice skiers, often lacking prudent judgment. They are also more likely to use equipment designed for adults or secondhand equipment. A study of young skiers in Sweden indicated that three fourths of the children who had accidents that resulted in lower extremity fractures were using bindings that did not release or released too late.[16] For young skiers, bindings should be adjusted to the needs of children, not to adult standards. The most common fractures of the lower extremity of young skiers include the usual boot-top fractures of the leg and occasional spiral fractures at the junction of the distal and middle thirds of the tibia. Variations unique to the young skier are buckle fractures occurring below the level of the boot top. Another variation of lower leg fractures in young skiers compared with adults is the rarity of coincidental fibular fractures, indicating a more lightweight, slower-moving participant. Knee injuries in young skiers are occurring with increasing frequency, secondary to higher-topped boots now in use (see Chapter 39). Sprains of the medial collateral and anterior cruciate ligaments lead the list. Any suspected ligament injury should have proper x-ray examinations to rule out epiphyseal plate disruption.

True skier's thumb or ulnar collateral ligament rupture is rare in children and adolescents, unless they are approaching adulthood (see Chapter 39). Though mimicking an ulnar collateral sprain, a fracture of the epiphyseal plate is more likely in the young skier.

Prevention of skiing injuries should include instructions at a qualified ski school for the novice skier. Bindings should be adjusted frequently and properly for the size and weight of the young skier. Children need to be cautioned against succumbing to peer pressure to ski beyond their capabilities on advanced slopes or to engage in "hot dog" activities. Lastly, the fatigued child is more prone to injury and needs to be ordered off the hill.

Ski Jumping

Studies done in Norway indicate that although there are a large number of jumpers under 12 years of age in that country, serious injuries were not found in this age group.[17] In the 15- to 17-year-old group, injury risk more than doubled, according to the study. Less serious injuries involving the shoulder girdle were caused by falling on the outstretched arm. Skiers landing off balance are subjected to twisting forces at the knee and ankle. Finally, overuse injuries found in the hip and knee cannot be overlooked, for the jumper must climb many steps to reach the top of the hill.

Although ski jumping is seen as a dangerous sport by many, in truth the young jumper is never far from the hill at any time during flight (see Chapters 33 through 36). Jumps for the young athletes are kept under 35 meters, with correspondingly low speeds. Injuries may occur on the inrun because of uneven snow conditions or on the outrun when one is landing beyond the knoll and sudden deceleration forces are caused by loose unprepared snow. More advanced jumpers are also apt to attempt jumps for which they are not technically prepared. This often occurs at the end of the season when the jumper is working for a new personal record. With good hill maintenance and with proper progression and supervision from the coach, ski jumping can provide the young athlete with an exhilarating yet safe experience.

Nordic Skiing

Enthusiasm for cross-country skiing is growing rapidly among young athletes. Unfortunately, traumatic and overuse injuries

are also increasing because of increased downhill speeds, faster skis and trails, and overtraining. Also, competitive skiers are now using the skating style (see Chapters 31 and 32). Unpublished data indicate skating as the major style used by young competitive skiers today.[12] This is especially true of junior National Team members who are skating as much as 95 percent of their training time. Early study results indicate that this technique may be responsible for increased numbers of overuse injuries involving the hip external rotators and the posterior tibialis. The associated double poling used with the skating technique is also causing upper extremity overuse injuries in the young skiers. In these cases, strains of the triceps and scapular stabilizing muscles occur.

Preseason conditioning plays a large role in prevention of injuries (see Chapter 2). For the young athlete this may include ski walking, hill bounding, and hill climbing with poles. Running programs as well as roller skiing and roller blading may also be part of the preparation for an injury-free winter season. Emphasis on upper body strength for "skaters" is also important.

Luge

Injuries seen in the young luger are caused by technique and driving errors, which are the result of inexperience and secondhand, poorly maintained equipment. Both lack of conditioning and strength as well as not maintaining proper head position against gravitation forces in the curves are important causes for loss of sled control. Accidents and injuries occur when young sledders progress to speeds that they are unable to handle.

Contusions are by far the most common injuries to the young lugers (see Chapter 41). Body parts not protected by the sled—elbows, hands, knees, and ankles—are those subjected to the icy walls. Concussions and facial lacerations are occasionally seen due to lightweight plastic helmets and face shields that are not shatterproof. Unfortunately, the development of good protective luge equipment lags behind many other winter sports.

SUMMARY

Caring for the young athlete in winter does not vary much from the guidelines established for caring for young athletes in general. The younger the athlete, the more of a supervisory role the coach and physicians must assume. Training programs for young athletes should center around teaching of basic skills and having fun. Strength training should be held off until the sports skills are mastered. Younger athletes need more conservative decisions in terms of when to be allowed to compete or to train following illness or injury. Prevention of illness or injury in these young people is often the key to a successful season.

The cold environment of many winter sports does present increased risk of hypothermia to young athletes, compared with their older counterparts. In children, there is little physiologic adaptation to exercise in the cold, and a decrease in body core temperature adversely affects physical performance. However, the risk of hypothermia can be virtually negated by proper supervision, including proper adjustments of clothing, nutrition, and hydration, along with paying careful attention to all weather conditions.

REFERENCES

1. Bar-Or, O: Metabolic response to acute exercise. In Bar-Or, O (ed): Pediatric Sports Medicine for the Practitioner. Springer-Verlag, New York, 1983, pp 1–18.
2. Benton, JW, Green, H, Elatherwick, J, Carr, J, Sutherland, GW, Grainer, LJ: Hockey optimizing performance and safety. The Physician and Sportsmedicine 11:73–83, 1983.
3. Cohen, HC, Faber, WM, et al: Altered serum lipoprotein profiles in male and female power lifters ingesting anabolic steroids. The Physician and Sportsmedicine 14:131–136, 1986.
4. Howarth, SM: Exercise in a cold environment. Exercise and Sports Science Review 9:221–263, 1981.
5. Howarth, SM, Freeman, A, Golden, H: Acclimatization to extreme cold. American Journal of Physiology 150: 38–40, 1947.
6. Inbar, O, Bar-Or, O: Anaerobic characteristics in male children and adolescents. Medicine and Science in Sports and Exercise 18:264–269, 1986.
7. Malina, R: Readiness for youth sport. Sport for Children and Youth. Human Kinetics, Champaign, IL, 1986.
8. Martens, R, Christina, R, Harvey, J, Sharkey, B: Coaching Young Athletes. Human Kinetics, Champaign, IL, 1981.
9. Micheli, L: Physiological and orthopedic considerations for strengthening the prepubescent athlete. National Strength and Conditioning Association 8:38–40, 1986.
10. Rowland, TW: Aerobic response to endurance training in prepubescent children: A critical analysis. Medicine and Science in Sports and Exercise 17:493–497, 1985.
11. Schneider, R, Kennedy, JC, Plant, ML: Sports Injuries and Mechanisms, Prevention and Treatment. Williams & Wilkins, Baltimore, 1985.
12. Schonning, JL and Harvey, J: Unpublished data, 1986.
13. Sharkey, B.: When should children begin competing? A physiological perspective. Sport for Children and Youth. Human Kinetics Press, Champaign, IL, 1986.
14. Smith, AD: Injuries in competitive figure skating. The Physician and Sportsmedicine 10:36–47, 1982.
15. Tottem, L: Practical consideration in strengthening the prepubescent athlete. National Strength and Conditioning Association Journal 8:38–40, 1986.
16. Ungerholm, S and Gustavsson, J: Skiing safety in children: A prospective study of downhill skiing injuries and their relation to the skier and his equipment. International Journal of Sports Medicine 6:353–358, 1985.
17. Wester, K: Serious ski jumping injuries in Norway. The American Journal of Sports Medicine 13:124–127, 1985.

CHAPTER 6

Women in Winter Sports

JOHN H. BLAND, M.D.

MURRAY JOSEPH CASEY, M.D.

The athletic prowess of women has been aptly recorded at least as early as the bull vaulters of the ancient Minoan civilization in the third millennium before the Christian era. But in modern times, except for such social diversions as lawn tennis and equestrian sports cultivated by the elite of Europe and 19th-century America, the involvement of women in strenuous sporting activities was not encouraged until our last 100 years, and the precisely developed competitive female athlete as known today has been truly a product of the present generation. Participation by women at all levels of sport, from the recreational to the intensive training required for world class performance, has paralleled an expansion of women's consciousness and the rise of a modern Olympic movement during the present century.

Following establishment of the first Olympic games of this modern era under the leadership of Baron Pierre de Coubertin at Athens in 1896, the first recorded participation by women was in the sport of archery during the IIIrd modern Olympiad held at St. Louis in 1904. It should be noted that Mrs. M. C. Howell of Cincinnati was the winner of the two individual archery championships and led the United States women to first place in the team competition. In 1908, the IVth Olympiad in London added lawn tennis to archery in the women's competitions, and women also competed in individual and pairs figure skating, the first of the "winter" sports to receive Olympic status.

The First Olympic Winter Games were established during the VIIIth Olympiad, in Paris, through retroactive recognition by the International Olympic Committee of a sports competition held at Chamonix during the winter of 1924. Following the introduction of women's and pairs figure skating in 1908, these events have been officially sanctioned in every Olympic competition. Then during the Lake Placid Olympics of 1932, women's speed skating was displayed as a demonstration sport. And in the 1936 Winter Olympics at Garmisch-Partenkirchen, Germany, official women's competitions in downhill and slalom skiing were held. Women's 10-kilometer cross-country skiing was added as an official Olympic sport during the 1948 games at St. Moritz, and a 3 × 5 kilometer cross-country ski relay was sanctioned at Cortina in 1956. However, it was not until the VIIIth Olympic Winter Games in 1960 at Squaw Valley, Idaho, that women's speed skating received Olympic recognition, with four events of 500 m to 3000 m in the competition. The thrilling women's "single seat" luge event and the beautiful sport of ice dancing were first sanctioned during the IXth Olympic Winter Games at Innsbruck in 1964.

Through this exciting history of Olympic competition, several outstanding women winter athletes deserve special mention for their remarkable accomplishments. These include Mrs. Syer of Great Britain, who won the very first women's figure skating competition in 1908; and Sonja Henie of Norway, who won the women's figure-skating titles in three successive Olympic Games—1928, 1932, and 1936. Speed skater Lydia Skoblikova of the Soviet Union, with six gold medals over two Winter Olympic Games, including all four women's competitions during 1964, has won more Olympic events than any other winter athlete, male or female. American Diane Holum won four speed skating medals during two Winter Olympic Games, including a gold medal in 1972. She then went on to coach the greatest speed skater of all time, Eric Heiden, who won five gold medals while setting five Olympic records during the Lake Placid games of 1980. These are but a few of the heroines of winter sport whose outstanding accomplishments give luminous visibility to the now overwhelming movement in women's sports. Over fifty million American women now actively engage in recreational and competitive sports, and large numbers of these women are involved with winter sports. The results are telling. Records set by men in ski racing and speed skating during the early decades of this century have been shattered by women during the 1970s and 1980s.

BIOLOGIC, PHYSIOLOGIC, AND PERFORMANCE POTENTIALS

That many of the top athletic performances of today's women equal or exceed those of men some 50 to 75 years ago is not to say that there are not biologic distinctions between the sexes. The differences between the performance levels of men and women in some sports will continue to be seen because clear-cut differences between the sexes in body composition and physiology do exist and can be scientifically measured. However, selection of the most talented athletes from an enlarging pool of women participants in both recreational and competitive sports, better conditioning, and improved coaching has and will continue to narrow the performance differences between men and women (Fig. 6–1).

ANATOMY AND PHYSIOLOGY

Nature has endowed the childbearing sex with special physical characteristics uniquely suited to that aspect of the generative function. Although there is considerable overlap between the male and female normal curves for virtually every measure of body composition, mature women do tend to smaller, less angular skeletons; higher body fat composition, with greater concentration in the thighs and buttocks; and smaller muscle mass and strength, especially in the upper body. The dominant female gynecoid pelvis, suited for parturition, results in medial angulation of the femurs. However, there is great variability among women in this physical feature, and evidence exists that those 15 to 30 percent of women with more narrow android type pelves may tend toward selection of the running sports.[43] Presently, we find no data as to selection or performance according to pelvic structure of the female participants in winter sports.

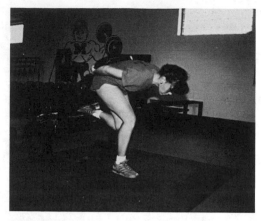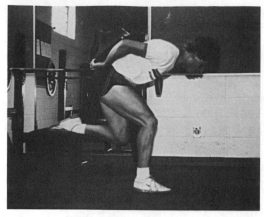

Figure 6–1. With heightened awareness and increased emphasis on skill training and conditioning by female athletes *(left)*, the margins of performance differences with male athletes *(right)* are narrowing in most winter sports. Elite women athletes of the future may well surpass the performance of their male counterparts in many sports.

On average, total body fat composition is between 22 and 27 percent in mature healthy young women, compared with about 15 percent total body fat composition in men. The difference of these averages is greatly narrowed when competitive athletes of both sexes are compared. Published data indicate average body fat composition of 15 to 22 percent in female Alpine and Nordic skiers, compared with 8 to 15[47] percent average body fat composition in their male counterparts. Our group found average body fat composition to be 16.5 percent among female candidates for the 1984 Olympic speed skating team, compared with 7.4 percent in the male candidates.[38]

Probably more significant to the present levels of performance that have been reached, however, are the differences between the sexes in muscle mass. Although studies have failed to show distinctions in the number of muscle fibers and the distribution of slow-twitch and fast-twitch fibers between male and female athletes,[19,39] the average muscle mass and strength of male athletes are considerably and significantly greater, especially in the arms and upper body.[30,48] These observed differences in strength have been attributed in the past to genetically larger frames and the effects of endogenous androgens on the musculature of postpubertal males. However, the potential for women to improve strength through training needs further evaluation.

Strength is related to both the number and size of muscle fibers, and weight-training programs with women have demonstrated very significant increases in strength over just 3 to 6 months of work.[47] Muscle hypertrophy, however, which was assessed by girth measurements, was considerably less in women than in comparably trained men,[6] so the importance of resistance training relative to the biologic determinants of frame size and hormonal milieu has not yet been fully defined. Nevertheless, the evidence of continued improvement on old records and the recent emergence of competitions in women's body building lead us to suspect that the female musculoskeletal system holds potential for athletic achievement that may go well beyond the levels of current realization.

Most differences between men and women in the measurements traditionally used by sports physiologists can be attributed to body size differences between the sexes. Cardiac output (heart rate $\times$ stroke volume) in untrained women exposed to subexertional work is maintained at levels closely coinciding with untrained male counterparts with larger cardiac volumes.[5] The observed increases of cardiac output in these untrained women were achieved by increased average heart rates in the tested women. However, an abundance of studies have shown that training can improve stroke volume and, therefore, cardiac output, without significant relative increases in heart rate of both men and women.[20,29]

A measurement of the amount of oxygen utilized by the body during a period of maximum work ($\dot{V}O_{2max}$) closely correlates with total endurance capacity. The $\dot{V}O_{2max}$ is dependent on many variables, including cardiac output and blood oxygen-carrying capacity.[2] Although a number of studies have demonstrated a significantly lower average $\dot{V}O_{2max}$ among women when compared with men, there is considerable overlap between the $\dot{V}O_{2max}$ normal curves of the two sexes, especially when trained athletes are compared.

Although there are significant differences between the reported average $\dot{V}O_{2max}$ of male and female athletes engaged in cross-country skiing, the most demanding competitive sport for cardiovascular conditioning,[41] the reported average $\dot{V}O_{2max}$ of female cross-country skiers significantly exceeds the average $\dot{V}O_{2max}$ of male ice hockey players and overlaps the normal curve of male speed skaters.[47] Moreover, when groups of male and female cross-country skiers engaged in the same training program were compared, the percentage improvements from baseline performances between men and women athletes were almost identical.[35]

When $\dot{V}O_{2max}$ in world class speed skaters was related to fat-free body weight, no significant differences were found between similarly trained male and female athletes.[38] However, the average body fat composition of female speed skaters (16.5 percent) significantly exceeded the body fat composition of male speed skaters (7.4 percent). The implications of these data are that $\dot{V}O_{2max}$ may be improved in women by conditioning to increase cardiovascular efficiency and to increase the proportion of lean body mass.

As mentioned earlier, $\dot{V}O_{2max}$ also depends on blood oxygen-carrying capacity, which in turn is related to hemoglobin concentration. In studying world class and junior speed skaters, we found significantly lower levels of hemoglobin and serum ferritin (a measure of total body iron) in female compared with male skaters.[15] We attributed these differences to the chronic demands of menstrual blood loss and inadequate dietary replacement of iron by the female skaters (see Chapter 4). Following a concerted effort to emphasize the importance of daily supple-

mental iron, we saw improvements in the hemoglobin levels of these skaters.

MENSTRUATION

In the United States and Europe, the onset of female puberty occurs normally before the 13th birthday, and menarche is experienced by 16 years of age or within 5 years of nipple budding. Once the young woman establishes her individual pattern of menstruation, usually at 21- to 45-day intervals, this characteristic cycle will normally continue until menopause in the fifth or sixth decade of life. During these reproductive years, regular cyclic menstruation depends upon a delicate balance between psychologic, neuroendocrine, and gonadal factors acting upon normally responsive uterine endometrium. The average blood loss with each normal menstrual cycle is between 30 and 100 ml, an amount that is insignificant in a healthy, well-nourished woman.[10] However, the demands of sport and intensive training, together with dietary insufficiencies sometimes seen even among elite athletes, may lead to relative iron deficiencies that require supplementation in order to maintain optimal levels of intracellular iron and circulating hemoglobin.

Much has been written about late menarchal age and menstrual irregularities among women who engage in intensive physical training. Compared with nonathletic controls, later age of menarche and more frequent occurrence of prolonged intervals between menstruation have been reported in runners, gymnasts, figure skaters, and ballet dancers.[3,32,33] In runners, the incidence of prolonged intervals (oligomenorrhea) and cessation of menstrual flow (amenorrhea) has been correlated with distances run; and in dancers, these menstrual disturbances have been related to the intensity of effort and training. Whereas the incidence of amenorrhea among swimmers and cyclists in one study significantly exceeded the incidence of amenorrhea in sedentary age-matched control women, the prevalence of this disorder in swimmers and cyclists did not increase with increasing intensities of training, as it did with runners.[42]

Although delayed menarche and a high incidence of amenorrhea are seen in distance runners, gymnasts, and ballerinas, these disturbances are infrequent among recreational runners, swimmers, cyclists, and those engaged in volleyball, softball, and basketball—all of whom tend to have greater proportions of fat in their body compositions.[33,42]

Observations such as these have led some investigators to believe that menarchal onset and the maintenance of regular cyclic ovulation and menstruation depend upon the achievement of minimal critical body fat composition.[24,43] Data that indicate menarche occurs at a critical weight were extrapolated to predict that at least 17 percent body fat composition is necessary for menarche.[24] Also, nomograms relating height, weight, and body fat composition were used to study the point at which menstruation was resumed in several young women who became amenorrheic with weight loss. It was concluded that about 22 percent body fat composition is necessary to maintain regular menstrual cycles.[24]

A number of factors with regard to body size, configuration, and tissue composition certainly must come into play not only in the onset and regulation of the menstrual cycle but also in the selection by young women of specific sports from among the various athletic pursuits available. Those with particular individual body types and skills will tend to select sports in which they are most likely to be successful. The long-limbed, narrow-hipped, late-maturing female is more likely to succeed as a runner, dancer, or figure skater than cohorts of the same age of shorter stature and greater body fat composition. For example, a study of Canadian athletes reported an average menarchal age of 14 years among Canadian figure skaters, compared with 12.9 years in Alpine skiers, an average menarchal age in the skiers which did not vary significantly from nonathletic student controls.[40] Moreover, when specific conclusions are based on measurements of body fat composition, the methodology is critical. By underwater weighing, several authors have found no differences in the body fat compositions of cyclically menstruating athletes, compared with irregularly menstruating athletes. In these studies, the overlaps of the normal curves between the two groups were observed to be so great that no absolute minimum percentage of body fat composition could be determined as being essential for regular menstruation.[43]

Using the underwater weighing method, we found no association of menstrual disruption with body fat composition among candidates for the United States Olympic Speed Skating Team.[14] However, among these elite speed skaters, we found that those who began athletic training before initiation of their menstrual cycles experienced delayed menarche and were subsequently prone to menstrual irregularities. Within this group, menstrual disruption was more closely associated with the commencement of vigorous exercise programs in late childhood than it was with their current weights, body fat compositions, or levels of training at the time of the study.

Others have documented delayed menarcheal age and increased incidences of amenorrhea in premenarche-trained runners and swimmers compared with teammates who began training after menarche.[24]

Recent investigations with athletes and control subjects are helping define the effects of exercise-induced inhibition of gonadotropin release in the hypothalamic-pituitary axis. Several studies have shown transient elevations in serum androgens as well as cortisol, norepinephrine, and other stress-related hormones following acute exercise.[3,4,44] Conflicting reports regarding the effects of exercise on levels of other circulating hormones may be a matter of inconsistency in the experimental designs or the failure of researchers to correlate their observed data with subjects' ovulatory status and/or ovarian cycles. Moreover, it is clear that female athletes, just as other women, may suffer menstrual disruptions because of various causes unrelated to their exercise programs and athletic pursuits. From a practical standpoint, it is important for coaches, team physicians, athletes, and their families to recognize three separate but easily classified disorders of menstruation: (1) delayed menarche, (2) disordered luteal phase, and (3) amenorrhea.

The team physician confronted with these problems needs guidelines for their management. We believe that women who have finally established individually typical 21- to 45-day menstrual cycles but then develop prolonged intervals, and those athletes in training whose intervals exceed 60 days, should be evaluated. Following a meticulous history and physical examination, we obtain an immunologic test for beta human chorionic gonadotropin (HCG) to rule out pregnancy. If this test is negative, serum is drawn in the fasting, resting state for determinations of thyroid-stimulating hormone (TSH), T_3 uptake, T_4, luteinizing hormone (LH), follicle-stimulating hormone (FSH), and prolactin. Serum levels of testosterone and cortisol should also be determined in those patients with detectable defeminization or hirsutism. The next step in our work-up is a progestogen challenge test performed by the oral administration of medroxyprogesterone acetate (Provera) 10 mg per day for 5 days. It is important to perform these steps sequentially because hormonal levels may be changed by the progestogen challenge. To interpret the results of these hormonal determinations satisfactorily, it is emphasized that the serum should be drawn in the morning while fasting and before exercise. Secretion of prolactin by the pituitary gland is extremely labile, and elevations may follow not only strenuous training exercise but even relatively mild physical and psychological stimulation. Finally, spontaneous menstruation occurring 1 to 3 weeks following the determination of pituitary gonadotropin (LH and FSH) levels lessen the validity of these tests, because they may be reflecting a midcycle ovulatory gonadotropin surge.

If, indeed, serum prolactin or TSH levels are elevated and galactorrhea is present, the patient should be evaluated forthwith to rule out a possible pituitary adenoma or primary hypothyroidism. Menstrual disturbances associated with elevations of TSH, even when T_3 uptake and T_4 determinations are normal, indicate probable active or impending hypothyroidism. Elevations of testosterone or cortisol levels need endocrinologic evaluation to rule out neoplasms and hypersecretory states of the gonads or adrenal glands. Those women with normal thyroid function tests and normal levels of gonadotropins and prolactin who experience withdrawal bleeding within a week following the progestogen challenge are probably experiencing exercise-induced anovulation, but they are probably producing sufficient estrogen to stimulate endometrial proliferation. However, the estrogen secretion may not be adequate to maintain bone mass and to prevent estrogen-dependent osteoporosis, which has been reported in some young amenorrheic runners,[9,23] changes that can lead to stress fractures in affected individuals.[34]

Failure of the patient to experience withdrawal bleeding following a progestogen challenge implies a significant problem for which reproductive endocrinologic evaluation is indicated, even when the determinations of serum hormone levels are reported to be within normal range. Normal to borderline low LH and FSH levels may be seen even in some cases of quite severe disruption of the hypothalamic pituitary axis, including anorexia nervosa and tumors or injuries of the brain or pituitary gland. Low gonadotropin levels indicate serious pituitary and/or hypothalamic disease, whereas persistent elevations of gonadotropin levels indicate primary ovarian failure. Elevations of the LH/FSH ratio is often seen in patients with anovulation on the basis of polycystic ovary syndrome; even though the absolute levels of one or both of these gonadotropins may remain within normal limits in patients with this disease.

In summary, when confronted with an athlete showing menstrual disturbance, the nongynecologic team physician is well advised to refer that patient for reproductive endocrinology evaluation when (1) menarche has not been achieved by the 16th birthday or within 2½ years following thelarche, (2) the forementioned serum hormone abnormalities are found on the screening evaluation, or (3) withdrawal bleeding does not occur in response to a progestogen challenge. When the screening tests are normal and withdrawal bleeding occurs, management is individualized. On one hand, simple reassurance and protection of the endometrium by progestogen stimulation and withdrawal at 1- to 3-month intervals is appropriate in those patients with good evidence of endogenous estrogenization on their physical examinations. On the other hand, patients who withdraw from the progestogen challenge with scanty flow and those whose Pap smear and vaginal mucosa show evidence of inadequate estrogen stimulation should be treated with the cyclic administration of exogenous estrogens for 25 days of each month and monthly progestogen during the last 10 to 12 days of each cycle. An alternative is to place these patients on a combined estrogen-progestogen oral contraceptive-type medication and to monitor clinical evidence for adequate estrogenization. In all cases of amenorrhea associated with athletic training, there should be special attention to determining the adequacy of dietary calcium intake. If this does not exceed 1000 milligrams of elemental calcium per day, supplementation is indicated.

Uterine bleeding at fewer than 21-day intervals is much less common than oligomenorrhea and amenorrhea in the serious athlete, but this more frequent bleeding can occur in any woman.[10] In the competitive or recreational sportswoman younger than 35 years of age, such bleeding usually results on the basis of anovulation or inadequate luteal phase (ovulation occurs but the ovarian hormonal secretion is insufficient to maintain the endometrial lining of the uterus). In such cases of "dysfunctional" bleeding, the blood loss can sometimes be quite abrupt and very heavy. In these situations the first priority is to check the flow of uterine blood loss.

Once anatomic pathology has been ruled out by a careful physical examination and pregnancy has been excluded with a negative immunologic test for beta HCG, dysfunctional bleeding can be almost always controlled by the administration of oral contraceptives that combine balanced dosages of an estrogen with a progestogen. If flow is heavy, the patient should be put to rest, and a combined oral contraceptive pill should be given every 6 hours until the bleeding stops. This will usually occur within 1 to 2 days after initiation of hormonal therapy. The oral contraceptive pill dosage can then be reduced to one tablet every 12 to 24 hours, usually without breakthrough bleeding. Oral iron replacement should be started immediately and then continued with oral contraceptives for an additional 21 to 28 days. The first withdrawal period is often heavy, and it may be necessary to reinstitute oral contraceptive pills once again to moderate the flow. In competitive athletes with this problem, we advise that they continue cycles of oral contraceptive pills until the season is over or at least for 3 months. Occasionally, the first acute bleeding is so severe as to require admission to an infirmary for intravenous administration of conjugated estrogens (Premarin) 25 mg and medroxyprogesterone acetate 10 mg every 12 to 24 hours. In these cases, a gynecologist usually should be called into attendance, because if bleeding does not abate, a dilatation and curettage should be considered to rule out intrauterine pathology. Women in their perimenopausal and postmenopausal years who experience abnormal uterine bleeding should *all* have histologic evaluation of their endometrial cavities.[12]

Sometimes young women will ovulate regularly but have inadequate luteal phase to maintain the endometrium. They may experience irregular or prolonged though scant menstrual-like uterine blood flow. When body iron stores are low (see Chapter 13), these patients should be placed on iron supplements. In those athletes for whom this menstrual disruption is psychologically disturbing, treatment should be considered with either cyclic combined oral contraceptive pills with hormonal dosage that is sufficient to maintain the endometrium without breakthrough bleeding, or, alternatively, medroxyprogesterone acetate 10 mg a day can be given for the last 10 days of each cycle. Either of these regimens should result in withdrawal bleeding that can be anticipated with regularity each month. Of course, any question of pregnancy should be ruled out before beginning hormonal medications in women during their reproductive years.

DYSMENORRHEA

Pelvic discomfort during menstruation, or dysmenorrhea, is reported by more than half of all women queried; but unless the pain is quite severe, it does not interfere with athletic performance. Fourteen of 21 speed skaters, ages 15 to 23 years, described mild cramping to significant pelvic pain with their menstrual periods.[13] However, only one of these young women experienced increased menstrual discomfort with rigorous exercise, and five actually noted lessening of their pelvic discomfort with intensive training and competition.

Dysmenorrhea can be classified as primary, when it begins at or soon after menarche, or as secondary, when dysmenorrhea begins later in life after several years or more of pain-free menstrual cycles. The discomfort of secondary dysmenorrhea is usually more severe than primary dysmenorrhea and is often due to actual anatomic disease entities, such as pelvic inflammation and endometriosis. The onset of secondary dysmenorrhea deserves gynecologic evaluation. Most cases of primary dysmenorrhea are believed to be the result of uterine prostaglandin release and can usually be controlled or significantly alleviated with salicylates or other mild prostaglandin inhibitors, such as ibuprofen in a dose of 200 to 400 milligrams every 4 to 6 hours, beginning on the day prior to expected menstruation. Because some people experience gastrointestinal upset with these medications, they should be given with or following the intake of at least a small amount of food.

CONTRACEPTION

Although oral contraceptive pills must be prescribed to recreational athletes with the same precautions as to nonathletes, the use of these medications in competitive athletes should also take into consideration their possible effects on performance. We have found that some athletes will experience disconcerting weight gain and tension with exogenous hormonal medications and will therefore eschew their use, especially during periods of intensive training and the competitive season. Use of oral contraceptive pills by many women clearly results in fluid retention, and recent studies with athletes have indicated that oral contraceptive pill use may be associated with decreases in strength, endurance, and $\dot{V}O_{2max}$.[21,36,49] We feel that in most cases, oral contraceptive pills should not be used to delay menstruation for competition in regularly cycling athletes unless the disability of severe dysmenorrhea or heavy flow would be likely to handicap or to interfere with performance. World class competitions and Olympic medals have been won in every phase of the menstrual cycle. And although there are clearly measurable physiologic and hormonal changes during various phases of the cycle, the majority of elite athletes report no noticeable deterioration or improvement in their performance during menstruation.

Although they are slightly less effective than combined oral estrogen-progestogen pills for contraception, barrier methods in combination with spermicides are nonetheless preferred by many sexually active athletes, especially those at the upper levels of competition. The effectiveness of any form of contraception is highly dependent upon

knowledgeable counseling and intelligent, motivated compliance.

MENSTRUAL HYGIENE

Vaginal tampon use has become the preferred method for menstrual hygiene of a large majority of active women. Commercial availability of tampons designed for appeal to many preferences has led to the increasing popularity of these devices. However, such products should not be used without some precautions. During the early 1980s, it was recognized that tampon use may be associated with a flulike syndrome characterized at the onset with high fevers, malaise and general myalgia, headaches, vomiting, and dizziness. Sore throat and a markedly red "strawberry" tongue and pharynx with an associated bright-red sunburn rash over the face and extremities may follow. Progression of the syndrome is marked with severe dehydrating diarrhea, lymphadenopathy, and headaches. The most severe cases are complicated by shock, respiratory distress, nephritis, hepatic decomposition, severe neurologic sequelae, and even death. Affected patients frequently report one, two, and sometimes three to five mild bouts with the syndrome during previous menstrual periods. Although each illness may be of equal severity, subsequent episodes tend to be more serious than the initial experience. There is ample evidence to implicate toxins from *Staphylococcus aureus* as the cause of toxic shock syndrome. Certain highly absorbent tampons are associated with an increased risk for this disease. Following withdrawal from the market of Proctor & Gamble Rely brand of superabsorbent tampons in 1980, there has been a progressive decline in the menstrual-related occurrence of this disease from all reporting sectors.

From October 1980 through January 1981, we saw four cases of toxic shock syndrome in young women between 16 and 26 years of age.[11] Although none of these young women was an athlete, two of the cases were directly related to tampon use, and one case followed a septic abortion. The other was associated with a staphylococcus infection following knee surgery. Since January 1981, we have seen no cases of this disease in an increasingly busy obstetric-gynecologic service. Also, during a follow-up of 13 United States

Speed Skating Team members who were instructed as to their use of tampons for menstrual hygiene, no cases of shock or prodromal symptoms have occurred. The decline in this disease may be due in large part to the nonavailability of Rely brand tampons, more restricted use of all superabsorbent tampons, a change in the biology or a decrease in the presence of *Staphylococcus aureus* in vaginal flora, or more careful attention to the hygienics of tampon use.

Women who use tampons are recommended to select those which are made of cottonlike materials. Tampons should be hygienically changed at least every 6 to 8 hours, and every effort should be made to restrict their use to when they are most needed, alternating tampons with sanitary napkins, which are preferably used during protracted bedtime hours. With this knowledge and following these precautions, the female athlete can use vaginal tampons with little risk of toxic shock syndrome. When early signs and symptoms of toxic shock syndrome develop, it is imperative that the physician act promptly to examine the patient and assure the absence of an intravaginal foreign body, culture the vaginal contents, begin rapid fluid replacements, and institute therapy with a penicillinase-resistant antibiotic.

PREGNANCY

Pregnancy is not a contraindication to exercise and sporting activities. A number of women have participated at the highest level of athletic competition while pregnant, and several have won Olympic medals. However, the physiologic stresses and bodily changes which accompany pregnancy, especially as it advances into the second and third trimesters, dictate moderation. Because of increases in both heart rate and stroke volume, cardiac output already begins to increase in the first trimester, reaching levels as high as 20 percent above nonpregnant norms. Cardiac output continues to rise in the second trimester to a maximum of about 40 percent above nonpregnant levels in the 25th to 28th week of gestation. Thereafter, as term is approached, cardiac output declines slightly, probably as a result of decreased circulating blood volume caused by blood pooling in the enlarging placenta and the mother's lower extremities.

Several mechanisms are responsible for the increased cardiac output seen during pregnancy. First, the changes in hormonal milieu are believed to cause generalized vascular dilation. Second, total blood volume enlarges due to increases in both red cell and plasma components. These changes lead in turn to increased stroke volume during the first trimester of more than 10 percent above nonpregnant levels. Finally, resting heart rate increases in response to the hormonal milieu and elevated metabolic rates. Therefore, abrupt, sustained vigorous activity during pregnancy can tax the reserves of an unconditioned heart.

Cardiac reserve (stroke volume × maximum heart rate − resting heart rate) can be improved through physical fitness programs that decrease resting heart rate. Such activities are best begun prior to pregnancy and then continued with moderation as gestation advances. In the trained pregnant athlete, cardiac output responds to light exercise with no impairment of the cardiac reserve because of the larger stroke volume and lower resting heart rate. But with more strenuous activity, heart rate increases faster than in the nonpregnant state.[45] Therefore, maximum heart rate is reached sooner, and cardiac reserve is less.[26]

Although measured $\dot{V}O_{2max}$ increases during early pregnancy, about half of the observed increase is due to the effects of fetal metabolism, and much of the rest corresponds to increases in maternal weight. During the third trimester, $\dot{V}O_{2max}$ decreases as term approaches. Planned moderate exercise programs have been shown to increase $\dot{V}O_{2max}$ during the second and third trimesters of pregnancy.[19]

The effects of exercise on labor and the outcome of pregnancy remain somewhat controversial. Programs of light to moderate exercise initiated during pregnancy have no effect on either the length of labor or the outcome of pregnancy.[18] On the other hand, elite athletes trained before pregnancy have been observed to have shorter labors, especially shorter average second stages from the time of full cervical dilation until expulsion of the newborn.[50] However, strenuous endurance-type exercise has been associated with earlier deliveries and decreased birth weights, factors that could account for the shorter labors in those who persist in serious training throughout pregnancy.

Although light exercise would seem to have no deleterious effect on the heart rate of an otherwise uncompromised fetus, studies have shown that more vigorous exercise late in pregnancy may sometimes result in transient fetal bradycardia for periods as long as 6 to 7 minutes.[1] Experimental investigations imply that these changes in fetal heart rate are probably the result of decreased uterine blood flow during exercise.[16,31] This may be no problem to a normal fetus; but to assure this, frequent assessment of fetal well-being should be undertaken throughout the second and third trimesters of pregnancy in women who engage in active exercise.

In cases of suspected or proven intrauterine growth retardation and in pregnancies complicated by severe maternal disease—such as diabetes, hypertension, and cardiac abnormalities—even light exercise may be contraindicated.

Elevated levels of the hormones relaxin, cortisone, and progesterone during pregnancy and the effect of the enlarging gravid uterus result in relaxation of supporting ligaments and shifts in the center of balance. During the latter half of pregnancy, these changes adversely affect performance and leave the gravid female prone to joint and musculoskeletal injuries. Activities that require deep flexion, extension, or sudden changes in direction should be proscribed during pregnancy. Although nature well protects the developing fetus within its fluid-filled amniotic sac, direct blows to the abdomen should be avoided. This precaution takes on special importance for winter athletes whose sports often require excellent balance and involve high speeds and the danger of impacts and falls.

It is wise to counsel sporting women that they should have pregnancy confirmed soon after the first missed menstrual period, and thereafter they should be followed by a competent obstetrician. The bulk of current opinion holds that unless there are complications, as previously noted, women may exercise and compete during early pregnancy with no known increased risk to self or fetus, and probably with no deterioration in perfor-

mance. Although it is likely that conditioning prior to conception may serve to well prepare women for the physiologic stresses of pregnancy, labor, and delivery, there is no evidence that strenuous training initiated during pregnancy has a favorable effect on outcome; in fact, the opposite may be true. As pregnancy advances, the exercise program should be moderated and the patient and her fetus carefully monitored. Weight gain—much of it obligatory breast and uterine enlargement, fat and fluid accumulation, and fetal-placental growth—is characteristic of a normal pregnancy. Healthful nutrition with iron and vitamin supplements is important to maintain maternal and fetal well-being. Weight gained during pregnancy will be rapidly shed after parturition. Following normal vaginal deliveries, serious training programs can usually begin within 4 to 6 weeks. Delivery by cesarean section may somewhat delay resumption of physical activities. In either case, most women can be at high levels of conditioning for recreational and competitive sports within 6 months after delivery.

MENOPAUSE AND POSTMENOPAUSE

Menopause is by definition the last postovulatory menstrual period at the termination of reproductive life. Naturally, this usually occurs during the fifth or early sixth decade. Occasionally, women may experience ovarian failure many years before this age. Early menopause may also result from surgery that has been done to remove or to correct a disease process. When menopause occurs prematurely before the expected natural age as a result of early ovarian failure or surgery, there is strong consensus among authorities that exogenous estrogen replacement therapy is indicated, unless there are complicating factors.[28] Hot flushes are prevented and atrophic changes of the vagina and urethra are retarded by estrogen replacement therapy. Studies have shown that prematurely postmenopausal women treated with estrogen replacement therapy less frequently suffer from hypertension, heart disease, strokes, and traumatic fractures.[7,27]

Until the sixth decade of life the incidence and incremental increase of coronary artery disease and myocardial infarction among American men far outstrip these parameters of heart disease in women of comparable ages. Following menopause, the incremental increase in coronary artery disease begins to rise in women until the incidence in women of the seventh and eighth decades approaches that of their male counterparts. Although some authorities impute the protective effect of endogenous estrogens from these observations, other sexual differences may predispose high-risk American men to fatal myocardial infarctions during their 30s and 40s, thereby skewing the data. Moreover, a number of authorities have raised concerns that increased activity of several coagulation factors observed in women undergoing replacement with some estrogen regimens might in fact lead to increased numbers of myocardial infarctions, cerebral vascular accidents, and thromboembolic disease. However, several longitudinal follow-up studies have failed to bear out these fears.[8,27] Estrogens have been shown also to elevate antithromboplastin activity, which may thereby counterbalance the estrogen effect on coagulation factors.[25] The bulk of available evidence gleaned mostly from longitudinal studies of women who were surgically castrated in the premenopausal years indicates that replacement with exogenous estrogens is protective against cardiovascular disease.[25,28]

Hypertension, thromboembolism, and strokes, as seen in younger women exposed to estrogens through combined estrogen-progestogen birth control pills, have not been seen in postmenopausal women on low-dose estrogen replacement therapy.[28] Recently, there has been an emphasis on superimposing cyclic progestogen therapy as a protection against endometrial cancer in postmenopausal women with intact uteri.[25] Although estrogens alone and estrogen-dominant birth control pills in younger women tend to lower serum cholesterol and increase high-density lipoprotein (HDL), effects which may be protective against coronary artery disease, high progestogen combined birth control pills have been observed to decrease the levels of HDL.

Cardiorespiratory reserve tends to diminish with aging. In the sedentary woman between 20 and 60 years of age, $\dot{V}O_{2max}$ declines as an inverse function with age. However, at least until menopause, more active women tend generally to maintain their $\dot{V}O_{2max}$ at levels in the order of sedentary 20-year-olds.[37] After 50 years of age, some studies have shown a sharp decline in the $\dot{V}O_{2max}$ of active women and then a gradual leveling off.[22] Studies on female masters runners (ages 45 to 49 years) generally showed $\dot{V}O_{2max}$ at levels comparable with many well-conditioned college-age female athletes.[46] The measure of differences in $\dot{V}O_{2max}$ between sedentary and active middle-age women is probably due not only to better cardiovascular conditioning but also to the leaner body builds of the more athletic women.

These observations on the cardiovascular effects of activity and conditioning and recent investigations that have shown that HDL can be increased through exercise programs emphasize the relative importance that conditioning may have on retarding the cardiovascular and respiratory compromises and disease which may accompany aging.

Osteoporosis

During the mid to late 30s, both men and women begin to lose bone mass. When this process leads to significant rarefaction and fragility of the bone, it is termed osteoporosis. For those with large skeletal frames and greater bone mass to spare at the beginning of this process, and for those who maintain adequate calcium, protein, and vitamin intake and engage in a lifelong program of weight-bearing exercise, osteoporosis is usually not a significant problem. But with aging, small-framed, sedentary, and poorly nourished women are susceptible to increased risk of fracture and vertebral collapse as a result of osteoporosis. Prior to menopause, estrogens produced by the ovaries have an antagonistic effect on the process of bone resorption, but after menopause the protective effects of these endogenous estrogens are lost.

There are three controllable factors known to retard bone loss following menopause: (1) resistance exercise, (2) adequate intake of vitamin D, calcium, and protein, and (3) estrogen replacement therapy.

To be effective in retarding bone loss, exercise must involve weight-bearing and resistance activities. Light to moderate weight lifting alternated with cross-country skiing or, in summer months, vigorous walking and mountain hiking for at least 45 to 60 minutes three to five times a week are forms of exercise readily available to most perimenopausal and postmenopausal women. The exercise programs of competitive master athletes will usually well exceed these recommendations. More casual participants in winter sports are advised to incorporate regimens such as these and stretching exercises into their recreational programs in order to maintain general physical fitness during the middle years.

Because there is evidence that gastrointestinal calcium absorption may decrease with age, and the diet of American women is so often deficient in this mineral, we feel that there should be a concerted effort to take in at least 1000 mg of dietary calcium each day before menopause and 1500 mg per day after menopause. When this fails, calcium supplementation is indicated. Several products are presently available that are both convenient and highly palatable.

In recent years, there has been a strong emphasis on estrogen replacement with exogenous estrogen medications in women who have premature menopause and in those undergoing natural menopause who are predisposed to pathologic osteoporosis.

When, with her gynecologist, the postmenopausal woman decides upon estrogen replacement therapy, we feel that an estrogen dose preferably equivalent to 0.625 mg of conjugated estrogen daily by mouth or 0.05 mg estradiol by transdermal patch should be used. Current standard practice in women with intact uteri is to superimpose exogenous progestogen, equivalent to medroxyprogesterone acetate 10 mg by mouth daily on the last 10 to 12 days of each monthly cycle. It may be unnecessary to interrupt the administration of estrogen at the end of monthly cycles; however, it has been our usual routine to carry out 25-day monthly cycles, leaving 3 to 6 days free of hormonal therapy, depending upon the month of the year. Occasionally, a few women will experience hot flushes during the 3 to 6 days that they are off of hormones each month. In these cases, we simply extend the period of hormonal administration to 27 days or more each month. Although available data indicate the probable protective effect of cyclic progesterone against endometrial cancer,[25] any abnormal bleeding that develops in the postmenopausal woman—whether or not they are on estrogen replacement therapy—should be thoroughly investigated.[12]

In those patients who have undergone hysterectomy, the use of progestogen cycles with estrogen replacement therapy is more controversial. We favor using progestogen with estrogen replacement in very young castrated women because of the observed protective effects of combined estrogen-progestogen birth control pills on benign breast disease.[25] The effects of various hormonal combinations on blood pressure, clotting factors, and serum lipids should be individually assessed and frequently monitored, especially in women in their middle and later years.

BREASTS

During the later phase of the ovulatory menstrual cycle, many women experience breast fullness, tenderness, and sensitivity. These symptoms are exaggerated as the breasts enlarge during pregnancy. Breast size and form are in large part genetically determined, but because these organs are predominantly composed of fat during the nonpregnant, nonlactating state, very thin highly trained women tend to be smaller-breasted than women who are overweight. Following menopause, both breast mass and the fine ligamentous supports of the breast tend to atrophy. Hormonal replacement therapy increases breast fullness through hyperstimulation but will not retard loss of natural support with aging. When exogenous estrogens are taken cyclically in the lower dosages appropriate for osteoporosis protection, there is currently no definitive evidence that estrogen replacement with or without progestogen either increases the risks of or prevents cancer of the breast.[25,28]

Nipple chafing and soreness due to dampness, cold, and rubbing are particular problems for women engaged in winter sports. Women using ultrathin one-piece speed suits during the winter have been particularly susceptible to these injuries, especially if a protective barrier is not used. Some of the newer fabrics allow the egress of body moisture while protecting against wind, rain, and snow and may be useful as either outer or inner garments. Application of a large Band-Aid or a thick layer of petroleum jelly to the nipples before engaging in activities that irritate the breasts can be protective against the extreme soreness that sometimes affects winter athletes.

Acute serious breast injuries are quite rare in winter sports, and usually they are the result of major accidents leading to lacerations. Minor contusions and abrasions can be handled conservatively. Significant hematomas should first be iced and then managed with warm applications and support until resolution. More common than acute injuries to the breast, however, is the tenderness of which many women complain when there is inadequate brassiere support and stabilization during athletic activities. Careful attention to the fitting of a good sports brassiere designed to support and to stabilize the breast against the chest wall, so as to prevent both up-and-down and rotary motion, will help prevent the constant vigorous breast motion that results in these discomforts. Although there is no clear evidence that breast support during younger years will prevent sagging in later life, since many factors are involved in the changes of breast conformation with age, it is reasonable to expect that these precautions by the younger woman athlete may prevent minor trauma to the fine ligaments and supporting tissues of the breast.

CONCLUSION

When Title IX, the Education Assistance Act, became US public law in 1972, female children, adolescents, and young adults were guaranteed an equal and fair share of federal tax dollars for their physical education. Legislation such as this and the establishment abroad of government- and committee-sponsored sports camps emphasizing physical education of the very young will continue to enlarge the pool of competitive female athletes and increase the interest of many other women in recreational sports and lifelong physical fitness. Scientific observations and studies of the developing female athlete will lead to greater understanding and knowledge of gynecology and human physiology. Access of females to professional coaching from an earlier age will improve performance, lessen the frequency of injuries, and

lead to new records and greater health and enjoyment of sport. Skiing, skating, sledding, and other outdoor winter activities are ideally suited to the task.

REFERENCES

1. Artal, R, Rutherford, S, Romem, Y, Kammula, RK, Dorey, FJ, and Wiswell, RA: Fetal heart rate responses to maternal exercise. Am J Obstet Gynecol 155:729–733, 1986.
2. Astrand, PO, Cuddy, TE, Saltin, B, and Stenborg, J: Cardiac output during submaximal and maximal work. J Appl Physiol 19:268–274, 1964.
3. Baker, ER: Menstrual dysfunction and hormonal status in athletic women: A review. Fertil Steril 36:691–696, 1981.
4. Baker, ER, Mathur, RS, Kirk, RF, Langrebe, SC, Moody, LO, and Williamson, HO: Plasma gonadotropins, prolactin, and steroid hormone concentrations in female runners immediately after a long-distance run. Fertil Steril 38:38–41, 1982.
5. Becklake, MR, Frank, H, Dagnenais, GR, Ostiguy, GL, and Guzman, CA: Influence of age and sex on exercise cardiac output. J Appl Physiol 20:938–947, 1965.
6. Brown, CH and Wilmore, JH: Effects of maximal resistance training on the strength and body composition of women athletes. Medicine and Science in Sports 6:174–177, 1974.
7. Burch, JC, Byrd, BF, and Vaughn, WK: Effects of long-term estrogen administration to women following hysterectomy. In van Keep, PA and Lauritzen, C (eds): Estrogens in the Post-menopause: Frontiers of Hormone Research. S. Karger, Basel, 1975, pp 208–211.
8. Burch, JC, Byrd, BF, and Vaughn, WK: Results of estrogen treatment in one thousand hysterectomized women for 14,318 years. In van Keep, PA, Greenblatt, RB, and Albeaux-Fernet, M (eds): Consensus on Menopause Research. MTP Press, Lancaster, England, 1976, pp 164–169.
9. Cann, CE, Martin, MC, Genant, HK, and Jaffe, RB: Decreased spinal mineral content in amenorrheic women. JAMA 251:626–629, 1984.
10. Casey, MJ: Abnormal genital bleeding. In Peckham, BM and Shapiro, SS (eds): Signs and Symptoms in Gynecology. JB Lippincott, Philadelphia, 1983, pp 384–418.
11. Casey, MJ: Toxic shock syndrome in young women. Presented at the 1983 Annual Sports Medicine Conference, March 7–10, Lake Placid, New York, 1983.
12. Casey, MJ: Postmenopausal bleeding. In Hofmeister, FJ (ed): Care of the Postmenopausal Patient. George F. Stickley, Philadelphia, 1985, pp 75–107.
13. Casey, MJ and Foster, C: Unpublished observations, 1988.
14. Casey, MJ, Jones, EC, Foster, C, Pollack, ML, and Du Bois, JA: Effect of the onset and intensity of training on menarchal age and menstrual irregularity among elite speedskaters. In Landers, DM (ed): Sport and Elite Performers. Human Kinetics, Champaigne, IL, 1984, pp 33–43.
15. Casey, MJ, Jones, EC, Foster, CF, Pollack, ML, and Hollum, D: Unpublished observations, 1983.

16. Clapp, J: Acute exercise in the pregnant ewe. Scientific Abstracts of the Society of Gynecological Investigation 26, 1979.
17. Clapp, JF, III and Dickstein, S: Endurance exercise and pregnancy outcome. Medicine and Science in Sports and Exercise 16:556–562, 1984.
18. Collings, CA, Curet, LB, and Mullin, JP: Maternal and fetal responses to a maternal aerobic exercise program. Am J Obstet Gynecol 145:702–707, 1982.
19. Costill, DL, Fink, WJ, Getchell, LH, Ivy, JL, and Witzmann, FA: Lipid metabolism in skeletal muscle of endurance trained males and females. J Appl Physiol 40:149–154, 1979.
20. Cunningham, DA and Hill, JS: Effect of training on cardiovascular response to exercise in women. J Appl Physiol 39:891–895, 1975.
21. Daggett, A, Davis, B, and Boobis, L: Physiological and biochemical response to exercise following oral contraceptive use. Medicine and Science in Sports and Exercise 15:174, 1983.
22. Drinkwater, BL, Horvath, SM, and Wells, CL: Aerobic power in females, ages 10–68. J Gerontol 30:385–394, 1975.
23. Drinkwater, BL, Nilson, K, Chestnut, CH, Bremner, WJ, Shainholtz, MS, and Southworth, MB: Bone mineral content of amenorrheic and eumenorrheic athletes. N Engl J Med 311:277–281, 1984.
24. Frisch, RE, Gotz-Welbergen, AV, McArthur, JW, Albright, T, Witschi, J, Bullen, B, Birnholz, J, Reed, RB, and Hermann, H: Delayed menarche and amenorrhea of college athletes in relation to age of onset of training. JAMA 246:1559–1563, 1981.
25. Gambrell, RD, Jr: The menopause: Benefits and risks of estrogen-progestogen replacement therapy. In Wallach, EE and Kempers, RD (eds): Modern Trends in Infertility and Conception Control, Vol 3. Year Book Medical Publishers, Chicago, 1985, pp 116–133.
26. Guzman, CA and Caplan, R: Cardiorespiratory response to exercise during pregnancy. Am J Obstet 108:600–605, 1970.
27. Hammond, CB, Jelovsek, FR, Lee, KL Creasman, WT, and Parker, RT: Effects of long-term estrogen replacement therapy. I. Metabolic effects. Am J Obstet Gynecol 133:525–536, 1979.
28. Hammond, CB and Maxson, WS: Current status of estrogen therapy for the menopause. In Wallach, EE and Kempers, RD (eds): Modern Trends in Infertility and Conception Control, Vol 3. Year Book Medical Publishers, Chicago, 1985, pp 95–115.
29. Kilbom, A: Physical training in women. Scandinavian Journal of Clinical and Laboratory Investigation 28(Suppl 119):7–34, 1971.
30. Laubach, L: Comparative muscular strength of men and women: A review of the literature. Aviation, Space, and Environmental Medicine 47:534–542, 1976.
31. Longo, L, Hewitt, CW, Lorijn, RHW, and Gilbert, RD: To what extent does maternal exercise affect fetal oxygenation and uterine blood flow? Fed Proc 37:905, 1978.
32. Loucks, AB and Horvath, SM: Athletic amenorrhea: A review. Medicine and Science in Sports and Exercise 17:56–72, 1985.
33. Malina, RM: Menarche in athletes: A synthesis and hypothesis. Ann Hum Biol 10:1–24, 1983.
34. Marcus, R, Cann, C, Madvig, P, Minkoff, J, Goddard, M, Bayer, M, Martin, M, Gaudiani, L, and Haskell, W: Menstrual function and bone mass in elite women distance runners: Endocrine and metabolic features. Ann Intern Med 102:158–163, 1985.
35. Niinimaa, V, Dyon, M, Shephard, RI: Performance and efficiency of intercollegiate cross-country skiers. Medicine and Science in Sports and Exercise 19:91–93, 1987.
36. Petrofsy, JS, LeDonne, DM, Rinehart, JS, and Lind AR: Isometric strength and endurance during the menstrual cycle. Europ J Appl Physiol 25:285–293, 1976.
37. Plowman, SA, Drinkwater, BL, and Horvath, SM: Age and aerboic power in women: A longitudinal study. J Gerontol 34:512–520, 1979.
38. Pollack, ML, Pells, AE, III, Foster, C, and Holum, D: Comparison of male and female Olympic speed-skating candidates. In Landers, DM (ed): Sport and Elite Performers. Human Kinetics, Champaign, IL, 1986, pp 143–152.
39. Prince, FP, Hikida, RS, and Hagerman, FC: Muscle fiber types in women athletes and non-athletes. Pflugers Archives 371:161–165, 1977.
40. Ross, WD, Brown, SR, Faulkner, RA, and Davage, MV: Age of menarche of elite Canadian skaters and skiers. Canadian Journal of Applied Sports Sciences 1:191–193, 1976.
41. Saltin, B and Astrand, DO: Maximal oxygen uptake in athletes. J Appl Physiol 23:353–358, 1967.
42. Sanborn, CF, Martin, BJ, and Wagner, WW Jr: Is athletic amenorrhea specific to runners? Am J Obstet Gynecol 143:859–861, 1982.
43. Scott, E and Johnston, FE: Critical fat, menarche, and the maintenance of menstrual cycles: A critical review. Journal of Adolescent Health Care 2:249–260, 1982.
44. Sutton, JR, Coleman, MJ, Casey, J, and Lazarus, L: Androgen responses during physical exercise. Br Med J 1:520–522, 1973.
45. Ueland, K, Novy, MJ, Peterson, EN, and Metcalfe, J: Maternal cardiovascular dynamics. IV. The influence of gestational age on the maternal cardiovascular response to posture and exercise. Am J Obstet Gynecol 104:856–864, 1969.
46. Vaccaro, P, Morris, AF, and Clarke, DH: Physiologic characteristics of masters female distance runners. The Physician and Sportsmedicine 9:105–108, 1981.
47. Wells, CL: Women, Sport and Performance. Human Kinetics, Champaign, IL, 1985.
48. Wilmore, JH: Alterations in strength, body composition and anthropometric measurements consequent to a 10-week weight training program. Medicine and Science in Sports 6:133–138, 1974.
49. Wirth, JC and Lohman, TG: Relationship of static muscle function to use of oral contraceptives. Medicine and Science in Sports and Exercise 14:16–20, 1982.
50. Zaharieva, E: Olympic participation by women: Effects on pregnancy and childbirth. JAMA 221:992–995, 1972.

CHAPTER 7

Orthotic Devices in Winter Sports

HUBERT F. RIEGLER, M.D.

Orthotic devices have a multitude of applications in winter sports activities. To properly understand and prescribe these devices, one must have a clear understanding of the biomechanics of the lower limb.

LOWER EXTREMITY BIOMECHANICS

It is impossible to discuss the biomechanics of the foot as a sole event. The pelvis and lower limbs are a series of interconnecting linkages. During the walking phase, the pelvis, femur, and tibia rotate in a transverse plane. The limb rotates internally during the swing phase and early stance phase. After 15 percent of the stance phase, external rotation begins and continues until after toe-off, at which point the rotation reverses. The knee axis is perpendicular to the axis of progression, with the ankle axis 20 to 30° externally rotated (Fig. 7–1).[16]

The longitudinal axis of the foot passes between the second and third toes, and in the normal foot, it is internally rotated 6°. The subtalar joint resembles an oblique hinge. Internal rotation of the leg will produce eversion of the calcaneus, and external rotation of the lower limb will produce inversion of the subtalar joint (Fig. 7–2). Proper subtalar motion is essential to avoid excessive stresses upon the ankle joint and knee joint. Subtalar motion toward the midline is inversion (up to 30°). The opposite is eversion (about 10°).[14,16] According to Wright,[27] during normal walking, subtalar inversion is 8°; whereas in flat feet, subtalar motion amounts to about 12° inversion. In normal walking,

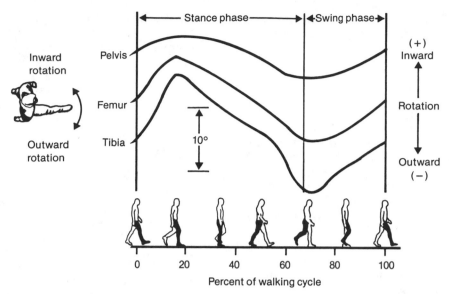

Figure 7–1. Transverse rotation of the pelvis, femur, and tibia during a normal walking cycle. Note that there is inward rotation until foot-flat at 15 percent of the cycle, after which there is progressive outward rotation until toe-off, when inward rotation once again begins. (From Mann, RA: Biomechanics of the foot. In AAOS: Atlas of Orthotics. CV Mosby, St. Louis, 1985, with permission.)

eversion of the subtalar joint takes place during the first 15 percent of the stance phase. Thereafter, inversion begins. This subtalar motion is passed on to the navicular and cuboid joints.[12] The navicular articulates with three cuneiforms and the medial three rays. The cuboid articulates with the lateral two rays. The ankle both dorsiflexes and plantar

flexes. Plantar flexion takes place at the time of heel strike. Progressive flexion then begins until about 40 percent of the cycle, at which point plantar flexion again occurs. During the swing phase, dorsiflexion occurs until heel strike. The amount of subtalar motion affects rotation of the knee and hip, and the converse is also true. With pes planus, there

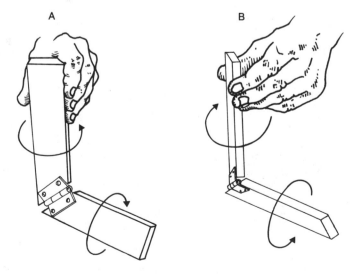

Figure 7–2. Analogy of the subtalar axes to an oblique hinge. (A) Outward rotation of the upper stick results in inward rotation of the lower stick. (B) Inward rotation of the upper stick results in outward rotation of the lower stick. (From Mann, RA: Biomechanics of the foot. In AAOS: Atlas of Orthotics. CV Mosby, St. Louis, 1985, with permission.)

is excessive subtalar motion and compensatory internal rotation of the tibia. Thus, orthotic devices stabilizing the subtalar joint will stabilize the knee and hip.[16]

The Walking Cycle

Heel strike begins the walking cycle. At 15 percent of the cycle, the ankle rapidly plantar flexes and the foot is flat on the ground. The limb internally rotates. The calcaneus through the subtalar joint everts while the forefoot remains flexible and adapts to the ground. At mid stance the lower limb externally rotates and the hindfoot inverts. From the beginning of this hindfoot inversion until toe-off occurs, there is progressive stabilization of the transverse tarsal joints and the longitudinal arch.[2,9,16]

During loading of the foot, the convex head of the talus is firmly seated in the concave navicular. Just prior to toe-off, the leg has reached maximum external rotation and the calcaneus is maximally inverted. All these mechanisms stabilize the longitudinal arch of the foot during toe-off. As soon as this happens, internal rotation of the lower segment begins and the calcaneus everts. The transverse tarsal joints and the longitudinal arch unlock; then the foot becomes flexible again. Internal rotation of the lower segment continues during the swing phase until foot-flat at 15 percent of the new walking cycle. The ground reaction force rarely exceeds 115 to 120 percent of body weight during walking.[17]

The Running Cycle

There are similarities and differences between walking and running. Running involves the whole body. It is cyclic and involves a sequence of support and airborne phases. Depending on the runner's weight, the ground reactive force is between three and eight times body weight.[2,6,14] Whereas a walker can usually cope with anatomic abnormalities, even the smallest deficiencies can have serious consequences to a runner. Joggers generally land on the side of the heel. Accomplished long-distance runners land on the ball of the foot and the heel instantaneously.[16]

Pronation-Supination

In a person walking at a normal pace, full pronation occurs within 150 milliseconds. In a runner during a 6-minute mile, this same event occurs in about 30 milliseconds.[5] As the foot strikes the ground, the calcaneus is slightly inverted and rapidly everts as it is loaded. As absorption of impact is continued and rapid pronation takes place, the foot adapts to the surface, supination locks the foot, and toe-off occurs. The foot stays in this position during the airborne phase.

The Q-angle changes with pronation and supination because of tibial rotation. Thus, anterior knee pain may be related to increased subtalar motion.[2,9,13,15] Medial supports (orthotic devices) decrease the amount of pronation and shorten the duration of the event, thereby decreasing rotation of the lower segment.[1,6,17,21]

The term *pronation* has been used and misused in the literature a great deal and in recent years has become an important term in the jargon of many athletes. Pronation is a normal function of the foot at the time of initial ground contact. As the body weight loads the subtalar joint, it collapses into a slightly everted position upon ground contact. The degree of pronation depends upon (1) the shape of the subtalar joints, (2) ligamentous supports, and (3) muscle strength.[13,16]

Abnormal pronation (hyperpronation) often leads to pathologic conditions in the foot and the joints above.[12] It may also affect the subtalar joint itself, or forefoot and the ankle joint.[3,4,13,14,25] It will produce abnormal knee rotation[2,9,13,15] and may alter spinal biomechanics. Brody[3] and others[7] have stated that hyperpronation may very well be a compensatory mechanism for tibia vara. It also may compensate for tight heel cords, midfoot varus, and forefoot varus. Furthermore, hyperpronation increases lower limb rotation with increased pelvic shear, which can also be stabilized by orthotic devices.[3]

It cannot be assumed that all athletes have abnormal pronation, and thus shoes, boots, or skates should not be produced with "varus wedges." Moderate heel stabilizers may often be appropriate.[20] Proper pronation deserves most careful evaluation by a skilled examiner. The extremities must be aligned properly, and required footwear and alterations of ski boots, skates, or running gear—including orthotic devices—should be prescribed based on careful, systematic, and consistently reproducible limb alignment.

INDICATIONS FOR ORTHOTIC DEVICES

Orthotic devices have been advocated for a multitude of pathologic conditions. In some instances, use of the device can be considered corrective, but in many instances it is supportive.

In a 1986 symposium on running, the question of orthotic devices and their effect on hindfoot motion was addressed.[17] A medial support when studied with high-speed motion cameras will bring about a decrease in the amount of eversion of the calcaneus and subsequent pronation. It becomes clear that orthotic devices control the foot by decreasing the amount of degrees as well as the rate of the pronation of the foot.[1,6,17,21]

Biomechanic aspects very similar to those of running take place during cross-country skiing and skating. Subtalar motion receives some control by rigidity of boots in skiing and skating, but, nevertheless, a significant amount of pronation and supination takes place even within these rigid boots.[22] Optimal positioning of the ski boot and cross-country boot with the respective ski can be achieved with appropriate alignment, the use of custom footbeds, and if necessary, corrective orthotic devices.

Alignment of the Lower Limb—"The Neutral Position"

There are three important parameters to be determined in aligning the lower segment properly with the foot:[9–11,13,26] (1) neutral subtalar joint, (2) heel-leg alignment (Fig. 7–3), (3) heel-forefoot alignment.

The neutral subtalar joint determination is made commonly with the patient in a prone position. The forefoot is rolled back and forth with one hand while the other hand feels the talar head protruding medially and laterally. When the talar head neither protrudes medially nor laterally, the foot is said to be in a "neutral position."[9,10,24] We believe that it is more physiologic to determine the neutral position in the stance phase. The athlete stands in a comfortable stance with the feet apart 10 to 15 cm. Most weight is borne on the leg not being examined in order to let the subtalar joint to be examined roll in and out of pronation with ease. At the same time, the talar head and talonavicular joint are palpated. When there is no prominence, or the same amount of prominence is felt medially and laterally, the foot is in "neutral position." It is agreed by most authors that the foot functions best at—or nearly at—its neutral position.[7,10,11,13,24,26]

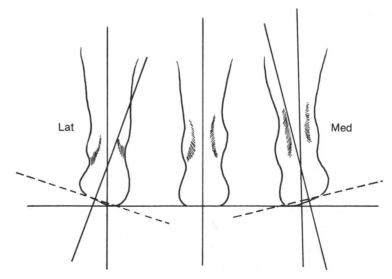

Figure 7–3. Heel-leg alignment *(left to right):* valgus, normal, varus.

Lat   Med

The same principle is applied when molding the foot for an orthotic device in a "neutral position" performance stance phase. Leg-heel alignment is evaluated by drawing a central axis from the lower segment to the center of the heel.[10,13,23]. Heel varus of 2 to 3° is within normal limits[2,10] (see Fig. 7–3).

The central calcaneal line should be perpendicular to the plane determined by the five metatarsal heads and is called the heel-forefoot alignment[2,10] (Fig. 7–4).

We believe that anatomic changes that take place in the foot between the unloaded, or partially loaded, and fully loaded mode are significant enough that orthotic devices designed to manage weight-bearing problems should be made from weight-bearing models.[18]

Thus the most appropriate system for fabricating and molding orthotic devices must allow for proper balancing, finding the neutral position of the subtalar joint, and for producing a weight-bearing mold in the desired corrective position in one simple and reproducible step.

Specific Orthotic Devices

There are three groups of orthotic devices currently in use. These are rigid, semiflexible, and soft. The latter is often an in-office or clinic-produced implant offering temporary relief for minor foot malalignments. It is also often used to produce a comfort footbed. It is of low cost and may later be replaced by a more permanent and lasting device. In the diabetic foot, the rheumatoid foot, or the foot with multiple deformities, this may be the product of choice. The major drawback is limited durability and early bottoming out.

The second group is semiflexible devices. These can be made in the office or in an orthotic laboratory from a cast or mold and require careful alignment of the limb in the neutral position with respect to the subtalar joint. Weight-bearing molding is preferred, and posting may be required if significant changes are to be made in the alignment. Thermoplastic materials are generally used. We have found this group to be the most useful and the most accepted among all device groups available. These semiflexible implants are more forgiving and seem to cause far fewer potential secondary problems than the rigid implants.[19,21]

We have used semiflexible thermoplastic stance molded implants in a prospective study in 235 patients. Follow-up of these patients ranged from 8 to 32 months. Questionnaires were obtained from 176 patients; 104 were female, and 72 were male. Ages ranged from 6 to 71 years, with an average age of 36 years. Eighty-six patients used their inserts in all footwear at all times. Ninety patients used the device for sports and in athletic shoes only. The most common diagnosis for which the devices were prescribed were pronation (83 patients), metatarsalgia (60 patients), and anterior knee pain with or without pronation (24 patients).

Of the patients who used their devices for athletics, 36 reported better performance, 16 better timing, and 20 patients reported an improved feeling for the playing surface.

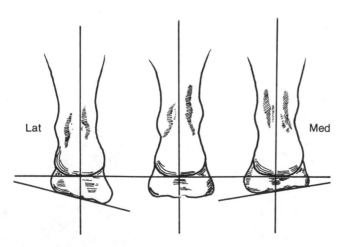

Figure 7–4. Heel-forefoot alignment *(left to right)*: valgus, normal, varus.

Table 7–1. IMPROVEMENT OF
SYMPTOMS WITH ORTHOTIC DEVICES

Improvement	Number of Patients	Percentage of Patients
None	12	6.8
25%	24	13.6
50%	52	29.5
75%	52	29.5
100%	36	20.5

Thirty-six patients had complete alleviation of their symptoms, 52 patients had 75 percent improvement, 52 had 50 percent improvement, 24 patients had 25 percent improvement, and 12 had no improvement of their symptoms and were dissatisfied with the product (Table 7–1).

Semiflexible implants are quite durable. It has been our experience that they will last approximately 12 months for runners averaging 20 to 25 miles per week, at least two seasons in cross-country skiers, and a minimum of three to four seasons in downhill skiers and skaters.

The third group of orthotic devices is the rigid type. These implants are made from plaster or thermoplastic imprint in a laboratory. The material used is generally acrylic (Rohadur) and very durable.

Rigid orthotic devices should be avoided if at all possible. Their use is primarily limited to severe foot deformities and at times indicated in very heavy athletes. Complications with these devices may include neuromas, stress fractures, and decreased shock absorption of the foot.[17,21]

Design Principles for Orthotic Devices

In creating an effective device for the foot, one must achieve the following:

1. Creation of an inner contour for the orthotic device that is capable of giving the foot architecture maximum passive support.

2. Positive stabilization of the device in the shoe to especially avoid valgus orientation or movement within the foot gear.[8]

3. Limited pronation/supination, which may be most desirable with specific sports activities; this can be controlled by orthotic devices.

Practitioners who initially produce plaster molds and then have final products made by a laboratory from these molds add an additional step and a source for error. Thermoplastic molds will produce the backbone of the final product. The laboratory should merely do the finishing job, and desired additional posting and correction—such as metatarsal cookies, medial or lateral wedging, hindfoot, midfoot, or forefoot, and any other desired changes—should be added.

A system using a plumb bob reproducibly fixed to the knee will allow for proper evaluation of lower segment alignment (knee to leg/heel axis and heel/forefoot alignment). Pillow systems under the thermoplastic molds will allow for correction of pronation and supination and should be sensitive to the weight of the patient.

Low-temperature thermoplastic molds must be used (230 to 250°F [110 to 121.1°C]), and the patient's foot must be insulated from the excessive temperature. Low-density plastic materials allow for some flexibility, which avoids the potential problems of rigid implants. Different densities of foam are supplied by the laboratory under the midfoot and are cemented together as layers for durability. The implant should have supports or activity-specific top covers available, depending upon the desire of the patient and prescription of the practitioner.

Specific Orthotic Devices in Winter Sports

Since 1979, we have had experience with over 40,000 athletes at all levels and in all disciplines of sport. Through this experience we have found that the demands of performance and comfort are specific for each sport. In working with many Olympic and National Team competitors we have come to certain conclusions regarding the fitting and alignment of orthotic devices to specifically meet the requirements of the various winter sports.

Alpine Skiing

Both upper and lower segments are forcefully internally and externally rotated in alpine skiing to produce steering and angulation in turning. Because the talus plantar flexes and dorsiflexes only at the ankle joint, this rotation translates into the subtalar joint,

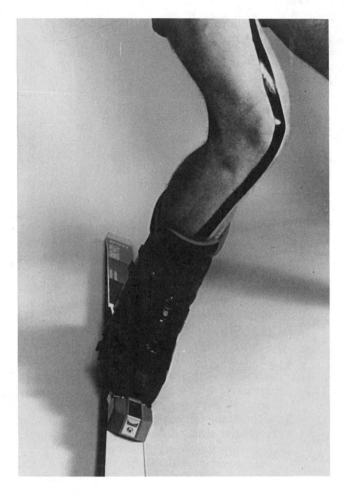

Figure 7–5. Excessive internal rotation of tibia and pronation prior to alignment and orthotics.

thus stressing this joint excessively. This in turn produces significant midfoot stress and subtalar pronation during a turn. To determine whether a skier needs only a custom-support footbed or whether a skiing orthotic will be required depends upon the skier's natural pronation and lower segment–foot alignment. The primary benefit of a *footbed* is custom support and comfort, and thus enhanced performance. The primary benefit of an *orthotic device* includes support, comfort, alignment, and correction of abnormal biomechanics and thus enhanced performance.

The properties of a skiing orthotic are very specific, and a running orthotic is not interchangeable with a skiing orthotic. Often, running orthotics contain heavy subtalar posting, which is undesirable for skiing.

Many of the currently available orthotic devices are very rigid and highly undesirable for skiers. The ski boot proper lends rigid support to the skier, and therefore the orthotic device must be semiflexible to allow normal motion of the foot during athletic events. The foot should never be "locked in" completely. Properly manufactured orthotic devices should respect the weight and performance levels of the athlete and the thermal demands of winter sports.

Alignment. For proper performance, the skier needs to have the boot shaft aligned to the lower segment. Most modern performance ski boots contain built-in shaft canting or alignment systems. These systems must be adjusted to accommodate the skier's natural varus and valgus of the tibia. These are the first steps in proper skiing alignment in which the skier's boot shaft now is properly aligned and the foot is accurately supported by an orthotic device or a custom-support footbed.

Skiing stance. A boot leveling system represents the final step in the alignment and support process. This system consists of a precision biomechanical measuring device designed to analyze the skiing stance appropriately. It incorporates principles of lower body biomechanics with the performance requirements of skiing and the design of today's ski boots by perfectly duplicating the skier's biomechanical relationship of knee position to a flat ski. Further fine tuning can be achieved for slalom and giant slalom skiers at high performance levels by building additional angulation into the system (Figs. 7–5, 7–6).

Ski Jumping

Important aspects during acceleration and especially at the time of takeoff are a flat ski position and even weight distribution on both lower limbs. Equally important, though, is the generation of power and lift at the time of takeoff.

In ski jumping, careful lower limb alignment must be performed and maintained with orthotic devices. Excessive pronation or supination is detrimental to the generation of speed and thrust, which determine distance.

Cross-Country Skiing

The two basic aspects of progression for the cross-country skier include gliding and skating. During gliding, the most efficient stance is that stance which allows a flat ski.

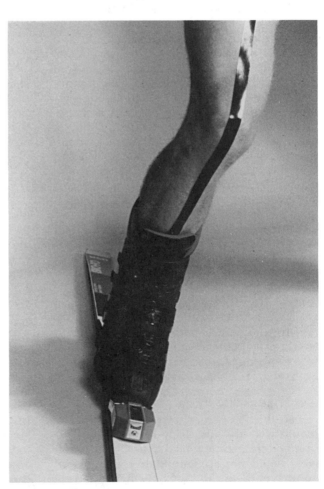

Figure 7–6. Improved stance with less stress on knee and better edge control after alignment and orthotic devices.

Excessive pronation or supination will put abnormal inside or outside pressures on the ski, resulting in loss of speed and distance with each stride. The second and probably more important aspect is skating. Abnormal foot biomechanics must be carefully analyzed, and excessive pronation and supination corrected appropriately. If these abnormal motions are allowed, excessive rotation of the lower segments will take place, resulting in the loss of energy and efficiency.[22]

Orthotic devices must be specific for the sport of cross-country skiing because of special design of the equipment. Cross-country skis are very narrow, and boots are extremely restrictive.

Hockey Skating

Hockey involves complex activities which include sudden stops and starts, tight turns, and acceleration with wide turns during forward and backward skating. Each of these skating skills places unique demands on the hockey player. Because of the tight fit and lacing desired by the competitor, a comfortable footbed is most desirable. Research at the McGill University[22] has clearly demonstrated that a high range of supination-pronation is undesirable for forward acceleration and maximum velocity. Thus, a "normal" foot with perfectly normal biomechanics will benefit from a custom footbed that concomitantly decreases pronation and supination. The "abnormal" foot with excessive pronation or supination needs to be balanced appropriately to give the player most advantageous alignment and to allow proper power skating and power glide.

We have had experience with National Hockey League professional teams and several college and top high school hockey teams. A prospective study was undertaken with a top-ranked college hockey team during the 1985–1986 hockey season. Twenty-two hockey players were equipped with custom footbeds of a semirigid type after careful limb alignment was achieved in a neutral stance phase. Ninety-four percent of the team was satisfied with the devices they received, but 6 percent were dissatisfied. The majority of the dissatisfied skaters had extremely tight-fitting boots, and their footwear could not accommodate the increased volume of the orthotic device. Eighty percent

of the players reported a better feel for the ice and improved proprioception. Seventy-five percent reported being less tired when using their custom footbeds, and 60 percent of the skaters were able to develop more speed and better pushoff.

This corresponds very well with the McGill study, in which several investigators concluded that improved performance can be achieved with maximum stabilization of the foot, which can, in turn, be accomplished only with custom footbeds and orthotic devices when lower segment alignment is abnormal.[22]

Figure Skating and Ice Dancing

Many of the demands a figure skater places upon the lower segments and feet are the same as those of the hockey player. Some aspects of figure skating, though, are quite different. Ultimate stability of the foot is essential to allow for precision landings after triple jumps and complex spins. A great deal of precision and sensitivity is required to perform school figures in a most precise fashion. When abnormal biomechanics exist in figure skaters, lower segment alignment will be useful to correct these conditions, and custom footbeds will aid in the performance of these events.

SUMMARY

Orthotic devices cannot be discussed without first understanding the biomechanics and alignment of the lower limb. Biomechanics of the foot is complex during the gait cycle and even more complex during high performance cycles. Minor biomechanic malalignment problems may not be of great significance during a sedentary style of living. However, these minor problems can cause significant problems during the high performance demands in winter sports and may produce injury or interfere with performance.

After careful examination, including limb and spine analysis in the stance phase, an orthotic device or a custom footbed produced in a balanced and neutrally aligned foot will generally give relief of symptoms secondary to the malalignment condition. Furthermore, a greater degree of comfort can be expected from a custom-made device. Enhanced performance can be expected when lower limb alignment is achieved for optimal performance due to precision alignment.

REFERENCES

1. Bates, BT, et al: Foot orthotic devices to modify selected aspects of lower extremity mechanics. Am J Sports Med 7:339, 1969.
2. Brody, DM: Running Injuries. Ciba Symposium 32(4), 1980.
3. Brody, DM: Techniques in the evaluation and treatment of the injured runner. Orthopedic Clin North Am 13(3):541–548, 1982.
4. Bruebaker, CE and James, SL: Injuries to runners. J Sports Med 2:189–198, 1974.
5. Cavanagh, PR, Clark, T, and Williams, K: An Evaluation of the Affect of Orthotic Force Distribution and Rearfoot Movement During Running. American Orthopaedic Society for Sports Medicine Meeting, Lake Placid, NY, 1978.
6. Cavanagh, PR and Lafortune, MA: Ground reaction forces in distance running. J Biomechanics 13:397–412, 1980.
7. Clement, DB, Taunton, DB, Smart, GW, and McNicol, KL: A survey of overuse running injuries. The Physician and Sportsmedicine 9:47–58, 1981.
8. Colson, MJ and Berglund, G: An effective orthotic design for controlling the unstable subtalar joint. Orthotics and Prosthetics 33:39–49, 1979.
9. D'Ambrosia, R: Orthotic devices in running injuries. Clin Sports Med 4:611–618, 1985.
10. D'Ambrosia, R and Drez, D: Prevention and Treatment of Running Injuries. CB Slack, Thorofare, NJ, 1982.
11. Drez, D: Running footwear. Am J Sports Med 8:140–141, 1980.
12. Elftman, H: The transverse tarsal joint and its control. Clinical Orthopedics and Related Research 16:41–46, 1960.
13. James, S, Bates, BT, and Osternig, LR: Injuries to runners. Am J Sports Med 6:40–50, 1978.
14. Kotwick, JE: Biomechanics of the foot and ankle. Clin Sports Med 1:19–34, 1982.
15. Lutter, L: Orthopedic management of runners. In Bateman and Trott (eds): Foot and Ankle. Thieme Stratton, New York, 1980, pp 155–158.
16. Mann, RA: Biomechanics of the foot. American Academy of Orthopedic Surgery, Atlas of Orthotics. CV Mosby, St Louis, 1985, pp 112–125.
17. Mann, RA, Baxter, DE, and Lutter, LD: Running Symposium. Foot and Ankle 1:191–226, 1981.
18. McGregor, RR: Personal communications, 1985.
19. Murphy, P: Orthoses: Not the sole solution for running ailments. The Physician and Sportsmedicine 14:164–170, 1986.
20. Rearfoot control, cushioning and shoe design. Nike Research Letter (2)1, 1983.
21. Effect of orthotics on rearfoot motion in running. Nike Research Letter (2)3, 1983.
22. High Performance Hockey Skates: Research Product Development. Warrington Products, Montreal, 1986.
23. Riegler, HF: Reconstruction for lateral instability of the ankle. J Bone Joint Surg 66-A:336–339, 1984.
24. Roy, S and Irwin, R: Sports Medicine. Prentice-Hall, Englewood Cliffs, NJ, 1983, pp 443–448.
25. Shaw, A: The effects of a forefoot post on gait and function. Journal of the American Podiatry Association 65:238–243, 1975.
26. Wernick, J and Langer, S: A Practical Manual for a Basic Approach to Biomechanics, Vol 1. Langer Acrylic Laboratory, Deer Park, NY, 1972.
27. Wright, DG: Action of the subtalar and ankle joint complex during the stance phase of walking. J Bone Joint Surgery 46A:361–367, 1964.

CHAPTER 8

Sport Psychology: Selected Considerations for Winter Sports

JAMES O. DAVIS, Ph.D.

The recent Winter Olympic Games focused even more attention on the psychology of the athlete and the role of sport psychology. Although many of the athletes openly described their psychology programs, the inevitable accidents and disappointments seemed to raise more speculation than ever about the mental states of the participants. At the same time, evening news programs found the controversial issues in sport psychology necessary to spice up their Olympic coverage, and thus not all the attention was flattering. Just what is sport psychology, and what is its role in the sport sciences and medicine? A brief historical view and progress notes on selected topics follow in these pages, in the effort to understand the mind of the athlete.

Early in this century, an experimental psychologist at the University of Illinois became interested in the role of motivation in sport. Making the assumption that pep talks, pep rallies, and attempts to "psych up" the athlete could be overarousing and could create problems, he corresponded with the famous Notre Dame football coach, Knute Rockne, who was often credited with giving emphatic talks before games. It is perhaps surprising that Rockne wrote in agreement with the psychologist's view, stating, "I do not make any effort to key them up, except on rare, exceptional occasions. I keyed them up for the Nebraska game this year, which was a mistake, as we had a reaction the following Saturday against Northwestern. I try to make our boys take the game less seriously than I presume some others do."[19]

The psychologist Coleman Roberts Griffith was to spend much of his career investigating the psychology of sport, more commonly through carefully controlled laboratory studies than through the collection of anecdotes. But whatever the source, he recognized the need to make this knowledge available to athletes and coaches. It is this model which is most often used in our contemporary efforts and which has won for Griffith the title "Father of Sport Psychology."

BEGINNINGS AND DIRECTIONS

By the early 1900s, American psychologists had turned their attention to sport in the laboratories at Harvard and Yale. Research, which revealed principles that still warrant attention today, was published as early as 1895 in journals such as *Psychology Review*. At the University of Illinois, C. R. Griffith accomplished one of his many "firsts" when the board of trustees approved his plans for the first North American sport psychology research facility. The next year he published his first text in sport psychology and followed it 2 years later with a second one.[19] Lack of financial support forced closure of the laboratory in 1932, but Griffith went on to become the first team psychologist when he was hired by P. K. Wrigley to work with the Chicago Cubs baseball team in 1938.[50]

Thereafter, general interest in sport psychology waned until a flood of enthusiasm during the 1960s led to the creation of the North American Society for the Psychology of Sport and Physical Activity in 1967. From this impetus has emerged a literature of applied psychology, which is found primarily in clinical journals. These have indicated that sport behavior responded to strategies that were originally developed for the management of personal problems.[13,23,42]

Today there are several professional organizations and scientific journals that advance the disciplined exploration of sport behavior, so it is not too surprising to learn that athletes and teams are increasingly coming into contact with practitioners. For example, Suinn[43] reports that there was only one official psychology contact with a US team at the Olympics in 1976; but by 1984 there were nearly a dozen similar contacts. In American universities, such contacts are even more frequent. One consequence is that more athletes, coaches, and organizations are demanding or considering the services of sport psychologists. The following discussion is an outline of some of the services commonly provided by the psychologists assigned to the 1984 and current US teams.

STRESS AND THE MANAGEMENT OF STRESS

Stress, anxiety, and autonomic arousal are all predicted to disrupt skilled performance and health. At least three investigations have reported a positive relationship between stressful life changes and injuries to athletes.[3,5,27] In these studies, life changes such as trouble with family members, outstanding personal achievements, and moving or purchasing a home were correlated with higher risk of athletic injury. In addition, May and his colleagues[27,28] report that preseason psychosocial factors were associated with subsequent health problems such as headaches, anxiety, weight changes, substance abuse, and musculoskeletal problems.

Stress is also predicted to affect performance during competition when the competition arousal levels are often higher and more uncomfortable than during practice or recreational conditions. Consistent with this are a number of studies, including the report that top international ski racers were 25 times more likely to be injured during racing than during practice.[25] However, the relationship between arousal and performance is not necessarily a simple one.

An early way of explaining the effect of stress on athletic performance has been called the inverted-U hypothesis. This position states that performance improves as arousal increases until an optimal level occurs; then any additional increase in arousal can be detrimental. Martens and Landers[26] successfully demonstrated the inverted-U function in a study that manipulated the arousal levels of junior high school subjects. More recently, Beuter and Duda[2] used video analysis of motion to document the detrimental effects of high arousal on motor performance. Eight-year-old boys performed three consecutive stepping motions over low obstacles without being aware that video equipment was recording their efforts. To enhance arousal, one of the investigators entered the room dressed as a doctor and announced that recording would be conducted, with a prize going to the best performer, and that this performance would be useful in predicting future athletic prowess. As expected, the boys were not as fluid in the high-arousal condition. The poorer performances during the high-arousal condition suggested that "what was once automatic and smooth in terms of the ankle joint now comes under more volitional control, which is less smooth and efficient."[2]

Oxendine[35] suggests that the inverted-U is not appropriate for very simple tasks, such as running straight for a goal or in football blocking, in which high levels of arousal may facilitate performance. On the other hand, reducing levels of stress is absolutely necessary for fine coordination tasks, such as archery, skating, or golf. Weinberg and Genuchi[48] found lowering arousal did help golfers; and Lanning and Hisanaga[20] reported the same was true for volleyball.

Still other factors may influence the role of arousal. Two studies reported that successful athletes were as anxious before competition as less successful athletes, but they reduced their anxiety more during competition.[24,31] Three studies of competitive wrestlers found no consistent patterns of anxiety in athletes with different levels of ability.[12,14,16] Suinn[47] suggests that some of the inconsistencies in these findings are due to the small sample sizes, different sports, different measures of anxiety, and the closeness of skills when athletes were sometimes defined as "unsuccessful" only because they "failed" to defeat their "successful" opponents. He further adds that we should not be surprised when the relationships prove to be complex or when we encounter cases that prove to be exceptions to the rule.

When an athlete presents a request for help in controlling stress, the psychologic strategies that are used will depend upon the sources of stress, the skills of the athlete, and the resources available. Commonly, these methods are based on behavioral and cognitive therapy interventions. The Jacobsen deep-muscle relaxation technique is widely used by North American psychologists. This method teaches the athlete to first tense and then relax muscle groups, progressing systematically through the body segments until the whole body is relaxed. Variations and extensions on this technique are common, including the learning of breathing, verbal, and imagery cues for controlling relaxation voluntarily before and during competition.

One illustration of the value of relaxation training involves a varsity swim team that was led through relaxation immediately after every evening workout, starting with preseason workouts and continuing to the end of the season.[6] Although caution must attend within group comparisons, the success of that season was nonetheless very satisfying. The prior season the team had finished third in their conference, placed 23rd in the NCAA Division II finals, and counted only one of their swimmers all-American. At the end of the season using relaxation for workout recoveries, they won their conference, placed seventh at their nationals, and boasted 12 all-American swimmers. One very interesting and provocative finding in that program was the reduction in injuries for the year compared to the year before. Fifty-two injuries were reported during the year before the relaxation, but only 25 occurred during the relaxation project. In an unpublished translation of Russian material,[41] there are several references to the use of relaxation for workout recovery, as well as to data collected from weight lifters that report faster recovery of heart rate, blood pressure, and skin temperature. Recovery and injury prevention deserve more attention as possible values of relaxation training.

In addition to the autonomic response component of arousal, there is a cognitive component. The athlete may report doubts, negative images, racing thoughts, or problems with attention. The procedure for changing the content of thoughts is called cognitive restructuring. This is based on the premise that thoughts, like overt behaviors, are governed by the principles of learning.[23,29,43] As an illustration of cognitive restructuring, consider the case of a decathlete who failed to clear any attempt at the high jump during an important national competition in which he had a very good chance of winning and scoring over 8000 points. He later explained that the failure was constantly on his mind, and he feared it would become a "mental block." In counseling, several suggestions were offered that might help change the imagery and the effect it could have on the athlete. One that was particularly effective was the suggestion that "failure" be renamed and remembered as a "dramatic detail." This manipulation was always attended by a sense of humor.

THE ROLE OF IMAGERY IN SPORT

The role of imagery in psychology was formally studied as early as 1897.[50] Essentially, it has been found that when an athlete rehearses an event mentally, visualizing and sensing the motor task, then the performance can be enhanced. Two corollaries to this are that when an athlete dwells on or anticipates failure or accident, then it may be a rehearsal for disaster. Many public examples of mental practice for sport exist, including accounts by Jean-Claude Killey, winner or all three Alpine skiing events, downhill racing, slalom, and giant slalom in the 1968 Winter Olympic Games at Grenoble. Reviews of the many studies of mental practice[4,36,37,44] draw these conclusions: Mental practice can facilitate performance, although it is not as effective as physical practice; and mental practice is more likely to be effective if alternated with physical practice.

In 1972, Suinn proposed combining relaxation with mental practice, calling the technique visual motor behavior rehearsal (VMBR). An important quality of VMBR is the emphasis placed on the vividness of imagery, which can be achieved by including details from nearly all the senses, including kinesthetic, proprioceptive, auditory, and emotional. With these refinements of mental practice, reports have been consistent in detailing successful applications of VMBR to sport.[8,18,33,34,39,40,49] Noel's careful study[34] involving tennis serves points to the importance of skill level in determining the value of mental practice. His results indicate that VMBR practice improved first-serve accuracy for skilled tennis players, but performance actually declined for novice players. This strongly indicated that the skilled players may have known what to practice, whereas the novices were simply rehearsing errors. This interpretation has been given support from a study with golfers by Woolfolk and coworkers.[51]

The illustration of choice for VMBR remains the first reported by Suinn.[42] Invited to help the Colorado State University ski team,

he divided skiers into two groups matched for racing ability. One group received the imagery training, and the other served as a control. The experimental group began reducing errors, learning courses better, and apparently impressing their coach, who began racing them and not the controls. The ski team won the men's, women's, and the overall league trophies. Other studies report similar results. Five projects with proper controls are reviewed by Greenspan and Feltz, who believe that VMBR is an efficacious procedure.[14a]

GOAL SETTING AND PERFORMANCE

Besides these applications of behavioral psychology to sports, the principles of other subareas of psychology have been used, including social psychology and industrial/organizational psychology. Goal setting represents one of these applications.

In a review of goal-setting studies conducted between 1969 and 1980, Locke and associates[22] found clear results that challenging goals will lead to higher performance than easy goals or no goals, and concrete goals are better than "do your best" goals. In their later interpretation of these findings, Locke and Latham[21] suggested that goal setting could be used to increase both the performance and the confidence of the athlete.

Although relatively few studies have been done with psychomotor or sport skills when compared with more than 100 studies reviewed from the areas of business and industry, the same principles seem to hold. Davis and Spennewyn[7] reported correlations between athletic success and goal-setting behavior in both swimmers and runners. Similar results were achieved with weight lifting[32] and with archers.[1]

OTHER CONSIDERATIONS

Although there have been considerable successes in transferring some of the principles of learning and cognition from psychology to sport, sport psychology has also created some impressive findings of its own that may well open doors for general interests.

One very exciting area of sport psychology is the finding that vigorous activity is often associated with psychologic changes generally regarded as salutary, including reduced levels of anxiety and depression, an enhanced sense of well-being, and improvements in cognition, perception, work, social skills, libido, self-concept, and body image.[11,38] So while it has long been accepted that the mind can influence the body, the complementary theorem that the body affects the mind is now widely accepted. Research has implicated the release of opiate-like peptides known as endorphins and has suggested that the effect is related to aerobic activity but not to isometric exercises alone.[30]

With the suggested benefits of sport being mental as well as physical, an interest in adherence to physical activity and compliance with health regimens is naturally enhanced. Dishman[9] reports that approximately half of the people who start a health-related exercise program will quit within the first 6 months. Some of the factors appear to be situational; for example, 17 percent of the participants who dropped out of a 20-week running program did so because of injuries created by the running. Personal characteristics also appear involved in the determination of adherence, with self-motivation[10] and ability to gain benefits from exercise[17] among them.

Currently there is a great deal of interest in the advances being made in the psychophysiology of sport. Hatfield and colleagues[15] reported that marksmen showed left-brain intellective activity while preparing their rifles, but this changed to right-brain dominance as they sighted the target. The role of right-hemisphere activity in perceptual, nonverbal tasks suggests a number of possibilities with reference to possible inherent talent, training strategies, and even gender differences. Might right-brain activity account for the state of consciousness in sport known as "flow"? The implications of these observations for biathalon, bobsledding, ice hockey, and figure skating are conspicuous.

CONCLUDING STATEMENTS

As with almost any advances in knowledge, sport psychology raises more questions than it finds answers. The truly exciting thing is that there are some answers, and the questions being raised are the right ones.

Sport is an integral part of our society, and it plays an important role in the socialization of our youth and the health of our people. It is most fitting that we pursue with relish the further understanding of what compels, attracts, and enriches us like little else in our world.

REFERENCES

1. Barnett, ML and Stancier, JA: Effects of goal setting on achievement in archery. Res Q 50:328–332, 1979.
2. Beuter, A and Duda, JL: Analysis of the arousal/motor performance relationship in children using movement kinematics. J Sport Psychol 7:229–243, 1985.
3. Bramwell, ST, Minoura, M, Wagner, NN, and Holmes, TH: Psychosocial factors in the development and application of the social and athletic readjustment rating scale (SARRS). J Hum Stress 1:6–20, 1975.
4. Corbin, C: Mental practice. In Morgan, W (ed): Ergogenic aids and muscular performance. Academic Press, New York, 1972.
5. Cryan, PD and Alles, WF: The relationship between stress and college football injuries. Journal of Sportsmedicine and Physical Fitness 23:52–58, 1983.
6. Davis, JO: Sports injuries and performance after a stress management program. Paper presented at Southwestern Psychological Association, Tulsa, April, 1988.
7. Davis, JO and Spennewayn, KC: Goal-setting and athletic success. Proceedings of the U.S. Olympic Academy XII, Texas Tech University, Lubbock, 1984.
8. Desiderato, O and Miller, I: Improving tennis performance by cognitive behavior modification techniques. Behavior Therapist 2:19, 1979.
9. Dishman, RK: Psychobiologic predicators of exercise behavior. In Partington, JT, Orlick, T, and Salmela, JH (eds): Sport in Perspective. Coaching Association of Canada, Ottawa, 1982.
10. Dishman, RK: Motivation and exercise adherence. In Silva, JM and Weinberg, RS (eds): Psychological Foundations of Sport. Human Kinetics, Champaign, IL, 1984.
11. Folkins, CH and Sime, WE: Physical fitness training and mental health. Am Psychol 36:373–389, 1981.
12. Gould, D, Horn, T, and Spreemen, J: Competitive anxiety in junior elite wrestlers. J Sport Psychol 5:58–71, 1983.
13. Gould, D and Weiss, M: The effects of model similarity and model talk on self-efficacy and muscular endurance. J Sport Psychol 3:17–29, 1981.
14. Gould, D, Weiss, M, and Weinberg, R: Psychological characteristics of successful and unsuccessful Big Ten wrestlers. J Sport Psychol 34:69–81, 1981.
14a. Greenspan, MJ and Feltz, DL: Psychological interventions with athletes in competitive situations: A review. The Sport Psychologist, in press.
15. Hatfield, B, Landers, D, and Ray, W: Cognitive processes during self-paced motor performance: An electroencephalographic profile of skilled marksmen. J Sport Psychol 65:42–59, 1984.
16. Highlen, P and Bennett, B: Psychological charac-

teristics of successful and unsuccessful elite wrestlers: An exploratory study. J Sport Psychol 1:123–137, 1979.

17. Ingjer, F and Dahl, HA: Dropouts from an endurance training program. Scand Sports Sci 1:20–22, 1979.

18. Kolonay, B: The effects of visuo-motor behavior rehearsal on athletic performance. Unpublished master's thesis, Hunter College, The City University of New York, 1977.

19. Kroll, W and Lewis, G: America's first sport psychologist. Quest 13:1–4, 1970.

20. Lanning, W and Hisanaga, B: A study of the relation between the reduction of competition anxiety and an increase in athletic performance. Int J Sport Psychol 14:219–227, 1983.

21. Locke, EA and Latham, GP: The application of goal setting to sports. J Sport Psychol 7:205–222, 1985.

22. Locke, EA, Shaw, KN, Sarri, LM, and Latham, GP: Goal setting and task performance: 1969–1980. Psychol Bull 90:125–152, 1981.

23. Mahoney, MJ: Cognitive skills and athletic performance. In Kendall, PC and Hollon SD (eds): Cognitive-Behavioral Intervention: Theory, Research, and Procedures. Academic Press, New York, 1979.

24. Mahoney, M and Avener, M: Psychology of the elite athlete: An exploratory study. Cog Ther Res 1:135–141, 1977.

25. Margreiter, R, Raas, E, and Lugger, LJ: The risk of injury in experienced Alpine skiers. Orthop Clin North Am 7:51–54, 1976.

26. Martens, R and Landers, D: Motor performance under stress: A test of the inverted-U hypothesis. J Personality Social Psychology 16:29–37, 1970.

27. May, JR, Veach, TL, Reed, MW, and Griffey, MS: A psychological study of health, injury, and performance in athletes on the U.S. alpine ski team. The Physician and Sportsmedicine 13:111–115, 1985.

28. May, JR, Veach, TL, Southard, SW, and Herring, MW: The effects of life change on injuries, illness, and performance in elite athletes. In Butts, NK, Gushiken, TT, and Zerins, B (eds): The Elite Athlete. Spectrum, New York, 1985.

29. Meichenbaum, D: Cognitive-Behavior Modification: An Integrative Approach. Plenum Press, New York, 1977.

30. Melchiond, AM, Clarkson, PM, Denko, C, Freedson, P, Graves, J, and Katch, F: The Physician and Sportsmedicine 12:4(9), 102–109, 1984.

31. Meyers, A, Cooke, C, Cullen, J, and Liles, L: Psychological aspects of athletic competitors: A replication across sports. Cog Ther Res 3:361–366, 1979.

32. Nelson, JK: Motivating effects of the use of norms and goals with endurance testing. Res Q 3:317–321, 1978.

33. Nideffer, RM and Beckner, CW: A case study of improved athletic performance following use of relaxation procedures. Perceptual and Motor Skills 30:821–822, 1970.

34. Noel, RC: The effect of visuo-motor behavior rehearsal on tennis performance. J Sport Psychol 2:220–226, 1980.

35. Oxendine, JB: Emotional arousal and motor performance. Quest 13:23–32, 1970.

36. Richardson, A: Mental practice: A review and discussion. Part I. Res Q 38:95–273, 1967.

37. Richardson, A: Mental practice: A review and discussion. Part II. Res Q 38:263–273, 1967.

38. Sachs, ML: Psychological well-being and vigorous physical activity. In Silva, JM, III and Weinberg, RS (eds): Psychological Foundations of Sport. Human Kinetics, Champaign, IL, 1984.

39. Schleser, R, Meyers, AW, and Montgomery, T: A cognitive behavioral intervention for improving basketball performance. Paper presented at the Association for the Advancement of Behavior Therapy, 18th Annual Convention, New York, November 1980.

40. Seabourne, T, Weinberg, R, Jackson, A, and Suinn, RM: Effect of individualized, non-individualized and package intervention strategies on karate performance. J Sport Psychol 7:40–50, 1985.

41. Seimuk, AA, Arkhangorodsky, ZS, and Zaitsev, YK: The role of autogenic training in the training loads of highly-qualified weight lifters. Unpublished document (no date). United States Olympic Committee Sports Science Program, Colorado Springs, CO.

42. Suinn, RM: Behavioral rehearsal training for ski racers. Behav Ther 3:519–520, 1972.

43. Suinn, RM: Psychology and sport performance: Principles and applications. In Staub, WF (ed): Sport Psychology: An Analysis of Athlete Behavior. McNaughton, Ann Arbor, MI, 1980.

44. Suinn, RM: Imagery and sports. In Sheikh, A (ed): Imagery, Current Theory, Research and Application. John Wiley & Sons, New York, 1982.

45. Suinn, RM: The 1984 Olympics and sport psychology. J Sport Psychol 7:321–329, 1985.

46. Suinn, RM: Behavioral approaches to stress management. In Asken, M and May, J (eds): Sport Psychology: The Psychological Health of the Athlete. Spectrum, New York, 1985.

47. Suinn, RM: Future directions in sport psychology research: Applied aspects. Paper presented at the Gatorade Conference, Tempe, AZ, February, 1986.

48. Weinberg, R and Genuchi, M: Relationship between competitive trait anxiety, state anxiety, and golf performance. J Sport Psychol 2:148–154, 1980.

49. Weinberg, R, Seabourne, T, and Jackson, A: Effects of visual-motor behavior rehearsal, relaxation, and imagery on karate performance. J Sport Psychol 3:228–238, 1981.

50. Wiggins, DK: The history of sport psychology in North America. In Silva, JM and Weinberg, RS (eds): Psychological Foundations of Sport. Human Kinetics, Champaign, IL, 1984.

51. Woolfolk, R, Parrish, M, and Murphy, S: The effects of positive and negative imagery on motor skill performance. Unpublished data, cited in Suinn.[47]

CHAPTER 9

Overtraining: Markers Associated with Overtraining

JAMES STRAY-GUNDERSEN, M.D.

METHODS
DISCUSSION

"Overtraining" is one of those words that is used frequently by many people who feel they have an intuitive sense for the meaning of the word. However, to define it in scientific terms becomes difficult. Clearly, "overtraining" produces poor performances, but so does "undertraining." Coaches also recognize "plateaus" in performance when athletes are training properly. Furthermore, the training principle of "hard/easy" or overload and recovery makes the judgment of performance problematic. There is also a time frame to consider. If an athlete trains very hard (overloads), he or she may be tired, for the moment, but then bounces back even stronger to achieve personal records after a short rest. However, occasionally an athlete will become overtrained to the extent that despite complete rest he or she is unable to compete for weeks, months, or the rest of the season. In the course of convalescence, the athlete becomes detrained as well. Thus, overtraining may be thought of as one end of a spectrum of negative adaptation, which is characterized retrospectively by the inability of the athlete to improve performance with a short period of rest. It is most likely brought about by training fractionally too much over many days and weeks. The other end of the spectrum is acute overwork, which is characterized by tiredness, soreness, and fatigue, but which responds quickly to a minimal amount of rest. Therefore, overtraining is a syndrome of chronic negative adaptation resulting in poor performance for a prolonged period of time in an athlete who is following a seemingly "reasonable" training program.

Previously, our only method to avoid overtraining was subjective. The coach would prescribe a training program based on his or her experience and knowledge and then watch and listen to see how the athletes were responding. The athlete would also "listen" to his or her body and communicate that information to the coach. This assumes that the coach has a good program, knows how to implement it, modifies it for the individual athletes, listens to them, understands what they are saying, and further modifies their conditioning programs accordingly. This method also assumes that the athlete has a coach, follows the program, understands what his or her body is saying and communicates this to the coach. When all these assumptions are valid, champions are produced from talented individuals.

Winter sports, particularly those like cross-country ski racing, biathlon, and combined, in which the race courses and the conditions vary widely, present an even greater challenge to the coach and athlete in attempting to avoid overtraining.

Several attempts have been made to provide objective data to aid in training athletes. Three avenues of testing have been employed. The most obvious is performance. If the athlete's performance in practice and competition continues to improve, then he or she is obviously responding positively to the training program. Secondly, testing in physiology laboratories has been used to monitor several important components of performance. Unfortunately, to date the testing has proved either too time consuming, too invasive, not specific enough, too infrequent, or too insensitive to be of much real value. The third avenue has been to follow markers that would lend objective information to subjective feelings. Resting heart rate has been used informally for many years. In 1982, Czajkowski[3] described a method in which he monitored supine and standing heart rates. The author felt this was a very effective way to monitor training, but how he reached this conclusion is unclear. Others have found resting heart rates to be an unreliable indicator of stress.[6]

A variety of markers have been suggested as indicators of overtraining on the basis of responses to severe acute exercise or to relatively short periods of very heavy training. These markers may be generally classified as shifts in the endocrine profile, muscle injury characterized by elevations in serum creatine kinase, and delayed muscle glycogen synthesis, which may lead to changes in serum lactate levels. These factors may be associated with muscle soreness, impaired performance, and/or unfavorable alterations in mood state. Little is known about the changes of overtraining parameters during more prolonged periods of severe training. Several investigators have described the response of testosterone and some other hormones to intense training.[4,10] A rise in serum creatine phosphokinase (CPK) has been associated with muscle soreness.[5,9]

The scientific study of anything implies studying the subject itself. With respect to overtraining, this becomes very difficult. The obvious cases are usually only apparent well after the initial onset and are relatively infrequent. It is also unethical to produce overtraining in a group of athletes whose life success depends on their present athletic success. Finally, it is not clear how best to produce overtraining.

Consequently, our group has developed a two-pronged approach to studying this problem.[8] We have purposefully overworked high-caliber recreational athletes for a 2-week period by adding four interval workouts to their usual routine. Secondly, we have monitored several parameters in elite athletes on the United States Nordic Ski Team.

METHODS

Group 1: Ten male recreational runners between the ages of 20 and 45 years of age were recruited. These men were running more than 40 miles per week and had recently completed 10 kilometers in 40 minutes or less. All were free of injuries or illness. The subjects were then entered into an initial 2-week baseline period, which consisted of their normal training plus a 5 kilometer time trial, a rest day, and a test day. Each evening their heart rates were recorded during sleep with the aid of a Quantum XL Heart Rate Monitor. The average heart rate was determined between 2 AM and 6 AM. After a day's rest and a 12-hour fast, the runners reported at 8 AM. Venous blood was

EXPERIMENTAL DESIGN

BASELINE—2 WKS
OVERTRAINING—2 WKS
RECOVERY—2 WKS

OVERTRAINING CONSISTS OF
ADDING FOUR INTERVAL (D)
WORKOUTS (20x440yds) TO
THE BASELINE WORKLOAD.

—WEEKLY 5K TIME TRIAL (A)
—WEEKLY VENOUS BLOOD SAMPLE (B)
—LABORATORY TESTING EVERY 2 WEEKS (C)
—HEART RATE DATA COLLECTION DAILY

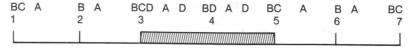

Figure 9–1. Experimental design.

drawn for determinations of free testosterone, cortisol, and CPK. This was followed by determination of height, weight, and percent body fat by hydrostatic weighing. Then the subject performed a bout of maximal exercise, during which maximal values for oxygen uptake, heart rate, and lactate were obtained by using standard open circuit spirometry, the heart rate monitor, and a Yellow Springs Lactate Analyser. The subjects then added four interval workouts to their baseline work during a 2-week period of "overtraining." The workouts consisted of 20 quarter-mile runs, reaching 90 percent of their maximal heart rates during the run. The athletes recovered until their heart rates reached 60 percent of maximum before beginning the next interval. The same protocol of rest and testing was followed as in the baseline period after the 2 weeks of overwork. This was followed by a 2-week recovery period in which the subjects resumed their normal training. The subjects then un-

derwent testing for a final time (Fig. 9–1). Data were subjected to a multiple analysis of variance with Neuman-Keuls post-hoc test applied where appropriate. Significance was set at $p < 0.05$.

In these runners, average sleeping heart rate increased, time-trial heart rate decreased, and maximal heart rate decreased significantly from baseline values in the overtraining period and returned to baseline values during the recovery period (Table 9–1, Fig. 9–2). Free testosterone concentration decreased and cortisol concentration in serum increased from baseline to the overtraining period and returned toward baseline values during the recovery period. However, the trend did not reach the level of significance. The ratio of the free testosterone value divided by the cortisol value decreased significantly during the overtraining period and returned toward baseline after the recovery period. The interaction statistic for the testosterone/cortisol (T/C) ratio was significant.

Table 9–1. EXPERIMENTAL RESULTS IN GROUP 1 OF TEN RUNNERS

	HRs* bpm	HR$_{5K}$* bpm	HR$_{max}$* bpm	T$_f$ pg/dl	C μg/dl	T/C*	CPK* U/liter
Base	44.8 ± 1.5	172 ± 4	181 ± 3	11.4 ± 1.3	17.1 ± 1.1	0.71 ± 0.11	161 ± 12
Overtraining	48.3 ± 1.5	166 ± 4	175 ± 3	9.5 ± 0.9	19.4 ± 0.9	0.49 ± 0.05	303 ± 41
Recovery	45.0 ± 1.6	170 ± 4	180 ± 3	11.1 ± 1.1	18.5 ± 1.1	0.60 ± 0.05	166 ± 15

HRs = heart rate sleeping beats per minute (bpm); HR$_{5K}$ = heart rate after 5 kilometer run; HR$_{max}$ = heart rate maximum; T$_f$ = free testosterone; C = cortisol; T/C = free testosterone (pg/dl) divided by cortisol (μg/dl); CPK = creatinine phosphokinase.
*Significant change during overtraining mean ± SE, $p < 0.05$

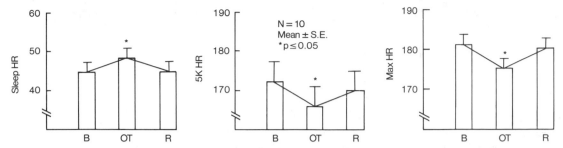

Figure 9–2. *(Left)* Sleep heart rate (beats per minute). *(Middle)* Five kilometer time trial heart rate (beats per minute). *(Right)* Maximal heart rate (beats per minute).

The CPK values rose significantly after the overtraining period and returned to baseline values after the recovery period (see Table 9–1, Fig. 9–3). No differences were noted in weight, percent body fat, maximal oxygen uptake, or maximal lactate concentration (Table 9–2).

Group 2: After a day of easy exercise, eight male members of the United States Nordic Ski Team had fasting morning blood samples drawn for testosterone and cortisol determinations on six occasions between May 1985 and March 1986. Concentrations of free testosterone and cortisol were determined by radioimmune assay from serum, and coaches and their athletes were informed of the results within 3 to 5 working days. The mean and standard error of the Group 2 data were determined. Variation within the same individual of Group 2 was noted, but no statistical analysis was applied.

The mean data from these skiers showed the lowest T/C ratio in November (Table 9–3). This was the time of greatest volume and intensity in their training programs and was performed during a month-long training camp at 6000 feet of altitude. In January, one of the eight athletes had a markedly reduced value for testosterone, and consequently his T/C ratio was also markedly reduced (Table 9–4). This value was obtained from a specimen drawn after the athlete was unable to compete in several races due to undue fatigue. The opinion of his coaches was that he was either sick or overtrained. Complete medical work-up revealed no detectable abnormalities other than the testosterone level.

DISCUSSION

These preliminary results suggest that monitoring heart rate, serum-free testoster-

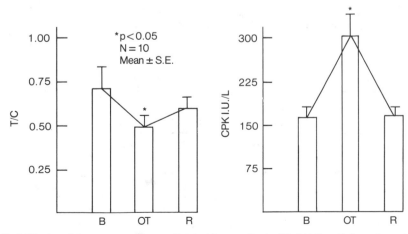

Figure 9–3. *(Left)* Ratio of free testosterone divided by cortisol. *(Right)* Creatinine phosphokinase (international units per liter).

Table 9–2. SUBJECT CHARACTERISTICS OF GROUP 1 OF TEN RUNNERS
(MEAN ± SE)

	Age (yr)	Height (cm)	Weight (kg)	% Body Fat	$\dot{V}O_{2max}$ (Liters/min)	$\dot{V}O_{2max}$ (ml/kg/min)	La (mM)
Base	33 ± 3	181 ± 1	74.3 ± 2.0	8.4 ± 1.1	4.73 ± 0.15	63.4 ± 1.7	10.8 ± 0.7
Overtraining			74.1 ± 1.9	7.9 ± 0.9	4.74 ± 0.13	64.2 ± 1.3	8.8 ± 0.8
Recovery			74.3 ± 1.9	7.7 ± 0.9	4.80 ± 0.14	64.6 ± 1.3	8.8 ± 1.2

$\dot{V}O_{2max}$ = maximal oxygen consumption; La = maximal blood lactate concentration following exercise.

one, and serum cortisol under controlled conditions may provide some objective information as to how athletes adapt to the stress of training. There are several aspects of this study that require more investigation. The runners group was "overworked" as opposed to "overtrained." The assumption is that by greatly overloading an athlete for a short period of time, similar physiologic changes to those produced by overtraining will occur. This assumption has not been conclusively shown to be true. For example, the performance of these runners during the 5-kilometer time trial was variable, with some subjects improving their performance and others showing reduced performance. This probably reflects the varying trainability of individual subjects. Although all subjects showed changes in the physiologic markers, at least some subjects were not overtrained by the interval workouts based on performance criteria.

The results from the Nordic skiers group are interesting. However, to establish convincingly a link between hormone data such as these and an athlete's response to training, data on the volume and intensity of training and the performance and heart rates under various conditions must be collected and analyzed. This work is ongoing in our laboratory.

A proposed mechanism for these changes follows. Training stimulates both anabolic and catabolic events in the cells involved with the training activity. If training causes a predominance of catabolic events in the tissues and this occurs for a sufficiently long period of time without recovery, negative adaptation follows, causing reduced performance, illness, or overuse injury. This negative adaptation is communicated to the central nervous sytem (CNS) by chemoreceptors via groups III and IV afferent fibers. These fibers synapse in the thalamus and the medulla, which in turn affects the output from the hypothalamus and the cardiovascular control center, among others. This activity modifies efferent activity, resulting in a myriad of changes in the organism. The heart rate response to a variety of conditions and hormonal production are among the many alterations that may be noted under controlled conditions.

Presently, this mechanism is conjecture.

Table 9–3. DATA, GROUP 2 OF EIGHT NORDIC SKIERS

	Date	T_f pg/dl	C µg/dl	T/C*
Group Data	May 20, 1985	35.3 ± 3.7	18.3 ± 1.6	1.99 ± 0.25
($\overline{X}$ ± SE, n = 9)	Jul 17, 1985	28.5 ± 2.7	18.1 ± 1.7	1.63 ± 0.16
	Sep 19, 1985	26.2 ± 2.0	19.7 ± 1.5	1.43 ± 0.19
	Nov 14, 1985	24.6 ± 2.7	19.9 ± 1.7	1.32 ± 0.17
	Dec 12, 1985	32.6 ± 3.5	22.6 ± 1.3	1.44 ± 0.14
	Mar 22, 1986	32.2 ± 2.0	22.0 ± 1.5	1.54 ± 0.12

T/C = free testosterone; C = cortisol.
*T/C = the value of free testosterone (pg/dl) divided by cortisol (µg/dl).

Table 9–4. DATA, AN INDIVIDUAL NORDIC
SKIER

	Date	T_f pg/dl	C μg/dl	T/C*
Individual A	May 20, 1985	48.9	25.0	1.96
	Jul 17, 1985	38.4	19.7	1.95
	Sep 19, 1985	28.9	22.9	1.26
	Nov 14, 1985	28.1	19.3	1.46
	Dec 12, 1986	50.5	25.2	2.00
	Jan 16, 1986	4.8	17.4	0.28
	Mar 22, 1986	30.5	30.0	1.02

T_f = free testosterone; C = cortisol
*T/C = the value of free testosterone (pg/dl) divided by cortisol (μg/dl).

However, there are several lines of evidence to support this contention. Peripheral chemoreceptors have been shown to modulate cardiovascular and pulmonary response under a variety of conditions.[7] Hormone levels have been shown to be altered by many different activities.[1,4,10,11] Furthermore, it has been shown that hormone levels are controlled by releasing or inhibiting factors from the hypothalamus,[2] which is presumably controlled by higher brain centers.

The efficacy of several objective physiologic markers under controlled conditions was investigated. Preliminary results suggest that heart rate and serum hormone levels under controlled conditions may reflect the ability of athletes to perform. Future work should concentrate on establishing the relationships between training stress and physiologic markers in recreational and elite athletes to provide accurate information aimed at discovering the mechanisms responsible for these observations.

REFERENCES

1. Adlercreutz, H, Harkonen, M, Juoppasalmi, K, Naveri, H, Huhtaniemi, I, Tikkanen, H, Remes, K, Dessypris, A, and Karvonen, J: Effect of training on plasma anabolic and catabolic steroid hormones and their response during physical exercise. Int J Sports Med 7:33–37, 1986.
2. Brobeck, JR (ed): Physiologic Basis of Medical Practice. Williams & Williams, Baltimore, 1973.
3. Czajkowski, W: A simple method to control fatigue in endurance training. In Komi, PV (ed): Exercise and Sport Biology. Champaign, IL, Human Kinetic Publishers, 1982, pp 207–212.
4. Dessypris, A, Kuoppasalmi, K, and Adlercreutz, H: Plasma cortisol, testosterone, androstenedione and luteinizing hormone (LH) in a non-competitive marathon run. Journal of Steroid Biochemistry 7:33–37, 1976.
5. Dressendorfer, R and Wade, C: The muscular overuse syndrome in long-distance runners. Phys Sportsmed 11:116–130, 1983.
6. Dressendorfer, R, Wade, C, and Amsterdam, E: Development of pseudoanemia in marathon runners during a 20-day road race. JAMA 246:1215–1218, 1981.
7. Mitchell, J and Schmidt, R: Cardiovascular reflex control by afferent fibers from skeletal muscle receptors. In Shepherd, JT and Abboud, FM: Handbook of Physiology, Section 2: The Cardiovascular System: Vol III: Peripheral Circulation, Part 2. Oxford University Press, New York, 1983, pp 623–658.
8. Stray-Gundersen, J, Videman, V, and Snell, PG: Changes in selected objective parameters during overtraining. Medicine and Science in Sports and Exercise 18(S):54, 1986.
9. Tiidus, PM and Ianuzzo, CD: Effects of intensity and duration of muscular exercise on delayed soreness and serum enzyme activities. Medicine and Science in Sports and Exercise 15:481–485, 1983.
10. Urhausen, A, Kallmer T, and Kinderman, W: A 7-week follow up study of the behavior of testosterone and cortisol during the competition period in rowers. Eur J Appl Physiol 56:528–533, 1987.
11. Villaneuva, AL, Schlosser, C, Hopper, B, Liu, JH, Hoffman, DI, and Rebar, RW: Increased cortisol production in women runners. J Clin Endocrinol Metab 65:133–136, 1986.

CHAPTER 10

Sports Vision Testing and Enhancement: Implications for Winter Sports

ARNOLD SHERMAN, O.D.

Winter sports involve the use of many vision skills that need to be well developed in order for the athlete to perform at maximum potential. Skills such as visual tracking, eye-body coordination, and dynamic visual acuity need to be tested and treated. The proper use of vision can make the difference between the winner and an also-ran.

This chapter discusses the importance of vision in performance and the need for proper evaluation, treatment, and enhancement for the athlete. Sports optometrists should be part of an overall sports medicine program.

It is generally agreed that vision is the primary sense modality used in obtaining information from our environment and in directing the activities of people. For an athlete, eyes should provide information that can be gathered, analyzed, processed, retrieved, and responded to quickly and efficiently with minimal effort and stress. The process of vision utilizes the eyes for input, the brain for integrating information from other senses (intersensory matching), and the action system of the body for output (response); feedback is built into the visual system for correction, adjustment, and refinement. The entire process constitutes the visual system which is not limited only to the external sense organs (eyes).

PRINCIPLES

1. Vision is the signal that directs the muscles of the body to respond, "the eyes lead the body."

2. Vision provides the athlete with information as to "where" and "when" to perform.

3. Vision is the athlete's time machine; and superior size, strength, speed, and agility cannot make up for inefficient processing of the information as to "where" and "when" to respond.

4. Most performances that fail are not due to the wrong physical movement but due to the movement being performed at the incorrect time or in the incorrect place.

5. The two eyes provide input data for central figure information, while the head maintains body orientation and balance for peripheral ground information. The head should remain still in the gathering of information (following the ball or puck) so as not to stimulate the semicircular canals, thereby necessitating a regain of balance.

6. Inner speech (talking to oneself) operates at the expense of awareness and does not belong on the field. It can only be used prior to or after the event as a checklist.

7. Normal visual findings are not enough for superior athletic performance. Superior visual skills are necessary, and even more important is the ability to use these skills efficiently.

8. Most vision skills are learned, and therefore they can be relearned and improved through training, but specific vision skills for individual sports must be isolated for enhancement.

9. Sports optometrists are concerned with visual enhancement in order to maximize the potential and performance of the athlete.

GENERAL SKILLS

Numerous visual skills have been cited as important in sports performance.[14] These include the following:

1. Visual acuity
2. Dynamic visual acuity
3. Ocular-motor skills
4. Eye–hand coordination
5. Depth perception and stereopsis
6. Accommodation
7. Central-peripheral awareness
8. Visual reaction time
9. Visual adjustability
10. Visualization

Other visual skills recently studied include glare recovery, contrast sensitivity, and perceptual styles, involving those which are field dependent and field independent.[2,5] A theoretical relationship between various sports and visual skills is presented in Table 10–1.

Since 1979, the Sports Vision Section of the American Optometric Association has participated with the United States Olympic Committee (USOC) at the National Sports Festival in testing visual performance of America's finest amateur athletes. In addition to classical tests of eye health, refractive condition, and visual acuity, the testing includes tests of visual performance. A similar testing program was utilized within the framework of the Elite Athlete Program in 1982–1984. Based on the results of these studies, visual training and enhancement programs were carried out with the US Olympic Archery, Fencing, Handball, Hockey, and Volleyball teams. It was interesting to note that failures on the eyesight parts of the evaluation ranged between 10 percent and 25 percent each; more than 50 percent of the athletes previously had never received an eye examination. Other studies with athletes have shown that 28 to 35 percent had reduced visual acuity that required prescription lenses.[1,4,8]

SPECIFIC SKILLS

Dynamic visual acuity (DVA) has been described as the ability to detect the detail of an object in the field of vision when there is relative movement between the person and the object. A test devised over three decades ago to assess would-be pilots[7] is useful for evaluating the DVA of athletes. In the DVA test, an object suddenly appears traveling at a constant angular velocity. The object is seen, and the central nervous system must estimate the direction and velocity of the movement. The brain must then send a message to the extraocular muscles, causing innervation appropriate to place and to hold the image of the object in the vicinity of the fovea for a sufficiently long period of time to

Table 10–1. SPORTS AND VISUAL SKILLS

	Visual acuity	Dynamic visual acuity	Ocular-motor skills	Eye/hand coordination	Binocular stereopsis	Accommodation	Central-peripheral awareness	Visual reaction time	Visual adjustability	Visualization
Archery	4	1	3	5	2	3	5	1	1	2
Baseball hit	4	5	5	5	5	5	5	5	5	5
Baseball pitch	3	2	3	4	3	3	5	1	3	5
Basketball	3	3	4	5	5	3	5	5	5	5
Bowling	2	1	3	5	3	2	4	1	3	4
Boxing	2	2	5	5	3	3	5	5	5	4
Football (Quarterback)	4	5	5	5	5	3	5	5	5	5
Golf	3	1	4	5	5	3	5	1	3	5
Gymnastics	1	3	3	5	5	3	5	5	5	5
Hockey (Goalie)	4	5	5	5	5	5	5	5	5	3
Pool	2	1	4	5	5	2	3	1	4	5
Race car driving	5	5	5	4	5	2	5	5	5	5
Racquetball	4	5	5	4	5	4	5	5	5	5
Running	1	1	2	1	1	1	4	3	1	4
Skiing	5	5	5	5	5	3	5	5	5	5
Soccer	3	4	5	5	5	3	5	5	5	5
Swimming	1	1	1	1	1	1	4	3	1	4
Tennis	4	5	5	5	5	5	5	5	5	5
Track — high jump	1	3	3	4	4	3	3	4	4	4
Track — pole vault	1	3	3	5	5	3	4	4	4	5
Wrestling	2	1	1	3	2	1	3	5	5	4

Arnold Sherman, O.D., Merrick, N.Y., is Chairman of the American Optometric Association's Sports Vision Section. Scoring: 1 — not related to 5 — extremely important

permit the resolution of the critical detail. It is the total efficiency of this complex process that is measured by the DVA test.

Kirshner[6] has described testing for DVA with an ocularotor device utilizing a Snellen chart projected into a rotating mirror with an arc diameter of 55 cm at a 10-foot testing distance. Sherman has devised a sports vision disc[18] (Fig. 10–1), which can be used to test and train dynamic visual acuity and ocular motor accuracy. The large letters are 20/60, and the small letters are 20/30 when tested at 10 feet. Using a children's phonograph, DVA can be scored at 78, 45, and 33 rpm. The norm established utilizing more than 1000 athletes is 20/30 acuity at 45 rpm. Dy-namic visual acuity is typically faster with hockey goalies, baseball hitters, and tennis players and considerably poorer in athletes whose sports do not require following fast-moving targets. Research by Sanderson and Whiting[11] indicates that DVA and catching performance were related, whereas static visual acuity was unrelated to both DVA and catching performance. It should be emphasized that the major factor involved in DVA is precise ocular-motor coordination.

Depth perception and stereopsis are related to precisely coordinating the two eyes together as a unit.[13] The ability to follow a rapidly moving target toward the observer is accomplished by the process of triangula-

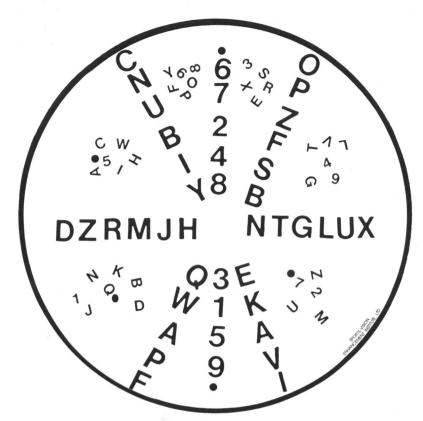

Figure 10–1. Sports vision disc designed by A. Sherman. See text for description and discussion.

tion; a triangle is formed by the moving target and the two eyes as it approaches. This process provides information as to where the target is at any given time and allows for the accurate hitting of a baseball and tennis ball or a save by a hockey goalie.

Numerous studies have shown better depth perception of the varsity athlete compared with that of the nonathlete, as well as better depth perception of more skilled players in specific sports. In a study of the 1984 US Olympic Volleyball Team, the primary difference in visual skills between the best players and the substitute players was depth perception speed of response on stereopsis testing.[12]

Peripheral vision also has been studied, and once again athletes were found to perform better than nonathletes. Using perimetry to determine size of visual fields, many studies indicate that better athletes tend to have larger peripheral fields than those who are less skilled and nonathletes.[10,16]

SPORTS VISION AVERAGE

Ocular-motor abilities, eye–hand coordination, and visual reaction time have been studied by numerous researchers. Clinical studies of eye-movement speed and accuracy as well as research reports indicate that the ocular movements of athletes are generally superior to those of nonathletes and do relate to athletic performance.[3,15,17] I have used the Saccadic Fixator (Fig. 10–2) with both amateur and professional athletes. A total of 371 athletes were tested for eye–hand coordination, visual proaction time (VPT), and visual reaction time (VRT), and a scoring system has been formulated to indicate their proficiencies. Results are obtained for each athlete by dividing the VRT by the VPT and multiplying by 100. This score has been labeled the Sports Vision Average (SVA).

$$SVA = (VRT/VPT) \times 100$$

Results indicate that the SVA is related to

specific sports as well as individual positions within that sport. Specific sports require specific visual abilities. I believe that successful players in sports requiring fast visual reactions to a moving object—such as hockey, baseball, and tennis—will tend to have higher SVAs than players in sports such as archery, gymnastics, golf, and bowling.

Procedure

The center of the Saccadic Fixator (see Fig. 10–2) is placed at approximately eye level. The habitual prescription for sports and normal overhead illumination are used.

Part I requires the athlete to press a button next to a red light. After this is done, the light moves randomly to another position on the board and remains there until the athlete hits that button. The number of "hits" in 30 seconds is recorded as the VPT.

Part II requires the athlete to perform the same task, with the exception that the red light is now programmed to move randomly at the rate of one light per second. If the athlete does not react quickly enough, the button will move to the next position on the board without a "hit" being recorded. The correct number of "hits" in 30 seconds is read off the fixator and recorded as the VRT.

Observations are made of behaviors such as head movement, use of two hands, and performance differences between right and left fields.

The SVA is then obtained for each player. For example, if on Part I the athlete scores 24 and in Part II scores 12, the athlete has obtained an SVA of 0.500

$$[VRT(PII)/VPT(PI)]$$
$$= (12/24) \times 100 = 0.500$$

A score of 27 on Part I and 18 on Part II indicates an SVA of 0.667. Data obtained from testing superior college athletes, athletes at the National Sports Festival in Colorado Springs, 1979, and professional tennis play-

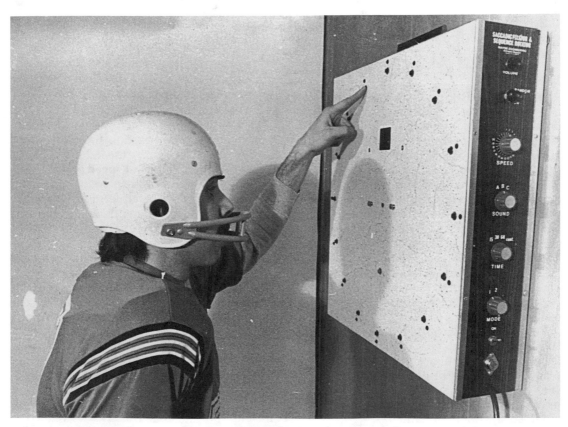

Figure 10–2. The Wayne Saccadic Fixator. (From Sherman,[15] with permission.)

Table 10–2. SPORTS VISION AVERAGES OF
ATHLETES ATTENDING NATIONAL SPORTS
FESTIVAL, COLORADO SPRINGS, 1979

Sport	Number	VPT	VRT	SVA
Archery	31	26.4	17.1	0.648
Baseball	11	23.6	20.9	0.886
Women's basketball	12	30.0	20.0	0.667
Boxing	11	26.0	14.6	0.562
Gymnastics	11	27.8	17.4	0.626
Team handball	43	28.0	19.0	0.679
Hockey (ice)	65	29.0	22.0	0.759
Modern pentathlon	17	28.0	19.0	0.679
Modern rhythmic gymnastics	9	25.7	13.0	0.506
Riflery	14	29.1	20.2	0.694
Table tennis	38	26.4	16	0.606
Water polo	30	29	21	0.724
Professional tennis	26	29.96	21.6	0.720
College basketball, men	15	25	14.7	0.588
College basketball, women	11	24.9	14.9	0.600
Baseball (college)	27	25.3	13.3	0.526

From Sherman,[15] with permission.

ers are summarized in Table 10–2. Averages were established for specific sports, and an overall average for all athletes examined is presented in Table 10–2.

IMPROVING SPORTS VISION SKILLS

Vision skills are learned and therefore improvable. Theoretically, if a vision skill is related to a specific sports performance and is a trainable skill, improvement in the sport should occur after a training program. Research studies are underway through the Vision Performance and Safety Committee of the USOC to determine this. Studies do indicate that vision skills such as ocular motility, depth perception, stereopsis, peripheral vision, reaction time, and eye–hand coordination can be improved.

A study of visualization on the free-throw scores of basketball players indicates that visualization is comparable to actual practice in improving free-throw percentage. Richardson[9] chose three random groups of basketball players, none of whom had ever previously practiced visualization. Group I practiced free throws every day for 20 days. Group II practiced on the first and 20th days, with no practice in between. Group III also practiced on the first and 20th days, but in addition, they spent 20 minutes a day visualizing sinking baskets and correcting their aim on the next shot if they mentally missed. The results showed that Group I, which actually had practiced shooting free throws, improved their averages by 24 percent. Group II, which had had no practice between the first and 20th days, did not improve at all. And Group II, which had visualized but also had had no practice, improved by 23 percent.

CONCLUSION

Comprehensive visual examination, diagnosis, and treatment of vision skills should be an integral part of the overall medical and training programs for all athletes participating in winter sports.

The vision evaluation should include tests that measure visual performance specifically related to the athlete's particular sport; for example, skiing and ice hockey require high-level performance in ocular motility, eye-body coordination, visual reaction time, and peripheral awareness of vision.

Visual enhancement, training, and calisthenics can often provide the extra edge for the athlete to maximize performance, to reach full potential, and to become a winner.

Finally, the judicious use of protective eye wear can prevent injuries to over 100,000 eyes each year (see Chapters 23, 24, and 29).[18] Special lenses are available to prevent snow glare and to eliminate harmful ultraviolet rays that are potential causes of keratitis, cataracts, and macula damage in winter sports participants.

REFERENCES

1. Bauscher, WA: Vision and the athlete. Optometry Weekly 59:21–25, 1968.
2. Cockerill, IM and MacGillivary, WW: Vision and Sports. Stanley Thornos, Cheltenham, England, 1981.
3. Falkowitz, C and Mendal, H: The role of visual skills in batting averages. Optometry Weekly 68:577–580, 1977.
4. Garner, AI: Visual aid prescribing for the athlete. California Optometry 3:18–19, 1977.
5. Hoffman, L, Polan, G, and Powell, J: The relationship of contrast sensitivity function to sports vision. Journal of the American Optometric Association 55:747–752, 1984.
6. Kirshner, AJ: Manual for the Oculorotor. Keystone View, Meadville, PA.
7. Ludvigh, EJ and Miller, JW: A study of dynamic visual acuity. (Joint Project N.M001075.01.01). United States School of Aviation Medicine, Pensacola, 1953.
8. Martin, WF: What the coach should know about the vision of athletes. Optometry Weekly 61:558–560, 1970.
9. Richardson, A: Mental Imagery. Springer-Verlag, New York, 1969.
10. Rudini, LM: Relationship between psychological functions tests and selected skills of boys in junior high school. Research Quarterly 39:674–683, 1968.
11. Sanderson, FH and Whiting, HTA: Dynamic visual acuity, a factor in catching performance. Journal of Motor Behavior 10:7–14, 1978.
12. Sanet, R and Getz, D: Personal communication, 1983.
13. Sherman, A: Overview of research information regarding vision and sports. Journal of the American Optometric Association 51:659–665, 1980.
14. Sherman, A: Prescribing for patients who play. Optometric Management 17:67–68, 1981.
15. Sherman, A: A method of evaluating eye-hand coordination and visual reaction time in athletes. Journal of the American Optometric Association 54:801–802, 1983.
16. Stroup, F: Relationship between measurements of field of motion perception and basketball ability in college men. Research Quarterly of the American Association of Health and Physical Education 39:674–683, 1968.
17. Trachtman, JN: The relationship between ocular motilities and batting average in little leaguers. American Journal of Optometry and Archives of the American Academy of Optometry 50:914–919, 1973.
18. Vinger, P: The eye and sports medicine. In Duane, TD (ed): Clinical Ophthalmology. JB Lippincott, Philadelphia, 1985, pp 1–51.

CHAPTER 11

Team Physician: Responsibilities for the World Class Winter Athlete

HOWARD M. SILBY, M.D.

This chapter reflects the author's personal experience with figure skaters, ranging from the grassroots to Olympic levels, as a "skating parent," as team physician, as Olympic team leader, and as chairman of the Sports Medicine Committee of the United States Figure Skating Association. It is hoped that at least some of this knowledge and these principles can be applied by others to their sports and help prepare medical professionals as they undertake their responsibilities as team physicians.

There are many physical, emotional, and athletic characteristics that distinguish the sport of figure skating and make the figure skating athlete unique. It is these very characteristics that have made the position of team physician in this sport an invigorating, rewarding experience. It is both refreshing and a change of pace to work with these goal-oriented, success-dedicated, physically and emotionally healthy athletes.

UNDERSTANDING THE ATHLETE

I think that in order to know what is expected of a team physician one needs to know something of the world class athlete. I do not have all the answers, but what I am going to say is based on my medical experience with skating athletes, plus my 16 years as a "skating parent" of two dedicated, figure skating daughters.

Psychologic Profile

I would like to emphasize the characteristics of goal orientation, constant striving for goal attainment, unusual initial trust and acceptance of people as they are or as they are said to be, and dogged determination. These athletes also tend to be extremely tense, especially at competition time, but they have an ability to cope emotionally with this tension. They are bright and generally extroverted, with a tremendous ability to concentrate and to learn, and they are generally tough both physically and emotionally. Thank goodness one does not need these characteristics to be a team doctor. The one negative characteristic is that these athletes tend to be unidimensional and naive; that is, they are usually extremely knowledgeable about their individual sport, but they have only a superficial knowledge of current events, great issues, and other cultural, social, and athletic events and activities. They are also insulated and isolated from the "real world" because they generally are exposed only to the finer and nicer aspects of life, both in their local communities as well as on the national and international scenes.

All of this is understandable in light of the very unique training schedule of the world class athlete, in particular of the figure skater, which includes 6 to 8 hours a day for skating, an additional 3 to 4 hours a day for school, and very close and intense relationships between skater, coach, and parent. Unlike many other athletic activities, this schedule is in operation at least 11 months of the year and for the most part occurs at a training center away from home. This puts additional strain on family ties, as well as both social and sexual peer relationships. Lastly, this is a solo sport, with none of the protections inherent in a team activity. When one is on the ice, one is all alone.

Physical Profile

These athletes are attractive, tough, well trained, and well disciplined. Scientific investigations are presently underway to study the physical conditioning, biomechanics, and psychologic profiles of these athletes. In particular, a research program has been developed over the last 2 years to study these areas. Known as "The Junior Elite Research Camp," it is a joint effort of the United States Figure Skating Association (USFSA) and the United States Olympic Committee (USOC), funded by a $200,000 Olympic Foundation grant.

Having the benefit of these observations, then, what are the prerequisites necessary to be a world team physician? Other than being a physician, I believe there are two: (1) understanding the athletic characteristics mentioned above and (2) understanding the sport itself, including the athletic tricks, the unique system of judging, and the structure and power of the USFSA and the International Skating Union (ISU).

UNDERSTANDING THE SPORT

In Figure 11–1 the administrative and political structure of the competitive figure skating world is shown, along with the position of the team physician within this schema. The broken lines indicate a loose relationship and responsibility between the areas noted. It is important to know and to understand the political and administrative structure so that you can interpret it for the skater, to be able to move within it freely and without making embarrassing mistakes, and to be able to follow its rules and regulations.

BEING A TEAM PHYSICIAN

Having a medical degree is not enough. Certain additional capabilities and qualities are needed:

1. *Think in terms of general medicine.* Specialty training is relatively unimportant and any M.D. could function as a team physician. As a neurologist, I had to suppress my very narrow focus and instead return to the thinking and philosophy that dominated my internship year. It is important to look at a problem not only with interest and an open mind but also to think in broad general terms and in more a "holistic" sense than a specialty one.

One also needs to function as a pharmacist as well, taking care not to give the athletes any banned drugs. Table 11–1 lists the drugs and supplies that I took with me. These drugs are carried in a shoulder bag or similar carry-on container. Not only are these drugs

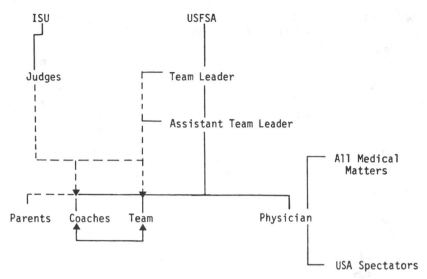

Figure 11–1. The administrative and political structure of the competitive figure skating world.

to be taken to and from all practice and competition events, but they are to be taken onto the airplane in case illness occurs during the long hours of international travel.

In addition to the usual medical tools, such as a stethoscope or ophthalmoscope, you must not forget to take the more nonstandard medical tools, such as batteries, flashlight bulbs, and so forth, which may be hard to find overseas (especially in an Eastern or Communist bloc country). Also, take a copy of your medical license and the document from your national governing body appointing you as team physician.

2. *Have a strong psychotherapeutic bias.* One does not need to know the history, mechanics, controversy, literature, or scientific basis of psychiatry—one only needs common sense, understanding, "tender loving care," and ability to listen. One must be careful, though, to give emotional advice only either when asked or when the vibrations are strong and clear that this is what is being requested. After all, it is not only the bodies of these athletes that are more agile than ours, but their minds as well. They have a very low tolerance for—and very efficient filter against—technical talk, nonsense, and generalities. However, they do need to ventilate, and giving them the opportunity and allowing it to happen is not always easy. One of the best and most efficient strategies is to ask, generally when alone and in a quiet area,

"How do you feel today?" It usually works like magic.

3. *Act as a cheerleader.* The tension and hype is enormous, and everyone is uptight. The physician, by virtue of his or her "neutral" position and noninvolvement in the political structure of the athletic organization, is not bound by the same rules of demeanor as the judges, coaches, and athletes. Thus, a good bit of enthusiasm in the form of verbal stroking, hand clapping, and upbeat mood strongly encourages the athletes and lets them know they have a friend. Even when a skater skates poorly, one can always find some move or maneuver that was well done and deserves a compliment.

4. *Do not play favorites.* There is a tendency to be biased toward one type of skating, such as dance or pairs or singles, or to have one particular skating athlete as a favorite. However, your time must be spent equally with all the athletes, not only individually but at their practice sessions as well. Even those who do not seem particularly friendly or who are quieter than others should be given the same amount of attention if possible.

5. *Get to know the coaches.* They are the final common pathway to the athletes and are the ones who are closest to them. They know almost everything there is to know, both physically and emotionally, about these very sensitive, finely tuned people and can

Table 11–1. MEDICATION AND MEDICAL SUPPLY LIST, UNITED STATES
FIGURE SKATING ASSOCIATION

Ophthaline Eye Drops, 15 ml	Procaine penicillin injection 3000,000, 10 ml
Corticosporin Ophthalmic Suspension 15	Adrenalin 1:1000 #6 ml
Corticosporin Otic Suspension, 10 ml	Benadryl, 50 mg/ml #10 ml
AVC Vaginal Suppositories #6	Compazine, 10 mb/ml #6 ml
Valisone Topical Ointment, 15 grams	Dramamine, 50 mg/ml #6 ml
Auralgen	Vitamin C, 500 mg #100
Tylenol #3, #50	Lomotil, 5 mg #100
Tylenol tablets #100	Valium, 5 mg #20
ASA #100	Multivitamins #100
Erythromycin, 250 mg #100	Actifed #50
Ampicillin, 250 mg #200	Dalmane, 30 mg #12
Tetracycline, 500 mg #100	Chlor-Trimeton, 4 mg #50
Darvocet N-100 #30	Robitussin Plain, 8 oz
Motrin, 600 mg #50	Pepto-Bismol, 16 oz
Benadryl, 25 mg #60	Campho-Phenique, 1 bottle
Prednisone, 10 mg #50	Hydrogen peroxide, 3%, 4 oz
Compazine suppositories, 25 mg #12	2″ × 2″ Gauze strips
Compazine tablets, 10 mg #20	Band-Aids
Dramamine, 50 mg #50	1″ Tape
Riopan Plus, #100	1 Sterile strip
Dulcolax tablets, #48	Alcohol swabs
Dulcolax suppositories #12	1 Swiss army knife
Tagamet, 300 mg #50	1 Magnifying glass
HCTZ, 50 mg #20	12 #3-ml Syringes
Throat lozenges	18 #22 or #23 ¾″ needles
Theophyl Tabs, 100 mg #30	
Naprosyn, 375 mg #50	

make the physician's job much easier. For example, a female skater might feel quite embarrassed to talk to the physician about a menstrual problem but quite at ease with having the coach knowledgeable of this plight. Remember, most of these athletes are in their mid to late teens, and so usually are not totally comfortable with physicians, especially male physicians they may have just met. Because the coach has such great influence on the skater, it is important to involve the coach in the medical problem and to make sure that the coach (even more so than the parent) is briefed on the diagnosis and the treatment plan. In my experience the coaches will not question your judgment and are almost always helpful in that they know a great deal more about the skater's personal past medical history than you do and they carry far greater weight in having the athlete accept and carry out the program you prescribe.

6. *Interact with the team leader.* The Junior World, the Senior World, and the Olympic skating teams all have a team leader and an assistant team leader. The team physician is the third member of this group. The national governing body is not allowed to send a physician to the Olympics; this is done only by the USOC. Although the team physician at world competitons is chief in all medical matters that relate to the team, he or she must comply in nonmedical matters and answer to the team leaders. It is here that the team physician can function as an "extra hand," and this is especially important because it is virtually impossible for the two team leaders to cover the four practice groups—men's singles, women's singles, pair, and dance—which frequently are going on simultaneously. Such a warm interaction, based on mutual respect, is felt by all the team members and sets up a very comfortable milieu in which they can operate.

7. *Maintain doping control.* Doping control is discussed a bit later in this chapter. Suffice it to say now that you, as a physician, are responsible for all drugs given to the athletes

and as such are responsible for making certain that they do not take banned drugs (see Chapter 12).

8. *Your mission.* In addition to the obvious official medical responsibility for the skating athlete, a few unofficial responsibilities await you. First, as an American physician in a foreign country you will find that some of the other country's team members will seek your advice and guidance, particularly if you have a specialty area. It is obviously important for international relations that these athletes be seen and treated to the best of your ability and knowledge.

Second, the accompanying American spectators, officials, and some non-Americans will seek you out for medical care and advice. The same guidelines mentioned above apply here. Of course, these are difficult decisions because of the potential medical malpractice uncertainties, and you will have to follow your own personal guidelines. However, being chosen to serve again as a team physician by the national governing body will depend upon many things, including what the official and unofficial entourage say and feel about you.

Last, while you are in a foreign country you are, of course, dependent on the local medical facilities. In a Western country, such as Denmark, these are quite good, new, and well equipped. In Communist bloc and poorer countries, such as Yugoslavia, they may be quite the opposite. It is important to get to know the organizing committee's physician immediately and to offer your expertise to him or her, as well as to thank him or her in advance for what he or she may do for your team members. In the same vein, interaction with other Western team physicians (especially the Canadian team physician) can be mutually beneficial since it is quite possible that you will have different specialties or that one of you will have a drug that the other needs but did not bring. Also, it is important to find out where the hospitals are located, to obtain their telephone numbers, and to find out how to get your athletes transported in case of emergency.

9. *Get to know the athletes and maintain visibility.* I have left these last two topics for the end because they are the most important and can be discussed together. The most important initial task of the team physician is to get to know every single athlete. Unfortu-

nately, there is very little time to do this, since many of the athletes are being met for the first time either at the international competitive site or on the plane going over to that site. One helpful strategy is to send out a letter, with the twofold purpose of introducing yourself as well as advising the athletes of your purpose. This is only partially effective, however. The most efficient and effective means is to establish rapport quickly. *The physician must take the initiative here*, introducing himself or herself to all the athletes, coaches, and parents, and letting them know that he or she is there to help them. One of the quickest and best ways of doing this is to take a very brief history from the athletes on a one-to-one basis and then to brief each one individually as to your mission. I had to learn what the pediatricians already know: In dealing with young people, concepts such as "medical confidence" and "Hippocratic oath" mean little, but being viewed as a "nice guy" means an awful lot.

After this initial introduction of yourself, *visibility* becomes the most important method of getting to know these athletes and getting them to view you as a friend. This means showing up at as many practice sessions as possible, snooping around the hallways and meal areas, and generally "hanging around"—not with them, necessarily, but, rather, where they are so they can see you and begin to feel comfortable with you. Remember, you are with the team to "be there." Sightseeing or long absences from the official hotel are to be avoided. If you want to travel around the country while at the competition, this is not the job for you. Being visible throughout the day every day, particularly during the first week of practice prior to the competitive event, will allow the athletes to view you as a friend and as someone truly interested in them.

All this is so important because of the tremendous stress these athletes are under, which is directly due to several forces acting upon them. In Figure 11–2 I have illustrated these forces in what I call the "pressure loop." Because most of these forces speak for themselves, I will not discuss each of them. (I must add that the pressure of physical illness is an additional threat that clearly worries the physician far more than it does the athlete.)

"PRESSURE LOOP"

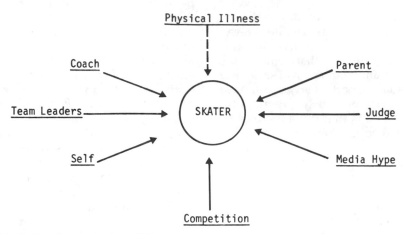

Figure 11–2. The "pressure loop." Forces to which the competitive figure skater is exposed.

DOPING CONTROL

The origin of the word "dope" apparently had its beginning in the Dutch word *doop*, which means a sauce or thick liquid. The definition of the phrase "to take drugs" had its origin between 1890 and 1900. If you look in any edition of Webster's International Dictionary, the word dope has many different definitions. Doping, for the athlete, is the ingestion of a drug designed to increase the athletic performance. Doping control consists of urinary testing for the presence of such drugs, with the expressed purpose of preventing their use.

The modern Olympic Winter Games first had organized ice skating in 1924 at Chamonix, France. However, it was not until the 1973 World Figure Skating competition in Bratislava that doping control was first done on figure skaters. Since then there has been only one instance of a positive result—that occurring in the 1983 Junior World Figure Skating championships in Sarajevo, when a female member of the French skating team was found with a banned substance. Their third-place finish was denied, and the medal was awarded to the fourth-place finisher, who happened to be an American.

Until recently, doping control was done only at Junior World, Senior World, and Olympic competitions. With the recent drug and doping scandals, however, the USOC has made testing mandatory at the National Sports Festival and the United States Nationals during an Olympic year. At the Olympic competitions, in addition, there is testing for sex typing.

The three basic categories of drugs that are banned are (1) sympathomimetic amines and other stimulants, (2) narcotics, and (3) anabolic steroids. In addition, several drug groups have been added in the past 2 years: caffeine, beta blockers, diuretics, and adrenal corticosteroids (see Chapter 12). Anyone found with a doping substance is subject to the loss of any medal earned and is banned from world competition for 15 months for a first offense and subject to a permanent world competitive ban for a second infraction. There are, naturally, extenuating circumstances and appeal processes that fall within the domain of the ISU in a non-Olympic event and of the International Olympic Committee (IOC) in an Olympic event. The function of the team physician is not only to understand the procedure involved but also to make sure that the athletes are thoroughly briefed as to the nature and consequences of any doping action. It has been the posture of the USFSA Sports Medicine Committee to keep hammering this theme away at the athletes, to the point at which they are basically checking with the physician before taking anything, even an aspirin. This is because so many over-the-counter drugs, eye drops, or topical creams may have banned substances in them; especially important in this regard are the nasal decongestants and cold and cough remedies. The physician must never forget the doping rules, in order to prevent inadvertently giving an athlete something that contains a banned drug. This is the reason, in treating these athletes, that I have stuck to antibiotics, aspirin, acetaminophen (Tylenol), anti-inflammatory medications, and multivitamins. I have relied a great deal on physical therapy, positive prognoses, reassurance about the problem, and a strategy of minimizing the significance of the illness. Once the competition is over, however, any drug that you feel is indicated can be used.

It must be remembered that the athletes are tested at the end of their long program except for single skaters, who are tested for beta blockers after the school figures. (School figures will not be performed in international competiton after 1990.) In a non-Olympic event, such as a world competition, the first four places are always tested, and on the day of the final competitive event an additional random placement is picked for testing by the ISU physician representative in charge of doping control. Some events, such as the pair events, are over early in the week; whereas others, such as senior ladies, may be delayed until the end of the competitive week. Thus a knowledge of the skating schedule is quite important in making decisions as to how to "carry" a patient with an illness that might require the use of a banned drug. I must admit that this has not been a problem to

date, and it has been quite easy to treat athletes without resorting to any of these banned substances. However, I stress that you would not want to reach "out of habit" for a decongestant or some similar medication that could cause an athlete to lose his or her medal, especially since the ultimate responsibility for this lies with you.

Details of the doping procedure are generally the same, whether at a World or Olympic event, and are best left to a more definitive treatment of the subject. Suffice it to say here that all of the administrative and technical work is done by the organizing committee responsible for the competition; your only responsibility, other than that stated above, is to make sure the athlete gets to the doping control station within 1 hour of the time he or she is picked for testing.

SUMMARY

Being a World Figure Skating team physician is work in the sense of the visibility it demands but is a breeze compared with everyday medical practice. It has many benefits, being unequivocally rewarding both emotionally and professionally—and it offers a chance to make new friends, a change of pace, and rejuvenation by the freshness, youth, athletic skill, and success that these athletes radiate. And best of all, there are no insurance forms.

I highly recommend that anyone who has a chance to go with any team or group involved in any type of elite competition do so. It is truly a rewarding experience.

CHAPTER 12

Prescribing for the Competitive Athlete

WILLIAM N. TAYLOR, M.D.

The use of medications by competitive athletes, for a variety of perceived reasons, has burgeoned to become a major area of focus in the 1980s. Medications are prescribed or provided to athletes or self-administered by athletes to enhance athletic performance, to treat injury or disease conditions, and for recreational and/or illicit purposes. In fact, the deaths of two professional athletes in the summer of 1986, caused by the illicit use of cocaine, has expedited the launch of a drug-control program with a four-corner approach to curbing medication abuse in athletics: drug education, drug testing, drug research, and newly proposed legislation for certain drugs.

The use of medications by competitive athletes, especially medications used to enhance athletic performance, is not a recent phenomenon. Past evidence of medication use by competitive athletes has relied heavily on personal interviews, hearsay, and other forms of anecdotal information. The lack of accurate, objective methods to ascertain this medication use has oftimes reinforced the belief that athletes could use a variety of drugs, even while competing, *safely* and *without detection or recourse*. This concept is incorrect.

The information provided within this chapter assumes that the competitive athlete will be subject to *accurate*, state-of-the-art urine drug testing immediately following competition. As of this writing, there are only two International Olympic Committee

(IOC) certified laboratories in the United States. These IOC-certified laboratories are the only centers that can accurately detect trace amounts of synthetic anabolic-androgenic steroid metabolites in the urine. Other laboratories within the United States that are seeking IOC certification have not yet mastered the methods necessary to detect trace amounts of the full range of anabolic-androgenic steroid metabolites in urine samples.

Prescribing or providing medications for the competitive athlete can be critical to the athlete in terms of the following parameters:

1. The health and well-being of the athlete
2. The recourse that the athlete *and* physician, coach, or trainer may face for detection of a banned substance in the urine of the competitive athlete
3. The recourse that the athlete's institution or country may face for the detection of a banned substance in the urine of the competitive athlete
4. The future financial impact on the athlete who is discovered using a banned substance
5. The "fair play" concept among competitive athletics
6. The impact on the broad scope of competitive athletics

With so much at stake, it is imperative that persons who are involved with providing medications to athletes should provide them correctly.

This chapter will provide brief topic discussions to assist in prescribing to the competitive athlete. However, no attempt is made to provide complete information on all the beneficial and adverse effects on athletic performance or the specific pharmacokinetics of the thousands of banned substances. It is hoped that this information will further the knowledge of the medication provider and delineate the responsibilities that go with providing medications to the competitive athlete. For questions beyond the scope of this text, the United States Olympic Committee (USOC) offers a drug hot line (1-800-233-0393) as a function of its drug control program to assist in the area of medication use by competitive athletes.

THE DEFINITION OF DOPING

In the past "doping" was widely considered to be a method used to introduce a foreign substance into an athlete in order to attain a *reduction* in athletic performance. For instance, a drug, such as a strong tranquilizer, could be slipped to a prize fighter in order to affect the outcome of a match. Such methods were linked to betting and financial rewards, and therefore they have cast negative rays on athletics.

More recently, sports medicine experts have acknowledged that some medications and methods have the potential to enhance athletic performance. Therefore, a more comprehensive definition of doping has been advanced in the USOC Drug Control Program Protocol[23]:

> Doping is the administration of or the use by a competing athlete of any substance foreign to the body or of any physiological substance taken in abnormal quantity or taken by an abnormal route of entry into the body, with the sole intention of increasing in an artificial and unfair manner his performance in competition. When necessity demands medical treatment with any substance which because of its nature, dosage, or application is able to boost the athlete's performance in competition in an artificial and unfair manner, this is to be regarded as doping.

THE ROLE OF THE MEDICATION PROVIDER

In the past a small number of sports medicine physicians and scientists have fancied themselves to be medical manipulators of athletes to subsequently aid these athletes to gain an unfair advantage over fellow competitors via doping techniques. Some of these physicians had complex, internal rationalization methods to justify their activities, such as "If I do not supply the drugs or blood for my athletes, they will just get them from the black market or use unsterile techniques." Some of these sports medicine physicians have earned the infamous title of "guru."

Within the past couple of years, nearly every doping method has been officially banned either by accurate, independent drug testing or by confirming evidence. Consequently, the roles of the sports medicine physician, coach, and trainer have been more clearly defined. The role of each individual dictates that no banned substances may be provided to competitive athletes for the purpose of enhancing their athletic performance. In fact, as detailed in the USOC Drug Control Program Protocol[23]:

> Any physician, coach, athletic trainer or other attendant to an athlete with a positive finding (urine drug-test for a banned substance), who is shown to have aided or abetted that offense, shall be suspended from the National Governing Body (NGB) and USOC programs by the NGB for at least the period that the athlete was suspended.

Moreover, the consequences to the physician of prescribing some of the banned substances may be even more severe than they are for the athlete. Even the physician's medical license may be in jeopardy. For instance, subsequent to a recent legislative session, changes in the Florida Medical Practice Act outlined grounds for discipline.[4] "Prescribing, ordering, dispensing, administering, supplying, selling, or giving growth hormones, testosterone or its analogs (anabolic steroids), human chorionic gonadotropin (HCG) or other hormones for the purpose of muscle building or to enhance athletic performance" is grounds for discipline. For a Florida physician who provides athletic patients with these substances, a subsequent positive finding on accurate urine testing may result in serious discipline.

In providing medications for a competitive athlete, the following parameters should be borne in mind:

1. The medication provider must assume the responsibilities for the medication prescribed for or provided to the competitive athlete.

2. The medication provider must become educated regarding what denotes a banned or safe medication, including many over-the-counter (OTC) preparations.

3. The medication provider must be familiar with the USOC's drug information service and use the hot line when assistance is needed.

4. The medication provider must become aware of state-of-the-art urine drug-testing

protocols and educate his or her athletes regarding the same.

5. The medication provider must not assist the competitive athlete in using doping medications or techniques; instead, he or she must discourage such activities.

6. The medication provider must become educated regarding the penalties that may be assessed when an athlete has been detected positive for a banned substance.

CATEGORIES OF BANNED SUBSTANCES

A substance is usually deemed to be banned if it can have detrimental effects on the health of the athlete or if it has the potential to enhance athletic performance or both. Essentially, the USOC observes the IOC list of banned substances:

1. Central nervous system stimulants
    a. Psychomotor stimulants
    b. Miscellaneous central nervous system stimulants
    c. Sympathomimetic amines
2. Narcotic analgesics
3. Anabolic steroids, testosterone, and growth hormone
4. Alcohol and beta blockers
5. Blood doping
6. Beta-agonists
7. Local anesthetics
8. Corticosteroids
9. Diuretics
10. Caffeine

CENTRAL NERVOUS SYSTEM STIMULANTS

The central nervous system (CNS) stimulants (Table 12–1) can result in psychologic and physical enhancement of athletic performance, but they can also cause detrimental mental and physical effects. Use of these substances produces aggressiveness, anxiety, and tremor. This can lead to poor judgment, which places the athlete at increased risk of injury. Potential complications from CNS stimulants include physical and psychologic dependence, personality changes and paranoia, cerebral hemorrhage (stroke), cardiac arrhythmias, and even cardiac arrest and death. During endurance events, especially

Table 12–1. EXAMPLES OF BANNED
CNS STIMULANTS

Psychomotor stimulants
  amphetamine
  benzphetamine
  chlorphentermine
  cocaine
  diethylpropion
  etilamfetamine
  fencamfine
  meclofenoxate and related compounds
  methylamphetamine
  methylphenidate
  norpseudoephedrine
  pemoline
  phendimetrazine
  phenmetrazine
  phentermine
  pipradol
Sympathomimetic amines
  clorprenaline
  ephedrine, epinephrine
  etafedrine
  methoxyphenamine
  metaproterenol
  isoetharine
  isoproterenol
Miscellaneous CNS stimulants
  amiphenazole
  doxapram
  ethamivan
  strychnine
  caffeine (over 12 mcg/ml urine)

and related compounds

in cold weather, the use of these drugs can greatly increase the risk for Raynaud's phenomenon, decreased blood flow to the distal extremities, and consequent frostbite.

Amphetamines

For over two decades, amphetamines have been used as ergogenic aids by athletes participating in a wide variety of sporting events.[6,7] Numerous studies have attempted to document the effects of amphetamines on human performance, with conflicting results.[11]

These stimulants have the potential for improving athletic performance in several ways, including perceived aggression enhancement, effort reduction, and endurance enhancement.[3] They have also been used as body fat reducing agents. Amphetamine use by athletes can increase their time to exhaustion and allow them to perform at higher levels of intensity for longer periods of time by mechanisms that seem to increase muscle efficiency and to decrease mental and neuromuscular fatigue.[11] However, they do so by masking pain and normal fatigue signals, thereby impairing judgment and increasing the athletes' risk for serious injury. Moreover, these drugs may cause the athlete to develop hypertension, tachycardia, nonlethal cardiac arrhythmias, insomnia, anorexia, restlessness, and severe personality changes. They may even lead to strokes and lethal cardiac arrhythmias.[11]

Among the amphetamine-induced personality changes are impulsive behavior, paranoia, explosive aggression, tendencies to violence, and frank paranoid schizophrenia. Amphetamine dependency and its withdrawal symptoms of depression can be recognized as apathy, premature fatiguing, and decreased athletic performance.[11] Some sports medicine physicians feel that amphetamine abuse by athletes may cause premature athletic "burnout." When employed, accurate drug testing has played a key role in eliminating amphetamine use during competitive athletic events.

Cocaine

Historically, cocaine has been generally considered to be a drug of recreation, addiction, and abuse rather than a performance-enhancing agent. However, cocaine's properties mimic a fast-acting, short-duration amphetamine that induces a seducing euphoria. Because of these characteristics, cocaine has a limited potential to enhance performance in certain athletic events.

Cocaine powder is snorted intranasally or injected intravenously, and because the free base is resistant to heat, the drug or a combination of the drug with bicarbonate of soda ("crack") may be smoked. The hydrochloride salt may be compounded with one or more of the following substances: mannitol, sucrose, lactose, caffeine, heroin, amphetamines, talc, phencyclidine (PCP), procaine, lidocaine, or strychnine.[5]

Within a minute or so of snorting cocaine,

the user feels "high." Then the search for more rapid effects with more intense "rushes" may lead to intravenous use and "free basing." The rate of absorption by injection or smoking free-base cocaine is increased about 10-fold over customary nasal snorting.[9] A comparison of intravenous injection with the smoking of free-base cocaine revealed that the free-base smoking induced more intense effects than injection, even when lower dosages of cocaine were taken by inhalation than injection.[9]

Like the amphetamines, cocaine stimulates the CNS, mimics the flight-or-fight response, and affects the medullary centers which control respiration, cardiovascular function, and heat regulation.[5] Therefore, the use of cocaine immediately prior to or subsequent to an intense bout of exercise could be extremely detrimental, causing respiratory difficulties, overstressing the cardiovascular system, and upsetting thermal regulation.[24] Adverse reactions to cocaine use, perhaps even with the initial experience, may include extreme hypertension, extreme hyperthermia, cardiac arrhythmias, myocardial infarction, and sudden death.[8]

Cocaine has several actions that are potentiating and make the concomitant administration of many other drugs hazardous. I believe that the simultaneous use of cocaine with anabolic steroids may increase the risks for heart attack, stroke, and sudden death in athletes.[21]

Like many other sympathomimetic drugs, cocaine basically prevents the neuronal reuptake of epinephrine and norepinephrine after they have been released. This results in a net increase in available neurotransmitters, which adds to their subsequent stimulatory effects. Also, cocaine may hasten the release of catecholamines from adrenergic nerve terminals. By this mechanism, the quantity of bound calcium may become more available in the nerve tissues after cocaine use, thereby enhancing the sensitivity of the receptors to neurotransmitters.[9]

The CNS responds to cocaine with cerebral effects of initial euphoria, followed by stimulation, and then loss of more primitive medullary functions. With overdoses, it is the loss of medullary functions that ultimately results in collapse and death.

The typical effect upon the user's CNS

after the euphoria ("rush") is a period of hyperactivity, which may be visibly manifested to observers. Pleasure gives way to negative sensations, particularly if the environment of the drug use is adverse. Emotional lability and paranoia are usual signs of impending advanced cocaine toxicity, as are tactile hallucinations (such as "cocaine bugs"), visual hallucinations (such as "snow lights"), and other sensory hallucinations which terminate in overt cocaine psychosis. Nausea, vertigo, and headache may precede later profound effects, such as tremors, tics, twitches, and jerks known as "cocaine leaps."[9] As with any drug, variables such as dosage, chronicity of use, route of administration, and individual susceptibility affect the actual pattern.

Advanced cocaine stimulation may result in generalized hyperreflexia, individual seizures, and status epilepticus even in the face of decreased responsiveness. Terminally, a depressive phase ensues, with the loss of reflexes, coma, and finally loss of vital functions, ending in death.[9]

Cocaine-induced cardiovascular effects include very early slowing of the pulse, followed by an increase in both pulse and blood pressure. Blood pressures may rise sufficiently high to cause intracranial hemorrhage or high-output congestive heart failure. Ventricular dysrhythmias may result from direct heart muscle damage, which promotes lethal arrhythmias, and death may ensue.[9]

Sinus, Diet, and Cold Medications

Many prescription and over-the-counter (OTC) medications contain drugs that are banned by the USOC and IOC. A number of medications used to alleviate symptoms of the common cold contain sympathomimetic amines, such as ephedrine, pseudoephedrine, phenylephrine, phenylpropanolamine, propylhexedrine, and others. Some of these chemicals are also included within the formulation of certain appetite-decreasing diet medications. Banned substances are present in almost all of the products with "decongestant" properties, whether by prescription or OTC. Some examples of OTC medications used for colds and sinus congestion that contain banned substances are listed in Table 12–2.

Table 12–2. EXAMPLES OF COLD AND SINUS PREPARATIONS CONTAINING
SUBSTANCES BANNED BY THE USOC AND THE IOC

Containing Ephedrine
 Bronkaid, Pazo Suppository, Wyanoids Suppository, Vatronol Nose Drops, Nyquil Nighttime Cold
  Medicine, Vick's Nighttime Cold Medicine, herbal teas and medicines containing "Ma Huang"
  (Chinese ephedra)
Containing Pseudoephedrine
 Actifed, Anamine, Afrinol, CoTylenol, Deconamine, Dimacol, Histalet, Historal, Isoclor, Novafed,
  Sudafed, Tussend, Chlor-Trimeton-DC, Drixoral, Polaramine, Rondec
Containing Phenylephrine
 Coricidin, Dristan, NTZ, Neo-Synephrine, Sinex
Containing Phenylpropanolamine
 ARM, Allerest, Contac, Dexatrim, Dietac, 4-Way Cold Tablets, Formula 44, Naldecon, Novahistine,
  Sine-aid, Sine-off, Sinutab, Triaminic
Containine Propylhexedrine
 Benzedrex Inhaler

Narcotic Analgesics

Narcotic analgesics may produce a sensation of euphoria, psychologic stimulation, perceptions of invincibility, and illusions of athletic prowess beyond the athlete's abilities—all of which are detrimental to the keen judgment required for top performance. They may also increase the pain threshold so that athletes may fail to recognize injuries and thus lead to more serious complications. Use of these drugs ultimately results in physical and psychologic dependence. Examples of banned narcotic analgesics are given in Table 12–3.

SYNTHETIC ANABOLIC-ANDROGENIC STEROIDS

Prior to 1983, accurate methods did not exist for the detection in urine of metabolites from the wide range of anabolic steroids that have been used by some athletes. Recent developments in laborious extraction techniques, mass spectrophotometer, gas-liquid chromography, computer-based "steroid maps," and closely supervised urine collection techniques have served to render the use of anabolic steroids by athletes highly detectable. Conservative estimates of athletes and fitness buffs who are using these drugs surpass one million.[18,19] Recent official estimates from the Federal Bureau of Investigation (FBI) indicate that the current black-market supply to athletes amounts to a $100 million annual business.[12]

Since testosterone was synthesized from cholesterol by independent scientists in Germany and Switzerland,[2,13] perhaps no drugs have been as controversial as testosterone and its analogs, the anabolic steroids. It is beyond the scope of this chapter to present a comprehensive discussion of all the potential effects of these drugs on athletic performance, but several books and documents are available to the reader who is seeking further

Table 12–3. EXAMPLES OF NARCOTIC
ANALGESICS BANNED BY THE USOC
AND THE IOC

anileridine
codeine
dextromethorphan
dextromoramide
dihydrocodeine
dipipanone
ethylmorphine
heroin
hydrocodone
hydromorphone
methadone
morphine
opium
oxycodone
oxymorphone
pentazocine
trimeperidine

Table 12–4. EXAMPLES OF ANABOLIC STEROIDS BANNED BY THE USOC

boldenone
costebol
dehydrochlormethyltestosterone
danazol
fluoxymesterone
mesterolone
metenolone
methandrostenolone
norethandrolone
oxandrolone
oxymesterone
oxymetholone
stanozolol
testosterone

and related compounds

information.[10,15,21] However, it can be concluded that these drugs may enhance muscle mass and strength in training athletes who are of proper nutritional status.[15] In 1984, the American College of Sports Medicine confirmed this in its official policy stand.[1]

Anabolic-androgenic steroids are substances banned by the USOC not only because they enhance athletic performance but also because they have potentially dangerous adverse effects. The major adverse conditions are in the behavioral system, where physical and psychologic addiction patterns and aggressive, hostile, violent, explosive, and criminal activities have been reported in heavy anabolic-steroid users.[16,17,21]

Other recent studies have indicated a plethora of evidence to show the potential for increased athrogenesis by these drugs, which could result in early cardiac disease, hypertension, and strokes.[21]

The urinary metabolites from anabolic steroids can be detected as long as several months after their use.[21] For this reason, some experts feel that frequent and random urine testing could help curb the black-market use of these drugs among competitive athletes. Examples of banned anabolic steroids are listed in Table 12–4.

ALCOHOL AND BETA BLOCKERS

Substances that have been used by athletes to "calm" the nerves have included al-cohol and beta blockers such as propranolol. Beta blockers are prescription drugs that are commonly used to treat hypertension, cardiac disease, alcohol and narcotic withdrawal, stage fright, migraine headaches, and tremors. They are used in sports such as pistol shooting to steady the trigger finger. Because they are believed to enhance athletic performance in this manner, beta blockers are substances banned by the USOC and the IOC.

BLOOD DOPING

The practice of blood doping (the intravenous injection of whole blood, packed red blood cells, or blood substitutes) (see Chapter 13) is banned by the USOC and the IOC. As yet, there is no applicable detection test for this practice. However, any evidence confirming the use of this technique to enhance performance will be cause for punitive action comparable to that for using a banned substance. This practice is banned because of its potential for enhancing performance,[14] and because of its potential to cause adverse effects such as thrombosis, sepsis, strokes, and allergic reactions to blood components.

BETA AGONISTS

The use of three beta agonists—terbutaline, salbuterol, and biltolterol—commonly prescribed to treat asthma conditions, is acceptable to the USOC under the following conditions:

The team physician must notify the head physician for the event beforehand as to which athletes on the team are asthmatics and are using, or may require the use of, any of these drugs. Notification must be in writing; and the drug, dose, and frequency of administration must be identified.

LOCAL ANESTHETICS

Certain local anesthetics have been approved for limited use under the following provisions:

1. Procaine, xylocaine, and carbocaine may be used, but not cocaine.
2. Only local injections can be used (intravenous injections are not permitted).
3. Use is medically justified only when it

permits the athlete to continue the competition without potential risk to his or her health.

Finally, the appropriate medical commission such as the IOC and/or USOC must be advised in writing by the head physician if the anesthetic has been administered with 24 hours of the competition.[23]

CORTICOSTEROIDS

The International Olympic Committee Medical Commission has become increasingly concerned by the misuse of corticosteroids in some sports.[23] Therefore the use of corticosteroids during Olympic competition has been restricted to only topical application or inhalation. Oral, intramuscular, and intravenous administrations are banned.

DIURETICS

The misuse of diuretics to effect rapid weight loss in certain sports—such as boxing, wrestling, and weight lifting—is potentially dangerous to the athlete. It also may give the athlete an advantage by placing him in a lower weight class for competiton. For these reasons, diuretics are now banned by the USOC.[23]

CAFFEINE

Caffeine has been shown to enhance athletic performance by both physical and psychologic mechanisms.[11] It has been arbitrarily determined that a caffeine concentration greater than 12 mcg/ml in an athlete's urine is defined as doping. At these levels, caffeine can potentiate cardiac arrhythmias and increase the risk of sudden death.[11] To reach this limit one would have to drink approximately six cups of coffee in a single sitting just prior to competition. However, other sources may contain caffeine, and it is possible to use enough of these caffeine-containing substances to reach the prescribed limit. For example,

- 2 cups of coffee = 3 to 6 mcg/ml urine caffeine concentration
- 2 colas = 1½ to 3 mcg/ml urine caffeine concentration
- 1 No-Doze tablet = 3 to 6 mcg/ml urine caffeine concentration

1 APC, Empirin, or Anacin tablet = 2 to 3 mcg/ml urine caffeine concentration.

GROWTH HORMONE

Available evidence suggests that the use of growth hormone has the potential of enhancing athletic performance.[16,22] Because there is no urine test at the present time that is capable of detecting exogenous growth hormone, the USOC is convinced that this substance will become abused in sport. Therefore, the USOC has established a policy that states that the use of growth hormone (human, animal, or synthetic) is prohibited, and any evidence confirming its use will be cause for punitive action comparable to that which will result from using a banned substance.[20] A recent congressional hearing was held regarding the reclassification of synthetic growth hormone as a schedule II substance under the Federal Controlled Substance Act.[21,22] Support for this bill came primarily from sports medicine physicians and scientists, the USOC, and other medical groups.[21]

CATEGORIES FOR ALLOWED SUBSTANCES

Table 12–5 provides a list of categories and examples within each category of substances that are *allowed* for IOC athletic competitions.

When there is any question, before prescribing a medication to an athlete prior to competition, the safest course is to have the medication verified by the official head physician for the event and a knowledgeable USOC medical staff member; for this purpose the athlete's physician is encouraged to use the USOC Drug Hot Line (1-800-233-0393).

CONCLUDING REMARKS

From the information provided in this chapter, it is obvious that drug prescribing and drug testing are linked. As long as drug testing is performed with the accurate methods available today and is not circumvented by cheaper, inaccurate, and ultimately litigation-producing equipment or staffs, this link between drug prescribing and drug testing should be a positive one for athletics.

Table 12–5. SUBSTANCES ALLOWED FOR IOC ATHLETIC COMPETITIONS

Analgesics	Mycelex
Acetaminophen	Tinactin
Aspirin	Zovirax
Nonsteroidal anti-inflammatory drugs	Antigouts
Easpirin	Colchicine
Ecotrin	Zyloprim
Antacids	Antihistamines
Amphogel	All antihistamines without decongestants
Maalox	Antinauseants and antiemetics (may be banned
Phazyme	in shooters)
Riopan	Combid Spansule
Antiasthma	Compazine
Aminophylline	Phenergan
Cromolyn sodium	Tigan
Nasalide	Vistaril
Theophylline	Antiulcers
Vancerase	Carafate
Vanceril	Tagamet
Antibiotics	Hemorrhoidal
All antibiotics	Anusol
Anticonvulsants	Anusol HC
Dilantin	Proctofoam-HC
Mysoline	Laxatives
Tegretol	Doxidan
Valium (except banned for shooters)	Fleet Enema
Antidiabetics	Metamucil
Diabinese	Modane
Micronase	Muscle relaxants
Insulins	Flexeril
Antidiarrheals	Norflex
Imodium	Robaxin
Kaopectate	Soma
Lomotil	Otic preparations
Antifungals and antibiotics (topical)	Auralgan
Bacitracin	Cerumenex
Betadine	Cortisporin
Kwell	Sedatives (may be banned in shooters)
Monistat	Halcion
Femstate	Restoril

Adapted from Voy.[23]

However, if shoddy or unscrupulous marketeers enter the realm of drug testing for athletic events, without the proper certification for these difficult tasks, then a quagmire of legal complications could destroy the advances that the members of the USOC's Drug Control Program have been able to accomplish. To obviate this, only certified competent medical staffs should be used to ensure proper collection of urine samples and the proper chain of custody of these specimens to independent IOC-certified laboratory facilities where they are meticulously logged and tested.

It is also apparent that continued drug education and drug legislation are going to play an important role in preventing the misuse of drugs in sports. Programs designed to offer educational programs along with drug testing will help ensure that every athlete gets an honest drug test and understands the reasons behind the testing.[23]

The necessity for new drug legislation for synthetic anabolic-androgenic steroids has recently become more apparent. It is strongly urged that these steroids be reclassified as controlled substances within the Federal Controlled Substance Act because of their habit-forming and violence-producing influences.[21]

Prescribing or providing medications to competitive athletes has become a complicated matter in the past few years. The provisions for prescribing, the accuracy for testing, and the importance of drug abuse in sports has provided the impetus to research for mechanisms to control drug use and abuse in competitive athletics. It is the responsibility of the medication provider to remain informed on these topics so that the athlete will attain a better understanding of the important issues.

REFERENCES

1. American College of Sports Medicine: Position stand on the use of anabolic-androgenic steroids in sports, revised. Sports Medicine Bulletin 19:13–18, 1984.
2. Buntenandt, A and Hanisch, G: Unwandlung des dehydroandrosterons in Androstendiol and Testosterone: ein weg sur darstellung des Testosterons aus Cholesterin. Ztschr für physiol Chemie 237:89, 1935.
3. Chandler, JV and Blair, SN: The effect of amphetamines on selected physiological components related to athletic success. Medicine and Science in Sports and Exercise 12:65–69, 1980.
4. Florida Board of Medical Examiners Newsletter. 4(2):1, 1986.
5. Gold, MS, Smith DE, and Olden, K: Cocaine: Helping patients avoid the end of the line. Emergency Medical Reports 6:17–23, 1985.
6. Heyrodt, H and Weissenstein, J: Uber Steigerung Korperlicher Leistungfahighkeit durch Pervitin. Archv fer Experimentelle Patholigie und Pharmakologie 195:273–275, 1940.
7. Karpovich, PV: Effect of amphetamine sulfate on athletic performance. JAMA 170:558–561, 1969.
8. Kossowsky, WA and Lyon, AF: Cocaine and acute myocardial infarction: A possible connection. Chest 85:729–731, 1984.
9. Kunkel, DB: Cocaine then and now. Part II. Of pharmacology and overdose. Emergency Medicine, July 15, 1986, 168–173.
10. Lamb, DR: Anabolic steroids in athletics: How well do they work and how dangerous are they? Am J Sports Med 12:31–37, 1984.
11. Lombardo, JA: Stimulants and athletic performance (part 1 of 2): Amphetamines and caffeine. Physician and Sportsmedicine 14:128–139, 1986.
12. Nightingale, SL: Illegal marketing of anabolic steroids to enhance performance charged (letter). JAMA 256:1851, 1986.
13. Ruzicka, L, Goldberg, MW, and Meyer, J: Uber die Synthese des Testikelhormons und Steroisomerer desselben durch Abbau hydrierter Sterine. Helv chim Acta 17:1934, 1935.
14. Sawka, MN, Young, AJ, Muza, S, Gonzales and Pandolf, KB: Erythrocyte reinfusion and maximal aerobic power. JAMA 257:1496–1499, 1987.
15. Taylor, WN: Anabolic Steroids and the Athlete. McFarland & Company, Jefferson, NC, 1982.
16. Taylor, WN: Hormonal Manipulation: A New Era of Monstrous Athletes. McFarland & Company, Jefferson, NC, 1985.
17. Taylor, WN: Super athletes made to order? Psychology Today 19:62–66, 1985.
18. Taylor, WN: Synthetic hGH should be calssified as a controlled substance to prevent abuse. Genetic Engineering News 6:4, 1986.
19. Taylor, WN: Human growth hormone: A controlled substance, proposal. Testimony to American Medical Association House of Delegates, Reference Committee E, June 16, 1986. Chicago, IL.
20. Taylor, WN: Will synthetic human growth hormone become the peril of genetic engineering? Annals of Sports Medicine 2:197–199, 1986.
21. Taylor, WN: Synthetic anabolic-androgenic steroids: A plea for controlled substance status. Physician and Sportsmedicine 15:140–150, 1987.
22. Taylor, WN: Potential abuses and illegal diversion of human growth hormone. Testimony to the U.S. House of Representatives, Subcommittee on Health and the Environment, April 8, 1987. Washington, DC.
23. Voy, RO: United States Olympic Committee Drug Control Program Protocol. U.S. Olympic House, Colorado Springs, CO, 1986.
24. Wooley, BH and Barnett, DW: The use and misuse of drugs by athletes. Houston Medical Journal 2:29–35, 1986.

CHAPTER 13

Sports Anemia and Blood Doping

ROBERT G. WESTPHAL, M.D.

Endurance-trained athletes adapt in many physiologic ways to the stresses of high performance. Hearts of athletes show morphologic and physiologic changes that reflect the ability to sustain increased cardiac output during prolonged competition. Increases in cardiac chamber diameter and in ventricular wall thickness compensate for chronic volume overload. A given stroke volume can be ejected with minimum work if contraction starts at a larger volume, and loss of energy is less when contraction occurs slowly. Consequently, a low heart rate is more efficient than a faster one.[8]

There are many other physiologic adaptations, including changes in blood volume. Before discussing the anemia—and the pseudoanemia—of sports it would be well to review the essentials of blood physiology. Most of the work in sports anemia and the adaptive physiology of endurance training has been done in distance runners or soldiers. But it does relate to winter sports in some specific areas (such as cross-country skiing, biathlon events, and speed skating) as well as in a general sense, since training for many sports involves running and other repetitive endurance activities.

BASIC PHYSIOLOGY

Red blood cells (RBCs) are made and mature in the hematopoietic bone marrow, which is found in the axial skeleton and to a lesser degree in the heads of the femurs. Under certain kinds of stress or in some disease states the hematopoietic marrow can expand into areas of fatty marrow. Under normal conditions the hematopoietic marrow is about 50 percent cellular. The formed elements of the blood all derive from pluripotential stem cells, which can become the progenitor of megakaryocytes (which produce platelets), granulocytes, or RBCs. Although some lymph follicles are present in normal marrow, lymphocytes are also made in the spleen and the lymph nodes.

Once a stem cell becomes committed to one cell line, it cannot change and produce something else. A committed RBC stem cell will produce about 10 RBCs in approximately 10 days. Regulation of the RBC mass is fairly complex. Cardiac output, arterial P_{O_2}, erythropoietin, and diphosphoglycerate (2,3-DPG) all play a role. Basically, however, the driving factor is tissue oxygenation, which modifies all of these other factors.

Erythropoietin, which is made in the kidney from a substrate manufactured in the liver, increases in response to a low tissue P_{O_2} occurring in specialized cells in the kidney. Erythropoietin has two major effects on the bone marrow. First, it increases the number of stem cells committed to the RBC line. Second, it tends to speed cells through the maturation process, shortening the time it takes for them to arrive in the circulation.

2,3-DPG is produced by the red cells during glucose metabolism. It decreases the affinity of oxygen for hemoglobin; thus, it tends to "offload" oxygen from the red cells to the tissues. Increases in 2,3-DPG will shift the oxygen dissociation curve to the right, just as will acidosis. The effect of shifting the curve to the right is to deliver more oxygen at any given level of P_{O_2}.

PSEUDOANEMIA

Studies in runners have shown an increase in red-cell 2,3-DPG, which, in favoring tissue oxygen delivery over long periods of exercise, reduces the stimulus for erythropoietin production and thus limits increases in circulating red-cell mass.[13] Measurement of the oxygen dissociation curve in runners, however, has not shown a corresponding shift to the right.[12] These studies were done on venous blood. Since acidosis will shift the curve to the right, it may be that the increased carbon dioxide production by laboring muscle causes a significant "local" aci-

dosis such that if one could measure the *local* oxygen dissociation curve it would be shifted; but enough buffering has occurred to normalize the curve in mixed venous blood. The facts that 2,3-DPG levels are increased, that blood volume is increased, and that there is enhanced oxygen extraction by muscles in trained athletes all support the concept that blood oxygen delivery in athletes is more efficient than in nonathletes. Less hemoglobin is needed to do the job, one might say.

Table 13–1 summarizes a study of Israeli soldiers on a forced 24-hour march.[2] Normally, plasma volume is about 40 ml/kg body weight in adult men and women; circulating red-cell mass is 30 ml/kg in men and 25 ml/kg in women. Plasma volume is controlled primarily by the renal regulation of salt and water excretion and by the various forces that determine intravascular versus extravascular fluid spaces. In this study one can see that prolonged exercise has the effect of increasing plasma volume by 16 percent, even 2 days after the march, thereby increasing total blood volume by about 8 percent. One would expect to see a hemoglobin of 13.5 at 8 hours; so the 13.8 hemoglobin seen in these soldiers probably reflects a slight but real increase in red-cell mass. Thus, although there is a drop in hemoglobin concentration, there is no drop in the actual circulating red-cell mass. This is an example of athletic "pseudoanemia."

SPORTS ANEMIA

A recent study of *acute* exercise (bicycle ergometer with a work-load increase every minute until exhaustion) showed an *immediate* hemoconcentration (sweat loss), and no anemia or increase in 2,3-DPG were noted even after 8 weeks of training. This suggests that hematopoietic responses seem to depend on the duration and kind of exercise and training intensity.[10]

Increased mechanical red-cell destruction, as in march hemoglobinuria, has been suggested as an explanation for the reduced levels of hemoglobin and serum haptoglobin and of the increased serum bilirubin seen during initial stages of prolonged severe exercise. However, frank hemoglobinuria was rare in runners during a 20-day road race;[4] and, except for the unusual, susceptible in-

Table 13–1. HEMATOLOGIC CHANGES IN TRAINED ATHLETES DURING AND AFTER A CONTINUOUS (120-km) 24-HOUR MARCH

	Baseline ($\overline{X}$)	9 hr ($\overline{X}$)	64 hr after Recovery
Hemoglobin (gm/dl)	14.6 ± 0.3	13.8 ± 0.4	—
Hematocrit (%)	45.2 ± 0.2	42.1 ± 1.1	—
Plasma volume, increase	—	16%	18%
Blood volume, increase	—	8%	10%

From Burstein et al,[2] with permission.

dividual, hemolysis is unlikely to provide a complete explanation for the observed reduction in hemoglobin concentration. The bone marrow could easily compensate for these small losses, unless iron (in the form of hemoglobinuria) was lost in large amounts as well.

However, one recent case study in a marathon runner showed that when he increased his mileage to 45 miles per week, the mean corpuscular volume (MCV) of his RBCs rose from 85 to 95, and his hemoglobin fell about 0.8 gm% over 5 years.[5] During this time the reticulocyte count was slightly higher and serum haptoglobin lower—particularly after a "hard marathon" race. In this runner, urinary hemosiderins were weakly positive, and ferritin fell. Although this athlete may be an extreme example, the implication was that some runners can have enough low-grade hemolysis to lose significant amounts of iron. Unfortunately, no other source of iron loss was investigated in this subject.

Iron deficiency believed secondary to gastrointestinal blood loss has been noted in long-distance runners. No specific mechanisms for the increase in fecal blood loss have been identified, but several possibilities have been suggested. These include intestinal ischemia, stress gastritis, underlying pathology, and drug-induced lesions. The latter point is important, because athletes may be using aspirin for a variety of reasons. However, in a study that showed that 7 of 32 marathon runners developed guaiac-positive stools after a race, there was no significant difference in recent drug use.[9] In that study, guaiac positivity correlated with younger age and with faster times.

There has been good documentation of iron loss in runners in several other investi-

gations. In one, a quantitative assay of fecal hemoglobin was used to measure stool blood loss in long-distance runners.[14] Controls were age and sex-matched. Neither controls nor runners took any medications or had any known gastrointestinal disease. Of 24 runners in this study, all but two had definite increases in fecal blood loss after finishing 10-km, 21-km, or 42-km runs. Table 13–2 shows the comparative data between runners and age- and sex-matched controls. Note that runners had lower levels of hemoglobin concentration and lower serum ferritins (ferritin levels are measures of iron stores in the body). Two of the 20 men and 2 of the 4 women were already iron-deficient, with ferritin levels of less than 12. Note also that the women appear to be more hypochromic than the femal controls or the men in either group.

These data may have implications for athletes in general; but particular attention should be given to the hemoglobin levels of athletes involved in endurance training and winter sports—such as cross-country skiers, speed skaters, and hockey players.

Some authorities do not feel iron studies are useful and that iron is moved from marrow to liver (by hemolysis) and by increased RBC mass.[7] However, I believe that iron deficiency can be a definite problem for some athletes.

BLOOD DOPING

In 1947 a study was published demonstrating the improved tolerance of hypoxia in normal men rendered polycythemic by homologous blood transfusion.[11] However, the current interest in blood doping probably stems from a 1972 article[6] in which physical work capacity was measured in athletes be-

Table 13–2. RED-CELL PARAMETERS AND IRON STORES IN 24 LONG-DISTANCE RUNNERS AND IN 24 AGE-/SEX-MATCHED CONTROLS

	Male Runners ($\overline{X}$) (N = 20)	Male Controls ($\overline{X}$) (N = 20)
Hemoglobin (gm/dl)	14 ± 0.6	15.2 ± 0.7
Hematocrit (%)	40.8 ± 2.1	45 ± 2.1
Ferritin (ng/ml)	69.6 ± 50	102 ± 86
	Female Runners ($\overline{X}$) (N = 4)	**Female Controls ($\overline{X}$) (N = 4)**
Hemoglobin (gm/dl)	12.4 ± 1.1	13.7 ± 0.8
Hematocrit (%)	36.5 ± 2.9	40.2 ± 1.8
Ferritin (ng/ml)	18 ± 18 (2 were iron deficient)	23.7 ± 6.8

From Stewart et al,[14] with permission.

fore and after removal of 800 ml of blood followed by reinfusion about 2 weeks later. There was a 13 percent increase in work capacity the day after reinfusion. Hemoglobin levels returned to normal in 14 days, but maximum work did not return to prephlebotomy levels until after reinfusion. However, most studies have shown that there is no consistency among performances after such procedures, although measurements of physiologic work do improve.

"Blood doping" has been much in the news lately, and—as it should be—the practice has been decried and banned by the United States Olympic Committee. There are many problems with blood doping. First, the removal of a unit or more of blood significantly jeopardizes the training status of athletes for 2 weeks or longer. Second, no controls have been used, such as the infusion of saline in the same amount. It may well be that simple volume expansion is the key to increased perfusion and improved performance. Third, if one uses homologous blood (blood from someone else), the attendant risks of transfusion-transmitted disease are significant, not to mention immediate or delayed transfusion reactions. Even if one used autologous blood (from self) there are real possibilities of mix-ups, contamination of the unit, improper storage with hemolysis, and so forth. Fourth, although some physiologic measurements have improved, there has been no published documentation of improved athletic performance until recently

(see below). Finally, and perhaps most importantly, the whole practice seems unsportsmanlike and unnecessary and represents an unwarranted intrusion of technology—unproven and risky technology, at that—into sports.

Recently, a study was published that did carefully look at actual athletic performance on the field.[1] Six trained, male distance runners ran a series of three 10-km races against one another (and themselves) before infusion (baseline), after infusion of 100 ml of saline, and after infusion of 400 ml (2 units) of previously frozen deglycerolized autologous red cells. The red-cell infusion led to significantly faster 10-km runs and to an increase in the packed-cell volume. There were no changes in p 50s or 2,3-DPG levels. Although the authors demonstrated improved performance using frozen, autologous red cells, they do not recommend it. Not only has it been declared "dishonest" by the International Olympic Committee, but also it does pose the real and dangerous risk of bacterial contamination, clerical error, or faulty storage.

A more reasonable approach would be to identify those athletes with iron deficiency and subject them to "iron doping." In a recent study from Chile,[15] 14 iron-deficient women athletes and 18 normal controls were evaluated in a cycloergometer and on a treadmill and then given either iron or placebo in a double-blind, crossover study. There were no significant differences in hemoglobin levels after 15 days of iron therapy; but in iron-deficient athletes there was improvement in oxygen consumption and a decrease in pulse rate, which indicate increased stroke volume efficiency. It may well be that in trained athletes, relative iron deficiency that has not yet progressed to anemia may hinder performance, and such performance may be improved by supplemental iron to replenish the stores.

RECOMBINANT-DNA PRODUCED ERYTHROPOIETIN

The whole topic of blood doping will soon become irrelevant and will be replaced by another controversy that is more closely related to the steroid problem; however, there will not be a simple test (or probably no test at all) to detect the presence of the drug involved.

Clinical trials are currently underway on a large scale to document the efficacy and safety of recombinant-DNA produced erythropoietin (rEPO). The gene for EPO has been spliced into the DNA of cultured human fibroblasts, from which large quantities of very pure hormone are harvested. In clinical trials to date, the use of rEPO has elevated hemoglobin levels in anemic patients with chronic renal disease from the 6 to 7 gm/dl range to levels of 10 to 12 gm/dl. Investigators are now accumulating data on the use of this drug to harvest increased quantities of autologous blood in normal adults, as well as its use in other anemias of chronic disease.

Although not currently available, it is quite likely that a "black market" for this drug will develop among high-performance athletes, their physicians, and their trainers. All people in the field of sports medicine should be alert to this problem and strongly resist the use of this substance. For one thing, dosage schedules and ultimate side effects on the hematopoietic system are not well known. Although the blood vessels of people with chronic renal failure are probably different from those of healthy young people, there have been disturbing reports of an increased incidence of stroke in those patients whose hemoglobin levels improved. There are no drugs, not even purified hormones, that do not have some deleterious effects. Not only should subterfuge and chicanery be resisted, we should not be giving potent drugs such as this to healthy young people for purposes of improving athletic performance.

IRON REPLACEMENT

Because iron in its elemental state is relatively toxic to tissues, the body has special means of transporting and storing it. Normally we absorb only about 10 percent of the food iron presented to the alimentary tract. The average North American diet contains about 6 mg of iron per 1000 calories. Thus, a 2500 calorie diet presents only about 15 mg of iron. Fish, meat, and poultry are all rich in absorbable iron. Eggs, spinach, and some other vegetable sources are also rich in iron, but it is poorly absorbed from such sources because it is bound to oxalates, phthalates, or other compounds. A consumption of about 15 mg of iron just about balances out with daily iron losses in men and may not be adequate for many women (see Chapters 4 and 6). During the first year of life and during puberty for women, iron needs exceed dietary iron intake. If one increases iron loss from prolonged endurance-type exercise, a negative iron balance may result (see Chapter 6). When laboratory data indicate significant iron loss, decreased stores, or low hemoglobin levels, iron supplementation is indicated. However, iron should *not* be used prophylactically. About 1 in 300 Americans are homozygous for the gene for hemachromatosis (iron overload disease), which may not manifest itself until later in life.

CONCLUSION

There are several factors at work that explain the "pseudoanemia" of high-performance athletes. First, increased levels of 2,3-DPG and improved oxygen extraction from the blood by trained muscles lower the heart rate and reduce the level of erythropoietin feedback. Because of salt and water retention, the plasma volume is increased significantly (approximately 15 percent), and the *concentration* of hemoglobin is proportionately lowered; however, the actual RBC mass is increased. The slightly lower hematocrit levels improve blood flow by decreasing blood viscosity. This results in better perfusion and may be the most important factor for improving work performance. It has been shown that perfusion—not necessarily oxygen extraction—is much better at hematocrit levels of 35 to 40 percent than at higher levels.

Except in unusual circumstances or in persons with underlying problems—such as SA hemoglobin—hemolysis is probably not as significant a factor as fecal iron loss in producing sports anemia. Fecal iron loss has been shown to increase in long-distance runners and may lead to iron-deficiency anemia, especially in women.

When hemoglobin concentrations measured at least 72 hours after strenuous exercise are less than 13 gm% in men and 12 gm% in women, they should be evaluated. Barring a history of hemoglobinuria, iron deficiency is the most likely cause. A mean corpuscular volume below $82u^3$ or a serum ferritin concentration lower than 12 ng/ml indicates serious iron deficiency, chronic inflammatory disease, or congenital hemoglobinopathy. Evaluation of bone marrow morphology and iron stores is indicated in confusing or complicated cases. Menstrual histories should be assessed. And, especially in older athletes, occult blood loss owing to primary gastrointestinal pathology must be ruled out.

Definitions and detection of a "latent" phase of iron deficiency are most difficult. However, no one should be treated with supplemental iron without appropriate evaluation of iron stores so as to avoid the danger of iron overload. It has been suggested that athletes with ferritin levels *below* 30 ng/ml should be treated with iron.[3] But treatment should not exceed 3 months without further evaluation of hemoglobin levels and iron stores. If iron supplement is used, timed-release or enteric-coated preparations should be avoided because they bypass the proximal duodenum, which is the site of primary iron absorption. Their major effect is to turn the stools black, not to increase the iron stores.

Emerging evidence indicates that athletic performance may be enhanced by improving hemoglobin levels in iron-deficient athletes through carefully monitored supplementation.

REFERENCES

1. Brien, AJ and Simon, TL: The effects of red blood cell infusion on 10-km race time. JAMA 257:2761–2765, 1987.
2. Burstein, R, Assia, E, and Epstein, Y: Sports anemia: A myth? Lancet 2:389, 1985.
3. Clement, D: The essential element. Runner's World, December 1985, pp 82–86.
4. Dressendorfer, RH, Wade, CE, and Amsterdam, EA: Development of pseudoanemia in marathon runners during a 20 day road race. JAMA 246:1215–1219, 1981.
5. Eichner, ER: Runner's macrocytosis and athlete's anemia (Abstract). Blood 64 (Suppl 1):45a, 1984.
6. Ekblon, B, Goldberg, AN, and Gullbring, B: Response to exercise after blood loss and reinfusion. J Appl Physiol 33:175–180, 1972.
7. Hallberg, L and Magnusson, B: The etiology of "sports anemia." Acta Med Scand 216:145–148, 1984.
8. Huston, TP, Puffer, JC, and Rodney, WM: The athletic heart syndrome. 313:24–32, 1985.
9. MacMahon, LF, Ryan, MJ, Larson, D, and Fisher, RL: Occult gastrointestinal blood loss in marathon runners. Ann Int Med 100:846–848, 1984.
10. Mairbaurl, H, Gaesser, G, Poole, D, and Tanaka, KR: Change in red cell metabolism before and after training. Blood 62(Suppl 1):26a, 1983.
11. Pace, N, Lozner, EL, Consolazio, WV, et al: The increase in hypoxia tolerance of normal men accompanying the polycythemia induced by transfusion of erythrocytes. Am J Physiol 148:152–163, 1947.
12. Ricci, G, Castaldi, G, Masotti, M, Lupi, G, and Bonetti, D: 2,3-diphosphoglycerate and P_{50} after exercise. Acta Haematologica 71:410–411, 1984.
13. Shappell, SD, Murray, JA, Bellingham, AJ, Woodson, RD, Detter, JC, and L'enfant, C: Adaptation to exercise: Role of hemoglobin affinity for oxygen and 2,3-diphosphoglycerate. J Appl Physiol 30:827–832, 1971.
14. Stewart, JG, Ahlquist, DA, McGill, DB, Ilstrup, DM, Schwartz, S, and Owen, RA: Gastrointestinal blood loss and anemia in runners. Ann Intern Med 100:843–845, 1984.
15. Walter, T, Donoso, H, Nunez, S, Chadred, P, and Stekel, A: Effect of treatment on physical work capacity of iron deficient female athletes: A double-blind, randomized, controlled study (Abstract). Blood 64(Suppl 1):43a, 1984.

PART II

Medical Problems Common to Winter Sports

CHAPTER 14

Infectious Diseases

MURRAY JOSEPH CASEY, M.D.

The major cause of morbidity at winter sporting events, like the major cause of morbidity whenever young people congregate, is infectious disease, primarily virus diseases of the upper respiratory tract.

Nearly two thirds of all visits to Medical Services by athletes, their coaches, and supporting staffs during the XIII Winter Olympic Games in Lake Placid in 1980 were for acute infections of the respiratory system and gastrointestinal tract.[1] Ninety-four percent of these infections (787 cases) were limited to the upper respiratory tract; whereas 16 cases of bronchitis and pneumonia were reported, and 39 cases of gastroenteritis were diagnosed. In addition, 10 patients were seen for nausea and vomiting, 6 for cough, and 10 for malaise and fatigue—all symptoms which may have been prodromal for respiratory infections or acute gastroenteritis.

Although the opportunity was lost to determine which specific agents were involved in those infections during the 1980 Winter Olympics, it behooves the physician who may be called to care for athletes and staff during similar events to be familiar with the most common causes and clinical courses of acute respiratory infection and gastroenteritis. Furthermore, extensive domestic and foreign travel, outdoor living, climateric extremes, fatigue, and crowding may render sporting participants more liable to contract respiratory and alimentary infections than those who are not subjected to such factors.

Knowledgeable coaching and support personnel are in a position to help prevent the lost time and illness associated with these infections by working with athletes and sports physicians to limit contagion and to improve care. Moreover, prompt treatment and an understanding of the importance of adequate rehabilitation and follow-up when infections do occur can limit the resulting morbidity and return the athlete to participation as soon as it is safe and reasonable.[2]

An indepth coverage of all infectious diseases that may befall the sports participant is beyond the scope of the present text. For this, the interested reader is referred to the various articles and books selected for citation by the authors of this section. Here our mission is to familiarize the reader with something of the etiologies, epidemiologies, and clinical presentations of those infections which we have found to affect athletes, travelers, and support personnel most frequently with an eye to preventing the occurrence of these illnesses and providing a rationale for differential diagnosis and management when they do occur (see also Chapter 45).

REFERENCES

1. Hart, GG: Final report, frequency of visits by ICD-9 diagnostic code. *Medical Report of the XIII Winter Olympic Games.* Lake Placid Olympic Organizing Committee Medical Services, Lake Placid, NY, 1980.
2. Roberts, JA: Virus illnesses and sports performance. Sports Medicine 3:296–303, 1986.

CHAPTER 15

Acute Respiratory Infections

MURRAY JOSEPH CASEY, M.D.

ELLIOT C. DICK, Ph.D.

Two thirds of acute respiratory infections among adults are caused by viruses. Most of these infections involve the upper tract alone. Among over 800 cases of respiratory infection treated by Medical Services during the 1980 Winter Olympics, only 11 cases of bronchitis and 5 cases of pneumonia were reported.[47] This chapter discusses the most frequent causes of acute respiratory infections in adult populations (Table 15–1).

VIRUS INFECTIONS

RNA Viruses

Rhinoviruses

In general epidemiologic studies, most upper respiratory infections are caused by RNA viruses, and among these, the rhinoviruses are the most frequent.[14,53] This group of small RNA viruses with more than 100 serotypes is the major cause of the common cold in adult populations.[44] Although the individual type can be identified by virus isolation and serotyping, it is unimportant and usually impractical to do so in the clinical setting. Since specific antibodies resulting from previous rhinovirus infections confer at least partial protection against that specific serotype, it is the plethora of other types that proves troublesome in preventing this disease. Moreover, antigenic variations occur over time.[14,21,44] For these reasons, rhinoviruses continue to account for about 40 per-

Table 15–1. ACUTE RESPIRATORY TRACT DISEASES (ARD) IN ADULTS

	Relative Frequency of Causative Agent*	
I. Unknown cause		40%†
II. Viruses		44%
A. RNA viruses		
1. Rhinoviruses	25%	
2. Coronavirus	3%	
3. Influenza virus	4%	
4. Parainfluenza viruses	4%	
5. Respiratory syncytial virus	4%	
6. Enteric RNA viruses	1%	
a. Coxsackie		
b. ECHO		
B. DNA viruses		
1. Herpes simplex virus	2%	
2. Adenoviruses	1%	
III. Mycoplasma		3%
Mycoplasma pneumoniae	3%	
IV. Chlamydia		3%
Chlamydia psittaci TWAR strain	3%	
V. Bacteria		10%
A. *Streptococcus pyogenes*	6%	
B. Bacterial pneumonias	4%	
1. *Streptococcus pneumoniae*	3%	
2. *Haemophilus influenzae*	<1%	
3. *Staphylococcus aureus*	<1%	
4. *Neisseria meningitidis*	<1%	
TOTALS	60%	100%

*This list includes all categories of ARD and will vary considerably with the diagnosis. Pharyngitis/tonsillitis may have a much higher bacterial component and more herpes simplex; clinical influenza during an influenza epidemic will be about 50 percent caused by influenza virus; common colds will be 30 to 40 percent caused by rhinovirus; atypical pneumonia may have a large mycoplasma and chlamydia component, and so forth.

†This may not mean that 40 percent of ARDs are caused by unknown agents. Probably 80 to 90 percent of all ARDs are caused by virus; however, many respiratory virus illnesses caused by known viruses are difficult to diagnose: serologic response may not occur and many viruses grow poorly in cell cultures, especially the coronaviruses and rhinoviruses.

cent of respiratory infections in adult populations.

Rhinovirus infections are characterized by the well-known symptoms of the common cold: nasal congestion, rhinorrhea, pharyngeal irritation and sore throat, malaise, and sometimes mild headache. Fever is rare, except in persons with asthma, who are especially susceptible to acute bronchitis. Symptoms begin after an incubation time of only 24 to 48 hours, are self-limited, and usually subside in less than a week. Virus shedding by nasal discharge begins before the onset of symptoms and may continue for 2 to 3 weeks thereafter. Rhinovirus may not be so highly contagious as previously believed.[21] Short-term, casual exposures have been shown to

result in the infection of only a small proportion of healthy young adults.[18] However, spread of rhinovirus infection is enhanced by crowded living conditions and extended periods of exposure. The virus appears to be disseminated by aerosol and, perhaps, by hand-to-hand contact.[21,23,46] Over 90 percent of a barrack's population was infected during a 4-week period.[75] The peak incidence of rhinovirus colds occurs during the fall and spring, but the infections also can be found during the winter months.

Coronaviruses

The second most frequent cause of common colds among adults are the coronaviruses.[51,66] They consist of two broad antigenic groups. Only two strains, one from each antigenic group, and their very close relatives have been grown in the laboratory. Therefore, diagnosis is almost exclusively serologic. It is known that some strain-specific immunity can be acquired, but there is evidently great antigenic heterogenicity and often very imperfect immunity. So repeated coronavirus infections are common. The greatest incidence of these infections has been reported in persons between the ages of 15 and 19 years.

Following infection by coronaviruses, the incubation period may be a day or so longer than the incubation time of a rhinovirus cold, but coronavirus respiratory illness is usually a bit shorter, ranging usually only 3 to 5 days. Coronavirus symptoms are similar to those experienced with rhinoviruses. Nasal congestion is the most common, followed in order by sneezing, cough, sore throat, and malaise. Chills and mild temperature elevations rarely occur in uncomplicated cases. The greatest frequency of coronavirus infection is in the late fall, winter, and early spring, and these viruses are considered to be the major cause of winter colds.

Transmission of Rhinoviruses and Coronaviruses

Although the incidence of common colds is highest during the winter months when they occur at least twice as frequently as during summer, experimental evidence suggests that it is not low temperatures per se that are responsible.[29,30] But the likelihood of their transmission is definitely increased by close contact over extended periods of time.[14,62] The environmental conditions that accompany winter weather, crowded classrooms, dormitories, and gymnasiums therefore serve to increase the exposure of persons to the responsible etiologic agents and account for the higher incidence of colds during the cooler months. Moreover, there is some evidence that strenuous exercise may decrease local nasal mucosa antibodies and thereby reduce resistance to respiratory infections;[79] whether the low temperatures to which the cross-country skiers taking part in this study were exposed played any causal role was not determined.

Transmission of both rhinoviruses and coronaviruses appears to result chiefly from inhaling infected droplets. For some years, it was thought that infection might be more efficiently transmitted through fomites and hands,[45,46] but recent data using a natural model for rhinovirus transmission suggest that aerosols are much more important.[21,23,36] So it is possible that the spread of infection with these two common cold viruses, and possibly other respiratory viruses as well, can be contained by careful attention to nasal sanitation[20] and good ventilation.[22,23,82] Self-inoculation of nasal mucosa and conjuctivae by fingers that have been in contact with virus-contaminated skin or plastic surfaces is another mode of possible cold virus transmission. Herein lies the possibility for limiting transmission. In clearing nasal passages, facial tissues should be used and care should be taken by team members to clear their respiratory passages gently, to prevent wide dissemination of the infected effluent.[20] Scrupulous hand washing, avoidance of direct skin-to-skin contact or contact with contaminated tissues, sporting equipment, and appliances also may help prevent infection with common cold viruses during periods of winter recreation and athletic training and competition. Towels should not be shared; paper handkerchiefs should be carefully used and disposed in closed plastic container bags; and commonly used washing facilities should be cleaned with Lysol or tincture of iodine before and after each use.

Influenza Viruses

Influenza viruses follow the cold viruses as the next most frequent cause of acute adult respiratory infections.[19,27,28,40a] These viruses take their name from an association with epidemics described by Italians of the 14th century as *influenzae di freddo* ("influence of the cold"). The RNA of these medium-size viruses is enclosed within a helical protein capsid surrounded by a lipid envelope from which project spikes that are responsible for viral attachment to host cells (hemagglutination antigen—HA) and other projections that serve to release newly formed virus from the host cells (neuraminidase antigen—NA). Three distinct types (A, B, and C) can be distinguished by the soluble complement-fixing antigen of the central ribonucleoprotein, and subtypes are determined by HA and NA antigenicity. Immunity to influenza viruses arises from previous infection or vaccination with specific subtypes.

Antigenic variation with influenza virus type A occurs by two mechanisms: (1) antigenic drift, and (2) antigenic shift.[28] Antigenic drift refers to changes in the HA, which result in reduced avidity of the old antibody to the new HA; so the individual will be less immune to the new mutant virus. These point mutations of HA occur often, sometimes yearly; and if the change is large enough, significant proportions of the population will be more susceptible to the new mutant. Antigenic drift also takes place in the NA, but this does not appear to be as important to immunity.

Antigenic shift is a much rarer event, occurring only every 10 to 15 years. Antigen shifts result from an actual reassortment of genes among the influenza A viruses. Antigen-determining genetic recombinations may occur between human and animal strains, such as birds and swine, because of double infections of the host. Recombinations seem to arise more frequently in the Orient where the proximity between man and domestic animals may be close and of long duration. When recombinations take place, the entire world population may be susceptible to the new virus subtypes, and influenza pandemics can result in much morbidity and loss of life. In this century, antigenic shifts occurred in 1918, 1929, 1947, 1957, 1968, and 1977, but because of protection conferred by previous influenza virus infection, not all have been accompanied by severe worldwide illness (Table 15–2). For instance, the HA and NA double shift that occurred in 1977 did not result in widespread severe illness because much of the middle-age and older population was partially immune from infection with a similar virus that was dominant between 1947 and 1957. The most serious influenza A pandemics of this century occurred in 1918, when more than 20 million lives were lost to this disease, and in 1957.

Influenza virus type B also can cause serious illness, but it does not have the pandemic potential of type A because it undergoes only antigenic drift and not the actual genetic recombinations responsible for antigenic shift. Antibody to type C influenza virus is widespread in the population, where it is the probable cause of mild flulike illnesses, especially among schoolchildren.[54]

Outbreaks of influenza usually occur during winter and early spring and are often found to follow introduction of the virus through a few sporadic cases. In circumscribed geographical areas, the extent of epidemics depends on the proportion of susceptible individuals. Because infection involves host contact via the respiratory route, this should be considered when young people are confined to crowded environments, such as schools and sports or military camps. Crowding during transportation to sporting events can also be the occasion for outbreaks of influenza.[57,69] Localized out-

Table 15–2. INFLUENZA TYPE A PANDEMICS OF THE 20th CENTURY

		Hemagglutinin and Neuraminidase Designations			
Common Name of Virus	Years of Prevalence	Old Subtype Names	New* Subtype Names	Prototype or Prominent Strains	Severity of Illness
Swine influenza†	1918–1928	$H_{sw}N1$	H1N1	A/swine/Iowa/15/30	Very severe
Influenza A	1929–1943	H0N1	H1N1	A/PR/8/32	Severe
A prime influenza	1947–1957	H1N1	H1N1	A/FM/1/47	Mild
Asian influenza	1957–1968	H2N2	H2N2	A/Singapore/1/57	Severe
Hong Kong influenza	1968–present	H3N2	H3N2	A/Hong Kong/1/68	Moderate
Russian influenza	1977–present	H1N1	H1N1	A/USSR/77	Mild

*Since 1980; see Douglas and Betts.[28]

†Influenza viruses could not be propagated until 1930, and the origin of the 1918–1928 "Spanish influenza" pandemic has been inferred from serologic studies.

breaks usually reach their peak within 2 to 3 weeks and then resolve within a month.[43]

Clinical influenza virus infection in susceptible individuals usually develops within 2 or 3 days following exposure. Mild prodromal symptoms, including nonproductive cough, malaise, headache, and a few chills, are often described. Influenza virus type A infections are usually more serious than type B infections, and influenza infections may be no more severe than a mild cold.

Classical epidemic influenza A may begin abruptly as a sudden shaking chill followed by temperature elevations as high as 104°F (40°C). In the absence of an evolving viral pneumonia or secondary bacterial infection, it is unlikely that these high temperatures will be sustained, and spontaneous defervescence, sometimes quite rapidly, with resolution of symptoms over 2 to 4 days is the rule in otherwise healthy young people. However, mortalities as high as 1000 per 100,000 population were noted in the 25- to 30-year-old age group during the devastating pandemic of 1918.[31] In both sporadic and epidemic influenza, sneezing, rhinorrhea, and conjunctivitis are common. Malaise and prostration are characteristic and many patients develop chest pain, but demonstrable pleurisy, pleural effusion, and auscultatory or x-ray evidence of pulmonary pathology are unusual. Hoarseness may be experienced, and the pharynx may appear injected, but no exudate is seen. Although gastrointestinal symptoms may occur in young children, they are uncommon in adults.

Complications. Although influenza infections are usually self-limited, it is important to be cognizant of the potentially serious complications that may follow. Primary viral pneumonia with rales and rhonchi on auscultation and increased vascular markings or patchy pulmonary infiltrates on x-ray examination may be associated with prostration of the patient for days or weeks. Young adults will usually recover without sequelae, but the disease may be fatal to aged individuals and to those with chronic cardiopulmonary diseases. Severe viral pneumonia should be managed in a hospital intensive care unit or inpatient pulmonary unit. Of special importance to athletes is the danger of viral myocarditis, which may occur more frequently than is generally realized.[35,60]

Potentially one of the most serious complications of influenza is secondary bacterial infection. *Staphylococcus aureus* and *Streptococcus pneumoniae* (pneumococcus) are the most common bacterial invaders. The former is characterized by necrotizing bronchopneumonia which may be followed by rapid vascular collapse. With *Staphylococcus* pneumonia, grapelike clusters of Gram-positive cocci will be found on examination of the sputum. Secondary pneumococcal pneumonitis results in alveolar exudates which show characteristic homogenous lobar densities on x-ray examination and readily identifiable Gram-positive cocci singly and in pairs on sputum examination. Less frequently, influenza may be complicated by *Haemophilus influenzae*, a Gram-negative bacterium, which may cause necrotizing tracheobronchobronchiolitis with pneumonitis. Simple, uncomplicated group A hemolytic streptococcus infection of the pharynx may complicate viral influenza, or this bacterial organism may rarely involve the lower respiratory tract and lungs.[59] (See discussion of *Streptococcus pneumoniae* later in this chapter.)

Most uncomplicated influenza infections will show continued improvement after the first 24 hours of illness. The pulse tends to be slow relative to temperature, cough is nonproductive, and white blood cell counts are normal to low. Persistent high fever, blood-tinged sputum, marked tachycardia, pulmonary findings by physical examination or on x-ray examination, and leukocytosis should alert the physician to the development of severe viral pneumonia or secondary bacterial invasion. Although there is no evidence that antibiotics are of value for either treatment or prophylaxis of uncomplicated influenza, these medications should be used without hesitation when bacterial superinfection is clearly suspected. Antibiotic treatment should be specific and should follow the accepted guidelines for the management of primary mycoplasma and bacterial pneumonias.

Prophylaxis. Recent studies have demonstrated the value of amantadine hydrochloride 100 mg twice daily as a prophylaxis against influenza A in persons not yet infected.[50] When this drug is begun at the onset of local epidemics and continued for the duration of the outbreak, it has been 90 percent effective in protecting against influenza illness with minimal side effects.[73] Amantadine is also apparently effective in diminishing the duration of fever and other symptoms of uncomplicated influenza A when treatment is begun early in the illness.[28] Because **amantadine is not effective against influenza type B infections,** consultation with local health authorities or laboratories of large hospitals capable of rapid virus typing is recommended before starting this drug. Significant side effects, including nervousness, difficulty concentrating, and insomnia, have been reported by 33 percent of students using this medication in a 4-week trial.[7]

Besides the potential use of amantadine, other drugs are on the horizon for the prophylaxis and treatment of influenza.[26,50,61] Otherwise, the treatment of influenza is aimed at reducing symptoms. (See discussion of symptomatic treatment later in this chapter.)

Although moderately effective influenza vaccines are now available and are used widely by the United States military, immunization of the civilian population is presently recommended only (1) for those persons in whom infection would represent a serious risk, such as persons over 65 years of age and those with chronic disorders of the cardiovascular or pulmonary systems, and (2) for those persons whose occupations cannot accommodate several days of incapacitation. Athletes may fall into this latter group. Because of the need to travel, to train, and to compete during possible epidemic influenza seasons, sports physicians and governing bodies should yearly study and weigh the availability of an effective vaccine and the possibility of prevention through vaccination of athletes and staffs versus the possible untoward effects of vaccination. During the "swine" flu vaccination program in the United States of 1976, an eightfold to tenfold increase in Guillain-Barré syndrome was reported among those who were vaccinated when compared with the unvaccinated population; albeit no increase in Guillain-Barré syndrome has been associated with influenza vaccine in subsequent years.[6,19,40a,58] Moreover, vaccination occasionally may result in febrile influenzalike illness and allergic reactions, including fatal anaphylaxis in those who are sensitive to egg proteins. When deciding whether or not to vaccinate the athlete, the potential impact of infection on competition and the possibility of avoid-

ing infection by strict regulation should also be considered. Health professionals working with competitive athletes are advised to seek current recommendations which appear on a regular basis in the *Morbidity and Mortality Weekly Report,* published by the United States Centers for Disease Control, Atlanta, Georgia, 30333.

Parainfluenza and Respiratory Syncytial Viruses

Parainfluenza viruses are important causes of severe respiratory illnesses, croup, bronchiolitis, and pneumonia in infants and young children.[11,71] Since most adults have been infected with one or more of the four known parainfluenza virus serotypes during childhood, reinfection in adults is usually followed only by an attenuated illness, manifested as mild upper respiratory symptoms.[24,65] In contrast to most uncomplicated rhinovirus and coronavirus infections, parainfluenza infections in adults are characterized by cough, hoarseness, sore throat, and swelling of the submandibular glands.

Like parainfluenza virus, the respiratory syncytial virus (RSV) is a large RNA virus of the Paramyxoviridae family, and it is an important respiratory pathogen in infants and children.[10,21] Although immunity is neither permanent nor complete following RSV infection, this virus rarely causes serious illness in adults. Nearly all adult cases occur as reinfections through exposure to infected children in their families or as teachers, nurses, and physicians. Adult infections are usually symptomatic, causing illness as mild as the common cold to fever and even prostration with rare influenzalike syndromes, which must be differentiated from mycoplasma pneumonia.

Both parainfluenza and RSV infections occur sporadically and epidemically, usually in the late fall, winter, and early spring. Infections are transmitted by direct contact with very small inoculae and by virus-contaminated aerosols from coughing and sneezing. Incubation of the Paramyxoviridae ranges from 3 to 4 days. Self-limited symptoms of uncomplicated parainfluenza infections in children generally last only 2 to 4 days, but symptoms from childhood RSV infections may persist for as long as 1 to 2 weeks.

Enteric RNA Viruses

Several of the enteric RNA viruses, including Coxsackie viruses and ECHO viruses may cause pharyngitis, pleurodynia, and the symptoms of common cold and even pneumonia in infants, children, and adolescents. Infections with these viruses usually occur during summer and autumn months, and they are probably not common causes of acute adult respiratory tract illness.[63] Transmission of the enteroviruses is usually through fecal contamination via the oral or nasal route. Because these viruses may continue to replicate in the intestinal tract for a month or longer, infected individuals may be contagious for many weeks, and the potential of flush toilets in disseminating infection may be substantial.

The chief importance of enterovirus infection for the athlete lies in the association of some ECHO virus and Coxsackie virus strains with myocarditis and aseptic meningitis.[76] Whether or not physical stress and exercise increase the risk of developing enterovirus cardiomyopathy,[8,78] it seems advisable to proscribe vigorous training and competition during acute illness and for several weeks of convalescence whenever such constitutional symptoms as significant fever, malaise, myalgia, fatigability, or lymphadenopathy accompany respiratory tract infections.

DNA Viruses

Herpes Simplex Virus

Acute exudative pharyngitis often follows primary exposure to herpes simplex virus infections in adults.[37,41] Most people experience their first exposure to herpes virus in early childhood. By adulthood, about 80 percent of the population show antibody evidence of past infection, but only about half of the college-age population is so protected. This reservoir of individuals susceptible to this DNA virus makes it an important cause of acute upper respiratory illness in young people. Either herpes simplex virus type 1 or type 2, distinguishable by monoclonal antibody tests, may cause oral-pharyngeal infections; but type 2 originally was reported to be associated only with genital lesions.

Primary upper respiratory herpes infections in young adults are characterized by symptoms of mild cold followed by shallow oropharyngeal ulcers, tonsillitis, pharyngeal inflammation and exudate, tender cervical and submandibular lymphadenopathy, and fever running between 100 and 102°F (37.8 to 39° C). The illness is self-limited, lasting usually only about 2 or 3 days. Herpes virus respiratory infections do not have a distinct seasonal peak. Clinically, primary herpes pharyngitis may be distinguishable from streptococcal infection by the former having generally milder systemic symptoms and lower fever. White blood cell counts tend to be near normal with herpes infections, whereas streptococcal pharyngitis tends to cause leukocytosis. Typical virus inclusion bodies can be found on cytologic smears of herpetic ulcers, and herpes virus can often be isolated from throat swabs if facilities for viral culture are available in the supporting laboratory. More often, it will be necessary to rule out the presence of streptococcal infection by negative bacterial cultures.

Exudative pharyngitis also may be seen with adenovirus infections and with the onset of mononucleosis, which is also most common in the late teens and college-age groups. There is considerable evidence available to link infectious mononucleosis to the Epstein-Barr virus, which was first isolated from African youngsters with Burkitt's lymphoma. The importance of recognizing this illness in athletes is that it is often accompanied by splenomegaly and occasionally by hepatomegaly. Spontaneous or traumatic rupture of the enlarged spleen may occur several weeks or more following onset of acute infectious mononucleosis, and some advisors recommend monitoring the size of the spleen until it returns to normal before returning athletes to training activities.[76]

Adenoviruses

Although adenoviruses are not common agents for illness in adult civilian populations, where adenovirus infections occur only sporadically, these moderate-size DNA viruses are one of the most common causes of acute respiratory disease among military recruits in North America.[2,3,39,64] These epidemics occur during winter and early spring months and may involve 15 percent to as many as 50 percent of the recruit population with clinical infections characterized by fever, pharyngitis, laryngeal inflammation, rhinorrhea, and hoarseness. The adenoviruses' incubation period of 6 to 9 days is longer than the incubation associated with most respiratory virus illnesses. About 10 percent of those infected with adenoviruses will develop chest rales and/or show patchy pulmonary infiltrates, usually unilateral, on roentgenography. Most adenovirus-caused acute respiratory disease in adults is self-limited to a clinical course of only 1 to 2 weeks, and bacterial superinfection is rare even when viral pneumonitis develops. However, adenovirus pneumonia may lead to the demise of as many as 15 percent of young children, and it is occasionally fatal in young adults. Tenfold more acute respiratory infections occur among military recruits during the winter compared with the summer months, and 72 percent of the winter infections are due to adenovirus, compared with 12 percent in the summer. Because of these observations there has been speculation regarding the role of crowding, cold weather, dampness, and fatigue for enhancing the susceptibility and spread of these infections among military personnel.

The usual transmission of adenovirus respiratory infection is by the respiratory route, but conjunctivitis is known to occur through infection with contaminated ophthalmologic preparations and equipment, towels, and inadequately chlorinated swimming pools. There are at least 41 adenovirus serotypes. The lower types 1, 2, 3, 5, and 6 are the serotypes most often associated with respiratory illness in children; whereas epidemic keratoconjunctivitis has been tracked chiefly to type 8. Types 3, 4, 7, 14, and 21 are the adenoviruses known to cause upper respiratory disease, pharyngitis, and pneumonia in adults. The first three of these serotypes are the most prevalent causes of infection in military recruits. For this reason, effective formalin-killed vaccines were developed and administered to military recruits over 20 years ago. However, when these viruses were found capable, alone or in combination with SV-40 virus, of causing sarcomas in laboratory animals and malignant transformation of cells cultured *in vitro*,[48,49,68] the vaccines were withdrawn and the incidence of acute respiratory disease in military training populations again began to increase. A live vaccine of adenovirus types 4 and 7 has subsequently been developed and was made available to the United States military.[67,80] However, this vaccine is not yet recommended for civilian populations because most individuals first experience the lower types of adenovirus as mild respiratory illness, pharyngoconjunctivitis, and diarrheal illness in childhood, and the occurrence of adenovirus infections among adult civilians is only sporadic. These viruses have never been shown to cause cancer in human beings, but they continue to be a major cause of morbidity and rare fatality in the military services. Avoidance of chills, dampness, fatigue, crowding, and the use of common towels, eye protectors, and facial equipment may help prevent the spread of adenovirus infections among susceptible young adults.

MYCOPLASMA INFECTIONS

In the early 1960s, *Mycoplasma pneumoniae*, one of the smallest life forms not requiring intracellular growth for replication, was confirmed to be the cause of atypical pneumonia, a generally mild form of pneumonitis which had been distinguished from typical bacterial pneumonias by its resistance to penicillin and the sulfonamides.[13] Subsequent investigations have further delineated the natural history of disease caused by this organism and its epidemiology.[4,15,16]

M. pneumoniae respiratory infections may be seen throughout the year, but outbreaks and small epidemics in colleges and military camps occur more often during the winter months.[38,64] However, *M. pneumoniae* outbreaks are not especially seasonal; for some years may be completely devoid of such infections, whereas many cases will occur in other years.[40,72] This organism is responsible for only about 6 percent of all respiratory illness in military recruits, affecting one out of 10, but it is responsible for about 50 percent of all pneumonia in that group.[15,16,64] Transmission is through respiratory droplets, and incubation takes from 1 to as many as 3 weeks. For this reason, outbreaks tend to be prolonged as the infection is passed from one individual to another. Shedding of the organism may begin several days before the onset of clinical illness and persist for several weeks following resolution, even when the disease has been treated successfully with antibiotics.

Symptoms of mycoplasma respiratory infection usually begin in the upper airway. Pharyngitis and tracheitis are more prominent than with rhinovirus and coronavirus infections. Malaise, a mild fever, and myalgia may be present, but these symptoms tend to be less severe than those associated with influenza and adenovirus infections, especially when the latter involves the lower respiratory tract. When mycoplasma infection extends to the bronchioles and lungs, the onset is usually insidious over 2 or 3 days, and symptoms and clinical findings are less striking than with adenovirus, influenza, and bacterial pneumonias. Furthermore, mycoplasma infections are almost invariably self-limited to 3 weeks or less, even without antibiotics. Cough is the most common symptom experienced with mycoplasma respiratory infection. When the pharynx and trachea are involved, patients may produce blood-tinged phlegm or blood-flecked sputum, but grossly purulent sputum, even with pneumonia, is rare with mycoplasma infection.

Roentgenographic findings often appear much more serious than the symptoms and the few fine rales on chest auscultation would predict. Multilobar infiltrates are seen, and about 50 percent of these are bilateral. Although the pulmonic infiltrates found with mycoplasma infections are usually at least as extensive as those associated with bacterial pneumonia, they are usually less dense. Large pleural effusions are rare with mycoplasma pneumonia, but blunting of the costophrenic angles on chest x-ray is not at all uncommon. X-ray findings and a nonproductive irritating cough may persist up to 3 weeks beyond the acute infection.

Raynaud's phenomenon (pain and blanching of the distal fingers and toes upon exposure to cold temperature) may follow mycoplasma infections in a few individuals (see Chapter 18). Although serious sequelae as a result of mycoplasma infections are rare, Stevens-Johnson syndrome (a bullous eruption of the mucous membranes, associated with constitutional symptoms), as well as pericarditis, myocarditis, and neurologic sequelae can occur.[12] When these complications are seen, prompt referral to the appropriate specialist is imperative to help prevent severe permanent disabilities or even fatal outcomes.

Although the definitive diagnosis of my-coplasma infection depends on demonstrating a rise of specific antibody titers or isolation of the causative organism, both tests require special laboratory facilities; mycoplasma pharyngitis, bronchitis, and pneumonia can be tentatively differentiated from virus infections and bacterial pneumonias by their epidemiology, onset, and symptoms when correlated with physical and laboratory findings. With mycoplasma infections, leukocytosis may be in the range of 8,000 to 15,000 white blood cells per cubic millimeter, and the erythrocyte sedimentation rate is elevated in two thirds of patients. The clinical impression of mycoplasma infection is further supported by the presence of cold agglutinins in the patient's serum. This is a nonspecific test that can be performed by placing 1 ml of fresh blood in a test tube containing anticoagulant. After chilling the tube on ice for 3 minutes, cold agglutinins will cause small blood clumps which can be observed with good lighting when the tube is gently rotated in a horizontal position. The presence of cold agglutinins is confirmed by warming the tube between one's hands and repeating the test a couple of times. Cold agglutinins may not occur with all acute mycoplasma infections, and they may be absent during the first week of symptoms; moreover, cold agglutinins may occur with adenovirus infections, but their incidence is lower.[3] However, their presence can be helpful in the differential diagnosis when more sophisticated laboratory tests are not available.

Infection with *Mycoplasma pneumoniae* confers at least transient partial immunity against reinfection, but recurrences have been observed after intervals of several years.[4] A nasally administered vaccine to *Mycoplasma pneumoniae* has been tried in military populations, but this showed only limited efficacy.[4,67]

Mycoplasma pneumoniae is highly susceptible to tetracycline and erythromycin but resistant to penicillins, cephalosporins, and the aminoglycosides usually used to treat bacterial pneumonias. Although mycoplasma infections are almost always self-limited, it is wise to treat the disease with antibiotics in order to lessen the symptoms and to shorten its clinical course. Antibiotic therapy should be continued for 2 weeks to help prevent relapses, which may occur in as many as 5 to

10 percent of patients with *Mycoplasma pneumoniae* infections.[4] Because the organism is often still present after clinical improvement occurs, it is important to administer a full therapeutic course of antibiotics. When there is any question of pneumococcus or Legionnaire's disease, erythromycin should be chosen because these organisms are not susceptible to tetracycline.[4]

CHLAMYDIAL INFECTIONS

Recently, a "new" *Chlamydia*, called strain TWAR after its laboratory designation, has been isolated, and it may be an important cause of respiratory disease in healthy young persons.[77] The genus *Chlamydia* contains two species of obligate intracellular bacteria-like organisms: *C. trachomatis* and *C. psittaci*. *C. trachomatis* is known to cause pneumonia in infants and also may be a pulmonary pathogen in immunocompromised adults. *C. psittaci* causes pneumonia in healthy adults, but it is almost universally contracted through exposure to infected birds—parrots, pigeons, poultry, and others. Person-to-person spread is exceedingly rare. In 1985, epidemics of mild *C. psittaci*-caused pneumonia were reported among young people (ages 13 to 32) in two northern Finnish villages, and the illnesses could not be linked to birds. Subsequently, similar *C. psittaci*-caused illnesses have been described in University of Washington students,[42] in hospitalized Nova Scotia adults, and in military trainees in Finland.[55] Biochemical characterization suggests that the TWAR chlamydia may be sufficiently distinct from *C. psittaci* to merit a separate taxonomic designation.[9] Apparently, the TWAR chlamydia represent an important "new" agent capable of causing widespread, human-to-human transmissible acute respiratory disease. It may have a predilection for young adults. No definite seasonal pattern has emerged.

In clinical presentation, most cases have appeared as a mild pneumonia, similar to mycoplasma pneumonia. Typically, the patient will first be seen several days after disease onset. Cough—usually without sputum—pulmonary rales, fever (37.5 to 39°C [99.5 to 102°F]), and rhinitis are usually found, and a chest radiograph almost universally reveals one or more focal infiltrates. A minority of patients have reported chest pain. The white blood cell count is usually normal and the erythrocyte sedimentation rate (ESR) elevated (21 to 75 mm/hr); the ESR may remain elevated for weeks. Typical of chlamydial infections, TWAR pneumonia may tend to chronicity and recurrence. There are reports of repeated TWAR infections.

The drugs of choice for chlamydia are the tetracyclines (for adults, 250 to 500 mg four times daily for 14 to 21 days), but since TWAR pneumonia is difficult to differentiate clinically from mycoplasma pneumonia, erythromycin (250 mg, perhaps 500 mg, four times daily) may be better initial therapy while awaiting results of diagnostic studies. TWAR is sensitive to erythromycin; erythromycin usually causes fewer gastrointestinal symptoms and provides better coverage of pneumococci and *Legionella*. The short (5-day) course of erythromycin has not been effective in that symptoms have often persisted or recurred, and a 2 to 3 week course may be more appropriate.

Specific serologic diagnosis of TWAR infection is not widely available and also may not be useful for acute illness because even IgM antibody is usually delayed for at least 21 days after onset of primary infections. However, *Mycoplasma pneumoniae* infection often may be indicated in the acute phase of illness by tests for cold agglutinins (see section on mycoplasma infections, earlier). If a diagnostic laboratory is available, tests for *M. pneumoniae* complement-fixing antibody also may be helpful.

BACTERIAL INFECTIONS

Streptococcus Pyogenes

Streptococcus pyogenes remains an important cause of acute pharyngitis, although its incidence and the severity of respiratory illnesses caused by this bacterium have decreased during the past 25 years.[56]

The streptococci are generally classified by their hemolytic effects in blood agar cultures. The pathogenic strains, which cause respiratory tract illnesses, are all limited to those which cause beta hemolysis, that is, a clear zone around colonies in culture. Beta-hemolytic streptococci are serologically differentiated by specific polysaccharide antigenic groups. Of these, group A are by far the most important cause of streptococcal pharyngitis and its sequelae; although groups C and G may cause pharyngitis of a milder form. Group A beta-hemolytic streptococci are subdivided on the basis of a surface protein antigen, the M antigen, into more than 70 strains, which produce a great variety of antigenic products such as streptolysin O, streptokinase, hyaluronidase, and others. Past infection with streptococcus, group A, probably renders longstanding resistance to reinfection. However, this immunity is type specific, and as noted, at least 70 distinct antigenic types are known to exist.

Acute rheumatic fever and glomerulonephritis have been intensely investigated and are known to be especially associated with Streptococcus group A infections of the M type. The incidence of acute rheumatic fever is highest following epidemics of severe pharyngitis with M types that elicit high titers of antistreptolysin O. Although there has been a dramatic decline in the incidence of acute rheumatic fever during the past 20 years, the continuance of intermittent outbreaks of this disease, especially in young people under crowded conditions,[5] calls for continued vigilance by those who care for winter athletes.

Streptococcal pharyngitis occurs more frequently during the winter months and is more common in colder climates. This is presumably due to the effect of closeness and crowding on transmission of the bacterium. Infection takes place through contact with the saliva or respiratory droplets of an infected individual. Because the contagiousness of streptococcus is rapidly suppressed by penicillin therapy, infection usually results from exposure to untreated individuals or asymptomatic carriers.

The incubation of streptococcus is between 2 and 4 days, following which there may be rapid onset of sore throat, fever often exceeding 39°C (102°F), headache, and severe myalgia and malaise. Examination will show the pharynx, uvula, and tonsils to be diffusely erythematous and edematous. In the posterior pharynx, lymphoid hyperplasia may be noted. The tonsils are enlarged, and in severe infections they are covered with diffuse or punctate yellowish or gray exudate. Milder infections may show only beefy red, edematous inflammation of the pharynx and tonsils, but tender anterior cervical nodes and pharyngeal adenopathy are almost always present.

Previously, streptococcal pharyngitis in childhood was not infrequently followed by scarlet fever, characterized by bright red "strawberry tongue" and generalized fine grainy pink skin eruption over the chest, neck, and upper trunk which then spread to the extremities. This was later followed by scaling of the face and desquamation of the trunk, palms, and soles. Since the advent of the antibiotic era this syndrome has been seen with progressively less frequency.

Streptococcus group A pneumonia was also at one time a not uncommon complication of influenza, but this, too, is now rarely seen. It was characterized by a rapidly progressive bronchopneumonia leading to consolidation of the lung, mediastinal involvement, and bacterial pericarditis. In the prepenicillin era, otitis media, mastoiditis, peritonsillar abscess ("Quinsy"), and suppurative cervical adenitis were quite common complications of streptococcal pharyngitis.

Since streptococcal pharyngitis has been widely treated with penicillin during the past generation, infections seem to be less frequent and milder, and acute rheumatic fever and glomerulonephritis have become uncommon. Although it is unclear whether glomerulonephritis is preventable with antibiotic treatment—and certainly other factors besides uncomplicated streptococcus infection are important in the etiology of rheumatic fever—most authorities continue to recommend treatment of culture-documented group A beta-hemolytic streptococcus pharyngitis with penicillin. If penicillin allergy is known or suspected, erythromycin may be substituted, but many strains are resistant to tetracycline, and sulfonamides are ineffective. Symptoms rapidly subside following the initiation of penicillin or erythromycin therapy, but treatment should be continued for 10 days as a prophylaxis against rheumatic fever. Individuals who have received antibiotic treatment for 24 hours are probably no longer infectious, even though streptococci sometimes may be cultured from their throats.

When suppurative infections or pneumonia is present, the patient should be hospitalized for intensive antibiotic treatment and support. Surgical drainage of bacterial sinusitis, otitis media, mastoiditis, and peritonsillar abscesses is often indicated; so otolaryngologic consultation should be obtained when these complications are diagnosed.

Because pharyngeal and tonsillar exudates are common with adenovirus infections, mononucleosis, and sometimes with herpetic pharyngitis, and because milder forms of streptococcus may be confused with these and other viral infections, it is imperative that throat cultures be obtained whenever streptococcus infection is suspected. On one hand, it is not appropriate to undertake even a small risk of allergic reaction or sensitization to penicillin unless the presence of significant streptococcus is confirmed by culture, while on the other hand, all beta-hemolytic streptococcus A infections should be treated to limit symptoms, to prevent sequelae, and to abate the spread of disease.[52]

Streptococcus Pneumoniae

Of the several bacterial pneumonias, only *Streptococcus pneumoniae* ("Pneumococcus") produces a primary illness which has been the cause of significant morbidity among those engaged in winter sports. The other major bacteria responsible for human pneumonia are almost always secondary invaders. When bacterial pneumonia complicates influenza, pneumococcus is the most frequent invader, followed by *Staphylococcus aureus* and *Haemophilus influenzae.*[27,59,70]

Rarely pneumococcus will suddenly and unexpectedly strike robust young adults with acute primary lobar pneumonia characterized by abrupt onset with a shaking chill and high fever, followed by cough, pleuritic chest pain, and symptoms of respiratory distress. However, only a small portion of pneumococcal pneumonias occur in otherwise healthy individuals, and these infections are seldom fatal.[70]

Streptococcus pneumoniae is a Gram-positive bacterium that is readily cultured on blood agar plates, especially in a carbon dioxide environment, because they are facultative anaerobes. They have an antigenic mucopolysaccharide capsule and more than 80 serotypes have been discovered. Many healthy people are found to harbor one or more types as part of their normal upper respiratory flora, and pneumonitis probably results only when there is a disturbance in host-defense mechanisms or if there has been a large inoculum of an unusually virulent type.[31] Just a few pneumococcus types apparently account for most of the clinical infections.[1,31]

Although minor outbreaks have been reported among military recruits, most cases of pneumococcal pneumonia occur sporadically during winter and early spring months.[83] Pneumococcal pneumonia usually follows a viral respiratory illness, and susceptibility to infection may be enhanced by fatigue and exposure to dampness and chilling.[83] Crowding may increase the likelihood of contracting a virulent strain, but in general the disease is not thought of as being highly contagious.[59,83]

Clinically, cough is the most common feature of pneumococcal pneumonia. The onset of high fever, often above 103°F (39.5°C), with sudden shaking or intermittent chills may be the first symptoms of which the patient is aware. Pleuritic chest pain, exacerbated by cough or deep breathing, may cause splinting of the ribs to reduce chest wall motion. As the disease progresses, thick bloody or rusty sputum will be produced by most patients. Illness is accompanied by severe malaise, myalgia and weakness, sometimes leading to prostration with severe infections, especially in previously debilitated patients.

On physical examination even the previously healthy individual will have a rapid pulse and show signs of some respiratory distress. Chest wall movements may be diminished, and dullness with decreased breath sounds will be found over pulmonary lobes which have been consolidated by the pneumonia. Harsh crackling rales and friction rubs may be heard with chest auscultation. Although an uncommon complication, pneumococcal meningitis may be heralded by nuchal rigidity, and this should be evaluated in examining every patient because of the serious implications of central nervous system involvement.

White blood cell counts with pneumococcal pneumonia will often be striking, usually in excess of 15,000 cells per cubic millimeter; however, leucopenia occasionally is the harbinger of a worsening prognosis in patients with severe infections. Although roentgenograms of the chest with pneumococcal pneumonia typically show homogenous opacity of one or more pulmonary segments or even entire lobes, some elderly or debilitated patients will develop bronchopneumonia with its characteristic patchy infiltrates evident on x-ray examination. The diagnosis of bacterial pneumonia is made by the clinical signs and symptoms, and pneumococcus may be differentiated by the finding of large numbers of Gram-positive ovoid diplococci mixed with white blood cells in rusty purulent sputum, which is distinguished from the thin blood-flecked sputum of virus and mycoplasma infections. Because bacterial pneumonias caused by *Haemophilus influenzae*, *Staphylococcus aureus*, *Neisseria meningitidis*, and *Streptococcus pyogenes* can present with clinical pictures similar to pneumococcus infection, the definitive diagnosis will require culture confirmation.[32,59]

When sputum cultures are obtained, it is wise to carry out antibiotic sensitivity testing, even when pneumococcus is found. Although more than 95 percent of the *Streptococcus pneumoniae* occurring in the United States of America is sensitive to penicillin, resistant strains have caused endemic illness abroad, and resistant strains are beginning to emerge in North America.[25,32,81,83] Cultures of the blood should also be taken in chronically ill patients and in those in whom severe bacterial pneumonia is diagnosed. Cerebral spinal fluid cultures should be obtained when there is nuchal rigidity or when neurologic signs are found.

Albeit bacterial pneumonitis is usually confined to those with chronic pulmonary or cardiovascular diseases, diabetes mellitus, and previous pneumonia infections, those who are involved in treating sporting injuries should also be attuned to the possibility of these complications occurring as a consequence of aspiration following trauma.

If pneumococcal pneumonia is clearly suspected in an otherwise healthy individual, current practice favors initiation of penicillin therapy in patients without allergic history while awaiting the results of sputum culture and sensitivity testing.[1,32,59,83] Cephalosporin or erythromycin can be used in individuals with known or suspected penicillin allergy.[1,32] Although the incidence of allergic cross-reaction between penicillin and cephalosporins is low, a scratch test with cephalosporin is recommended before it is administered to anyone with a history of penicillin reaction, and then the first dose should be given with great care.[32] Unless complicated by an extrapulmonary nidus of infection, response of pneumococcal pneumonia to therapy with antibiotics is usually rapid, with defervescence in 24 hours or less. While most pneumococcal pleural effusions respond to antibiotic treatment, empyema requiring surgical drainage will develop in a few patients. Therefore, clinical signs and chest x-ray examinations should be followed until resolution has been ascertained.

Aspiration Pneumonia

Physicians, nurses, coaches, and emergency medicine technicians caring for sporting participants who are susceptible to trauma must be militant in their effort to recognize and promptly treat aspiration pneumonitis.[74] This syndrome may be initiated by inhalation of acidic gastric contents or vomitus, blood, and foreign bodies—such as a broken tooth—especially when the athlete is in a state of unconsciousness. The stomachs of recreational and even competitive athletes may contain small amounts of nonobstructing ingested materials or obstructing particulate food matter because of delayed emptying times related to the excitement of competition or because of injudicious eating shortly before participation. From an iatrogenic standpoint, traumatic emergency tracheal intubation may, itself, cause bleeding, which irritates the bronchial and alveolar linings leading to pulmonary inflammation and edema.

Tachypnea, wheezing, rales, fever, intractable cough, or severe dyspnea following head and upper body trauma should alert the health care provider to the possibility of aspiration. A localized lung infiltrate, collapse, or overinflation may be the key to recognizing mechanical bronchial obstruction. Aspiration of nonparticulate gastric contents and blood tends to cause more diffuse pulmonary infiltrations; but clotted blood can also lead to endobronchial obstruction.

When the diagnosis of aspiration is made, emergency hospitalization is mandatory for cultures, monitoring, and respiratory support. Some authorities recommend immediate high-dose intravenous corticosteroids to lessen pulmonary injury by decreasing the inflammatory response to aspiration. However, it is the consensus that steroids are of no value for preventing pneumonitis when they are administered more than an hour or two following aspiration, and they should not be continued for more than 24 hours.[74] Moreover, most acutely administered high-dose intravenous corticosteroids will be cleared within 1 week. Therefore, in view of the consequences of pulmonary aspiration, such treatment, if judged to be prophylactically beneficial, should not be withheld because of protocol considerations (see Chapter 12). In the unusual case in which an athlete may be in a position to compete shortly after such treatment, the managing physician should supply a letter detailing the accident and reasons for acutely administering intravenous corticosteroids. This should be presented by the athlete to the sport's governing body when medical declarations are made prior to competition. Individual consideration can then be applied to the situation if the athlete shows some minimal residual metabolites with drug testing.

Anaerobic and mixed anaerobic-aerobic infections tend to dominate in community-acquired aspiration pneumonias, because of the bacterial flora which are inhaled from the oropharynx and upper respiratory passages. Prophylactic antibiotics are probably useless for preventing aspiration pneumonia, but when temperature spikes, pulmonary infiltration increases, or putrid malodorous sputum develops several days following known or suspected aspiration, intensive antibiotic therapy with anaerobic coverage should be instituted after sputum cultures have been obtained.[74] In these cases, the physician should be alert to the possible presence of a previously unrecognized endobronchial obstruction or developing pulmonary abscess. High dosages of penicillin with clindamycin and an aminoglycoside is an acceptable initial antibiotic regimen, pending the results of bacterial culture and sensitivity studies.

SYMPTOMATIC TREATMENT

Virtually all mild upper respiratory infections can be symptomatically relieved with ephedrine-type decongestants and cough suppression with codeine or one of its analogs. However, athletes competing in United States Olympic Committee (USOC) and International Olympic Committee sanctioned events and events sponsored by other national governing bodies and international athletic federations are *precluded by protocol* from using these drugs. Presently, there is no USOC proscription against the use of topical oxymetrazoline as nasal drops or spray or against systemic chlorpheniramine maleate antihistamines alone for relief of congestion, rhinorrhea, and sneezing. Inhalation of the vapors from menthol, camphor, and eucalyptus oil containing preparations applied to the throat and chest have decongestant and antitussive effects; and pure eucalyptus, menthol, and guaifenesin expectorants are useful for the relief of cough and minor throat irritation. More severe sore throat can be relieved with warm saline solution gargles, hexylresorcinol lozenges, and lozenges or pharyngeal sprays containing phenol and sodium phenolate. Warm neck packs can relieve muscle tension and the pain of pharyngitis and cervical lymphadenitis. The recuperative powers of warmth, rest, sleep, and fluids cannot be overemphasized. Acetaminophen can be used as an antipyretic and for relief of headaches, myalgia, and general malaise. Reye's syndrome (fatty liver necrosis and encephalopathy) has been associated with salicylate treatment of children and adolescents with influenza and other viral infections.[84] Therefore, pediatricians and other physicians treating young people are advised against using aspirin and all forms of salicylate-containing medications in patients with viral disease. Because drugs banned by the USOC are incorporated into the formulations of many over-the-counter cough and cold preparations, athletes and their coaches and physicians are well advised to remain current regarding the regulations of their ruling bodies. When there is any doubt regarding the acceptability of a specific medication, athletes or their staffs should contact the USOC Drug Control Hotline at 1-800-233-0393 or the appropriate athletic federation.

Finally, much has been written in the popular health literature about the possible effectiveness of large doses of ascorbic acid (vitamin C) and more recently about zinc ion for prevention or treatment of the common cold.[17,33,34] Presently, there is little scientific evidence that megadoses of vitamin C will reduce the likelihood of contracting viral respiratory infections or reduce the severity of their symptoms. However, the jury is still out on the question as to whether either ascorbic acid or zinc may reduce the number of days of disability caused by colds.[34,53]

CONCLUSION

Upper respiratory infections are the most frequent cause of acute illness among those engaged in winter sports, but as we have seen in our discussion, careful attention to hygiene and to facility and equipment use may be effective in preventing spread of the most common etiologic agents. Respiratory infections with rhinoviruses, coronaviruses, parainfluenza, respiratory syncytial virus, and the enteric RNA viruses are self-limited and only moderately symptomatic. They can be effectively treated with prescribed and over-the-counter medications and simple remedies. More severe respiratory infections in otherwise healthy adults are unusual, and these, too, are generally highly responsive to promptly instituted appropriate therapy. Accurate and timely diagnosis, knowledgeable management, adequate convalescence, and careful follow-up are the keys to limiting discomfort and disability from respiratory infections in winter athletes and staffs.

REFERENCES

1. Austrian, R: Pneumococcal infections. In Braunwald, E, Isselbacher, KJ, Petersdorf, RG, Wilson, JD, Martin, JB, and Fauci, AS (eds): *Harrison's Principles of Internal Medicine*, ed 11. McGraw-Hill, New York, 1987, pp 533–537.
2. Baum, SG: Adenovirus. In Mandell, GL, Douglas, RG Jr, and Bennett, JE (eds): Principles and Practice of Infectious Diseases, ed 2. John Wiley & Sons, New York, 1985, pp 988–994.
3. Baum, SG: Adenovirus diseases. In Wyngaarden, JB and Smith, LH Jr (eds): Cecil Textbook of Medicine, ed 18. WB Saunders, Philadelphia, 1988, pp 1767–1768.
4. Baum, SG: Mycoplasmal infections. In Wyngaarden, JB and Smith, LH Jr (eds): Cecil Textbook of Medicine, ed 18. WB Saunders, Philadelphia, 1988, pp 1561–1565.
5. Bisno, AL: Acute rheumatic fever: Forgotten but not gone. N Engl J Med 316:476–478, 1987.
6. Breman, JG and Hayner, NS: Guillain-Barre syndrome and its relationship to swine influenza vaccination in Michigan, 1976–1977. Am J Epidemiol 119:880–889, 1984.
7. Bryson, YJ, Monahan, C, Pollack, M, and Shields, WD: A prospective double-blind study of side effects associated with the administration of amantadine for influenza A virus prophylaxis. J Infect Dis 141:543–547, 1980.
8. Burch, GE: Viral diseases of the heart. Acta Cardiol 34:5–9, 1979.
9. Campbell, LA, Kuo, CC, and Grayston, T: Characterization of the new *Chlamydia* agent, TWAR, as a unique organism by restriction endonuclease analysis and DNA-DNA hybridization. J Clin Microbiol 25:1911–1916, 1987.
10. Chanock, RM: Respiratory syncytial virus. In Wyngaarden, JB and Smith, LH Jr (eds): Cecil Textbook of Medicine, ed 18. WB Saunders, Philadelphia, 1988, pp 1758–1760.
11. Chanock, RM: Parainfluenza viral diseases. In Wyngaarden, JB and Smith, LH Jr (eds): Cecil Textbook of Medicine, ed 18. WB Saunders, Philadelphia, 1988, pp 1760–1762.
12. Chen, S, Tsai, CC, and Nouri, S: Carditis associated with *Mycoplasma pneumoniae* infection. Am J Dis Child 140:471–472, 1986.
13. Clyde, WA, Jr: Mycoplasma infections. In Braunwald, E, Isselbacher, KJ, Petersdorf, RG, Wilson, JD, Martin, JB, and Fauci, AS (eds): Harrison's Principles of Internal Medicine, ed 11. McGraw-Hill, New York, 1987, pp 757–759.
14. Couch, RB: The common cold: Control? J Infect Dis 150:167–173, 1984.
15. Couch, RB: Mycoplasma pneumonia (primary atypical pneumonia). In Mandell, GL, Douglas, RG Jr, and Bennett, JE (eds): Principles and Practice of Infectious Diseases, ed 2. John Wiley & Sons, New York, 1985, pp 1065–1076.
16. Couch, RB: Mycoplasma pneumoniae. In Knight, V (ed): Viral and Mycoplasmal Infections of the Respiratory Tract. Lea & Febiger, Philadelphia, 1973, pp 217–235.
17. Coulehan, JL, Eberhard, S, Kapner, L, Taylor, F, Rogers, K, and Garry, P: Vitamin C and acute illness in Navajo schoolchildren. N Engl J Med 295:973–977, 1976.
18. D'Alessio, DJ, Meschievitz, CK, Peterson, JA, Dick, CR, and Dick, EC: Short-duration exposure and the transmission of rhinoviral colds. J Infect Dis 150:189–194, 1984.
19. Davenport, FM: Influenza viruses. In Evans, AS (ed): Viral Infections of Humans: Epidemiology and Control, ed 2. Plenum Press, New York, 1982, pp 373–396.
20. Dick, EC, Hossain, SU, Mink, KA, Meschievitz, CK, Schultz, SB, Raynor, WJ, and Inhorn, SL: Interruption of transmission of rhinovirus colds among human volunteers using virucidal paper handkerchiefs. J Infect Dis 153:352–356, 1986.
21. Dick, EC and Inhorn, SL. Rhinoviruses. In Feigin, RD, and Cherry, JD (eds): Textbook of Pediatric Infectious Diseases, ed 2. WB Saunders, Philadelphia, 1987, pp 1539–1558.
22. Dick, EC, Jennings, LC, Meschievitz, CK, MacMillin, D, and Goodrum, J: Possible modification of the normal winter fly-in respiratory disease outbreak at McMurdo Station. Antarctic Journal of the United States 15:173–174, 1980.
23. Dick, EC, Jennings, LC, Mink, KA, Wartgow, CD, and Inhorn, SL: Aerosol transmission of rhinovirus colds. J Infect Dis 156:442–448, 1987.
24. Dick, EC, Mogabgab, WJ, Holmes, B: Characteristics of para-influenza 1 (HA-2) virus: Incidence of infection and clinical features in adults. Am J Hygiene 73:263–272, 1961.

25. Dixon, JMS, Lipinski, AE, and Graham, MEP: Detection and prevalence of pneumococci with increased resistance to penicillin. Can Med Assoc J 117:1159–1161, 1977.

26. Dolin, R, Reichman, RC, Madore, HP, Maynard, R, Linton, PN, and Webber-Jones, J: A controlled trial of amantadine and rimantadine in the prophylaxis of influenza A infection. N Engl J Med 307:580–584, 1982.

27. Douglas, RG, Jr: Influenza. In Wyngaarden, JB and Smith LH Jr (eds): Cecil Textbook of Medicine, ed. 18. WB Saunders, Philadelphia, 1988, pp 1762–1767.

28. Douglas, RG, Jr and Betts, RF: Influenza virus. In Mandell, GL, Douglas, RG Jr and Bennett, JE (eds): Principles and Practice of Infectious Diseases, ed 2. John Wiley & Sons, New York, 1985, pp 846–866.

29. Douglas, RG, Jr, Lindgren, KM, and Couch, RB: Exposure to cold environment and rhinovirus common cold. N Engl J Med 279:742–747, 1968.

30. Dowling, HF, Jackson, GG, Spiesman, IG, and Inouye, T: Transmission of the common cold to volunteers under controlled conditions. Am J Hygiene 68:59–65, 1958.

31. Dull, HB, Kendal, AP, and Patriarca, PA: Influenza. In Last, JM (ed): Maxcy-Rosenau Public Health and Preventive Medicine, ed 12. Appleton-Century-Crofts, Norwalk, CT, 1986, pp 138–147.

32. Durack, DT: Pneumococcal pneumonia. In Wyngaarden, JB and Smith, LH Jr (eds): Cecil Textbook of Medicine, ed 18. WB Saunders, Philadelphia, 1988, pp 1554–1561.

33. Dykes, MHM and Meier, P: Ascorbic acid and the common cold. JAMA 231:1073–1079, 1975.

34. Eby, GA, Davis, DR, and Halcomb, WW: Reduction in duration of common colds by zinc gluconate lozenges in a double-blind study. Antimicrobial Agents and Chemotherapy 25:20–24, 1984.

35. Edelen, JS, Bender, TR, and Chin, TDY: Encephalopathy and pericarditis during an outbreak of influenza. Am J Epidemiol 100:79–84, 1974.

36. Editorial. Splints don't stop colds—surprising! Lancet 1:277–278, 1988.

37. Evans, AS and Dick, EC: Acute pharyngitis and tonsillitis in University of Wisconsin Students. JAMA 190:699–708, 1964.

38. Evatt, BL, Dowdle, WR, Johnson, M Jr, and Heath, CW Jr: Epidemic mycoplasma pneumonia. N Engl J Med 285:374–378, 1971.

39. Foy, HM: Adenoviruses. In Evans, AS (ed): Viral Infections of Humans: Epidemiology and Control, ed 3. Plenum Publishing Corporation, New York, 1989, pp 77–94.

40. Foy, HM, Kenny, GE, Cooney, MK, and Allan, ID: Long-term epidemiology of infections with *Mycoplasma pneumoniae.* J Infect Dis 139:681–687, 1979.

40a. Glezen, WP, and Couch, RB: Influenza viruses. In Evans, AS (ed): Viral Infections of Humans: Epidemiology and Control, ed 3. Plenum Publishing Corporation, New York, 1989, pp 419–449.

41. Glezen, WP, Fernald, GW, and Lohr, JA: Acute respiratory disease of university students with special reference to the etiologic role of *Herpesvirus hominis.* Am J Epidemiol 101:111–121, 1975.

42. Grayston, JT, Kuo, CC, Wang, SP, and Altman, J: A new *Chlamydia psittaci* strain, TWAR, isolated in acute respiratory tract infections. N Engl J Med 315:161–168, 1986.

43. Greenberg, SB, Couch, RB, and Kasel, JA: An outbreak of an influenza type A variant in a closed population: The effect of homologous and heterologous antibody on infection and illness. Am J Epidemiol 100:209–215, 1974.

44. Gwaltney, JM, Jr.: Rhinoviruses. In Evans, AS (ed): Viral Infections of Humans: Epidemiology and control, ed 3. Plenum Publishing Corporation, New York, 1989, pp 593–615.

45. Gwaltney, JM, Jr, and Hendley, JO: Transmission of experimental rhinovirus infection by contaminated surfaces. Am J Epidemiol 116:828–833, 1982.

46. Gwaltney, JM, Jr, and Moskalski, PB, and Hendley, JO: Hand-to-hand transmission of rhinovirus colds. Ann Int Med 88:463–467, 1978.

47. Hart, GG: Final Report, Frequency of Visits by ICD-9 Diagnostic Code: Medical Report of the XIII Winter Olympic Games. Lake Placid Olympic Organizing Committee, Lake Placid, NY, 1980.

48. Huebner, RJ, Casey, MJ, Chanock, RM, and Schell, K: Tumors induced in hamsters by a strain of adenovirus type 3. Proc Natl Acad Sci 54:381–388, 1965.

49. Huebner, RJ, Chanock, RM, Rubin, BA, and Casey, MJ: Induction by adenovirus type 7 of tumors in hamsters having antigenic characteristics of SV-40 virus. Proc Natl Acad Sci 52:1333–1340, 1964.

50. Immunization Practice Advisory Committee, Centers for Disease Control: Prevention and control of influenza. MMWR 36:373–387, 1987.

51. Inhorn, SL, and Dick, EC: Coronaviruses. In Feigin, RD and Cherry JD (eds): Textbook of Pediatric Infectious Diseases, ed 2. WB Saunders, Philadelphia, 1987, pp 1531–1539.

52. Komaroff, AL: A management strategy for sore throat. JAMA 239:1429–1432, 1978.

53. Kapikian, AZ: The common cold. In Wyngaarden, JB and Smith, LH Jr (eds): Cecil Textbook of Medicine, ed 18. WB Saunders, Philadelphia, 1988, pp 1753–1757.

54. Katagiri, S, Ohizumi, A, and Homma, M: An outbreak of type C influenza in a children's home. J Infect Dis 148:51–56, 1983.

55. Kleemola, M, Saikku, P, Visakorpi, R, Wang, SP, and Grayston, JT: Epidemics of pneumonia caused by TWAR, a new *Chlamydia* organism, in military trainees in Finland. J Infect Dis 157:230–236, 1988.

56. Krause, RM: Streptococcal diseases. In Wyngaarden, JB and Smith, LH Jr (eds): Cecil Textbook of Medicine, ed 18. WB Saunders, Philadelphia, 1988, pp 1572–1580.

57. Ksiazek, TG, Olson, JG, Irving, GS, Settle, CS, White R, Petrusso, R: An influenza outbreak due to A/USSR/77-like (H₁N₁) virus aboard a US Navy ship. Am J Epidemiol 112:487–494, 1980.

58. Langmuir, AD, Bregman, DJ, Kurland, LT, Nathanson, N, and Victor, M: An epidemiologic and clinical evaluation of Guillain-Barre syndrome reported in association with the administration of swine influenza vaccines. Am J Epidemiol 119:841–879, 1984.

59. Lerner, AM and Jankauskas, K: The classic bacterial pneumonias. In Disease-a-Month. Year Book Medical Publishers, Chicago, IL, 1975, pp 1–46.

60. Lewes, D: Viral myocarditis. The Practitioner 216:281–287, 1976.

61. McClung, HW, Knight, V, Gilbert, BE, Wilson, SZ, Quarles, JM, and Divine, GW: Ribavirin aerosol treatment of influenza B virus infection. JAMA 249:2671–2674, 1983.

62. Meschievitz, CK, Schultz, SB, and Dick, EC: A model for obtaining predictable natural transmission of rhinoviruses in human volunteers. J Infect Dis 150:195–201, 1984.

63. Modlin, JF: Coxsackievirus and echovirus. In Mandell, GL, Douglas, RG, Jr, and Bennett, JE (eds): Principles and Practice of Infectious Diseases, ed 2. John Wiley and Sons, New York, 1985, pp 814–825.

64. Mogabgab, WJ: Acute respiratory illnesses in university (1962–1966), military and industrial (1962–1963) populations. American Review of Respiratory Disease 98:359–379, 1968.

65. Monto, AS: The Tecumseh study of respiratory illness. V. Patterns of infection with the parainfluenzaviruses. Am J Epidemiol 97:338–348, 1973.

66. Monto, AS: Coronaviruses. In Evans, AS (ed): Viral Infections of Humans: Epidemiology and Control, ed 3. Plenum Publishing Corporation, New York, 1989, pp 153–167.

67. Monto, AS: Acute respiratory infection. In Last, JM (ed): Maxcy-Rosenau Public Health and Preventive Medicine, ed 12. Appleton-Century-Crofts, Norwalk, CT, 1986, pp 147–154.

68. Morris, JA, Casey, MJ, Eddy, BE, Lane, WT, and Huebner, RJ: Occurrence of SV-40 neoplastic and antigenic information in vaccine strains of adenovirus type 3. Proc Soc Exp Biol Med 122:679–684, 1966.

69. Moser, MR, Bender, TR, Margolis, HS, Noble, GR, Kendal, AP, and Ritter, DG: An outbreak of influenza aboard a commercial airliner. Am J Epidemiol 110:1–6, 1979.

70. Mufson, MA: Pneumococcal infections. JAMA 246:1942–1948, 1981.

71. Mufson, MA: Viral pharyngitis, laryngitis, croup and bronchitis. In Wyngaarden JB and Smith, LH Jr (eds): Cecil Textbook of Medicine, ed 18. WB Saunders, Philadelphia, 1988, pp 1757–1758.

72. Murphy, TF, Henderson, FW, Clyde, WA, Jr, Collier, AM, Denny, FW: Pneumonia: An eleven-year study in a pediatric practice. Am J Epidemiol 113:12–21, 1981.

73. Payler, DK and Purdham, PA: Influenza A prophylaxis with amantadine in a boarding school. Lancet 1:502–504, 1984.

74. Reynolds, HY: Aspiration pneumonia. In Wyngaarden, JB and Smith, LH Jr (eds): Cecil Textbook of Medicine, ed 17. WB Saunders, Philadelphia, 1985, pp 1513–1516.

75. Rosenbaum, MJ, Deberry, P, Sullivan EJ, Pierce, WE, Mueller, RE, and Peckinpaugh, RO: Epidemiology of the common cold in military recruits with emphasis on infections by rhinovirus types 1A, 2 and two unclassified rhinoviruses. Am J Epidemiol 93:183–193, 1971.

76. Roberts, JA: Viral illnesses and sports performance. Sports Medicine 3:296–303, 1986.

77. Schachter, J: *Chlamydia psittaci*—"Reemergence" of a forgotten pathogen. N Engl J Med 315:189–191, 1986.

78. Sutton, GC, Harding, HB, Trueheart, RP, and Clark, HP: Coxsackie B_4 myocarditis in an adult: Successful isolation of virus from ventricular myocardium. Aerospace Medicine 38:66–69, 1967.

79. Tomasi, TB, Trudeau, FB, Czerwinski, D, and Erredge, S: Immune parameters in athletes before and after strenuous exercise. J Clin Immunol 2:173–178, 1982.

80. Top, FH, Jr, Grossman, RA, Bartellone, PJ, Segal, HE, Dudding, BA, Russell, PK, and Buescher, EL: Immunization with live type 7 and 4 adenovirus vaccines. J Infect Dis 124:148–154, 1971.

81. Ward, J: Antibiotic-resistant *Streptococcus pneumoniae:* Clinical and epidemiologic aspects. Rev Infect Dis 3:254–266, 1981.

82. Warshauer, DM, Dick, EC, Mandel, AD, Flynn, TC, and Jerde, RS: Rhinovirus infections in an isolated Antarctic station: Transmission of the viruses and susceptibility of the population. Am J Epidemiol 129:319–340, 1989.

83. White, FMM: Pneumococcal infection. In Last, JM (ed): Maxcy-Rosenau Public Health and Preventive Medicine, ed 2. Appleton-Century-Crofts, Norwalk, CT, 1986, pp 218–222.

84. Willis, J: Study verifies association of aspirin with Reye syndrome. FDA Drug Bulletin 17:29, 1987.

CHAPTER 16

Acute Gastrointestinal Infections

DAVID R. HILL, M.D.

Infectious gastrointestinal syndromes affect persons of all ages throughout the world. In developed countries, such as the United States, diarrheal illness is second only to respiratory infections as a cause of illness in most families. Throughout the developing world, diarrheal diseases constitute the greatest single cause of morbidity and mortality, especially affecting infants and young children. For the more than eight million individuals who travel annually to the developing world for business, pleasure, athletics, or adventure, traveler's diarrhea may affect 30 to 50 percent of them, potentially preventing the individual from participating in their planned activities for several days. Indeed, throughout the years, several athletic performances have been adversely affected by debilitating diarrhea. Because of the potential impact of a diarrheal illness on an athlete's performance, whether the event occurs in the United States or in locations throughout the world, it is important that athletes, their physicians, and support staffs are able to prevent, to diagnose, and more importantly, to manage diarrhea to allow the athlete to return quickly to the event.

GENERAL PRINCIPLES

Gastrointestinal syndromes cover a wide range of clinical pictures that reflect specific bacterial, viral, or parasitic etiologies and their pathogenic mechanisms. In individual cases, interaction of the host with the infectious agent is also important in determining the outcome of these infections.

129

Pathogenic Mechanisms

The gastrointestinal tract is a remarkable secretory and absorptive system. It is estimated that at least 8 liters of fluid a day are exchanged across the intestinal mucosa; the majority of this occurs in the small intestine. This delicate balance can be disrupted by agents that cause "noninflammatory" diarrhea by producing increases in fluid and electrolyte secretion into the small bowel via enterotoxins, or by agents that cause "inflammatory" diarrhea through destruction of the mucosa in the ileum and colon by direct invasion or the production of cytotoxins. Infectious agents that exhibit close adherence to intestinal epithelial cells may cause diarrhea by other, as yet undefined, mechanisms. However, recognition of the different pathogenic mechanisms is important in differentiating the several clinical syndromes.[12] Thus, agents that produce enterotoxins cause predominantly noninflammatory watery diarrhea, whereas those which are invasive or which produce cytotoxins give the symptoms of inflammatory diarrhea and dysentery (tenesmus; abdominal pain; and frequent bloody, mucoid stools).

The classic enterotoxin cause of noninflammatory diarrhea is that which is elaborated by *Vibrio cholerae*. Cholera toxin binds to specific ganglioside receptors on intestinal epithelial cells and through the activation of intracellular enzymes results in increased secretion of anions and water. Nowadays, cholera is a rare cause of diarrhea in developed countries. Another cause of noninflammatory diarrhea is toxin-producing *Escherichia coli*, which is the most common etiologic agent of diarrhea in travelers. Enterotoxigenic *E. coli* (ETEC) elaborates two toxins, a heat-labile (LT) and a heat-stable (ST) toxin. Heat-labile toxin works through mechanisms similar to those for cholera toxin; whereas ST activates other enzymes that cause increased intestinal secretions.

Examples of the pathogens of "inflammatory" diarrhea are *Shigella* and invasive *E. coli*. These bacteria exert their effects predominantly by destroying colonic epithelial cells, thereby promoting a profound inflammatory response in the bowel wall. *Salmonella, Campylobacter, Yersinia*, and certain of the *Vibrios* may also produce diarrhea by invasion of the intestinal mucosa. Another agent that produces a potent cytotoxin is *Clostridium difficile*.

Close adherence to intestinal epithelial cells, usually in the small bowel, is the mechanism of diarrhea production by some strains of *E. coli*. *Giardia lamblia*, which also adheres closely to the mucosal brush border, probably produces diarrhea by interfering with the delicate absorptive mechanisms of the intestine. A newly recognized protozoan, *Cryptosporidium*, may also cause diarrhea through close adherence. Viral agents such as rotavirus and Norwalk-like viruses attach to the villus tips of the small bowel, destroying these cells and leaving a predominance of crypt cells which results in increased intestinal secretions.

Finally, the mucosal inflammatory response of the host, as it attempts to clear an enteric agent, may result in further mucosal damage and diarrhea. With this complexity of the host-pathogen relationship, it is likely that multiple mechanisms, including some that are yet to be discovered, participate in the production of symptoms with acute gastrointestinal infections.

Evaluation of the Patient

A careful clinical history is critical to the complete assessment of patients with a gastrointestinal illness. Questions should be asked that concern not only the nature of the diarrhea—whether it is nocturnal, watery, bloody, or formed—but also what has been the patient's food exposure, travel, previous antibiotic use, or sexual contact (Table 16–1). Also are there close associates with a similar illness? These areas are important because certain infectious agents may be epidemiologically linked with each of these historical features.[12] As examples, diarrhea that lasts for more than 1 to 2 weeks or that occurs after ingestion of water in the wilderness is often caused by the intestinal parasite *Giardia lamblia*. Diarrhea occurring after ingesting seafood may be associated with *Vibrio* infection. Several people who become ill a day or two after a common food exposure may be infected with *Salmonella*. Finally, diarrhea that occurs while someone is taking antibiotics may be caused by *Clostridium difficile*.

A particularly differentiating feature is the distinction between "inflammatory" and "noninflammatory" diarrhea, as described.

Table 16–1. HISTORICAL FEATURES TO CONSIDER IN A DIARRHEAL ILLNESS

Characteristics of diarrhea
  watery
  gross or occult blood, or mucus
  formed stool
Duration of illness
Type of illness
  fever
  nausea and vomiting
  cramping, tenesmus
Food or untreated water exposure
Others with a similar illness
Travel (cruise ship, seacoast, developing world,
  wilderness)
Antibiotic use
Sexual contact

Noninflammatory diarrhea is usually caused by pathogens of the small bowel, whereas inflammatory diarrhea is caused by pathogens of the colon and terminal ileum. Inflammatory diarrhea is often associated with more severe symptoms and potential complications and may require specific diagnostic measures with subsequent antimicrobial therapy. Clinically, patients with inflammatory diarrhea have a history of more than three liquid stools per day, often with gross blood or mucus present, a fever greater than 38.5°C (101°F), crampy abdominal pain, and some signs of systemic toxicity. Further differentiation can be made on the basis of a stool examination. These syndromes are summarized in Table 16–2.

A physical examination should be performed with particular attention to the patient's degree of hydration by measuring orthostatic changes of pulse and blood pressure and by assessing mucous membranes and skin turgor. The stool should then be examined to confirm if it is grossly watery, mucoid, or bloody; a sample can be examined for occult blood and for the presence of inflammatory cells.

The presence of fecal leukocytes has been helpful for many years, dating back to World War I, when the Royal Army Medical Corps set up field stations for running these tests to distinguish between "simple diarrhea" and bacillary dysentery due to *Shigella*. The technique involves taking a sample of stool (including mucus if present), placing it on a glass slide, mixing it with a drop of methylene blue dye, and then—after covering it with a cover slip—microscopically examining the specimen under a high-dry objective.

Table 16–2. DIFFERENTIATION OF DIARRHEAS AND THEIR ETIOLOGIC AGENTS

	Noninflammatory	Inflammatory
Mechanism	Small bowel—enterotoxin or adherence	Colon—invasion or cytotoxin
Syndrome	Temperature <38.5°C (101.3°F)	Fever >38.5°C (101.3°F)
	Watery diarrhea	Diarrhea with gross blood or mucus
	Mild cramping	Severe cramping and tenesmus
Agents	Bacteria	Bacteria
	Enterotoxigenic *E. coli*	*Campylobacter jejuni*
	Vibrio cholerae	*Salmonella enteritidis*
	Salmonella enteritidis	*Shigella*
	Vibrio parahemolyticus	Invasive *E. coli*
		Vibrio parahemolyticus
		Yersinia enterocolitica
		Clostridium difficile
	Protozoa	Protozoa
	Giardia lamblia	*Entamoeba histolytica*
	Cryptosporidium	
	Viruses	
	Rotavirus	
	Norwalk-like agents	

The finding of numerous sheets of polymorphonuclear cells places the diarrhea in the inflammatory category. The highest yield from stool culture will come from stools that contain blood or polymorphonuclear cells.

CLINICAL SYNDROMES

Acute Food Poisoning Secondary to Infectious Agents that Occurs Within Sixteen Hours

In this section the discussion is limited to food poisoning with predominantly gastrointestinal symptoms that is caused by infectious agents and has an incubation period of 16 hours or less.[18] Food-borne infectious agents, including *Salmonella*, with predominantly longer incubation periods will be covered in subsequent sections. Food poisoning secondary to chemical agents or associated with neurologic symptoms will not be discussed, and the reader is referred to the references.[18]

Nausea and abdominal pain, followed by vomiting and diarrhea which occur within 6 hours of ingestion of food is usually due to *Staphylococcus aureus* or *Bacillus cereus*. These diseases are caused by toxins already elaborated by the bacteria, thereby accounting for the short incubation period. There are several heat-stable enterotoxins of *S. aureus* that can cause the syndrome; although in recent years most disease in the United States has been due to type A. The foods most commonly associated with *Staphylococcus* contamination are potato salads, cream-filled pastries, and high-protein foods such as ham and poultry. As with many of the food poisoning illnesses, this has resulted from contamination by a food handler of previously cooked food followed by maintenance of the food for several hours at temperatures that allow multiplication of the pathogenic bacteria and production of enterotoxins.

B. cereus causes a clinical picture very similar to staphylococcus, although diarrhea may be seen less frequently. *B. cereus* elaborates a heat-stable toxin. The food source is often fried or boiled rice, which has been cooked and then held at ambient temperatures.

Diarrhea and abdominal cramping that occur 8 to 16 hours after food ingestion is usually due to *Clostridium perfringens* (type A strains) or to long-incubation *B. cereus*. Nausea and vomiting occur in 30 percent or fewer of the individuals who ingest *C. perfringens* or long-incubation *B. cereus*, unlike the short-incubation syndromes in which these symptoms are more frequent. With *C. perfringens* food poisoning, it is usually a beef product that has been stored improperly and allowed to sit at room temperature, thereby allowing the anaerobic bacterium to germinate. Once the food has been ingested, the vegetative bacteria sporulate and produce their heat-labile enterotoxin in the alkaline environment of the small bowel. The type A *Clostridium* enterotoxin causes sodium and chloride ions and fluid to be secreted into the intestinal lumen. There also may be some toxic damage to the villus tips. *B. cereus* also produces a heat-labile toxin and results in a similar clinical illness.

The specific etiologic diagnosis of the bacterium responsible for acute food poisoning is often difficult and requires isolating the organism from the suspected food source and also from ill patients. Occasionally the toxin of *S. aureus* can be identified in food.

The prevention of illness requires the basic measures of proper handling, cooking, and storage of food. Food should be prepared by persons only after careful hand washing, and then the food should be fully cooked. Cooked foods should be eaten promptly and not stored for prolonged periods at warm or ambient temperatures. When food is stored, it should be cooled quickly to temperatures lower than 7°C (45°F). One can prevent *C. perfringens* and *B. cereus* food poisoning by adequately reheating foods to at least 75°C (170°F) to destroy the vegetative bacteria and their toxins.

Noninflammatory Diarrhea

Noninflammatory diarrhea is characterized by nausea and vomiting with watery diarrhea, but the stool does not contain polymorphonuclear cells or blood.[14] A low-grade fever is often present.

Noninflammatory diarrhea is caused by viral, bacterial, and parasitic organisms that usually exert their pathogenic mechanisms in the upper intestine (see Table 16–2). The mainstay of management of these patients is symptomatic.

Viral Agents

The majority of noninflammatory diarrhea in the United States is due to viruses.[1] The syndrome that they produce is commonly termed "intestinal flu." In adults, the main agents are Norwalk-like viruses,[20] which account for up to 40 percent of all nonbacterial gastroenteritis. These viruses are so named because they have both structural and clinical similarity to the Norwalk virus which was first identified in an outbreak of gastrointestinal illness in Norwalk, Ohio, during the late 1960s. Epidemiologic studies have determined that outbreaks are associated with food, water, and person-to-person transmission of the infectious virus. Secondary attack rates are high, especially among children. The incubation period is usually 1 or 2 days. Illness is characterized by nausea, vomiting, abdominal cramps, diarrhea, and headache. Diarrhea is more common in adults, and vomiting is more often seen in children. Low-grade fever is reported in about a third of the cases. Illness is usually mild and self-limited, lasting 24 to 60 hours in most instances.

The other major viral agent of diarrhea is rotavirus. In the United States and the developing world, rotavirus appears to be an important cause of dehydrating diarrheal illness, predominantly in the pediatric age group. Up to 15 percent of diarrhea illnesses among international travelers is caused by either rotavirus or Norwalk agents.

Bacterial Agents

The classic cause of noninflammatory bacterial diarrhea is *Vibrio cholerae*.[14] Clinical illness with *V. cholerae* is limited predominantly to the developing world. Enterotoxigenic *E. coli* (ETEC) is the most frequent cause of diarrhea in the international traveler and will be discussed at greater length in the section on traveler's diarrhea. Although *Salmonella* and other bacterial agents (see Table 16–2) can overlap in their syndromes, they usually cause inflammatory diarrhea and are therefore discussed in that part of this chapter.

Parasitic Agents

Giardia lamblia, a pathogenic enteric protozoan, is the most frequently identified intestinal parasite in the United States, and it is an important cause of diarrhea throughout the developing world.[11,15] Transmission of *Giardia* infection is usually via fecally contaminated water; however, person-to-person transmission occurs among young children in day-care centers and between sexually active homosexual males. A wide range of animal reservoirs act as sources for contamination of natural freshwater supplies. Therefore, in the United States many *Giardia* outbreaks and sporadic cases have occurred when persons ingest untreated surface water. In this country, *Giardia* is the leading identified cause of waterborne diarrhea. Waters in the mountains of the Colorado Rockies, Pacific Northwest, and Northeastern United States have been the souces of *Giardia* infection for many hikers and campers.

The parasite has two stages in its life cycle: the cyst stage and the trophozoite stage. The trophozoite is the form that is active in the intestine. The organism then encysts before being passed via the feces into the environment. Infection may occur after ingestion of as few as ten *Giardia* cysts. Excystation occurs, and the upper small bowel of the new host is colonized by the trophozoites.

Clinical giardiasis can range from an acute self-limited illness to a syndrome of chronic diarrhea, malabsorption, and weight loss. In individuals with symptomatic giardiasis, illness occurs after an incubation period of 1 to 2 weeks and is characterized by the acute onset of diarrhea, abdominal cramps, bloating, and flatulence. Malaise, nausea, and anorexia are common; but vomiting, fever, and tenesmus are not. Stools range from watery to greasy and are usually foul smelling. Gross blood is not seen. Weight loss of more than 10 pounds often accompanies giardiasis, and lactase deficiency is common. The most important distinguishing feature of giardiasis is the duration of diarrhea, which lasts for at least 7 to 10 days from the time of onset. Therefore, giardiasis should be considered in all patients with prolonged diarrhea or malabsorption. Because of the long incubation period, the first symptoms of giardiasis in a traveler often do not occur until the person has returned from overseas. Diagnosis of the disease is confirmed by the demonstration of *Giardia* cysts or trophozoites in stool specimens. Duodenal contents may also be sampled for trophozoites. All patients with symptomatic giardiasis should be treated.[21,23]

Inflammatory Diarrhea

Bacterial Agents

Campylobacter jejuni, Salmonella, and *Shigella* are the most common causes of invasive bacterial diarrhea.[13] Until several years ago, *Campylobacter* was not even recognized as an agent of diarrhea, whereas now it is one of the leading causes of invasive bacterial diarrheas.[2,3] *Campylobacter jejuni* is a fastidious Gram-negative rod that grows best at 42°C (107.6°F) in an atmosphere of increased carbon dioxide. On Gram stain *Campylobacter* has the curved, seagull appearance of the Vibrios. The organism is found throughout the animal kingdom, where it frequently infects poultry. Patients usually acquire *Campylobacter* infections through contaminated foodstuffs. Mountain water has also been a source of infection to hikers.

Clinical *Campylobacter* illness occurs after an incubation period of 2 or more days and may be initiated by a prodrome of fever, malaise, and headache. Most patients progress to have a dysenteric syndrome of bloody diarrhea, abdominal pain and tenesmus (rectal urgency). Fever and nausea are usually present, but vomiting is less common. Diagnosis is made by culturing *Campylobacter* from the stool. The organism may also be identified with dark-field microscopy or modified acid-fast staining of the stool.

Illness with *Campylobacter* is usually self-limited, with symptoms abating by 7 days. Although treatment may not alter the clinical course, especially if started a few days into the illness, it is often indicated to eradicate fecal shedding of the organism and to prevent the occasional relapse of infection and person-to-person spread.

The species *Salmonella enteritidis* has more than 2000 serotypes; the most frequent cause of diarrhea is *Salmonella enteritidis* subspecies *typhimurium. Salmonella* produces an enterocolitis that ranges from mild self-limited diarrhea to a dehydrating dysenteric syndrome.[17] *Salmonella* enterocolitis is occasionally complicated by extraintestinal infection. *Salmonella,* like *Campylobacter,* are widely distributed in animal species, especially poultry, which then become sources for human infection. *Salmonella* is the most common cause of documented food-borne outbreaks of diarrheal illness. As with other causes of acute food poisoning, improper storage of food is often implicated.

Gastrointestinal symptoms begin within 2 days of *Salmonella* infection. Nausea, vomiting, abdominal cramps, and diarrhea are the most common symptoms. Fever occurs in about 50 percent of patients. The diarrhea associated with *Salmonella* infection is usually profuse and watery and may be dysenteric. In uncomplicated cases, which is the usual situation in healthy adults, symptoms subside within 48 to 72 hours and recovery is uneventful. In hosts compromised by the extremes of age or by underlying illness, infection can be complicated by bacteremia and localization to extraintestinal sites (such as bone or the meninges). For the normal host with uncomplicated illness, antibiotic therapy is usually not necessary because treatment may not affect the clinical course and may prolong the duration of convalescent excretion of the organism.

Shigella species (*dysenteriae, flexneri, boydii,* and *sonnei*) are the traditional causes of "bacillary dysentery."[6] Because humans are the only reservoir of *Shigella,* infection occurs after person-to-person contact or fecal-oral spread. This is a particular problem with young children in day-care settings, in custodial institutions, and among sexually active homosexual men. Most infections with *Shigella* in the United States are limited to these groups, with the highest frequency occurring in children less than 10 years of age. However, in the developing world, *Shigella* may occur in many age groups and becomes a risk for the international traveler. The spread between individuals is also aided by the low inoculum needed for infection—often only 200 organisms or less.

Within 3 days after infection with *Shigella,* clinical illness occurs and is characterized by fever and abdominal cramping, initially associated with watery diarrhea and then dysenteric stools. Rectal urgency and tenesmus are usually seen. In small children, hyperpyrexia and seizures may occur. Although illness with *Shigella* may be self-limited, antimicrobial therapy is indicated to shorten the duration of diarrhea and fever and to prevent further fecal-oral spread of the pathogen.

Other bacterial causes of inflammatory diarrhea include specific serotypes of invasive *E. coli*.[13] These may be difficult to identify because most persons excrete *E. coli* in their stools. A new syndrome of hemorrhagic diarrhea has been associated with *E. coli*, serotype 0157:H7, which has been seen after ingestion of improperly cooked meats, often in fast-food chains. Several other vibrios besides *Vibrio cholerae*, particularly *Vibrio parahemolyticus*, have been associated with gastrointestinal illness after the ingestion of inadequately cooked seafood. Outbreaks of *V. parahemolyticus* have been documented on cruise ships, in coastal communities, and in Japan. The disease is usually fairly mild and limited to about 3 days.

Yersinia enterocolitica can produce inflammatory diarrhea in adults or children, a syndrome of mesenteric adenitis in adolescents that mimics appendicitis, and a systemic illness similar to typhoid fever. Diagnosis of *Yersinia* is difficult because isolation of the organism requires special culture techniques. If *Yersinia* occurs in an outbreak and it can be recognized, antimicrobial therapy is often helpful in limiting the illness.

Pseudomembranous colitis is a syndrome caused by the anaerobe *Clostridium difficile*. It has been most commonly associated with previous or concomitant antibiotic use, which alters the normal enteric flora, allowing pathogenic *C. difficile* to overgrow and to cause disease. Pseudomembranous colitis occurs in about 1 percent of individuals taking the antibiotic clindamycin. This syndrome also has occurred with many other antibiotics. The patient usually experiences fever, abdominal pain, and diarrhea, which is frequently bloody. When the disease is suspected, sigmoidoscopy should be performed. Pseudomembranous colitis is characterized by the finding of multiple yellow-white mucosal plaques which may become confluent. The diagnosis is confirmed by the detection of *C. difficile* toxin in stool samples. In many cases, diarrhea will improve once the incriminating antibiotic is discontinued; however, in other cases it will be necessary to administer vancomycin or metronidazole.

Parasitic Agents

Entamoeba histolytica is an enteric protozoan responsible for most dysentery secondary to parasites.[22,26] Of the several amoebas that inhabit humans, *E. histolytica* is the only important pathogen. It has a worldwide distribution. *Entamoeba* cyst prevalence ranges from 3 to 4 percent in the United States to as high as 30 to 50 percent in tropical areas. As many as 450 million persons are infected worldwide, with the majority being asymptomatic carriers of the organism. Transmission of *Entamoeba* is usually through fecally contaminated foodstuffs, but it may also occur through contaminated water and by person-to-person transfer. This latter mode is important in the United States between sexually active homosexual men and within custodial institutions. Because humans are the only reservoir of infection, the chronic carrier is an important link in the epidemiology of amoebiasis.

Infection occurs after ingestion of the *Entamoeba* cyst form and enteric release of trophozoites which infect the colon and occasionally the terminal ileum. The pathogenicity of amoebae relates to strain virulence, host resistance, and local intestinal conditions.

Although *E. histolytica* usually produces only intestinal disease, extraintestinal amoebiasis (primarily hepatic abscesses) occurs in about 5 percent of all cases. Intestinal *Entamoeba* infection ranges from asymptomatic cyst passage (90 percent of cases) in most individuals to mild, intermittent diarrhea in some and even to dysenteric colitis in a few. Dysenteric colitis is characterized by frequent, small, blood-tinged stools. These are usually accompanied by abdominal pain, weight loss, and fever. Amoebic disease may resolve spontaneously, or it may last for weeks and even become fulminating and lead to intestinal perforation and death. Patients with an amoebic liver abscess often give a history of low-grade fever and chronic pain in the right upper abdominal quadrant with local tenderness on palpation.

The diagnosis of amoebiasis should be suspected in the differential diagnosis of dysentery and ulcerative colitis and in individuals with diarrhea who give an appropriate exposure history. Diagnosis of *Entamoeba* intestinal disease is confirmed by the demonstration of trophozoites in the stools or ulcer scrapings obtained by sigmoidoscopy. Sigmoidoscopy also will often reveal numerous discrete ulcerations covered by a yellowish necrotic film. Serologic testing is helpful if stools are negative. About 85 percent of persons with invasive *Entamoeba* intestinal disease and over 95 percent of patients with amoebic liver abscesses will have antibodies to the organism. Patients with amoebic liver abscesses usually will not have concomitant dysentery. When amoebiasis is diagnosed, the disease should be treated (see discussion of treatment later in this chapter).

Traveler's Diarrhea

Traveler's diarrhea is an illness that affects 30 to 50 percent of Americans who travel to developing countries.[5] Although the illness is usually mild and lasts for only a few days, it can alter one's planned activities significantly, be they athletic, recreational, or business. Many an athlete's performance has been adversely affected by a debilitating gastrointestinal illness. Travelers to Latin America, Africa, the Middle East, and Asia are at highest risk. Areas with intermediate risk are some of the Caribbean islands and southern Europe. The disease occurs after the traveler ingests food or water that has been fecally contaminated. Commonly contaminated foods include raw fruits and vegetables, uncooked meat, and fresh seafood. For travelers to the developing countries it is good to remember the old adage: "If you can't boil it, cook it, or peel it, forget it."

The etiologies of traveler's diarrhea are listed in Table 16–3. There are probably other, as yet undescribed, causes, since in only 50 to 70 percent of cases is the causative agent identified. Enterotoxigenic *E. coli* is the most common cause of traveler's diarrhea,

Table 16–3. ETIOLOGIES OF TRAVELER'S DIARRHEA

Enterotoxigenic *E. coli*
Shigella
Salmonella
Campylobacter jejuni
Aeromonas hydrophila
Vibrios
Rotavirus
Norwalk agent
Giardia lamblia
Entamoeba histolytica
Cryptosporidium

accounting for about 50 percent of cases. Another 10 to 20 percent of the cases are caused by *Shigella* or *Salmonella*. *Aeromonas, Campylobacter*, and *Vibrios* are some of the other bacteria which are less common causes of traveler's diarrhea. The Norwalk virus and rotavirus cause diarrhea in 5 to 15 percent of travelers. Of the parasitic agents that infect travelers, giardiasis occurs in about 5 percent of individuals, and amoebiasis occurs even less frequently. As noted previously in this chapter, travelers who acquire *Giardia* may not become symptomatic until after they return home. In the early 1970s, travelers to Leningrad were found to have an increased risk of acquiring *Giardia*, a risk that may still continue to this time. *Cryptosporidum* is a newly recognized protozoan of humans that has been found to be a rare cause of watery diarrhea in travelers.[24] Another unusual parasitic cause of diarrhea is *Strongyloides stercoralis*, which is limited to long-term travelers in an endemic area, particularly the developing world.

Traveler's diarrhea usually occurs within the first week of arrival in a new country (median 6 to 13 days). Diarrhea and abdominal cramps are accompanied by nausea and malaise in 50 percent of persons. Fever up to 38°C (100.4°F) occurs in 10 to 20 percent of affected individuals. Vomiting is less common. Bloody stools or dysentery are also seen infrequently (2 to 10 percent). For most travelers affected with diarrhea, the duration of illness is usually only 3 to 4 days, and 60 percent of individuals will be better in less than 48 hours. Although there has been much interest in the prevention of traveler's diarrhea by pharmacologic agents, the potential complications of this preventative therapy have shifted attention to the exercise of greater caution with food and water.

Enteric Fever

Enteric fever is a systemic illness that occurs primarily in the developing countries. It is characterized by sustained fever; headache; profound malaise; and abdominal pain, tenderness, and distention. Typhoid fever, the most common enteric fever, is caused by *Salmonella typhi*, which is transmitted through the ingestion of food or water contaminated by the feces or the urine of an infected patient.[9] After an incubation period of

10 to 14 days, fever usually rises in a step-wise fashion and then becomes sustained over several days. Although diarrhea may be present initially, constipation is more likely in the later stages of disease. Unless antimicrobial therapy intervenes, the sustained toxicity of typhoid fever over a 2- to 3-week period can profoundly exhaust the patient and lead to multiple complications, such as pneumonia, gastrointestinal hemorrhage, and perforation. Additional, less common causes of enteric fever are *Yersinia enterocolitica*, *Campylobacter fetus*, and other *Salmonella* bacteria.

MANAGEMENT

Fluid and Electrolytes

The most important therapeutic modality in the treatment of diarrhea is the replacement of fluids and electrolytes lost in the diarrheal stools.[12,14] In many cases this is the only treatment necessary, because the diarrheal illness will be self-limited and of short duration. In most diarrheas in which the pathogen involves the upper small bowel or colon, glucose-coupled sodium and water absorption remains intact. The classic example of this is in toxigenic diarrheas, either from *V. cholerae* or enterotoxigenic *E. coli*, in which the volume lost in stools may be replaced simply by an equal oral volume of glucose, salt, and water. In most cases, rehydration can occur via the oral route, except when rapid reversal of dehydration is required or when there is significant vomiting.

Table 16–4 lists two formulas for the preparation of rehydration fluids.[4,12] Oral rehydration can be accomplished by ingesting potable fruit juices, caffeine-free soft drinks, broths, and bouillons. These may be supplemented with salted crackers, rice, or toast. In general, dairy products initially should be avoided because there might be an associated lactose intolerance. Products with caffeine, very cold or very hot drinks, spicy or fatty foods, and roughage also should be avoided because they may worsen symptoms. As the patient improves, the diet may be gradually increased to bland solids, such as bananas, chicken, potatoes, and pasta given in frequent small feedings.

Nonantimicrobial Agents

Prevention

There has been much interest in the use of both antimotility agents, such as loperamide (Imodium) and diphenoxylate (Lomotil), and nonspecific agents, such as bismuth subsali-

Table 16–4. ORAL REHYDRATION FLUIDS

Chemical Formula	*grams/liter*
glucose	20
potassium chloride (KCl)	1.5
sodium chloride (NaCl)	3.5
sodium citrate*	2.9

General Formula†

Drink alternately between glasses until thirst is quenched. These liquids may be supplemented with other caffeine-free liquids as needed. Salted crackers may be added. The diet may be slowly advanced to contain lactose-free, bland foods which are given in frequent small meals as tolerated.

Glass No. 1	*Amount*
Orange, apple, or other potable fruit juice (rich in potassium)	8 ounces
Honey or corn syrup (contains glucose necessary for absorption of salts; table sugar [1 tbsp.] may be substituted)	½ teaspoon
Table salt (sodium and chloride)	1 pinch
Glass No. 2	
Potable water	8 ounces
Baking soda (contains sodium bicarbonate)	¼ teaspoon

*Sodium bicarbonate, 2.5 grams/liter, may be substituted.
†Modified from Centers for Disease Control,[4] p 148.

cylate (Pepto-Bismol) and kaolin/pectin (KaoPectate), in the prevention of diarrhea.[5] Unfortunately, the antiperistaltic agents have not proven to be effective in the prevention of traveler's diarrhea. And although studies have demonstrated reduction in the incidence of diarrhea in international travelers by the prophylactic use of bismuth subsalicylate, the protection remains only modest. Also, in certain individuals, long-term bismuth ingestion may lead to toxicities, particularly in those persons on high-dose aspirin therapy.

Treatment

Once the illness has developed, antimotility agents, including both loperamide and diphenoxylate, and natural opiates (paragoric, tincture of opium, and codeine) generally afford some control of diarrhea and relief of abdominal cramping. So the use of these medications may often make it possible for infected individuals to participate in their planned activities. One should be cautious, however, in the use of these agents. When there is fever in excess of 38.5°C (101°F) and blood and mucus in the stool, antimotility drugs may obscure the symptoms of inflammatory diarrhea. In shigellosis, antiperistaltic agents have been demonstrated to prolong both the clinical illness and the excretion of infectious organisms. Pepto-Bismol tablets will accomplish a modest reduction in traveler's diarrhea, according to some reports.[7]

In those few cases of acute infectious gastroenteritis marked by severe vomiting, parenteral antiemetics also may be required. In the adult with persistent vomiting, prochlorperazine (Compazine) may be administered orally (5 to 10 mg, 3 or 4 times daily), via rectal suppository (25 mg twice daily), or by intramuscular injection (5 to 10 mg every 4 hours as needed). Promethazine hydrochloride (Phenergan) also may be used orally (25 mg every 4 to 6 hours), by suppository or intramuscularly in the same dosages.

A special note should be made when dealing with competitive athletes to meticulously consult the rules of the specific sport's governing body concerning banned medications (see Chapter 12). As of this writing, the antimotility agents loperamide (Imodium) and diphenoxylate (Lomotil) are acceptable for use by competitors in International Olympic Committee (IOC) sanctioned events; whereas paragoric, tincture of opium, and codeine *are not.* And although prochlorperazine (Compazine) and promethazine hydrochloride (Phenergan) antiemetics may be used by most athletes competing in IOC events, these drugs may be banned for shooters. Whenever any doubt about the use of a drug exists, it is wise to consult the United States Olympic Committee Drug Control Hotline 1-800-233-0393.

Antimicrobial Agents

Prevention

Numerous antibacterials have also been studied for the prevention of diarrhea while traveling. Among them are doxycycline, trimethoprim, and trimethoprim with sulfamethoxazole. Although these antibacterials decrease the incidence of diarrhea to 5 to 15 percent for the short-term trip of 3 weeks or less, this is probably just about the same incidence of diarrhea found in travelers who simply exercise due caution about their food and water ingestion. Prophylactic antibacterial medications may cause serious allergic reactions in a small number of individuals, and adverse drug side effects, such as photosensitivity from doxycycline, may occur in others. Furthermore, other infections such as vaginal candidiasis and pseudomembranous colitis can develop in patients on antibacterial drugs; and the treatment of those individuals who do develop diarrheal illness while on a prophylactic antibacterial agent becomes complex. Therefore, a consensus panel on traveler's diarrhea found that the average traveler should not take antibacterial medications prophylactically to prevent what is usually only a mild illness.[5] On the other hand, antimicrobial prophylaxis can be considered after the potential risks are explained to short-term travelers on particularly important trips; for instance, athletes engaged in competition and those with medical conditions that would be adversely affected by diarrhea.

Treatment

Table 16–5 lists the agents used for the antimicrobial treatment of diarrhea caused by several of the most common pathogens. *Campylobacter* is the most common etiology of inflammatory diarrhea in the adult resid-

Table 16–5. ANTIMICROBIAL THERAPY OF DIARRHEAS

Enteric Agent	Antimicrobial†	Dosage*	
		Adult‡	Pediatric§
Campylobacter	Erythromycin	250 mg qid × 5–7 d	40–50 mg/kg/d in 4 doses × 5–10 d
Shigella	Ampicillin	2–4 g/d in 4 doses × 5–7 d	50 mg/kg/d in 4 doses × 5 d
	Trimethoprim (TMP)/ Sulfamethoxazole (SMX)	1 double strength (d.s.) tab (160 mg TMP/800 mg SMX) bid × 5 d	5 mg (TMP)/kg q 12 h × 5 d
	Tetracycline	2.5 g in a single dose	Not used in children
Salmonella	Ampicillin	See *Shigella*	See *Shigella*
	TMP/SMX	See *Shigella*	See *Shigella*
Traveler's diarrhea	SMX/TMP	1 d.s. tab bid × 3–5 d	4 mg (TMP)/kg bid × 3–5 d
	Trimethoprim	200 mg bid × 3–5 d	4 mg/kg bid × 3–5 d
	Doxycycline	100 mg bid × 3–5 d	Not used in children
	Ciprofloxacin	500 mg bid × 3–5 d	Not used in children
Giardia lamblia	Quinacrine	100 mg tid × 5–7 d	2 mg/kg tid × 5–7 d
	Metronidazole	250 mg tid × 7 d	5 mg/kg tid × 7 d
	Furazolidone	100 mg qid × 7–10 d	2 mg/kg qid × 10 d
Entamoeba histolytica¶ (invasive)	Metronidazole PLUS	750 mg tid × 10 d	35–50 mg/kg/d in 3 doses × 10 d
	Diiodohydroxyquine	650 mg tid × 20 d	30–40 mg/kg/d in 3 doses × 20 d
(carrier)	Diiodohydroxyquine	650 mg tid × 20 d	30–40 mg/kg/d in 3 doses × 20 d

*All doses are for oral administration.
†Each medication has important potential side effects and contraindications. Full prescribing information should be consulted.
‡The letter d indicates day.
§Pediatric doses should not exceed the adult dose.
¶Please refer to the references for alternative regimens.[23,27]

ing in the United States and will constitute the majority of the cases of this syndrome that present acutely to a physician's office or emergency room. Therefore erythromycin therapy can be administered to the patient empirically for *Campylobacter* while awaiting return of the cultures. However, if the patient has a travel-related dysentery or is in a risk category for *Shigella* infection (i.e., sexually active homosexual men, residents of custodial institutions), therapy for *Shigella* should be started. Trimethoprim/sulfamethoxazole is the treatment of choice for shigellosis when microbial susceptibility is unknown and when *Shigella* isolates are commonly resistant to ampicillin and tetracycline.[6] Ampicillin or tetracycline can be used in the treatment of shigellosis when the organism is sensitive to these drugs. A new class of an-

tibiotics, the quinolones, may help avoid the difficulty of deciding which antibiotic to initiate, because the quinolones cover both *Campylobacter* and *Shigella*.[10] Norfloxacin (400 mg by mouth twice daily for 5 days)—although it has not yet been approved by the Food and Drug Administration (FDA) for treatment of diarrhea—and ciprofloxacin (500 mg by mouth twice daily for 5 days) are two quinolones currently available.

As discussed earlier, most *Salmonella* infections in the healthy young adult do not require antimicrobial therapy. (*Salmonella* infections should be treated, however, in immunocompromised hosts and patients at the extremes of age.)

Traveler's diarrhea that is moderate to severe can be treated with 3 to 5 days of trimethoprim/sulfamethoxazole, trimethoprim alone, doxycycline, or a quinolone.[7,10,17] Therapy will shorten the duration of this illness to 1 or 2 days.

Parasitic diarrheas should be identified and then treated. The treatment of choice for giardiasis in adults is either quinacrine for 5 days or metronidazole for 7 days. These regimens have 80 to 95 percent efficacy rates. Furazolidone is an alternative for children because it comes in a liquid suspension.[21] Paromomycin has been used successfully in pregnant patients without known untoward effects.

There are many treatment regimens for amoebiasis which depend upon preference of the physician and the location of the parasite in the host, whether the bowel lumen, intestinal submucosa, or extraintestinal site.[23] Tissue disease (invasive intestinal and hepatic amoebiasis) is usually treated with metronidazole. This drug is combined with or followed by an intraluminal agent, usually diiodohydroxyquine, to prevent relapse of the amoebic infection. Before any of these antimicrobials are used, the contraindications and potential side effects should be considered.

PREVENTION

The basic prevention measure for enteric infections is interruption of the fecal-oral transmission of bacteria, viruses, and protozoa. This requires the provision of potable water and the proper disposal of sewage. For the individual, excellent personal hygiene is necessary, with frequent washing of hands especially for food handlers. Chlorination of water may not be sufficient to kill *Giardia* cysts; so municipal water supplies should be subjected to flocculation, sedimentation, and filtration, as well as chlorination. To prevent food-borne illnesses, foods should be completely cooked and not allowed to sit for long periods at room temperature before being eaten. For individuals in the field, water for personal use should be brought to a boil or treated with fresh chlorine or iodine preparations such as Halazone or Potable Aqua. One method for field treatment of water is to make a saturated solution of crystalline iodine. Twelve and one half milliliters of this solution is added to a 1 liter poly bottle of the water to be purified and allowed to stand for 30 minutes.[19] Adjustments must be made for turbid or extremely cold water (see Chapter 45).

SUMMARY

Diarrheal illness is a major problem both in the United States and in the developing world. Differentiation of the several clinical syndromes and proper recognition of the offending infectious agents will go a long way toward decreasing the considerable morbidity from this illness.

Several points emerge in the management of patients with infectious gastrointestinal syndromes. The first is the distinction of inflammatory from noninflammatory diarrhea. Inflammatory diarrhea, associated with invasive infectious agents, usually requires specific intervention, including stool cultures, antimicrobial therapy, and close observation of the patient. Noninflammatory diarrhea is most often self-limited and can be treated with symptomatic therapy. For all diarrheal syndromes, patients should be adequately hydrated until the disease subsides. Fortunately, this can most often be done by administering balanced salt/glucose solutions orally.

Traveler's diarrhea can be prevented most effectively by exercising care when ingesting food and beverages in the developing world. Both antibiotics and judicious use of antimotility agents may be indicated to treat this syndrome.

Finally, there are some unique syndromes to which the clinician should be alert. Giardiasis should be considered in those persons who have diarrhea lasting for more than 10 to 14 days. A stool for ova and parasites will need to be ordered to make this diagnosis.

Effective management of diarrheal illnesses will lead in almost all cases to prompt recovery with a minimum of interruption of travel schedules and sporting activities.

REFERENCES

1. Blacklow, NR and Cukor, G: Viral gastroenteritis. N Engl J Med 304:397–406, 1981.
2. Blaser, MJ and Reller, LB: Campylobacter enteritis. N Engl J Med 305:1444–1452, 1981.
3. Blaser, MJ, Wells, JG, Feldman, RA, Pollard, RA, and Allen, JR: Campylobacter enteritis in the United States: A multicenter study. Ann Int Med 98:360–366, 1983.
4. Centers for Disease Control: Health Information for

International Travel. HHS Publication No. (CDC) 88-8280, May 1988. (Write Superintendent of Documents, US Government Printing Office, Washington, DC 20402, or telephone (202) 783-3238.)

5. Consensus Development Conference Statement: Traveler's diarrhea. Rev Infect Dis 8:S227–S233, 1986.

6. DuPont, HL: Shigella species (Bacillary dysentery). In Mandell, GL, Douglas, RG, and Bennett, JE (eds): Principles and Practice of Infectious Diseases, ed 2. John Wiley & Sons, New York, 1985, pp 1269–1274.

7. DuPont, HL, Ericsson, CD, and Johnson, PC: Chemotherapy and chemoprophylaxis of traveler's diarrhea. Ann Int Med 102:260–261, 1985.

8. DuPont, HL, Reves, RR, Galindo, E, Sullivan, PS, Wood, LV, and Mendiola, JG: Treatment of traveler's diarrhea with trimethoprim/sulfamethoxazole and with trimethoprim alone. N Engl J Med 307:841–844, 1982.

9. Edelman, R and Levine, MM: Summary of an international workshop on typhoid fever. Rev Infect Dis 8:329–349, 1986.

10. Ericsson, CD, Johnson, PC, DuPont, HL, Morgan, DR, Bitsura, JA, and de la Cabada, FJ: Ciprofloxacin or trimethoprim-sulfamethoxazole as initial therapy for traveler's diarrhea. Ann Int Med 106:216–220, 1987.

11. Erlandsen, SL and Meyer, EA (eds): Giardia and Giardiasis. Plenum Press, New York, 1984.

12. Guerrant, RL: Principles and definitions of syndromes. In Mandell, GL, Douglas, RG, and Bennett, JE (eds): Principles and Practice of Infectious Diseases, ed 2. John Wiley & Sons, New York, pp 635–646.

13. Guerrant, RL: Inflammatory enteritides. In Mandell, GL, Douglas, RG, and Bennett, JE (eds): Principles and Practice of Infectious Diseases, ed 2. John Wiley & Sons, New York, 1985, pp 660–669.

14. Guerrant, RL and Hughes, JM: Nausea, vomiting and noninflammatory diarrhea. In Mandell, GL, Douglas, RG, and Bennett, JE (eds): Principles and Practice of Infectious Diseases, ed 2. John Wiley & Sons, New York, 1985, pp 646–655.

15. Hill, DR: Giardia lamblia. In Mandell, GL, Douglas, RG, and Bennett, JE (eds): Principles and Practice of Infectious Diseases, ed 2. John Wiley & Sons, New York, 1985, pp 1552–1556.

16. Hill, DR and Pearson, RD: Health advice for international travel. Ann Intern Med 108:839–852, 1988.

17. Hook, EW: Salmonella species (including typhoid fever). In Mandell, GL, Douglas, RG, and Bennett, JE (eds): Principles and Practice of Infectious Diseases, ed 2. John Wiley & Sons, New York, 1985, pp 1256–1269.

18. Hughes, JM: Food Poisoning. In Mandell, GL, Douglas, RG, and Bennett, JE (eds): Principles and Practice of Infectious Diseases, ed 2. John Wiley & Sons, New York, 1985, pp 680–689.

19. Kahn, FH and Visscher, BR: Water disinfection in the wilderness. West J Med 122:450–453, 1975.

20. Kaplan, JE, Gary, GW, Baron, RC, Singh, N, Schonberger, LB, Feldman, R, and Greenberg, HB: Epidemiology of Norwalk gastroenteritis and the role of Norwalk virus in outbreaks of nonbacterial gastroenteritis. Ann Int Med 96:(Part 1):756–761, 1982.

21. Lerman, SJ and Walker, RA: Treatment of giardiasis. Literature review and recommendations. Clin Pediatr 21:409–414, 1982.

22. Martinez-Palomo, A and Martinez-Baez, M: Selective primary health care: Strategies for control of disease in the developing world. X. Amebiasis. Rev Infect Dis 5:1093–1102, 1983.

23. Drugs for parasitic infections. Medical Letter 30:15–22, 1988.

24. Navin, TR and Juranek, DD: Cryptosporidiosis: Clinical, epidemiologic and parasitologic review. Rev Infect Dis 6:313–327, 1984.

25. Pichler, HET, et al: Clinical efficacy of ciprofloxacin compared with placebo in bacterial diarrhea. Am J Med 82 (Suppl 4A):329–332, 1987.

26. Ravdin, JI (ed): Amebiasis: Human Infection by Entamoeba Histolytica. John Wiley & Sons, New York, 1988.

27. Strickland, GT (ed): Hunter's Tropical Medicine, ed 6. WB Saunders, Philadelphia, 1984.

CHAPTER 17

Skin Problems in Winter Sports

RODNEY S. W. BASLER, M.D.

The skin, positioned at the anatomic and functional interface between the organism and its environment, is subjected to a number of stress factors in the course of winter sports. Many of these factors are experienced by athletes and participants in other settings as well,[2,4] but some result from the specific climatic conditions of cold, ice, and snow. Protective measures can prevent many of the common forms of cutaneous injury observed in winter sports, and other pathologic states are easily observed and rarely require lengthy cessation of activities when treated appropriately.

PHOTOINJURY

Although seemingly paradoxical, some of the more troublesome cutaneous problems encountered during the winter months are actually due to overexposure to the sun. Many winter sports are outdoor activities; therefore, open-air enthusiasts from ice skaters to mountain climbers must be mindful of the continuous exposure they may receive from direct, absorbed, and reflected sunlight.[2] In addition, the midday light hours with the most intense sun rays are those which are often sought for these activities because of their relative warmth.[1] Incident sun rays reflected from ice and snow to the anterior neck and under the chin can result in burns to these areas which usually do not have the toughening effect of frequent exposure. Furthermore, most hats and many other head coverings used in recreational sports offer no protection against reflected rays from below. Acute sunburn of the neck is commonly seen in unprotected skiers (Fig. 17–1).

A potentiating factor for sunburn, seen particularly in skiing and mountain climbing, is the intensification of sunlight with altitude. Ultraviolet rays from the sun have 20 percent greater potential for causing cutaneous injury at 5000 feet altitude than at sea level.[8]

When planning winter outings, the athlete should be mindful of the need to protect against photoinjury. Fortunately, there are a wide variety of commercially available chemical sunscreens from which to choose. Each is rated for its "sun-protective factor," or SPF. This rating, which ranges from 2 to 15, represents the multiple of the unit of time that skin can be exposed to sunlight after application of the product and still show the same biologic effect as unprotected skin.[5] For example, one can be exposed to the sun twice as long for the same reaction using a sunscreen of SPF 2, or six times longer with one of SPF 6. Generally, sunscreens with an SPF of 10 to 15 are recommended for lengthy outdoor winter activity. Special care must be taken to cover all exposed areas evenly to

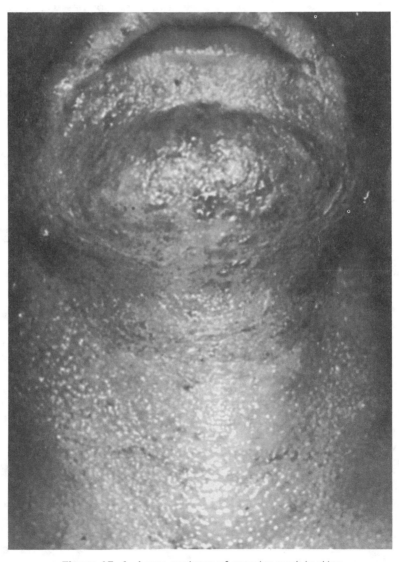

Figure 17–1. Acute sunburn of anterior neck in skier.

prevent the often surprising appearance of sunburn "islands."[3] If perspiration should be a problem, a sunscreen with superior ability to maintain efficacy while subjected to moisture (a property termed "substantivity") should be used.[3]

Treatment of acute sunburn depends upon the severity of the photoinjury. In most instances mild to moderate cutaneous inflammation will abate in 24 to 48 hours without treatment. Emollient moisturizers and internal anti-inflammatory drugs are of some palliative benefit. In more severe cases of photoinjury with vesicle or bulla formation, topical and even systemic corticosteroids may be indicated.[1]

WIND

Wind is a consistent environmental factor that confronts outdoor-sports enthusiasts and may be magnified in winter sports. Harsh cold winds can potentiate other winter factors and add to the discomfort and sometimes injury of the skin. The damaging effects of sunlight are intensified by wind, as are the deleterious effects of cold. Wind also contributes significantly to skin dehydration, causing the familiar winter dryness which results in erythema, scaling, and other eczematous changes of exposed areas; and dry, parched, cracked lips and nostrils. To minimize these consequences, heavy applications of oil-based ointments and emollients are recommended before and after skiing, skating, climbing, and ice fishing in harsh winter winds.

JOGGING EXPOSURE

With the popularity of jogging carried over to the winter months and with the importance of this activity in training programs, we are beginning to see dermatologic problems in runners caused by exposure to the windy, cold environment. Many of the problems can be avoided by proper preparation for cold-weather jogging.

In dressing for winter jogging, multiple layers of light clothing should be worn. Air trapped between the layers retains body heat and acts as an insulator against the cold. Special precautions must be made to cover the anterior neck, sometimes referred to as the most vulnerable square inch of skin on the human body. To protect the neck, turtleneck sweaters and wool scarves are commonly employed but are often a bad choice. Heat and perspiration sensitize the neck, making it particularly susceptible to irritation from wool and synthetic fibers found in most scarves and sweaters. A much better approach is wrapping a terry cloth towel around the neck. This fabric is less irritating and much more absorbent, while offering an equivalent barrier against cold. It is important that all areas of the body be afforded equal protection from clothing. The much distressing injury of penile frostbite may occur when the jogger is protected below the waist by only polyester pants and underwear with an anterior opening[7] (see Chapters 18 and 27).

Another simple recommendation for winter joggers and all other outdoor-sports enthusiasts is to postpone shaving and washing exposed areas from the morning until after facing the elements, because natural sebum offers a certain degree of protection against wind and cold. The application of oils in the form of lotions and ointments contributes to an additional insulating effect. Although the use of such ointments over the nose and cheeks may seem somewhat messy, it is considerably less of an inconvenience to most joggers than wearing a ski mask. The application of a creamy sunscreen is a practical means of defending simultaneously against two potential forms of injury.

SKIER'S TOES

Discoloration of the nailbeds of the great toes, usually bilateral, is seen in skiers who have a habit of leaning forward. This tender phenomenon, referred to as "skier's toe" (Fig. 17–2), is due to subungual hemorrhage caused by lateral shearing of the superficial nailbed capillaries as the plate is forced into the anterior portion of the ski boot. Although this condition is more likely with the use of ill-fitting equipment, even skiers with properly fitting boots may suffer from it. A simple precaution for those who are prone to this injury is the paring of the nail plate as far proximally as possible without pain. Acute care includes penetrating the nail with a hot object, such as a cautery point or the time-honored red-hot paper clip. Warm-water soaks will, in time, bring relief to those without the

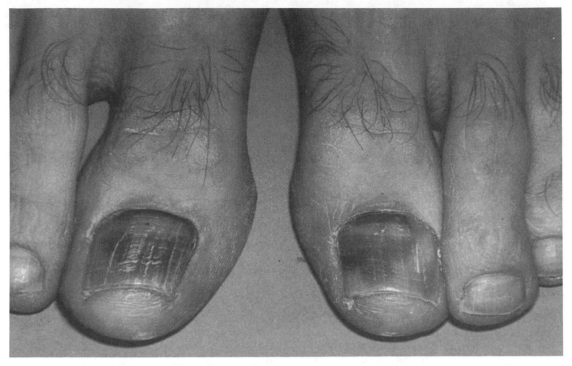

Figure 17–2. "Skier's toes."

necessary equipment or fortitude to carry out the aforementioned procedures.

CHILBLAINS

Chilblains, or pernio, is a relatively uncommon but distressful cutaneous problem that develops during periods of exposure to cold, damp environments (see Chapter 18). This form of cold injury is characterized by the appearance of exquisitely tender pruritic and painful red to violaceous discolorations of the skin. Young adults, especially women, are most commonly affected. The distal digits, particularly the toes, are now the most frequently affected areas. Historically, chilblains was associated with work and life in the cold damp climates of northern Europe. Now the onset often coincides with ski trips and other outings of unusual exposure to cold and high humidity.

The fact that resolution of chilblains can be expected spontaneously as summer, with its sustained warmth, approaches offers little solace to the winter athlete. In those who are afflicted with this condition, every effort must be made to keep the extremities warm at all times—not only when outdoors. Heavy woolen stockings should be worn when inside, even while sleeping. Careful attention should be given to prevent constriction of the feet and hands from tightly fitting boots or gloves. Vasodilators, such as nitroglycerin, and low-potency topical corticosteroids to relieve inflammation may be of some value in the treatment of chilblains.

FRICTION BLISTERS

One of the more common skin injuries encountered by cross-country skiers, winter hikers, and especially mountain climbers is the friction blister. Even minor friction, continuously applied, can result in the separation of the epidermis from the dermis with the resulting accumulation of tissue exudate in the dead space. This process is accentuated in those sports which have been specifically mentioned, because the terrain, if acceptably challenging, is never even. In climbing up, the heels usually suffer; while climbing down, the toes suffer.[9] Ill-fitting boots, impossible to exchange in the deserted wilderness, can prove disastrous on even a short weekend excursion.

Properly fitted boots with absorbent stockings are the best defense against friction blisters. Foot powders and double stockings, each of a different fabric, will diminish the friction applied directly to the foot. If blisters have formed, they are best treated by draining the collected fluid or blood three times within the first 24 hours and permitting the overlying epidermis to remain in place until it sloughs naturally.[6]

HOT-TUB INFECTIONS

One of the more pleasurable experiences associated with winter outings is a dip in the hot tub at the end of the day. Unfortunately, the warm, damp environment of the tub provides an overwhelmingly more hospitable environment for infectious organisms than the stark winter landscape. Of primary concern are the bacteria, particularly *Pseudomonas*, which thrive in the tepid water if the pH and chemical additives are not carefully regulated.

In addition, extended immersion in the hot tub, particularly while wearing a tightly fitting composition swimsuit, can lead to an occlusive folliculitis of the inferior buttocks, referred to as "bikini bottom."[4] Prevention of this irritating infection can be as simple as removing the suit for short periods and allowing the skin to dry completely before returning to the tub, or, in appropriate settings, eliminating it all together. Treatment with systemic antibiotics and topical antibiotic acne preparations, such as clindamycin and erythromycin solutions, usually results in rapid resolution of the condition.

OTHER BACTERIAL INFECTIONS

Regardless of the venue, exertion of any type is predictably associated with perspiration. Elevation of the body's core temperature in a well-bundled and insulated winter athlete will result in a similar degree of sweating to that seen in a summer jogger running in the briefest of uniforms. The negative effect of the moisture—namely, softening and maceration of the stratum corneum—is actually compounded by the

occlusion of the heavy clothing. Because the skin's primary defense against invasion by infective organisms is the desiccating effect of a dry, intact stratum corneum, maceration through occluded perspiration contributes to various types of infection. Bacteria and fungi find especially excellent breeding grounds in the warm damp skin under heavy winter clothing.

Bacterial folliculitis can occur over nearly any hair-bearing area of the body, but it is more commonly seen over the upper back, anterior thighs, and lower buttocks where the concentration of hair follicles is most dense. Crops of tender papules and small pustules develop in the affected areas and usually produce significant concomitant pruritus. Wearing absorbent cotton clothing next to the skin, such as a cotton T-shirt under jogging or ski gear, affords some measure of prevention. Treatment includes antibacterial cleansers, topical antibiotic solutions (such as clindamycin or erythromycin acne preparations), and occasionally systemic antibiotics.

FUNGAL INFECTIONS

The intimate association between athletes and fungi is evidenced by such North American colloquialisms as "athlete's foot" and "jock itch."[2] The macerating effect of occluded perspiration renders the skin vulnerable to penetration by ubiquitous fungi. The intertriginous parts of the body, especially the axillae, groin, and toe webs, are especially at risk from strains of both dermatophytes and yeasts. Consistent attention to elimination of moisture build-up is critical in preventing chronic irritation of this type of infection. Frequent changes of clean absorbent stockings and underclothing, as well as the application of foot and body powders, are of significant benefit. Although cornstarch is often used as a cheap, readily available substitute for powder, the nutrient effect of this preparation may actually promote microbial growth in some instances. Definitive treatment of fungal infection is difficult, and in many cases permanent cure is impossible. Topical and systemic agents, such as clotrimazole, tolnaftate, griseofulvin, and ketoconazole, may bring about temporary eradication but rarely lead to permanent resolution if conditions for the growth of organisms remain favorable. Nonetheless, significant symptomatic relief can almost always be achieved.

PHYSICAL URTICARIAS

Certain systemic conditions with cutaneous manifestations may be aggravated by physical factors inherent in winter sports participation. The most potentially disabling of these disorders are categorized as physical urticarias. Vascular reactions, such as acute hives and angioedema, mediated by histamine, are seen in this group, and their occurrence during otherwise pleasurable athletic endeavors may discourage an individual from further pursuing a specific activity. Cholinergic urticaria, cold urticaria, and mechanical urticaria are particularly irritating to the winter sports enthusiast, who might seek professional help because of the appearance of intensely pruritic, erythematous papules during outdoor activities. Treatment or prevention of the physical urticarias is usually only marginally successful, although it is not uncommon for the problem to ''burn out'' over time. H_2 antihistamines are more beneficial than H_1 antagonists in the management of most types of physical urticarias. H_2 antihistamines many be even more effective in combination with antiserotonin preparations. Systemic corticosteroids may be used prophylactically to provide relief in severely affected individuals when prescribed on a long-term, alternate-day basis, but use of these medications is banned for athletes participating in events sanctioned by the International Olympic Committee, the United States Olympic Committee, and many other sports governing bodies (see Chapter 12).

CONCLUSION

The special requirements and demands of the various winter sporting activities and the particular indoor and outdoor environments of the season supply the conditions for developing a number of dermatologic problems which can mildly or severely curtail these activities. Fortunately, many of these problems can be prevented with appropriate precautionary measures. Skin problems that do occur in association with winter sports are usually easily diagnosed, and in most cases they can be readily and effectively treated and relieved.

REFERENCES

1. Basler, RSW: Damaging effects of sunlight on human skin. Nebraska Medical Journal 63:337–340, 1978.
2. Basler, RSW: Skin lesions related to sports activity. Primary Care 10:479–494, 1983.
3. Basler, RSW: Sunscreens. Nebraska Medical Journal 68:162–165, 1983.
4. Basler, RSW: Dermatologic aspects of sports participation. Current Concepts in Skin Disorders 6:15–19, 1985.
5. Basler, RSW and Rheim, E: Sunlight and skin. Journal of Dermatology and Allergy 5:23–27, 1982.
6. Cortese, TA, Fukuyama, K, Epstein, WL, and Fulzberger, MB: Treatment of friction blisters. Arch Dermatol 97:717–721, 1968.
7. Hershkowitz, M: Penile frostbite, an unforeseen hazard of jogging. N Engl J Med 296:178, 1977.
8. Levine, N: Dermatologic aspects of sports medicine. J Am Acad Dermatol 3:415–424, 1980.
9. Mikelionis, J: Mountains, snow and skin. Cutis 20:346–347, 1977.

CHAPTER 18

Cold Injuries, Raynaud's Disease, and Hypothermia

MURRAY P. HAMLET, D.V.M.

With the great increase in outdoor activities, cold injury poses a rising threat for a large segment of the population in winter sports.

Traditionally, people involved in outdoor winter activities were hearty, thoughtful people who had some knowledge of protecting themselves from the cold.[32] With the increase in popularity of outdoor recreation, there has also been an increase in naiveté about the threat of cold-weather injuries. Moreover, people tend not to think about the risk of exposure to the cold for causing injuries while jogging or being run off the road while on a bicycle. If the injured runner or cyclist is not found in the winter, only a few minutes of exposure may result in significant risk for cold injury.

Although frostbite remains the single greatest cold-injury threat, cold also plays a role in other injuries. Because running has become such a popular sport with all ages and both sexes, it may be important to start this discussion on the threat of cold injury to runners. Runners, because of their high activity, tend to wear limited amounts of clothing with only wind protection. Cold-injury prevention is, in fact, the rational use of clothing. Exposed areas of the body—such as the face, ears, and hands—tend to be the highest risk areas. Protection of these parts is relatively simple. However, the sweat produced in running tends to collect in stocking caps, mittens, and gloves where it can freeze. An even greater threat to runners is being injured in the cold. Runners are often reclusive individuals, and their training areas are often isolated and remote. A slip and fall injury in the cold with the minimal protection usually worn for running then becomes a high-threat situation for that individual. There is often little likelihood of being found in a short time, and they are therefore subject to frostbite of the hands and feet.

Sports that increase the windchill factor also increase the risk of cold injury to exposed flesh.[3] Skiing, biking, and running increase the air flow over the face and, therefore, in cold weather increase the likelihood of frostbite. Protection of these exposed areas can take many forms. The use of topical medications to prevent injury has been widely touted, but there have been no solid research studies to verify this advocacy. There is little doubt that these oils, greases, and emollients prevent the drying and chapping of skin in the cold/dry air, but whether or not they protect the skin from frostbite is still open to question. Some of these materials definitely change one's perception of cold, but they may not change the freezing rate of skin. We have recently completed a study utilizing some of these compounds with a pig skin model. Although the data indicate that two of these compounds can slow the freezing rate of skin, the freezing is very superficial and when the skin does freeze, it is a more serious injury. So while a chemical like dimethyl sulfoxide (DMSO) does change the freezing rate of skin, it has limited usefulness in preventing cold injuries in sports.[12]

The question of whether or not beards prevent cold injury is frequently asked. Beards and mustaches do not protect against cold injury except for the cheeks, which are injured usually in a relatively minor way. The main advantage to having a beard in cold weather involves avoiding shaving. Shaving removes oils and the superficial epithelial layer of the skin, rendering the face more likely to dry and to crack in the cold. Wearing a beard keeps the face hydrated, leaves oils on the skin, and helps prevent chafing of the face caused by rubbing against clothing, parka hoods, and so forth.

PERFORMANCE IN THE COLD

Although it seems performance times in the cold tend to be slower than at warm temperatures, there have been few scientific studies on why this occurs. One can theorize that the relatively avascular joints cool rapidly when exposed to cold. As the joint fluid viscosity increases, more force is required to bend those joints, particularly the knee. Some loss in nerve conduction across the joints may also play a role in performance decrements.

CHILBLAINS

Chilblains is a localized itching and painful erythema seen in individuals subjected to working long periods in cold, damp environments (see Chapter 17). Although this was a common problem in the past, the present social structure in the United States tends to reduce this kind of injury.

In most cases, the effect of chilblains is short lived, and recovery is almost always complete. The swelling, itching, and tenderness of exposed flesh often recede within a few hours or overnight. Chilblains usually occurs in climates that are moderately cold with high humidity. Although the face and ears may be involved with chilblains, the hands, legs, and especially the feet and toes are most frequently affected. Tissue affected with chilblains appears red and swollen, and it is quite tender and hot to the touch. If vasoconstriction from cold alternating with vasodilation occurs chronically, the tissue becomes tense and purple, and blister formation may occur. Initial itching may be followed some days later by pain. In its acute form, chilblains is considered nothing more than an aggravation, but in the chronic form it can be mildly disabling, producing necrosis of the skin, ulcers, and scarring.

IMMERSION FOOT OR TRENCHFOOT

Immersion foot and trenchfoot are physiologically the same injury. They are caused by having cold wet extremities for an extended period of time. Immersion foot usually refers to a situation following shipwreck, when the extremity of an individual is immersed in water unable to get dry while the individual is sitting in a life raft. Whole body cooling is a significant part of the immersion injury. This is a time/temperature injury. The warmer the temperature, the longer the time required to produce immersion injury; but colder temperatures require shorter durations. Although this injury may be a threat to ocean travel, sailing, and perhaps wind surfing, the reporting of this injury in civilian literature is extremely rare. Even in peacetime military experience, immersion foot is rare. Shipwrecked individuals are usually found quickly or lost, and survivors are not exposed long enough to produce this injury. Trenchfoot involves cold wet exposure on land and is quite similar to immersion foot. Immobilization and dependency of cold, wet limbs combine with the blunt trauma of walking to produce this injury.

Although some immersion-type pathology can occur in as little as 12 hours of exposure to the wet and cold, most serious injuries are produced after 3 days or more of exposure. This injury goes through three phases of different durations and different severities: prehyperemic, hyperemic, and posthyperemic phases. There is a difference in tissue susceptibility to immersion injuries. The skin is quite resistant; but muscles and nerves are extremely susceptible to this cold, wet injury. Diagnosis of immersion injury and trenchfoot is by history and by the physical appearance of the extremity. Treatment consists of anti-inflammatory medications, elevation of the limb, mild cooling with a fan, and prevention of systemic infections. It should be noted that very little therapeutic value occurs from treatment of this injury. Generally the management is to wait and see the extent of injury, and then surgical debridement or amputation will be needed.

FROSTBITE

Frostbite results from actual freezing, causing ice crystal formation within the tissues. Frostbite injury is the most common cold injury during winter sporting events.

Pathophysiology

As tissue cools, the blood vessels constrict, decreasing blood flow.[18] This constriction may be circumferential in the digits, but it can occur also in bare areas of skin, such as the face. A combination of cooling and ischemia anesthetizes nerve endings, allowing tissue to freeze in a relatively painless manner.[27] Many individuals do not perceive themselves getting a frostbite injury and notice this only after the fact, when the skin is white, hard, and insensitive. This injury often progresses without discomfort for minutes or hours, thereby increasing the amount of frozen tissue and allowing the freezing front to advance proximally up the fingers or toes. Although tissue freezing is often anesthetic when it occurs, rewarming produces extreme pain. With warming, an initial rapid hyperemia occurs. This is followed within minutes by a sudden drop in blood flow, which results in ischemia of the extremity with subsequent cooling. The extent and severity of the frostbite injury now defines the amount of tissue that will be lost, and a line of demarcation will form in the next few days. Minor frostbite injuries recover with only mild hyperemia, swelling, and minimal pain. Deeper injuries involve full skin thickness damage, ischemia, cyanosis, blister formation, and eventual mummification of the necrotic tissue. As the injury progresses in severity, the line of demarcation becomes more obvious, occurs more quickly, and forms a 1 or 2 millimeter line of liquefaction between viable tissue and the mummifying eschar. In many cases this line of demarcation may occur quite early, but in other cases it may take weeks to clearly differentiate viable from nonviable tissue. Nonintervention in this process is an important part of frostbite therapy.

Treatment

Mild frostbite injuries of the face can be warmed with the palm of the hand or the back of a mitten. Although injuries to the face can initially be quite painful on rewarming, major tissue loss is uncommon. If the cartilage of the ear freezes, however, it will mummify and slough. Direct rubbing of the frozen tissue is contraindicated because damage to superficial epithelium may result. Injuries to extremities are more severe and pose greater clinical difficulties in management.[28–30] Frostbite to the hands and feet can pose a significant threat for loss of digits. Rewarming the frozen part is best accomplished either with body heat or warm water between 40 and 43°C (104 to 109°F).[1,2] Although rapid rewarming in water produces the greatest pain, it also produces the best tissue salvage. Temperatures over 43°C (109°F) can produce more injury; excessive heat during rewarming can produce devastating results. Physicians will seldom see solid frozen extremities because some degree of thaw has almost always occurred prior to hospitalization. Once rewarming has begun, it is ill advised to subsequently place the extremities in a warming bath. Twice daily whirlpooling at approximately 35°C (95°F) in water to which Betadine has been added is the treatment of choice. Complete range of motion exercise should be initiated immediately to preclude flexion contractures. If the frostbite injury is perceived to be deep, the use of intra-arterial reserpine appears to give the best long-lasting result.[5,33,34,36] Injection of reserpine 0.5 mg intra-arterially into each affected limb produces immediate vasodilation which may last throughout the entire treatment process. Subsequent injections may be necessary if vasospasm recurs. If the reserpine injection is done intra-arterially, no systemic blood pressure changes or tranquilization occurs. In order to prevent early infection, care should be taken not to rupture skin blisters which occur after rewarming. In most cases, blisters will slough spontaneously without any major infection problems several days into the treatment. Although the initial pain during rewarming may require some analgesia, most patients do not require pain medication for very long. Pulsatile pain late in treatment is best managed with intra-arterial reserpine. Although infections are rare, culture, sensitivity, and appropriate antibiotic therapy combined with reserpine will serve to heal them promptly. Early surgical intervention should be avoided. Severe frostbite injuries should be allowed to demarcate and mummify prior to undertaking any surgical procedure. This allows a clear demarcation of viable tissue, and if major amputation is indicated, it provides a good granular stump with fewer retraction problems and fewer cases of phantom limb. Little benefit has been shown with other medications, but low-molecular-weight dextran in severe injuries prevents sludging of the blood and improves distal circulation.[9,31] Heparin and aspirin have not been shown to produce major improvement in tissue salvage.

Unusual Frostbite Injuries

Although penile frostbite has been reported in runners, cross-country skiers, and speed skaters with thin racing suits (see Chapter 27), it is usually easily prevented by adding layers of insulation in the groin area. Penile frostbite is usually not a severe injury, but even superficial injuries in this area can be extremely painful.

Freezing of the lips, tongue, or hands to bare cold metal surfaces generally occurs in children, often as the result of horseplay, but this can occur also in adults who handle supercooled metal objects. The initial pain frequently results from stripping away the superficial epithelium when the tissue part is removed from the metal. If this occurs to the tongue or lips it can be quite painful, but usually it is not a deep injury.

Drinking supercooled beverages with high alcohol content can result in freezing of the lips, tongue, and esophagus. Although rare, this can be a fatal injury.

Corneal frostbite injuries are reported in cross-country skiers and snow mobilers. The use of goggles will prevent such an injury. These injuries may require corneal transplant, and no known treatment other than warming and patching has proven to be effective. Use of corticosteroids is contraindicated in this injury.

Postinjury Sequelae

As the severity of frostbite injury increases, postinjury sequelae also increase. Cold sensitivity along with peripheral constriction is the most common complaint after frostbite. This may be severe enough to limit outdoor activities and may later produce Raynaud's disease with tingling, paresthesia, and hyperhydrosis. Management of these complaints is difficult. Pavlovian conditioning to relieve the peripheral constriction has proven to be effective, and in the future, selective peripheral serotonin blockade may be available.[21] Other medical approaches have not been effective and provide only short-term relief of symptomatology. Biofeedback techniques, although initially effective, extinguish quickly and do not stand up to significant cold challenge.[22]

RAYNAUD'S DISEASE

Raynaud's disease is an abnormal bilateral peripheral constriction of the small arteries and arterioles of the hands and feet associated with either emotional stress, cold exposure, or combination thereof. Although occupational Raynaud's disease may arise from the use of vibratory tools, the etiology of idiopathic Raynaud's disease remains a mystery. Raynaud's disease is also sometimes associated with autoimmune disease, with severe results. Although Raynaud's disease may occur at any age and in either sex, the syndrome is uncommon before puberty and much more frequent in women than in men.

The peripheral reaction sequence to cold is as follows: Skin temperature receptors perceive cold temperature. This message then is relayed through the peripheral nerves to the central nervous system, which initiates peripheral vasoconstriction in order to preserve core heat. This mechanism works essentially the same for both cold-sensitive and normal individuals, and the rate is essentially the same. However, the centrally mediated impulse to peripherally vasoconstrict lasts only a short time, probably less than 2 minutes. Cold-sensitive individuals will vasoconstrict at the same rate as normal individuals, but cold-sensitive individuals often will cool the extremities to lower temperatures than normal. The centrally mediated constriction message then disappears, and peripheral constriction is subsequently maintained by a peripheral constrictor. If the cold is severe or long-lasting enough, the peripheral constrictor normally will be relieved by a cold-induced vasodilation reaction in about 11 to 15 minutes. We believe that Raynaud's disease results from abnormal maintenance of the initial peripheral constriction (i.e., a lack of the cold-induced vasodilation response to intense or prolonged cold). According to this hypothesis, Raynaud's disease is a problem of the peripheral constrictor-vasodilator response rather than a centrally mediated disease. This is why centrally acting drugs have been ineffective in dealing with Raynaud's symptoms over the long term. Investigators in our institute have developed techniques utilizing Pavlovian conditioning procedures to dislink the central from the peripheral constrictors and to condition the peripheral constrictor to dilate rather than to constrict in response to cold. Although the procedure has gone through a number of iterations, it is essentially Pavlovian conditioning of the peripheral constrictor.[20]

The technique requires a cold outdoor temperature or chamber (0 to 5°C [32 to 42°F]) and an insulated container for hot water. The procedure is as follows: The cold-sensitive individual with Raynaud's disease is dressed lightly and put in a warm room (about 22 to 24°C [72 to 75°F]). The patient then immerses the hands in hot water to just above the wrists. This water should be as hot as the patient can stand—roughly, 42°C (108°F). The hands are left immersed approximately 3 to 5 minutes, at which time they are taken out of the water and wrapped in a towel. Then the individual proceeds outdoors or into the cold room. When in the cold, the hands are unwrapped and immediately placed in an insulated hot-water pail (42°C [108°F]). At this point, the patient's torso begins to chill. The patient is kept in the cold for approximately 8 to 10 minutes. Then the hands are again wrapped in the towel and the patient is taken back into the warm room to again immerse the hands in hot water. The patient stays in the warm room roughly 3 to 5 minutes until the torso warms up.

In this procedure, the hands remain hot and dilated, but the torso goes from warm to cold to warm. Although the cold temperature initiates a centrally mediated message to constrict peripherally, the hands stay dilated because of being immersed in hot water. This training procedure conditions the hands to dilate rather than to constrict in response to a cold stimulus. The routine is repeated 3 to 6 times a day every other day for approximately 50 to 60 treatments. Some people require more training than others. We have obtained good results in most patients with Raynaud's disease within about 50 treatments.

This procedure appears to have fairly long-lasting benefits, giving good responses for up to 3 to 4 years. However, retraining may be necessary on a yearly basis. Using these conditioning methods, we have seen both the relief of symptomatology and an improvement in peripheral blood flow, but these findings may not directly correlate. We have also seen the healing of Raynaud's disease induced ulcers within a 2-week time span. Patients have been extremely enthusiastic about the results of these methods; albeit many are quite skeptical when they start the conditioning.

HYPOTHERMIA

Hypothermia is whole-body cooling sufficient to cause depression of the core temperature. In a sports setting, this occurs usually from an accident or injury that renders the individual incapable of getting back to a warm environment. Exercise hypothermia can occur in marathon skiers or runners shortly after the race when the individual is hypoglycemic, hypovolemic, and peripherally dilated for maximum heat dissipation. More commonly, hypothermia occurs during recreational hiking in the mountains where a combination of events, weather changes, and physical capabilities place individuals in a high-threat setting. Poorly equipped, inexperienced hikers going for a pleasant walk in the hills are often confronted with sudden weather changes. Rain, wind, and overexertion combine to get them into trouble. Hypothermia can occur rapidly from unexpected plunges into freezing water[8,23,24] while snowmobiling, ice fishing, skiing, skating, or hiking. Wet clothing is devastating to the conservation of heat. Winter hikers and climbers should prepare for the worst weather contingency, be trained in the rational use of clothing, be alert for changes in the weather, and be aware that accidents in remote areas can lead to serious hypothermic experiences. Leaders should be aware that dehydration plays a major role in hypothermia. Individuals should be encouraged to drink in the absence of thirst in order to prevent peripheral and central dehydration. Peripheral dehydration is a compensatory process that occurs from mild dehydration combined with peripheral vasoconstriction from cold exposure. Cold-induced vasodilation is blunted, resulting in long-term ischemia of the extremities.

Management of Hypothermia

Field Management

The most important single factor in the treatment of hypothermia is to recognize that individuals—even comatose, asystolic individuals—may be resuscitated successfully.[13] Treatment is different for conscious and unconscious individuals.

Conscious hypothermic persons should have their wet clothing removed and then should be insulated with added garments, sleeping bags, blankets, or whatever warming materials are available. They should be encouraged to drink warm, sweet liquids in large volumes to improve circulating volume and to provide an energy source for exercise. Once insulated and hydrated, they should be encouraged to exercise to increase muscle activity and heat production. If possible, they should be put in a warm building or provided with a warm shower. Although hypothermic individuals may appear to be drunken, stumbling and shivering uncontrollably, they generally respond to peripheral rewarming procedures without harm.

On the other hand, comatose hypothermic persons in a field setting offer a much greater challenge. These individuals should be handled very carefully, insulated, and transported as quickly as possible to adequate medical facilities. Positive-pressure respiration is advisable during evacuation, but cardiopulmonary resuscitation (CPR) remains controversial. Verification of ventricular fibrillation is extremely difficult in a field setting, and chest compression will almost surely produce asystole. Delays for CPR also can compromise the rescue effort. Field rewarming procedures are generally not effective and also lengthen the time required to get the patient to definitive medical care. If available, heated humidified oxygen can be used, but this measure should not be perceived as a major rewarming technique. Intravenous fluids can be lifesaving, but they are extremely difficult to start in a field setting.

Hospital Management

The general treatment of hypothermia is a five-step process.[37] This process can be summarized as follows: (1) rapid core rewarming, (2) prevention of arrhythmias, (3) replacement of circulating volume with intravenous fluids, (4) respiratory support, and (5) pH and electrolyte management. Although mildly hypothermic persons can be managed rather simply with warming blankets and bedrest, severe hypothermic persons require significant intervention to bring them back to normothermia. For readers who are interested in greater detail, a review of the physiology of cooling can be found elsewhere.[10] Specifics of clinical management will be covered here.[15–17]

Rewarming. Patients who are conscious

and have a core temperature above 32°C (90°F) can be managed with external methods of rewarming only. They are usually lucid, able to describe their experience, and able to carry on a reasonable conversation. Warm blankets are often sufficient to return them to normal core temperature. Patients with core temperatures below 32°C (90°F) may be either conscious or unconscious. Clinical thermometers generally available do not record temperatures below 32°C (90°F). However, Zeal low-reading thermometers for use in the field and resuscitation center are available from Scotia Instrument Company (100 Leiblin Drive, Halifax, Nova Scotia B3R1NS; telephone 902-447-4835). Conscious patients with temperatures below 32°C (90°F) are generally incoordinate, incoherent, and unable to recite simple phrases. They require a little more aggressive rewarming, and heated humidified oxygen or immersion of the torso in warm water is advisable. Unconscious patients with temperatures below 32°C (90°F) require specific rewarming techniques. Patients who are unconscious with temperatures between 26° and 32°C (79° and 90°F) should be considered for internal methods of rewarming.[6,14,25,26] Peritoneal dialysis[11,19,35] and torso immersion are generally the most acceptable techniques. Patients with temperatures below 25°C (77°F) should generally be considered for femoral-femoral bypass rewarming. Although many patients have been rewarmed with other techniques, bypass appears to give the greatest chance for survival. The coldest successful resuscitation appears to be near 15°C (59°F). Emergency room staffs should be trained to recognize hypothermic patients and to know the options for rewarming.

Rewarming techniques. Warm blankets are sufficient for conscious individuals but provide very little total heating input and only prevent further heat loss. Heated humidified oxygen produces small total heat input and should not be considered a major rewarming technique. Dry land hypothermic persons, who are volume depleted because of long-term cold diuresis and long-term cooling, can generally manage the precipitation of water in the lungs from heat transfer with this process. However, normovolemic hypothermic individuals, such as those exposed to icy waters, will not tolerate airway rewarming techniques. Rewarming rates are slow with this procedure, and it should be considered only as an adjunct to other rewarming methods. Hypothermia rewarming blankets which contain circulating fluid are often available now in hospital surgical suites. These blankets are convenient and do provide a significant amount of heat input in a controlled setting. The patient's torso should be wrapped with these blankets, but the limbs should be left out in the room air.

Warm-water immersion is used extensively for rewarming hypothermic persons and provides a significant heat input, but it does pose some specific problems. Total body immersion produces peripheral vasodilation in the limbs. During the hypothermic experience, large volumes of blood are sequestered in the limbs which become colder than the core and also become severely acidotic from shivering. Third-space fluid contains a significant amount of potassium from the loss of the sodium pump in the muscle cells. Immersing these limbs during warming procedures causes peripheral vasodilation with return of this colder hyperkalemic, acidotic blood to the core. The sudden loss of blood pressure, acidosis, and hyperkalemia can produce major cardiac arrhythmias and may cause cardiac standstill or fibrillation. For that reason, it is wise to immerse only the torso. The arms, legs, and the head are kept out of the rewarming bath.

Warm peritoneal dialysis is another rewarming method that is growing in acceptance. Dialysis provides significant heat input to the core because of the large peritoneal surface area that is available for heat exchange. Warm peritoneal dialysis can be done easily and readily in an emergency room. The technique also provides some control over pH and electrolytes and may remove drugs and alcohol from the hypothermic individual.

Extracorporeal circulation utilizing cardiac bypass—specifically femoral-femoral bypass—is used on extremely cold patients, but this technique requires surgical intervention and considerable hospital staff support. Extracorporeal blood warming provides a method for rapid return of heat and circulation to the severely hypothermic patient. One major problem involved in extracorporeal blood warming relates to trying to raise the central venous pressure too rapidly. Endothelial cells below 30°C (86°F) are unable to hold fluid in the vascular space. Attempting to raise the central venous pressure too early will cause extensive leakage into extravascular spaces with devastating results. Circulation should be maintained at low venous pressures about 3.0 cm H_2O. Clear indications of the ability of the vascular system to hold fluid should be seen before slowly raising central venous pressure.

Cardiac arrhythmias. The major cause of problems in rewarming hypothermic patients is cardiac arrhythmias, fibrillation, and arrest. Dramatic cardiac rhythm disturbances may be present during hypothermia, but it should be recognized that many of these arrhythmias are physiologically normal for the individual patient at that particular low temperature. So, it should be cautioned that manipulating the hypothermic patient may precipitate ventricular fibrillation because the fibrillatory threshold is decreased by cold. Although cardiac arrhythmias during hypothermia do not respond well to chemical intervention, most will disappear during rewarming. Dose-response curves for the standard antiarrhythmic drugs have not been well worked out in conditions of hypothermia, and if these medications are given to subjects when they are cold, toxic effects may occur on rewarming. A variety of factors contribute to the arrhythmias seen in hypothermia, including acidosis, decreased cellular oxygen concentration, blood volume depletion, and the direct effect of low temperature on tissues. Attempts at cardioversion, therefore, are not usually successful in the fibrillating heart below 30°C (86°F). When cardiac arrest occurs in patients with core temperatures below 30°C (86°F), some method of core rewarming and management of the physiologic needs should be combined with half-rate cardiopulmonary resuscitation. Once body temperature is above 30°C (86°F), cardioversion can be attempted, but one should not give up too soon. Although most antiarrhythmic drugs have not been effective in treating hypothermic cardiac arrest, bretylium tosylate at slightly larger than normothermic dosage appears to be of some value.[4,7] Again, it should be noted that cardiopulmonary resuscitation of the hypothermic heart can produce ventricular fibrillation or standstill, so electrocardiographic proof of asystole or fibrillation must be obtained before cardiopulmonary resuscitation is initiated. Electrocardiography, pulse, respirator, and blood pressure monitoring are indicated throughout the process of rewarming and resuscitation.

Intravenous fluid replacement. The administration of intravenous fluids to the hypothermic patient can be lifesaving. By decreasing blood viscosity, general circulation is improved and cardiac output is increased. Replacement fluids should be potassium free and lactate free. Crystalloid solutions with glucose are probably the safest and easiest to use. Dilution of the intravascular contents alone decreases the concentration of potassium, increases the pH, and improves the peripheral blood flow. Rapid correction of pH should be avoided, and the patient should be kept mildly acidotic throughout the entire rewarming process. To correct severe acidosis, early administration of sodium bicarbonate may be necessary, but the use of continuous bicarbonate should be avoided. Extremely elevated serum potassium levels can be managed initially with intravenous glucose and insulin. However, the use of insulin must be carefully monitored, because rapid shifts in blood glucose may occur during the rewarming process when rebound pancreatic production of insulin may drive potassium dangerously low. Absolute blood glucose levels and electrolyte concentrations, particularly potassium, should be determined frequently. Potassium concentrations in the range of 30 mEq/ml have been recorded with subsequently successful resuscitations.

Respiratory support. In general, some initial small-volume positive-pressure respiration is indicated in the comatose hypothermic patient. However, the volume should be kept small to prevent overstimulation of the heart. Many hypothermic patients will start gasping respiration if small-volume respiratory support is initiated. Spontaneous respiration will improve during rewarming and will have a major impact on pH management throughout the process. Supplemental oxygen, about 50 percent concentration, is indicated during early resuscitation to lower the fibrillatory threshold. When arterial P_{O_2} and P_{CO_2} determinations are made to assist in the management of hypothermic patients, it is probably not necessary to correct these values for temperature. The utilization of positive-end expiratory pressure may be required to treat acute pulmonary edema; this technique usually need not be used during hypothermic resuscitation. Intubation may be necessary, and bronchorrhea may require meticulous airway management to prevent obstruction. Hyperventilation should be avoided to prevent respiratory alkalosis and ventricular fibrillation.

Aftercare of Hypothermia

The most common problem following a hypothermic experience is bacterial pneumonia, which follows hypostatic pulmonary congestion and bronchorrhea. Good cleansing respiratory therapy is advised, and the patient should be followed with sequential chest x-ray examinations until clear. Although the pancreas is generally the only parenchymal organ to show petechial lesions in hypothermia, internally rewarmed patients do not develop pancreatitis. And complications with pulmonary edema, acute tubular necrosis, disseminated intravascular coagulation, and bleeding gastric ulcers have been reported. Immediately following a hypothermic experience patients have trouble controlling blood pressure and temperature regulation, but these mechanisms will return to normal over a period of weeks.

CONCLUSION

By their very nature and the climates in which they are conducted, winter sports pose a susceptibility to cold injury. Fortunately, because of the controlled conditions under which most winter training and competitions are held, serious cold injuries are not common. Planning, protection, good sense, and good supervision can prevent virtually all such cold injuries associated with winter sports, with the possible exception of those which result from accidents to mountain skiers, climbers, and hikers and those which result from unexpected immersion in cold water. Of these, frostbite and hypothermia are the most significant.

A cardinal rule in dealing with severe frostbite is not to rewarm the part when there is any danger whatsoever of refreezing. The injury can be greatly enhanced by freezing, thawing, and refreezing the tissue. It is better to "walk them out of the woods" on a frozen limb than begin warming where there is no facility for continued thawing and definitive treatment.

All hypothermic patients deserve an attempt at rewarming and resuscitation. The hypothermic response to cold is a protection of the body against the threat of reduced circulation. Resuscitation of the hypothermic person is quite straightforward as long as the basic needs of getting heat to the body core, tempering cardiac arrhythmias, supporting respiration by judicious cardiopulmonary resuscitation as outlined, and slowly returning the circulation are borne in mind. Overzealous use of medications, surgically opening the chest for direct cardiac massage, and attempts to quickly return serum electrolyte concentrations and other physiologic parameters to normal usually result in failure or complications. Dramatic procedures such as cardiac bypass are reserved for severe (15 to 21°C [59 to 70°F]) hypothermia, often with asystole. Successful resuscitations are becoming more common as the medical profession understands the physiology of hypothermia.

REFERENCES

1. Bangs, CC: Disturbances due to cold. In Conn, HF (ed): Current Therapy. WB Saunders, Philadelphia, 1981, pp 981–988.
2. Bangs, CC, Boswick, JA, Hamlet, MP, Sumner, DS, and Weatherley-White, RCA: When your patient suffers frostbite. Patient Care 11:132–156, 1977.
3. Boswick, JA, Thompson, JD, and Jonas, RA: The epidemiology of cold injuries. Surgery, Gynecology and Obstetrics 149:326–332, 1979.
4. Buckley, J, Bosch, OD, and Bacaner, MD: Prevention of ventricular fibrillation during hypothermia with bretylium tosylate. Anesthesia Analgesia 50:587–593, 1971.
5. Burns, JH and Rand, MJ: Noradrenaline in artery walls and its dispersal by reserpine. Br Med J 1:903–908, 1958.
6. Collis, MD, Steinman, AM, and Chaney, RD: Accidental hypothermia: An experimental study of practical rewarming methods. Aviation, Space and Environmental Medicine 48:625–632, 1977.
7. Danzl, DF, Sowers, MB, and Vicario, SJ: Chemical ventricular defibrillation in severe accidental hypothermia. Annals of Emergency Medicine 11:698–699, 1982.
8. Golden, F, St C: Recognition and treatment of immersion hypothermia. Proc Royal Soc Med 66:1058–1061, 1973.
9. Goodhead, B: The comparative value of low molecular weight dextran and sympathectomy in the treatment of experimental frost-bite. Br J Surg 53:1060–1062, 1966.

10. Gregory, RT and Doolittle, WH: Accidental hypothermia. Part II. Clinical implications of experimental studies. Alaska Medicine 15:48–52, 1973.
11. Grossheim, RL: Hypothermia and frostbite treated with peritoneal dialysis. Alaska Medicine 15:53–55, 1973.
12. Hamlet, MP, Ahle, N, and Schoning, P: Unpublished data, 1987.
13. Harnett, RM, O'Brien, EM, Sias, FR, and Pruit, JR: Initial treatment of profound accidental hypothermia. Aviation, Space and Environmental Medicine 51:680–687, 1980.
14. Hayward, JS and Steinman, AM: Accidental hypothermia: An experimental study of inhalation rewarming. Aviation, Space and Environmental Medicine 46:1236–1240, 1975.
15. Hunter, WC: Accidental hypothermia. Part I. Northwest Medicine 67:569–573, 1968.
16. Hunter, WC: Accidental hypothermia. Part II. Northwest Medicine 67:735–739, 1968.
17. Hunter, WC: Accidental hypothermia. Part III. Northwest Medicine 67:837–844, 1968.
18. Jarrett, F: Frostbite: Current concepts of pathogenesis and treatment. Rev Surg 31:71–74, 1974.
19. Jessen, K and Hagelsten, JO: Peritoneal dialysis in the treatment of profound accidental hypothermia. Aviation, Space and Environmental Medicine 49:426–429, 1978.
20. Jobe, JB, Beetham, WP, Jr, Roberts, DE, Silver, GR, Larsen, RF, Hamlet, MP, and Sampson, JB: Induced vasodilation as a home treatment for Raynaud's disease. J Rheumatol 12:953–956, 1985.
21. Jobe, JB, Sampson, JB, Roberts, DE, and Beetham, WP, Jr: Induced vasodilation as treatment for Raynaud's disease. Ann Int Med 97:706–709, 1982.
22. Jobe, JB, Sampson, JB, Roberts, DE, and Kelly, JA: Comparison of behavioral treatments for Raynaud's disease. J Behav Med 9:89–96, 1986.
23. Keatinge, WR: Survival in Cold Water. Blackwell Scientific Publications, Oxford, 1969.
24. Keatinge, WR: Accidental immersion hypothermia and drowning. Symposium on Environmental Problems 219:183–187, 1977.
25. Leadingham, McA, Routh, GS, Couglas, IHW, and MacDonald, AM: Central rewarming system for treatment of hypothermia. Lancet 1:1168–1169, 1980.
26. Lloyd, EL: Accidental hypothermia treated with central rewarming through the airway. Br J Anaesthesia 45:41–47, 1973.
27. Merryman, HT: Mechanism of freezing injury in clinical frostbite. In Vierech, E (ed): Proceedings of the Symposium on Arctic Medicine and Biology. IV. Frostbite. Arctic Aeromedical Laboratory, Fort Wainwright, AK, 1964, pp 1–7.
28. Mills, WJ, Jr: Clinical aspects of frostbite injury. In Vierech, E (ed): Proceedings of the Symposium on Arctic Medicine and Biology. IV. Frostbite. Arctic Aeromedical Laboratory, Fort Wainwright, AK, 1964, pp 149–196.
29. Mills, WJ, Jr: Summary of treatment of the cold-injured patient. Alaska Medicine 15:56–57, 1973.
30. Mills, WJ, Jr: Frostbite. Alaska Medicine 15:27–47, 1973.
31. Mundth, ED, Long, DM, and Brown, RB: Treatment of experimental frostbite with low molecular weight dextran. J Trauma 4:246–257, 1964.
32. Orr, KD and Fainer, DC: Cold injuries in Korea during winter of 1950–51. Army Medical Research Laboratory, Fort Knox, KY, 1951.
33. Porter, JM and Reiney, CG: Effect of low dose intra-arterial reserpine on vascular wall norepinephrine content. Ann Surg 183:50–55, 1975.
34. Rakower, SR, Shahgoli, S, and Wong, SL: Doppler ultrasound and digital plethysmography to determine the need for sympathetic blockade after frostbite. J Trauma 18:713–718, 1978.
35. Reuler, JB and Parker, RA: Peritoneal dialysis: The management of hypothermia. JAMA 240:2289–2291, 1978.
36. Snider, RW and Porter, JM: Treatment of experimental frostbite with intra-arterial sympathetic blocking drugs. Surgery 77:557–561, 1975.
37. US Army Research Institute of Environmental Medicine: Resuscitation of Accidental Hypothermia Victims. (Report No. T42/76.) United States Army Medical Research and Development Command, Natick, MA, 1976.

CHAPTER 19

Exercise-Induced Bronchospasm in Winter Sports

WILLIAM E. PIERSON, M.D.

ROBERT O. VOY, M.D.

Exercise-induced bronchospasm (EIB) has affected athletes as early as the first games in Olympia, Greece. Shortness of breath following exercise, which is the hallmark of EIB, was described by Arateus the Capedocian in 200 AD.[32] Many athletes have struggled in training and competition without knowledge of why they were having respiratory difficulties.[16] The handicap of EIB has been largely overlooked until the last decade when more physicians and athletes began to recognize the disorder.[1] Exercise-induced bronchospasm was very costly to a competitor from the XXI Olympiad in Munich, who had to relinquish his gold medals when it was discovered that he was using a banned drug for the treatment of his EIB.[8] Only in the past decade has EIB been studied in any systematic fashion with regard to its prevalence, physiologic changes, and pharmacologic management.

As we begin to understand the mechanisms of EIB, its relevance becomes obvious for athletes engaged in winter sports performed at high altitudes and often subzero temperatures or in cold, dry ozone-filled ice rinks.

DESCRIPTION

Exercise-induced bronchospasm represents a transient increase in airways responsiveness, with air flow obstruction following

3 to 8 minutes of strenuous exercise.[5] This phenomenon is characterized by moderate to severe airways obstruction occurring 5 to 15 minutes following strenuous exercise. These changes take place in both the large and the small airways, and individuals have varying degrees of involvement, depending upon the predominant site of air flow obstruction. The major changes with EIB are bronchoconstriction and smooth muscle contraction. More recently, late-phase changes which result in significant small and large airways obstruction have been described at 6 to 10 hours following initial airways obstruction.[7]

DEFINITION

Individuals with EIB usually experience a mild degree of bronchodilation during early periods of exercise and subsequently develop moderate to severe bronchoconstriction in both large and small airways following cessation of exercise. Maximum airway obstruction occurs between 5 and 15 minutes following completion of vigorous exercise, and spontaneous recovery usually occurs over a period of 30 minutes to 2 hours later.[19] The severity of obstruction is directly proportional to bronchial hyperresponsiveness. Generally, the degree of obstruction following exercise is proportional to methacholine bronchial sensitivity, although that relationship is nonlinear.[11] This is due in large part to the fact that EIB is dependent upon more than simple bronchial hyperresponsiveness. In the large airways, changes can occur that are characterized by a decrease in forced expiratory volume in one second (FEV_1) or peak expiratory flow rate (PEFR), causing decreases in the order of 10 percent or more from pre-exercise baseline levels. Changes have also been noted in the forced expiratory flow at 25 to 75 percent of vital capacity (FEF_{25-75}) or at mid maximum expiratory flow rate (MMEF), and those changes are usually abnormal if they are 20 percent or greater decreases from the baseline resting airway function. Other changes have been shown in airway resistance and specific airway conductance and in total vital capacity.

ETIOLOGIC FACTORS

Several different factors have been described as the etiologic stimulus for producing EIB. McFadden and colleagues[24,25] have described heat loss from the upper airway as the major etiologic mechanism for EIB. These studies showed that breathing subfreezing dry air caused the same amount of bronchospasm with the same characteristics of bronchial responsiveness as exercise challenge testing. These conclusions were based upon measurement of retrotracheal temperature changes and, ultimately, direct airway changes in the first six or seven generations of bronchi where heating and humidification occur.[24] The inspired air inhaled at rest is usually warmed and humidified to 100 percent relative humidity in the first five to seven generations of bronchi. However, strenuous exercise causes the nasal air conditioning to be bypassed as minute ventilation exceeds the capacity of nasal breathing, and mouth breathing is initiated; then cooling of the upper airway becomes significant with high levels of ventilation. This is accentuated when dry air is inhaled because of a net water loss from the airway. Under normal circumstances of relative humidity in the range from 30 to 50 percent, water content is somewhere between 6 and 11 milligrams per liter of inspired air. However, when the air temperature is increased to 37°C (98.6°F) at the alveolar level, the water content is increased to 44 milligrams of water per liter of air. This water is usually extracted from the fluid-phase mucous layer lining the respiratory tract to the alveoli. Calculations on adults have shown that approximately 350 square centimeters of surface area of the first seven generations of bronchi contain a volume of somewhere between 0.25 and 0.42 ml of fluid.[18] To accomplish vaporization of 1.5 to 3.0 ml per minute with heavy breathing, it is apparent that a great deal of water is extracted from the fluid phase of the upper respiratory tract.

This has given rise to the more recent hypothesis, which expands our concept of the etiologic basis of EIB as being secondary to water loss from the airway. Accordingly, water loss causes subsequent increase in osmolarity of the fluid interface of the respiratory epithelium and airway mast cells.[3] Eggleston and others[14] have shown that hyperosmolar fluids surrounding mast cells trigger the release of inflammatory mediators, including histamine and aracidonic acid metabolites. These, along with other well-described inflammatory mediators, cause the airflow obstruction that is characteristic of EIB.

This hypothesis has been strengthened by the studies of Anderson and colleagues,[2] who have shown that inhaling water-saturated air diminishes the effect of EIB and hyperventilation-induced asthma. The inhalation of saturated air diminishes the net water loss from the lining fluid phase of the respiratory tract. And it has been shown that airway responsiveness is inversely related to the water content of inspired air; drier air at the same temperature, whether or not it is hot or subfreezing, causes an increase in EIB.[4]

It has been shown by Deal,[10] however, that retrotracheal temperature reduction is directly proportional to the reduction in FEV_1 following exercise. This is complicated by the necessity for hyperventilation at high exercise rates of work. Since Anderson and others[2] have shown that children with EIB can have decreases in lung function as great as 40 percent or more following the inhalation of warm (37°C [98.6°F]) dry air, more than airway cooling alone must be necessary as an inciting stimulus of EIB. Also, they found that the expired air temperature was as high as 35°C (95°F), thereby revealing that little if any airway cooling had occurred.

Recently, investigators have shown that bronchospasm was induced by inhalation of hyperosmolar solutions.[36] This indirectly indicates that with significant water loss from the respiratory tract and subsequent hyperosmolar changes in the fluid interface, the mast cells and other cells could be exposed to the induction of inflammatory mediator release and the cascade of immunologic events that follows the liberation of these mediators into the airway.

PATHOPHYSIOLOGY

Several different factors that have been alluded to above will now be discussed in greater depth as they relate to the pathophysiology of EIB. Following heat and/or water loss, the subsequent development of a hyperosmolar fluid interface along the respiratory tract leads to several events. These include the release of inflammatory mediators—including histamine, prostaglandin, leukotrines, and other aracidonic acid metab-

olites—which may act directly upon smooth muscle cells, resulting in the rapid onset of bronchospasm and other vascular events that are slow in onset but profound in their duration. Also, vagal bronchoconstriction from afferent irritant nerve receptors in the airway can follow the inflammatory changes noted with chemical mediator released from mast cells and respiratory epithelial cells. These irritant receptors cause vagal afferent nerve fibers to induce an increase in bronchomotor tone secondary to reflex bronchoconstriction.

In addition, mast cells have been shown to discharge high-molecular-weight chemo-attractants, such as neutrophil chemotactic factor, which recruit neutrophils and induce a prolonged inflammatory response.[26] This causes several secondary biochemical and cellular reactions, including epithelial cellular damage with decrease in epithelial cell joint integrity, which thereby can significantly change the action of cilia and mucociliary transport. These cellular events are more common in the late-phase reactions that characterize asthmas and, in particular, the late-phase response of EIB. Epithelial cells can also produce aracidonic acid byproducts which can serve as inflammatory mediators which also worsen the epithelial junction damage as well as affect mucociliary clearance. With the epithelial cellular damage, it is possible that increased exposure of irritant receptors occurs and subsequently induces bronchoconstriction by hyperventilation.

Finally, alpha-adrenergic receptors are thought to reside in either the cholinergic ganglia or in the postganglionic nerve fibers that innervate the bronchopulmonary smooth muscle. These are important because they can be stimulated by noradrenalin (NAD), which can be discharged by sympathetic nerve fibers passing to the vascular tree contiguous with these ganglia and/or postganglionic nerve fibers.[31] It is of real interest that a patient who has just undergone EIB remains refractory to bronchospasm for about 2 hours when subsequently challenged with exercise testing. However, they remain very responsive to methacholine, histamine, or allergen rechallenge—any of which can induce severe bronchospasm immediately after EIB. These observations suggest that exercise is a specific stimulus that results in ventilatory changes that cause hyperosmolarity and/or cooling of the upper airways and the subsequent chain of events resulting in inflammatory mediatory release and bronchoconstriction both in the initial 5- to 10-minute phase following exercise and again in the 4- to 6-hour course following initial bronchoconstriction.[6]

PULMONARY PHYSIOLOGIC CHANGES

Classically, EIB follows a significant exercise challenge of 3 to 8 minutes, during which there is initial bronchodilation.[15] (See Fig. 19–1.) After termination of the exercise challenge, moderate to severe airflow obstruction occurs either in the large airways or in the small airways and sometimes in both. This has been well documented by spirometry that shows changes in FEV_1 and FVC as well as FEF_{25-75} that signify small airways obstruction.[9] Other tests, including specific airways conductants, have shown significant rises in airway resistance and obstruction that usually peak from 5 to 15 minutes following exercise challenge testing. These changes gradually resolve and can be followed with a late-phase reaction somewhere between 4 and 6 hours following the initial bronchoconstriction from exercise. Those patients who have the most severe early changes are at the highest risk of developing

late-phase reactions.[22] It has been noted that these changes are initially accompanied by release of histamine and/or other mast cell mediators. During the 4- to 6-hour late-phase responses, these are followed by late-phase reactants, including high-molecular-weight neutrophil chemotactic factor and aracidonic acid metabolites. Early- and late-phase responses are deferentially susceptible to pharmacologic modification. The early-phase reactions are quite responsive to beta-adrenergic agents and, indeed, $beta_2$ agents are highly effective in blocking the early response. On the other hand, corticosteroids are ineffective in blocking early-phase response but are quite effective in blocking the 4- to 6-hour late-phase response. Sodium cromoglycate (cromolyn), however, has the capacity to block *both* early- and late-phase responses, probably attesting to the multiplicity of cromolyn's pharmacologic actions.

PREVALENCE

Exercise-induced bronchospasm has been noted in a significant proportion of high-performance athletes.[17] The Australians have noted a 5 to 14 percent rate of asthma or EIB among their last five Olympic teams.[16] In a study of Division 1 intercollegiate athletes at the University of Washington, Rice and associates[30] found an EIB rate of 2.8 percent. Six percent (8/126) of the 1984 United States

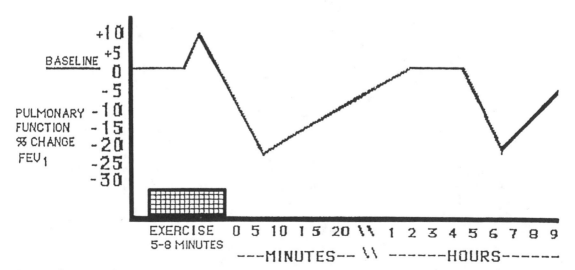

Figure 19–1. Typical graphic response illustrates initial improvement and subsequent fall at 7 minutes after exercise, recovery 20–120 minutes to baseline, and the late-phase reaction in subset of subjects with EIB. (The late-phase exercise-related reaction is less severe than the initial EIB experience.)

Winter Olympic Team and 11 percent (67/597) of the 1984 United States Summer Olympic Team were found to have EIB.[29] This suggests that the prevalence rate of EIB among athletes can be estimated conservatively in the range of 3 to 10 percent and that it is common even among highly trained athletes.

DIAGNOSIS

The diagnosis of EIB is aided by history and exercise challenge testing. The clinical history for EIB usually is characterized by coughing, chest tightness, wheezing, and difficult breathing following exercise. The degree of reliability of a history for EIB is variable; many athletes who deny symptoms of EIB will show a significant degree of bronchospasm when tested.

The United States Olympic Committee has used a questionnaire for the detection of athletes with EIB and has refined the precision of the history by noting other signs and symptoms of respiratory allergic disease which correlate with athletes who have bronchial hyperresponsiveness manifested by EIB.

Several exercise challenge tests have been used, including free-range running, treadmill, and various ergometric systems such as cycloergometer and rowing ergometer.[13] The free-range running test is the most asthmagenic of all of the challenge tests and gives the highest rate of responsiveness. It is a test that is relatively easy to perform, requiring only a track, hallway, or stairs where athletes can run for a minimum period of 3 to 8 minutes. The treadmill test has been a more standardized test for the detection and study of EIB, and it can be varied by elevation of the treadmill and the speed at which the treadmill is run. In highly trained athletes, it is sometimes very difficult to give the maximum exercise challenge required to induce EIB. Ergometric systems, including cycloergometers and rowing ergometers, are less asthmagenic than either the treadmill or free-range running, but they have been widely used in various laboratories as standarized exercise challenge tests.

In all these tests, it is necessary to document pulmonary function studies with either spirometry or peak-flow meters during exercise and at 5-minute intervals for 30 minutes following the exercise challenge. It is becoming apparent that tests in the 4- to 12-hour period after exercise are also important to detect the late-phase asthmatic response.

MANAGEMENT

Pharmacologic Management

Sodium cromoglycate (cromolyn) has been used in the past to block EIB.[20] Initially, it was taught that the action of cromolyn was mast cell wall stabilization, deriving specifically from its effect on mast cell membrane with subsequent inflammatory mediator release. However, cromolyn has other properties, including action on postganglionic cholinergic fibers. Cromolyn has also been shown to increase the airway resistance induced by cold air in abnormal subjects and to prevent EIB in nonatopic individuals. These observations would suggest that mast cells are not the sole site of cromolyn action. Cromolyn has been shown to change the dose-response curve for inhaled histamine; it is thought that this may occur by inhibition of vagal efferent fibers passing through the cholinergic nervous system. Finally, synergistic protection against both cold-induced bronchospasm and hyperventilation bronchospasm has been noted with cromolyn and a beta$_2$-adrenergic agonist.[21]

In another major drug class, ipratroprium bromide, which is an antimuscarinic agent, has been shown to alter exercise-induced bronchoconstriction but not to the degree of cromolyn or beta$_2$-agonist aerosols. It has been hypothesized that this drug works through blockade of alpha-adrenergic receptors and/or antimuscarinic action. The primary activity of ipratroprium bromide has been bronchodilation, by which it is successful in blocking EIB but not with the same potency as the beta-adrenergic drugs.[37]

The beta-adrenergic drugs (Table 19–1), especially when administered by aerosol, have been shown to be potent blockers of EIB.[35] These drugs include albuterol, terbutaline, fenoterol, metaproterenol, and procaterol. Each of these adrenergic agents causes significant bronchodilation and subsequently blocks exercise-induced bronchoconstriction. It is clear that a host of pharmacologic probes are effective in altering EIB. Recently, calcium channel blockers have been shown to

Table 19–1. PHARMACOLOGIC MANAGEMENT OF EXERCISE-INDUCED
BRONCHOSPASM

I. Normal resting pulmonary function tests (PFTs)
   A. Beta$_2$ agonist aerosol
      1. Albuterol* MDI: 2–3 puffs 10 minutes before exercise
      2. Metaproterenol MDI: 2–3 puffs 10–15 minutes before exercise
      3. Terbutaline* MDI: 2 puffs 10–15 minutes before exercise
      4. Pirbuterol MDI: 2 puffs 10–15 minutes before exercise
   B. Beta$_2$ agonist syrup or tablets
      1. Albuterol* (Proventil, Ventolin)
         Syrup: 5–7.5 ml 1 hour before exercise
         Tablets: 4 mg 1–2 hours before exercise
      2. Metaproterenol (Alupent, Metaprel)
         Syrup: 10–20 ml 1 hour before exercise
         Tablets: 10–20 mg 2 hours before exercise
      3. Terbutaline (Brethine, Bricanyl)
         Tablets: 2.5–5 mg 2 hours before exercise
   C. Cromolyn sodium* (Intal)
      1. MDI: 2–4 puffs 10–15 minutes prior to exercise
      2. Solution by nebulizer: 20–40 mg 15 minutes prior to exercise
   D. Theophylline* (rapid release) (Slo-Phyllin): 5 mg/kg by mouth 1 hour before exercise
   E. Ipratroprium bromide (Atrovent): 2–3 puffs 20–30 minutes before exercise
   F. Terfenadine (Seldane): 120 mg 1 hour before exercise
II. Abnormal resting pulmonary function tests (PFTs). This therapeutic strategy is twofold: stabilize
    and correct abnormal airway function to normal status, then pretreat before exercise.
   A. Stabilization of abnormal airways
      1. Cromolyn sodium (Intal) MDI: 2 puffs bid to qid, TAKEN REGULARLY
      2. Theophylline (sustained release): adequate dosage to maintain serum level of 7.5 to 20 mcg/
         ml, TAKEN REGULARLY
         Range: Dosing must be individually titrated (5–20 mg/kg ideal body weight)
      3. Corticosteroids (topical) MDI: 2–3 puffs bid to qid REGULARLY
      4. Anticholinergic agents (Atrovent): 2–3 puffs tid REGULARLY
   B. Preexercise treatment
      1. Beta$_2$ agonist aerosol
         a. Albuterol* MDI: 2–3 puffs 10–15 minutes before exercise
         b. Metaproterenol MDI: 2–3 puffs 10–15 minutes before exercise
         c. Terbutaline* MDI: 2 puffs 10–15 minutes before exercise
      2. Beta$_2$ agonist syrup or tablets
         a. Albuterol* (Proventil, Ventolin)
            Syrup: 5–7.5 ml 1 hour before exercise
            Tablets: 4 mg 1–2 hours before exercise
         b. Metaproterenol (Alupent, Metaprel)
            Syrup: 10–20 ml 1 hour before exercise
            Tablets: 10–20 mg 2 hours before exercise
         c. Terbutaline (Brethine, Bricanyl)
            Tablets: 2.5–5 mg 2 hours before exercise
      3. Cromolyn sodium* (Intal)
         MDI: 2–4 puffs 10–15 minutes prior to exercise
         Solution by nebulizer: 20–40 mg 15 minutes prior to exercise
      4. Theophylline* (rapid release) (Slo-Phyllin): 5 mg/kg by mouth 1 hour before exercise
      5. Ipratroprium bromide (Atrovent): 2–3 puffs 20–30 minutes before exercise
      6. Terfenadine (Seldane): 120 mg 1 hour before exercise

*Approved for use by athletes competing in United States Olympic Committee sanctioned events.

be fairly potent blockers of EIB. This finding is consistent with the hypothesis that the calcium-dependent phase of mast cell mediator release can be blocked by calcium ion blocking agents. It also serves as evidence of a calcium-dependent phase of EIB, which is most likely related to inflammatory mediator release from airway mast cells.[27]

Nonpharmacologic Management

Several modalities exist for the nonpharmacologic management of EIB.

Warm Humid Air

The inhalation of warm humid air causes far less bronchoconstriction during the same amount of exercise as breathing dry air, especially dry cold air. Thus, if susceptible athletes are encouraged to undertake water sports such as swimming, water polo, and other water-related activities, they will have less likelihood for EIB.

Face Masks

The use of face masks for rebreathing warm air and modest rebreathing of expiratory carbon dioxide, which has been shown to be a bronchodilator, will actually diminish the degree of EIB that occurs in athletes under vigorous exercise conditions.[33]

Circular Exercises

Circular exercises and other passive exercising have been described as warm-up activities that result in less EIB.

Vigorous Warm-Up Exercises

Some athletes actually undertake vigorous warm-up exercises to induce their maximum EIB. Following this, they will be relatively refractory to further EIB for the next 2 to 3 hours. This strategy can be employed by athletes who have the opportunity for a vigorous warm-up.[38]

Diet

It has been shown that the ingestion of food 2 hours prior to exercise can significantly increase the likelihood of exercise-induced anaphylaxis and the attendant bronchospasm that accompanies that syndrome. Specific foods that have been shown to be related to EIB and/or anaphylaxis include shrimp, celery, and melon.[23]

Physical Training

Vigorous physical training has been shown to increase resting airway function and allows an athlete a larger margin of vital capacity prior to participating in an event that can cause EIB. The highly conditioned athlete may have EIB, but its impact will be less than on those who are in poor physical condition.

COMPLICATING FACTORS

Several factors have been noted to cause significant changes in bronchial hyperresponsiveness, especially in persons who have EIB as a manifestation of that hyperresponsive state.

Upper respiratory tract infections from various viral agents have been shown to elevate bronchial hyperresponsiveness and susceptibility to EIB. Several authors have reported significantly increased bronchial hyperresponsiveness in patients with paranasal sinusitis, which may result as a complication of upper respiratory tract infection or chronic nasal allergic disease.[34] The importance of this observation is that treatment of EIB will not be successful unless the paranasal sinus disease is also adequately treated and cleared.

It has also been noted that pollens and other aeroallergens can increase bronchial hyperresponsiveness in sensitive patients. Therefore, EIB may be more severe during the pollen season if the athlete is sensitive to airborne pollens.[12] Athletes with nasal allergic disease, including pollen hayfever and perennial allergic rhinitis, have increased rates of EIB. Control of nasal allergic disease, therefore, is one important factor in diminishing EIB.

Air pollutants have also been demonstrated to increase EIB. Sulfur dioxide, gas or aerosol, has been shown to cause significantly increased exercise-induced bronchoconstriction of both small and large airways.[28] Ozone will also increase bronchial hyperresponsiveness to exercise.

SUMMARY

The cold, dry air of winter and mountainous altitudes is particularly conducive to the development of EIB in susceptible individuals. However, early recognition and appropriate management of EIB can allow many athletes so affected to participate fully in winter sports. The diagnosis of EIB by the history of chest congestion, coughing, and decreasing performance with exercise is helpful, but it can be aided by a more systematic questionnaire that will detect EIB in otherwise "normal" athletes. The diagnosis of EIB is confirmed by performance of exercise challenge tests, such as a treadmill or cycloergometer, to verify the induction of bronchospasm by exercise. Management of EIB may entail such nonpharmacologic means as an early vigorous warm-up routine to induce refractoriness, gentle circular exercises, the use of a face mask for rebreathing warmed air, and participation in a physical training program to increase anaerobic fitness. Pharmacologic management includes the appropriate use of sodium cromoglycate, beta-adrenergic agonists, theophylline, ipratropium bromide, and calcium channel blocking agents. In addition, the antihistamine terfenadine can be used effectively to block EIB. These pharmacologic agents can be used in both national and international competitions when approved in advance by the appropriate national governing body and/or the United States Olympic Committee and the International Olympic Committee (see Chapter 12).

REFERENCES

1. Anderson, SD: Current concepts of exercise-induced asthma. Allergy 38:289–302, 1983.
2. Anderson, SD, Daviskas, E, and Schoeffel, RE: Prevention of severe exercise-induced asthmas with hot humid air. Lancet 2:629, 1979.
3. Anderson, SD, Schoeffel, RE, Black, JL, and Daviskas, E: Airway cooling as the stimulus to exercise-induced asthma: A re-evaluation. Eur J Respir Dis 67: 20–30, 1985.
4. Anderson, SD, Schoeffel, RE, Follet, R, Perry, CP, Daviskas, E, and Kendall, M: Sensitivity to heat and water loss at rest and during exercise in asthmatic patients. Eur J Respir Dis 63:459–471, 1982.
5. Bar-Yishay, E and Godfrey, S: Mechanisms of exercise-induced asthma. Lung 162:195–204, 1984.
6. Bhagat, RG, Strunk, RC, and Larsen, GL: The late asthmatic response. Ann Allerg 54:272; 297–301, 1985.
7. Bierman, CW: A comparison of late reactions to antigen and exercise. J Allerg Clin Immunol 73:654–659, 1984.
8. Clarke, KS: Sports medicine and drug control programs of the U.S. Olympic Committee. International Symposium on Special Problems and Management of Allergic Athletes. J Allerg Clin Immunol 73(5); 2(Suppl):740–744, 1984.
9. Cropp, GJA: Relative sensitivity of different pulmonary function tests in the evaluation of exercise-induced asthma. Pediatrics 56(Suppl):860–867, 1975.
10. Deal, EC, Jr, McFadden, ER, Jr, Ingram, RH, Jr, and Jaeger, JJ: Hyperpnea heat flux: Initial reaction sequence in exercise-induced asthma. J Appl Physiol 46:476–483, 1979.
11. Eggleston, PA: A comparison of the asthmatic response to methacholine and exercise. J Allerg Clin Immunol 63:104–110, 1979.
12. Eggleston, PA: Methods of exercise challenge. International Symposium on Special Problems and Management of Allergic Athletes. J Allerg Clin Immunol 73; (Suppl):666, 1984.
13. Eggleston, PA and Guerrant, JL: A standardized method of evaluating exercise-induced asthma. J Allerg Clin Immunol 58:414–425, 1976.
14. Eggleston, PA, Kagey-Sobotka, A, Schleimer, RP, and Lichtenstein, LM: Interaction between hyperosmolar and IgE-mediated histamine release from basophils and mast cells. Am Rev Respir Dis 130:86, 1984.
15. Eggleston, PA, Rosenthal, RR, Anderson, SA, Anderton, R, Bierman, CW, Bleeker, ER, Chai, H, Cropp, GJA, Johnson, JD, Konig, P, Morse, J, Smith, LJ, Summers, RJ, and Trautlein, JJ: Guidelines for the methodology of exercise challenge testing of asthmatics: Study Group on Exercise Challenge, Bronchoprovocation Committee, American Academy of Allergy. J Allerg Clin Immunol 64:642–645, 1979.
16. Fitch, KD and Godfrey, S: Asthma and athletic performance. JAMA 236:152–157, 1976.
17. Godfrey, S: Symposium on special problems and management of allergic athletes. International Symposium on Special Problems and Management of Allergic Athletes. J Allerg Clin Immunol 73; (Suppl):630–633, 1984.
18. Hahn, AG, Anderson, SD, Morton, AR, Black, JL, and Fitch, KD: A reinterpretation of the effect of temperature and water content of the inspired air in exercise-induced asthma. Am Rev Respir Dis 130:575–579, 1984.
19. Kawabori, I, Pierson, WE, Conquest, LL, and Bierman, EW: Incidence of exercise-induced asthma in children. Pediatrics 56:847–850, 1975.
20. Konig, P: The use of cromolyn in the management of hyperractive airways and exercise. J Allerg Clin Immunol 73:686–689, 1984.
21. Latimer, KM, O'Byrne, PM, Morris, MM, Roberts, R, and Hargreave, FE: Bronchoconstriction stimulated by airway cooling: better protection with combined inhalation of terbutaline sulphate and cromolyn sodium than with either alone. Am Rev Respir Dis 128:440–443, 1983.
22. Lee, TH, Nagakura, T, Papegeorgiou, N, Iikura, Y, and Kay, AB: Exercise-induced late asthmatic reactions with neutrophil chemotactic activity. N Engl J Med 308:1502–1505, 1983.
23. Maulitz, RB, Pratt, DS, and Schocket, AL: Exercise-induced anaphylactic reaction to shellfish. J Allerg Clin Immunol 63:433–434, 1984.
24. McFadden, ER, Jr, Denison, DM, Waller, JF, Assoufi, B, Peacock, A, and Sopwith, T: Direct recordings of the temperatures in the tracheobronchial tree in normal man. J Clin Invest 69:700–705, 1982.
25. McFadden, ER, Jr and Ingram, RH, Jr: Exercise-induced asthma: Observations on the initiating stimulus. N Engl J Med 301:763–769, 1979.
26. Nagakura, T, Lee, TH, Assoufi, BK, Denison, DM, Newman-Taylor, AJ, and Kay, AB: Neutrophil chemotactic factor in exercise and hyperventilation-induced asthma. Am Rev Respir Dis 128:294–296, 1983.
27. Patel, KR: The effect of calcium antagonist, nifedipine in exercise-induced asthma. Clin Allerg 11:429–432, 1981.
28. Pierson, WE, Covert, DS, and Koenig, JQ: Air pollutants, bronchial hyperreactivity and exercise. J Allerg Clin Immunol 73:717–721, 1984.

29. Pierson, WE and Voy RO: Exercise-induced bronchospasm in the XXIII summer Olympic games. New England Regional Allergy Proceedings (in press).

30. Rice, SG, Bierman, CW, Shapiro, GG, Furukawa, CT, and Pierson, WE: Identification of exercise-induced asthma among intercollegiate athletes. Ann Allerg 55:790–793, 1985.

31. Richardson, J and Beland, J: Nonadrenergic inhibitory nervous system in human airways. J Appl Physiol 41:764–771, 1976.

32. Samter, M (ed): The extant works of the Cappadocian. In Excerpts from Classics in Allergy. Ross Laboratories, Columbus, OH, 1969, pp 2–4.

33. Schachter, EN, Lach, E, and Lee, M: The protective effect of a cold weather mask on exercise-induced asthma. Ann Allerg 46:12–16, 1981.

34. Slavin, RG: Sinusitis. International Symposium on Special Problems and Management of Allergic Athletes. J Allerg Clin Immunol 73; part 2(Suppl):712–716, 1984.

35. Sly, RM: Management of exercise-induced asthma. Drug Therapy 12:95–99, 102, 1982.

36. Smith, CM and Anderson, SD: Hyperosmolarity as the stimulus to hyperventilation asthma. J Allerg Clin Immunol 75:143, 1985.

37. Thomson, NC, Patel, KR, and Kerr, JW: Sodium cromoglycate and ipratropium bromide in exercise-induced asthma. Thorax 33:694–699, 1979.

38. Yazigi, R, Sly, RM, and Frazer, M: Effect of triamcinolone acetonide aerosol upon exercise-induced asthma. Ann Allerg 40:322–325, 1978.

CHAPTER 20

Headache in Winter Sports: Benign Exertional Headache

WILLIAM J. MULLALLY, M.D.

Headache remains the most common pain experienced by humans. It has been estimated by the National Migraine Foundation that each year, 42,000,000 Americans present to physicians for diagnosis and treatment of their headaches.

Headache is the most common neurologic disease. The history of this disorder can be traced from ancient to modern times. References to headaches have been found as early as 3000 BC in a Sumerian poem and Babylonian literature from the same period.[8]

For those who suffer from recurrent headaches, the pain represents more than transient disruptions of normal daily patterns. Headaches often consume the lives of the afflicted, dictating changes in their behaviors and their routines.

For the athlete, headaches provoked by exertion may represent the barrier to success. Headaches actually may limit the amount of time that can be devoted to practice, and, in certain instances, may adversely affect the level of performance during competition.

THE CLASSIFICATION OF HEADACHES

The basic classification of headaches involves three main groups: (1) traction and inflammatory, (2) muscle contraction, and (3) vascular syndromes.[4]

167

Table 20–1. TRACTION AND INFLAMMATORY HEADACHE

  I. Headache from changes in intracranial pressure
   A. Mass lesions (tumor, hematoma or abscess)
   B. Hydrocephalus
   C. Venous sinus thrombosis
   D. Increased venous pressure (mediastinal obstruction, emphysema)
   E. Cerebral edema from other causes (pseudotumor cerebri, hypertensive encephalopathy, Addison's disease, postcraniotomy, hypocalcemia, acute nephritis)
   F. Postlumbar puncture producing reduced intracranial pressure
 II. Headache from inflammation
   A. Immunologic diseases and angiitis
   B. Meningeal infection (meningitis, meningoencephalitis)
   C. Compression or inflammation of the cranial nerves
   D. Sinus infection
III. Headache of cerebrovascular disease
   A. Subarachnoid hemorrhage
   B. Cerebral infarction
   C. Transient ischemic attacks
 IV. Cervical arthritis
  V. Temporomandibular joint dysfunction
 VI. Head trauma
VII. Idiopathic cranial neuralgia (tic douloureux, glossopharyngeal neuralgia, geniculate neuralgia)
VIII. Atypical facial pain
 IX. Other (glaucoma, eye strain, postherpetic neuralgia, retrobulbar neuritis, dental abscess, postmyelographic reaction, postconvulsive headache)

TRACTION AND INFLAMMATORY HEADACHES

Traction and inflammatory headaches (Table 20–1) include those headaches which are evoked by organic diseases of the skull or its components. As the name implies, pain is produced by either traction and/or inflammation of the pain-sensitive structures of the head. The parenchyma of the brain is insensitive to pain. Intracranial structures that are sensitive to pain include cranial sinuses and afferent veins, arteries of the dura mater, arteries of the base of the brain and their major branches, and parts of the dura mater in the vicinity of the large vessels. The extracranial structures that are sensitive to pain include skin, scalp, fascia, muscles, mucosa, and arteries. The skull itself is relatively insensitive to pain. Pain pathways for structures above the tentorium cerebelli are contained in the fifth cranial nerve, the trigeminal nerve. Referred pain from these structures is usually appreciated in the temporal, frontal, and parietal regions. For structures below the tentorium cerebelli, pain pathways are contained in the upper cervical spinal roots and, to a lesser extent, the glossopharyngeal and vagus nerves. Referred pain from these regions is usually felt in the occipital area. Included in the category of traction and inflammatory headaches are mass lesions of the brain, infection, and subarachnoid hemorrhage.[4,9] Headaches in this category are thankfully uncommon.

MUSCLE CONTRACTION HEADACHES

The muscle contraction headaches are often referred to as "tension headaches." This group is the most common type of headache. At least 70 percent of the population has experienced a muscle contraction headache at one time or another during their lives. It is usually described as a dull, band-like sensation; tightness; or a pressure sensation involving the entire head and radiating into the neck. It may range from an infrequent occurrence to a persistent pain, which may last for days, months, or years. It is often related to stress. The head pain of muscle contraction headache was previously believed to be caused by persistent contraction of the muscles of the head, neck, and face. However, studies have shown that contraction of these muscles need not be present for the discomfort to be felt. Chronic muscle contraction headaches are frequently seen in association with depression.[4,9]

VASCULAR HEADACHES

Vascular headaches (Table 20–2) include migraine and all variants, cluster headache, and a number of other types of headaches that are also considered vascular-type headaches. One of these is the exercise-induced headache, which is the focus of our discussion.

Migraine Headache

Migraine is best described as a "sick headache." The pain is characteristically throbbing in character and is usually accompanied by nausea and vomiting. Although the pain is unilateral in the majority of instances, approximately 30 percent of migraine attacks are bilateral. Interestingly, the term migraine is derived from the Greek word "hemicrania," which means "half-head." Photophobia and sensitivity to sound usually accompany the migraine headache, and the patient may wish to lie perfectly still in a dark, quiet room in order to lessen the discomfort. Common migraine, which comprises 80 to 90 percent of these headaches, is not accompanied by distinct neurologic signs or symptoms. Mood disturbances, however, such as depression, euphoria, and nonspecific symptoms such as a craving for sweets may precede this type of headache. Classic migraine is preceded by frank neurologic symptoms such as visual disturbances, including scotomata or blind spots, hemianopia, teichopsia or fortification spectra, flashing lights or photopsia. Less common symptoms include numbness and paresthesias, unilateral blindness, lateralizing weakness, vertigo, diplopia, ataxia, aphasia, and even syncope. The symptoms characteristically precede the headache by approximately 10 to 20 minutes and are collectively referred to as an aura. Auras usually abate by the time that the headache appears, but occasionally, they may persist into and beyond the headache. The pain of migraine headaches may last from hours to days. Migraine usually begins in the second or third decade of life. A positive family history of migraine is obtained in approximately 70 percent of affected individuals. Migraine is more common in women. It has been estimated that 20 percent of the female population and 10 to 15 percent of the male population suffer from migraine.[4,9]

Cluster Headache

Cluster headache is so termed because afflicted patients may experience one to several headaches per day for a period of 3 to 6 weeks, and then remain headache free from 9 to 12 months or longer. Spring and fall are the most common times for this type of headache to occur. The pain of cluster headache is more intense than that of migraine but lasts for a shorter period of time. Cluster

---

Table 20–2. VASCULAR HEADACHE

  I. Migraine
   A. Common
   B. Classic
   C. Variants (retinal migraine, vertebrobasilar migraine, hemiplegic migraine, ophthalmoplegic migraine, facial migraine, cervical migraine, complicated migraine, migraine accompaniment)
 II. Cluster headache
   A. Episodic
   B. Chronic
   C. Cluster headache variants, including chronic paroxysmal hemicrania
III. Toxic vascular headache
IV. Benign exertional headache (effort headache, cough headache, orgasmic headache)
 V. Altitudinal headache
IV. Decompression headache
VII. Hypertensive headache
VIII. Headache and pheochromocytoma

---

headache is unilateral in location and usually found in or around the eye. It is often described as a constant, severe pain, as if a "hot poker were being pushed into the eye." The sufferer is often awakened from sleep, usually 1 to 2 hours after the onset of sleep, and unlike the person suffering from migraine, will pace the floor rather than lie still. Nausea and vomiting are uncommon, but most sufferers experience increased lacrimation and nasal congestion or discharge on the side of the headache. The pain of cluster headache usually lasts for less than 1 hour, with the range being 5 minutes to 4 hours. Cluster headaches are uncommon, occurring in less than 1 percent of the population. Unlike migraine, 80 to 90 percent of cluster headaches occur in men.[9] No genetic predisposition has been found.

Exertional Headache

The first recorded reference to the exertional headache can be traced to Hippocrates in approximately 460 BC. Hippocrates stated that "one should be able to recognize those who have headaches from gymnastic exercises or running or walking or hunting, or any other unseasonable labor or from immoderate venery."[1] Tinel,[16] a French physician, provided us with the first description of exertional headache in 1932 with a report on patients who developed headaches from maneuvers that increased intrathoracic pressure. He described one patient as being unable to cough, to blow his nose, to hold his breath, to laugh, to cry, to bend his head, or to make any minor muscular effort without feeling pain. The headache that was produced was brief, lasting from a few seconds to minutes, and was compared with a sharply localized hammer-blow. In 1965, E. Jokl[5] provided an excellent description of his own headache which occurred after exercise. When he was a freshman in medical school, he ran as an anchorman on the mile relay team of his university in Germany. A few minutes after his race in a German track championship, he stated that his happiness over the victory was interrupted by an attack of headache accompanied by nausea, vomiting, and weakness, which lasted for 15 minutes. None of his professors were able to explain what occurred, and he was unable to find an appropriate reference to such a disorder in any of his textbooks of physiology or medicine. Jokl and Jokl[6] reported on several athletes who, after their event in the Mexico City Olympics, developed severe, unilateral, retro-orbital headaches, accompanied by nausea, vomiting, and scotomata. These headaches occurred after prolonged running, rather than after sprinting, and lasted approximately 1 hour. In some cases, a striking prostration occurred.

In 1968, Rooke[14] reported following 103 patients with exertional headaches for 3 years or longer. He defined exertional headache as "one that transiently interrupts complete comfort in response to exertional activities such as running, bending, coughing, sneezing, heaving, lifting, or straining at stool. Onset is prompt, and its duration is usually brief." Rooke was a student of Sir Charles Symonds who in the 1950s reported a high incidence of organic disease in patients who experienced a form of exertional headache—"the cough headache." Up until Rooke's report, it was commonly believed that headaches that were produced by efforts that increased intrathoracic pressure, such as coughing, sneezing, straining or exercising, were an indication of organic intracranial disease. Of the 103 patients that Rooke followed, 10 were later found to have organic disease, usually at the base of the brain. (Three patients had basilar impression. Two each had platybasia, subdural hematoma, and benign tumors. And one had Arnold-Chiari syndrome.) The headache was more common in men than in women at a ratio of 4:1 and twice as common in patients over 40 than in young patients. Hypertension was noted in 16 of the 103 patients, but it was never severe. Rooke was not able to determine an exact cause for these headaches. He postulated that prior respiratory infections may have resulted in diffuse inflammatory meningeal reactions. However, cerebrospinal fluid studies in 36 patients were unrevealing. Dental infection was also considered, but never found. Rooke concluded that the Valsalva maneuver was possibly the common denominator that produced these headaches. He believed that the transient increase in cranial blood pressure from the Valsalva maneuver resulted in dilatation of the venous sinuses and that this might trigger the exertional headaches. Long-term follow-up revealed that 10 percent of Rooke's patients were free of the headache after the first year, 30 percent after 5 years, and over 70 percent after 10 years.

In 1982, Diamond expanded on the concept of exertional headache and described a number of patients who experienced exercise-induced, vascular-type headaches of longer duration.[3] He observed eight women and seven men ranging between 22 and 72 years of age. Five of the patients developed headaches only during physical activity. The remaining patients experienced headaches both during exercise and also with activities such as coughing, shouting, and sneezing. The location of the headache was variable but remained consistent in each patient. Nine patients had bilateral headaches. In five patients headaches were unilateral, and in one patient the headaches alternated from side to side. The duration of these headaches ranged from 15 minutes to 16 hours, with a mean of 4 hours. The character was throbbing in eight, stabbing in six, and pressure-like in one. Six of the patients also had headaches unrelated to exertion but similar to the pain produced by exertion. Four of the patients had common migraine, and two experienced cluster headaches. Two patients experienced muscle contraction headaches, which were distinct from their exertional headaches. Dr. Diamond[3] described several factors that he believed might be responsible for exercise-induced headache. These included raised intrathoracic pressure, sudden rises in systemic blood pressure, and maneuvers that would cause traction on the pain-sensitive structures of the head. He also postulated that vasoactive chemicals might be involved.

In 1982, Massey[11] noted that headaches experiencd by runners had many features in common with altitudinal headache. Massey believed that hyperventilation during exercise as well as at high altitudes produced hypocapnia, which removed the dilator response to carbon dioxide, thereby precipitating the headache. He also stated that exertion could produce a rise in systemic blood pressure with resultant extracranial vasodilatation and headache.

Headache on exertion implies that physical activity has produced the head pain. Several authors have attempted to distinguish between the headache that occurs in response to activities such as weightlifting and bowling from headaches that occur in response to aerobic sports, such as cross-country skiing, ice skating, running, and swimming. They term the latter headache "effort migraine."[2] In my opinion, such distinction and terminology unnecessarily complicate the topic. All headaches that occur as the direct result of physical activity are exertional headaches. Cough headache is included in this category. Headaches occurring on exertion that are found to be secondary to organic disease are obviously not to be included in the category of benign exertional headache. Headaches that occur secondary to traumatic injury to the head and neck are also not to be included in the category of exertional headaches. Rather, posttraumatic headaches represent a distinct entity.

The stimuli that precipitate exertional headaches may differ, but the head pain itself is very often migrainelike and for the purpose of classification is considered a type of vascular headache. A typical muscle contraction headache may also occur as a result of exercise, emphasizing the inherent difficulty in the categorization of headaches in light of the neurogenic theory of migraine. Many experts believe that there is no true distinction between the muscle contraction headache and common migraine. The exertional headache is often sharp or throbbing in character and may be accompanied by nausea and vomiting. Elementary neurologic signs such as visual disturbance, weakness, aphasia, and sensory deficit have been described in association with exercise-induced headaches, even in people with no previous history of migraine. The headache may be bilateral or unilateral. It characteristically lasts from minutes to several hours. Luge athletes have described a headache that persisted for days following a luge run.

The amount of exertion necessary to precipitate the headache varies from person to person. In aerobic sports, it has been postulated that doubling the pulse for at least 10 seconds is necessary to provide an adequate stimulus for headache. In well-conditioned athletes, much longer periods of exertion time may be required to induce headaches. Activities that increase intrathoracic pressure and, secondarily, intracranial pressure, produce headaches by a different mechanism; albeit the character of the pain may be quite similar to that experienced by athletes competing in aerobic sports. The frequency of the benign exertional headache varies with the sport. Although exact figures are not available, it occurs often in long-distance runners and cross-country skiers, and participants in alpine skiing have been known to complain of headaches related to their sport as well.

In luge sledding, virtually every participant experiences headaches, which they associate with the sport (see Chapter 41). From 1985 to 1986, we examined four male and four female members of the United States National Luge Team, ranging from 16 to 30 years of age.[13] All eight members of the team reported having headaches that were directly related to their luge runs. These headaches were usually bilateral, varying from a mild ache to a severe, incapacitating, throbbing pain. Neck pain was not a significant complaint. The duration of the headaches ranged from less than 1 hour to days, the usual duration being several hours. Two athletes experienced common migraine in addition to their luge-related headaches. One of these sledders also had a family history of migraine. The luge-associated headaches were more severe early in the training season and were said to be aggravated by rough or bumpy tracks. Fast tracks also seemed to provide more of a stimulus to these headaches. As we followed the luge athletes, the severity of their headaches definitely lessened toward the end of their competitive season.

Exertional headache is pervasive in the world of sports. The percentage of participants who suffer from headaches varies, depending on the type of sport in which they are involved. Although exact numbers are not available, we know that the frequency may range from an uncommon occurrence in some sports to an almost universal experience in others. To the athlete who suffers from exercise-induced headaches the problem is paramount and must be addressed.

Mechanism of Exertional Headache

The classic teaching has been that the pain of the vascular headache results from dilatation of intracranial or extracranial blood vessels, producing the characteristic throbbing pain, which is often accompanied by nausea and vomiting. The aura of classic migraine was believed to be the result of constriction of intracranial blood vessels occurring before the dilatation. Recent research has shown that the mechanism appears to involve changes in monoamine transmission in the central nervous system. Inhibition of transmission in pain pathways by enkephalins is known to be regulated by serotonergic neurons originating in the brainstem raphe nuclei. Noradrenergic neurons originating in the locus ceruleus of the brainstem are intimately involved with this system. Migraine and most other benign headaches appear to result from a defective central monoaminergic transmission in a system that extends from the upper cervical spinal cord through the brainstem and hypothalamus to the cortex. Vascular changes that do occur are the result of the neural stimulation from these pathways. Characteristic changes in certain blood elements, such as platelet aggregation and serotonin release, appear to be induced by specific releasing factors which are mobilized by direct neurogenic stimulation. Other manifestations, including sterile inflammation around cranial blood vessels, appear to be secondary to stimulation or inhibition of specific central pathways as well.[8,10,12]

The trigeminal nerve contains the pain pathways for structures above the tentorium cerebelli. Fibers from the trigeminal nerve descend in the spinal tract to the level of the second cervical segment. Upper segments of the spinal cord form an important center for the relay of head pain. Sensory fibers from the upper three cervical roots make synaptic contact with trigeminal neurons in the spinal tract and nucleus.[9] Significant overlap exists between the cervical and trigeminal distributions. Patients with headaches often suffer from pain in the cervical region. In addition, patients suffering from disease of both the upper and the lower cervical spine often experience headaches. It is well known that patients suffering from flexion-extension injuries of the cervical spine develop headaches more than 60 percent of the time.[9]

The cluster headache variant, chronic paroxysmal hemicrania, which has been described by Sjaastad and colleagues,[15] is pertinent to this discussion. This vascular headache, which occurs most commonly in women, is always unilateral and is described as a severe pain, unaccompanied by nausea and vomiting, that can occur 6 to 24 times a day with each attack usually lasting less than

15 minutes. The headaches are uniformly precipitated by flexion of the neck. Body flexion will not produce an episode. After a 5- to 15-second latency, the patient will experience a pulsating sensation on the side of the neck where the headache will develop, followed by the severe, unilateral headache, which is located periorbitally. Rotation of the head may also produce the headache with a latency of approximately 30 seconds. A partial Horner's syndrome often accompanies the pain. Arteriographic studies in patients suffering from this disorder have shown that the carotid arteries are not occluded when the neck is flexed. Various mechanisms have been proposed to explain this disorder, including a neurochemical hypothesis. Because of the short latency, however, it is now generally believed that autonomic mechanisms might be involved, specifically the sympathetic nervous system.[15] The hypothalamus, which is the source of the autonomic nervous system, is intimately involved in the central monoaminergic system which I have described previously in this chapter. Control of the monoaminergic transmission may be induced by the hypothalamus directly, or indirectly, as a result of impulses received from the cortex or thalamus. Cluster headaches probably originate in the hypothalamus.

I postulate that the exercise-induced headache occurs through stimulation of the central monoaminergic system, which results in the enhancement or diminution of monoamine transmission in different pathways. Stimulation may affect the system anywhere along its course, ranging from the upper cervical region through the brainstem to the hypothalamus, thalamus, and cortex. The various mechanisms that have been proposed for the production of the exertional headache may indeed be valid in that they affect the central monoaminergic system. It can readily be seen that susceptibility to headaches would vary from individual to individual. The well-documented lower susceptibility of well-conditioned athletes to exercise-induced headache results because the central pathways have had time to adapt to the exertion of their sports. The incidence of headaches among luge athletes can be readily explained by repeated stimulation of the central pathways at the cervical level. The neck of the luge athlete is persistently flexed

against strong gravitational pull during a luge run. A bumpy track produces repeated jolts, thereby enhancing the stimulation presented to the cervical pathways. Furthermore, sports that produce increased intrathoracic pressure by the Valsalva maneuver result in increased intracranial pressure which may then stimulate the central pathways in certain individuals. Although the Valsalva maneuver may come into play with the luge-related headache, it is usually avoided by well-trained athletes, and this may also help explain the declining experience with headaches as the sledding season progresses.

Aerobic exercise may provide stimulation at an entirely different level of the central monoaminergic system, but with the same result. The mechanism for stimulation of the central pathways during aerobic activities is unclear. Hypocapnia, as postulated by Massey,[11] may be implicated. Other considerations include neurochemical release and possibly stimulation of the hypothalamus through prolonged exercise. Cervical stimulation may also be a factor but to a lesser extent than in sports such as luge and bobsledding.

Dehydration, hypoglycemia, and altitude above 5000 to 6000 feet (see Chapters 44 and 45) probably increase the susceptibility to exercise-induced headaches.[2]

Treatment of Exertional Headaches

Treatment of benign exertional headache should be multifaceted. Proper conditioning is imperative, and it also appears that a warm-up period prior to competition might be helpful to reduce stimulation of the sympathetic nervous system and resultant activation of the hypothalamus.[7] Exercises designed to increase the strength of the cervical musculature should be instituted. This may serve to provide some protection against overstimulation of the cervical pathways. For the luge athlete, research is under way to develop a cervical support that would be attached to a thoracic corset. This could greatly lessen the amount of stimulation to the neck of the sledder during a run.

For the athlete who does not respond to conservative measures, medication may be necessary. Nonsteroidal anti-inflammatory drugs, specifically indomethacin, have been shown to be effective treatment for patients suffering from exercise-induced headaches. Diamond reported that 13 out of 15 patients who experienced prolonged exertional headaches improved on indomethacin. When they were taken off this medication, the headaches returned. Although indomethacin is a potent inhibitor of prostaglandin synthesis and a vasoconstrictor that also decreases cerebrospinal fluid pressure, the exact mechanism by which the drug relieves exercise-induced headaches remains unknown.

The dosage of indomethacin that was found to be effective in treating exercise-induced headaches is 25 mg, three times a day.[3] It is interesting that the pain of chronic paroxysmal hemicrania is also alleviated with indomethacin. I have found other anti-inflammatory medication to be effective, including naproxen, 500 mg, twice daily; naproxen sodium, 550 mg, twice daily; and ibuprofen, 800 mg, four times daily. The beta blockers such as propranolol are also useful in situations in which the athlete experiences headaches each time he or she participates in the sport.

Some authors have suggested that the use of ergotamine or methysergide before exercise may help prevent exertional headache. However, these medications, although effective, are on the list of drugs banned by the International Olympic Committee; so they must be avoided by athletes involved in Olympic and World Cup competitions. Nonsteroidal anti-inflammatory medications, however, may be used unless a medical contraindication exists (see Chapter 12).

Differential Diagnosis of Headaches

All patients who experience exercise-induced headaches should be examined by a physician. Although the presence of organic disease is not common, it does occur often enough to warrant a thorough evaluation. In the study by Rooke,[14] approximately 10 percent of patients were later found to have organic disease. Intracranial lesions, such as posterior fossa tumors and foramen magnum syndromes may produce exercise-induced headaches. Subarachnoid hemorrhage should always be considered and ruled out as an etiologic possibility, as should subdural and epidural hematomas. Cervical spine disease must also be considered. A detailed medical history should be taken, followed by a complete medical and neurologic examination. Further diagnostic work-up is performed, depending on the preliminary findings and index of suspicion of the examiner. These studies might include skull and cervical x-ray examinations, contrast-enhanced computerized tomography scans with views of the foramen magnum, and magnetic resonance imaging of the head and cervical regions.

The presence of dental occlusive disease as a cause of the temporomandibular joint (TMJ) syndrome is highly touted as a frequent cause of headache. In my experience, it is uncommon and overdiagnosed. Headache that may occur as a result of TMJ disease is usually of moderate intensity and located at the vertex, occiput, or in the face, overlying the joint itself. Head pain that is produced by TMJ syndrome emanates primarily from muscular tension. Vascular headaches do not occur as a result of dental disease or TMJ dysfunction. Individuals who experience the type of pain ascribed to TMJ disease should be evaluated by a dentist who is knowledgeable in this field. Application of dental splints may prove helpful to alleviating these symptoms (see Chapter 41).

CONCLUSION

Exercise-induced benign exertional headache is a vascular-type headache that afflicts many athletes, particularly those engaged in aerobic sports. Among winter athletes, sledders are especially susceptible to exertional headache, which must be differentiated from other types of vascular headache and from headaches caused by traction, inflammation, and posttrauma. Exercise-induced headaches can be lessened with conditioning and training and managed with appropriate medication.

REFERENCES

1. Adams, F: The Genuine Works of Hippocrates. Williams & Wilkins, Baltimore, 1939.
2. Appenzeller, O: Cerebrovascular aspects of headache. Med Clin North Am 62:467–480, 1978.
3. Diamond, S: Prolonged benign exertional headache; its clinical characteristics and response to indomethacin. Headache 22:96–98, 1982.
4. Diamond, S and Dalessio, D: The Practicing Physician's Approach to Headache, ed 3. Williams & Wilkins, Baltimore, 1982.
5. Jokl, E: Indisposition after running. Medicina Dello Sport 5:363, 1965.
6. Jokl, E and Jokl, P: Der Beitrag der Sportmedizin zur klinischen Kardiologie—das Sportherz. In Altern

Leistungsfahigkeit Rehabilitation. F.K. Schattauer Verlag, 1977, pp 47–56.

7. Lambert, RW, Jr and Purnet, DL: Prevention of exercise induced migraine by quantitative warm-up. Headache 25:317–319, 1985.

8. Lance, JW: Headache. Ann Neurol 10:1–10, 1986.

9. Lance, JW: Mechanism and Management of Headache, ed 4. Butterworth, London, 1982.

10. Lance, JW, Lambert, GA, Goadsby, PJ, and Duckworth, JW: Brainstem influences on the cephalic circulation: Experimental data from cat and monkey of relevance to the mechanism of migraine. Headache 23:258–265, 1983.

11. Massey, WE: Effort Headache in Runners. Headache 22: 99–100, 1982.

12. Moskowitz, MA: The neurobiology of vascular head pain. Ann Neurol 16:157–168, 1984.

13. Mullally, WJ and Livingston, IR: Luge Headache. Presented at the American Association for the Study of Headache Annual Meeting, San Francisco, June 1988.

14. Rooke, ED: Benign exertional headache. Med Clin North Am 52:801–808, 1968.

15. Sjaastad, O, Egge, K, Horven, I, Kayed, K, Lund-Roland, L, Russell, D, and Slordahl Conradi, I: Chronic paroxysmal hemicrania: Mechanical precipitation of attacks. Headache 19:31–36, 1979.

16. Tinel, J: Un syndrome dialgie vein euse intracranierc: la cephalee a l'effort. La Pratique Medicale Francaise 13:113–119, 1932.

PART III

Injuries Common to Winter Sports

CHAPTER 21

Initial Assessment and Management of Acute Winter Sports Injuries

DAVID R. WEBB, M.D., F.A.C.S.M.

There always seems to be a sense of urgency in taking care of injured athletes. Invariably, the athlete—in addition to the coach, parents, sportswriters—asks, "How long will I be out? When can I go back?" Under the right circumstances—which may be just before the family ski vacation, the hockey league championship, or the Olympic trials—even a mild sprain can loom as an "emergency."

Occasionally, injuries occur in winter sports that do require immediate medical intervention to save life, limb, or sight. More frequently, injuries occur that, although not immediately life or limb threatening, merit timely treatment. In either case, true emergency or urgency, successful outcome may depend largely on the skillful initial assessment and management of the injury by the primary physician.

This chapter presents a practical approach to the athlete whose injuries require emergent or urgent attention. Although treatment of such injuries may involve surgery and almost certainly will involve diligent rehabilitation, the present discussion is limited to the initial assessment and management of the injuries. Emphasis will be given to the key decisions to be made by the physician on the firing line and the pitfalls to be avoided.

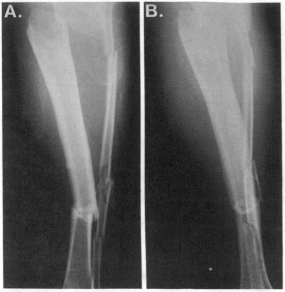

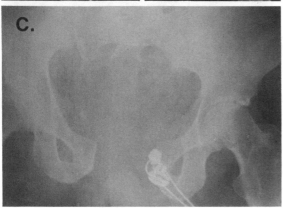

Figure 21–1. (*A, B*) AP and lateral radiographs of the leg of a downhill skier who collided at high speed with a fixed metal route marker. The comminuted, severely deformed tibia-fibula fracture was an immediately evident problem. (*C*) AP radiograph of the pelvis of the same individual. Hemorrhagic shock associated with this pelvic fracture was the more urgent problem. Indeed, the patient nearly died in the emergency department, and in the course of his hospital stay he required transfusion of over 40 units of whole blood before hemodynamic stabilization was achieved.

APPROACH TO THE SEVERELY OR MULTIPLY INJURED ATHLETE

Acute injury is a familiar occurrence in winter sports. Most of these injuries—the skier's dislocated shoulder or the hockey player's facial fracture, for example—are isolated, obvious injuries. With multiple trauma, however, the most obvious and familiar injuries may actually be the least urgent of the athlete's problems (Fig. 21–1). It is precisely because multiple, severe injuries occur infrequently in sports that the fundamentals of trauma care merit review.

There are some important "do's and don't's" that apply to carrying out the ABCs of life support (Airway, Breathing, Circulation) in a trauma situation, and sports can pose additional particular problems. For ex-

ample, in managing the airway of a head-injured athlete, using the basic life support head-tilt-neck-lift maneuver to open the airway would be contraindicated, and airway access might be restricted by the athlete's helmet and face mask (Fig. 21–2).

Of paramount importance is to have an efficient, prioritized plan for initial assessment and management of the injured athlete. In a critical situation, the standard "take a history, do a physical examination, make an assessment, come up with a treatment plan" approach to patient care is obviously inappropriate. My preference is the primary survey, resuscitation, secondary survey, definitive care approach recommended by the Committee on Trauma of the American College of Surgeons.[7]

The primary survey is simply a rapid as-

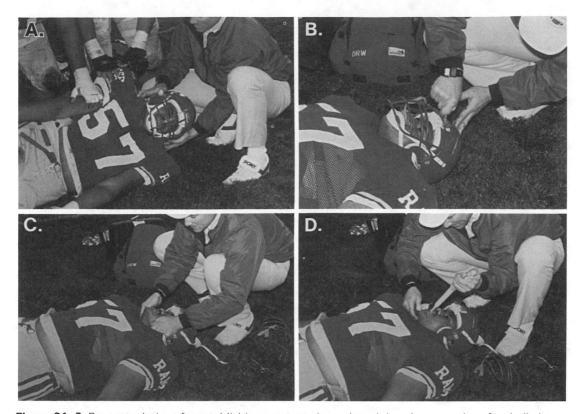

Figure 21–2. Proper technique for establishing a patent airway in an injured, unconscious football player. (Quite similar considerations may apply in other sports, e.g., snowmobiling, bobsledding.) (*A*) Log-rolling the athlete to the supine position. *It takes only a few extra seconds to protect the spine; whereas cord injury lasts a lifetime.* Four persons are required. The leader controls the head and neck and directs the other three who are positioned at the shoulders, hips, and legs. The leader's hands are crossed initially and unwind as the athlete is turned by the three assistants. The objective is to roll the athlete's body as a unit, keeping the spine immobile. Thereafter, an assistant maintains secure immobilization of the head and neck. (*B*) Preferably, access to the airway is gained by removing the mask, not the helmet. The mask is entirely removed. Cage-type masks are removed by cutting the plastic hinges. A scalpel can be used, but a stout, sharp knife works better. The cuts are made on the side of the hinge away from the face. Older bar-type masks are removed with a bolt cutter. A full wrap-around helmet such as that sometimes worn by snowmobilers may necessitate removal of the helmet at the scene. To do so without moving the neck is a difficult trick at best, worth learning and practicing if you're going to be in that type of situation. In the emergency room, it is much simpler just to cut off the wrap-around part of the helmet with a cast saw. (*C*) The athlete's chin strap is unfastened, the mouthguard is removed, and the airway is opened with a chin-pull or jaw-thrust maneuver. *A head-tilt-neck-lift maneuver to open the airway is contraindicated.* If immediate access to the airway is not required (i.e., if C-spine protection is the only consideration), the chin strap is left fastened. (*D*) The airway is cleared of any secretions, vomitus, blood, and so forth which may be present. A cook's basting syringe can be used for this purpose. This item, which can probably be procured from most kitchens, is the portable suction device par excellence. Thereafter, the position of the jaw is maintained and the suctioning repeated as necessary. (From Garrick and Webb,[3] with permission.)

sessment of vital functions. The idea is to find out what is about to kill the patient. Resuscitation is what is done to prevent that from happening. It is begun simultaneously with identification of airway, ventilatory, or circulatory problems in the primary survey (see the following section). The secondary survey is a head-to-toe assessment of the patient. The idea is to identify all the problems that will eventually require definitive treatment of some sort. Providing such treatment may require referral to a specialist and/or transportation to a trauma center.

Primary Survey

The ABCs represent the assessment/treatment priorities, that is, the order in which the primary survey/resuscitation is to be carried out. An appropriate mnemonic for the sports trauma situation is 1 A B C D E H (a modification of the standard Advanced Trauma Life Support mnemonic to make it more applicable to "at the scene," as well as "in the emergency room," situations).

1. *First, do no harm.* The most important thing in this regard is to ascertain that the cervical spine is protected until spinal injury has been ruled out. Do not permit any unnecessary manipulation of the neck, such as removal of a helmet. When it is necessary to turn or to move the athlete, use the proper log-roll technique (see Fig. 21–2).

A. *Airway.* As the highest treatment priority, airway patency must either be ruled in or obtained. Simply asking the athlete a question ("Annie, Annie, are you OK?") is a useful way to begin assessing both the airway and the level of consciousness (see below). In the athlete with an apparent airway problem, use the chin lift or jaw thrust maneuver and a suction device first. Do not use a head-tilt-neck-lift maneuver (see Fig. 21–2).

If unsuccessful in clearing the airway, proceed quickly to nasotracheal intubation or cricothyroidotomy. In children, you may attempt orotracheal intubation with an assistant carefully immobilizing the head and neck. Do not attempt tracheostomy as an emergency procedure.

B. *Breathing.* Next, adequate ventilation must be assured. Provide positive-pressure ventilation if indicated. Relieve tension pneumothorax if present.

Under ideal circumstances, the chest would be completely exposed to permit proper inspection, palpation, and auscultation. In a snow bank halfway up the mountain, it may be better just to slide your hands under the victim's outer clothing. By simple palpation, you should be able to ascertain whether or not the thorax expands and contracts appropriately with respiration, and you should be able to detect a gross flail chest or marked subcutaneous emphysema.

C. *Circulation.*
1. Identify and control external hemorrhage. Use direct pressure over the wound.
2. Assess adequacy of cardiac output by checking pulse(s), skin color, and capillary refill. Palpable radial, femoral, and carotid pulses imply systolic blood pressures of at least 80, 70, and 60 mmHg, respectively. Thumbnail capillary refill in the time it takes to say "capillary refill" suggests normovolemia. (Obviously, with cold exposure, skin color and capillary refill are less than perfectly reliable diagnostic signs.)

D. *Disability.* Carry out a brief, baseline neurologic (disability) assessment. Check the size and reactivity of the pupils. Use the AVPU mnemonic as follows to describe the level of consciousness:

A—Alert
V—Responds to verbal stimuli
P—Responds to painful stimuli
U—Unresponsive

E. *Exposure.* The aphorism in the emergency room is "undress to assess"—reflecting the importance of a thorough examination so as not to miss anything important. This obviously has limited at-the-scene applicability in most winter sports situations, in which too much "exposure" may already be a major problem. Still, a judicious look at a particular injury may be appropriate. For example, you do not want to wait until blood has soaked through 4 inches of down clothing before you perceive the need to control the hemorrhage associated with an open fracture.

H. *Help.* Upon completion of the primary survey, the extent of the life-threatening injuries and the requirements for further management of those injuries should be apparent. Obtain help and arrange for transportation as appropriate. Then proceed with further resuscitation, stabilization, and secondary assessment.

Fundamental as these concepts would seem to be, they are sometimes forgotten or ignored in "the heat of battle." If indeed there are no life-threatening problems, following the above protocol "wastes" only a few seconds of your time. If, however, there is a life-threatening problem, following the protocol can keep you and your patient out of a lot of unnecessary trouble and may help you save your patient's life.

Resuscitation

As you proceed with resuscitation, you will endeavor to repair and to stabilize the identified life-threatening problems. The extent to which you are able to do this will obviously depend upon the circumstances (e.g., whether you're still on the mountainside, or in a community hospital emergency room, or in a major trauma center). However, the basic plan remains the same. Resuscitative measures begun during the primary survey are continued, and specific treatment for shock, hypothermia, cardiac dysrhythmias, and so forth is initiated as indicated. The adequacy of resuscitation is continually and quantitatively assessed. *Vital signs are vital.* In the winter sports situation, monitoring the core temperature is particularly important (see Chapter 18).

Secondary Survey

As you go on to the secondary survey, keep in mind that your objective is simply to obtain a sufficient database for making a safe and appropriate disposition. It is not necessary to make definitive diagnoses, but, rather, it is necessary and sufficient only to identify problems that require further treatment. Indeed, *it is inappropriate to continue a work-up that would delay an obviously indicated disposition.* For example, a patient with abdominal trauma and peritoneal signs requires hemodynamic stabilization and transfer to a surgical service. It is not necessary for you to determine that the patient has a ruptured spleen, or even a hemoperitoneum. It would be contraindicated to delay transport in order to obtain an intravenous pyelogram (IVP).[2]

Definitive Care

For the injured athlete, "definitive care" comprises not just the definitive surgical treatment of the injuries, but all of the care required to enable him or her to return safely to athletic participation. This may include surgery, casting, bracing, medical treatment, physical therapy, rehabilitation, and modified sport-specific training.

A more complete discussion of the evaluation and treatment, and especially the definitive care, of the severely injured athlete is beyond the scope of this chapter. The interested reader is referred to the several articles and texts cited at the end of this chapter.[3,7,10]

APPROACH TO THE ATHLETE WITH POSSIBLE SPINAL INJURY

Although uncommon, spinal fractures, dislocations, and cord injuries do occur in sports. In fact, sports account for some 10 to 15 percent of all severe spinal injuries.[6] Among winter sports, both downhill skiing and ice hockey have been implicated.[4,6,8,9]

If anything in sports is more tragic than catastrophic spinal injury, it is the severe injury made catastrophic by improper treatment. This is not just a theoretic concern. In one series of spinal cord injuries, some 10 percent of patients had onset or worsening of neurologic deficit after the original injuries had occurred.[5] There are numerous accounts of patients who became quadriplegic after having been able to ambulate or to move their limbs at the scenes of accidents. In my own practice, I have had a patient walk in with an unstable neck fracture 2 weeks after having been bucked off his horse and landing on his head. Another presented with a complaint of neck pain several hours after a bicycle accident in which he had landed on his head with sufficient force to break his helmet in two. He had actually been referred from the emergency department for another problem without immobilization or radiographic examination of his cervical spine.

The caveats remain. *Apparent absence of neurologic deficit does not rule out spinal injury. Anyone who has sustained substantial trauma to the head or neck is presumed to have an unstable injury of the cervical spine until that possibility has been ruled out.*[7] To do so clinically, one must demonstrate sequentially that the patient is fully alert, that there is no neck pain, tenderness, or deformity; that there is no neurologic deficit; and finally, that there is a full and pain-free range of active neck motion. If any one of these criteria is not met, then immobilization and radiographic examination are required[7,11,12] (Fig. 21–3). It is better to be a stickler for spine protection and be "wrong" 99 percent of the time than to be cavalier about it and be "right" 99 percent of the time.

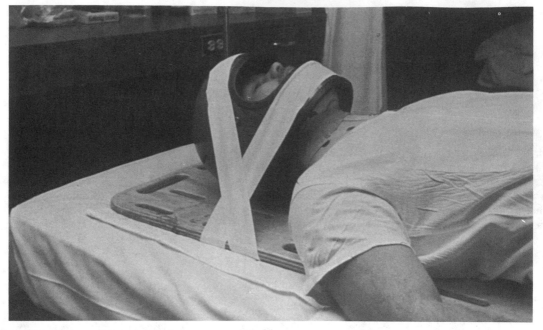

Figure 21–3. Proper technique of spine immobilization. The patient has been log-rolled onto a long spine board as shown in Figure 21–2. Manual control of the cervical spine is maintained, the torso and limbs are strapped to the board, and a rigid or semirigid (Philadelphia) cervical collar is applied. Sandbags, IV bags, or the like can be used to provide additional stabilization of the cervical spine. Finally, the head and neck are secured to the spine board with tape, gauze rolls, velcro straps, and so forth.

APPROACH TO THE ATHLETE WITH EXTREMITY INJURY

As with multiple system injuries, there are certain assessment/treatment priorities with extremity injuries. Of highest priority (greatest urgency) are control of hemorrhage, prevention of further injury, and restoration of blood flow to the injured limb. Of next greatest urgency are reduction of joint dislocations, wound care (especially in the case of open fractures or dislocations), and replantation of amputated parts. Of least urgency are such things as definitive treatment of fractures; repair of tendons, ligaments, and peripheral nerves; and treatment of meniscal tears. The aphorism that "a fracture is a soft tissue injury complicated by a broken bone" helps keep things in proper perspective.

The examiner must beware of certain pitfalls. In the skeletally immature, for example, "just a sprain" may in fact be a physeal injury—more protection is usually required. "Just a bruise" of the arm (biceps, brachialis) or thigh (quadriceps) may lead to myositis ossificans—protection from further injury is essential. "Just a bruise" of the leg may in fact be an acute compartment syndrome—a condition that must be diagnosed and treated urgently. Manifestations of a "wrist sprain" may reflect more serious local trauma—carpal fracture must be ruled out by physical examination and bone scan. ("Negative x-rays" do not rule out this diagnosis.) An "isolated" fracture of a paired bone, e.g., radius and ulna, may not be—look for a fracture or dislocation of the other. Do not undertreat an acute shoulder subluxation—it should be treated exactly as a dislocation. Do not mistake peroneal tendon dislocation for a lateral ankle sprain—the former requires surgical treatment, the latter does not. Do not treat (gamekeeper's) thumb sprains lightly—careful examination, protection, and sometimes surgical treatment are required.

To a large extent, preventing further injury means properly padding and splinting the injured limb before moving the patient. The general rule "Splint 'em as they lie" particularly applies to fractures involving the spine, shoulder, elbow, wrist, and knee. With angulated long-bone fractures, however, it is usually best to "straighten" the limb prior to splinting, especially if there is any neurovascular impairment and/or extreme tenting of the skin. Satisfactory alignment can usually be accomplished by first applying gentle in-line traction on the limb (with an assistant providing countertraction as necessary) and then gently bringing the distal part back into its normal anatomic position. While traction is maintained, the neurovascular status of the limb is reassessed (and documented), and then the appropriate splint is applied and/or secured. (Injury-specific splinting techniques are summarized in Table 21–1.)

Virtually anything that provides some stability can be used as a splint. This includes adjacent body parts, rolled-up or folded-up blankets, clothing, pillows, and so forth, as well as specifically designed splinting devices. The "most appropriate" splint will depend on the specific injury and circumstances.

Air splints are ubiquitous and in the multiple trauma situation are certainly expe-

Table 21–1. IMMOBILIZATION OF SPECIFIC INJURIES

Site	Injury	Suggested Immobilization
SC joint	Dislocation or sprain	Figure-of-eight clavicle strap and sling
Clavicle	Fracture	
	Proximal and middle thirds	Sling and swath or figure-of-eight strap and sling
	Distal third	Sling and swath
AC joint	"Separation" or sprain	Sling and swath
Shoulder	Dislocation	
	Anterior	Unreduced, splint "as is"
		Postreduction, sling and swath or shoulder immobilizer
	Posterior	Sling and swath "as is"
Humerus	Fracture	
	Shaft	Rigid splint, sling and swath
	Supracondylar	Splint "as is" (or as required to restore distal blood flow)
Elbow	Fracture or dislocation	Splint "as is," sling
Forearm	Fracture	Rigid splint, air splint, or pillow splint and sling
Wrist	Fracture or dislocation	Splint "as is," sling
Hand	Any severe injury	Bandage and splint in "intrinsic plus" position (MCPs flexed, IPs extended)
Finger	Volar plate injury	Splint PIPJ in 30° of flexion
	All other	Splint in "intrinsic plus" position
Thumb	UCL sprain	Abduction-limiting splint or thumb spica cast
Pelvis	Fracture	MAST, spine board
Hip	Fracture	Traction splint, rigid splint, or splint to uninjured limb, and spine board
	Dislocation	Spine board and support injured limb with pillows
Femur	Fracture (shaft)	Traction splint and/or MAST
Knee	Any severe injury	Splint "as is" (or as required to restore distal blood flow); use knee immobilizer, Jones' compression splint, or traction-type splint without traction
Tibia/fibula	Fractures	Rigid splint, Jones' compression splint, traction splint with some traction, or air splint
TendoAchilles	Grade III strain	Splint in full plantar flexion with Jones' compression splint
Ankle and foot	Any severe injury	"Posterior" splint, Jones' compression splint, air splint, or pillow splint
Toe	Fracture or dislocation	Tape to adjacent toe

Adapted from Caroline.[1]

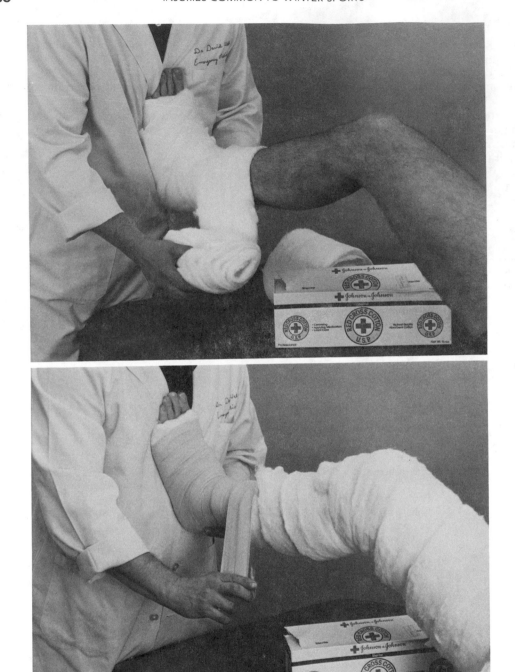

Figure 21–4. Application of a Jones' compression splint. The limb is first wrapped with thick cotton sheet wadding. Then, either layers or elastic bandages and plaster strips or, more simply, just an elasticized plaster bandage is applied. (From Garrick and Webb,[3] with permission.)

dient. They are used mainly for distal extremity fractures. They do provide some compression for control of swelling and bleeding, but the pressure can vary considerably with changes in altitude and temperature, and excessive pressure can cause neurovascular impairment. In transport, they can be quite hot and uncomfortable, and they certainly do not immobilize as well as rigid splints. These drawbacks ought to preclude their use except when expediency is the paramount concern.

Medical (originally military) antishock trousers (MAST) are a special type of air splint. They are used to splint pelvic fractures and other lower limb injuries and to tamponade abdominal, pelvic, and lower limb bleeding. Any of the problems associated with air splints can occur with the use of MAST pants, although most versions now feature pop-off valves which limit excessive pressure build-up. Congestive heart failure/pulmonary edema can be made worse by MAST pants and is thus a contraindication to their use. The major problem with MAST pants, however, is the hypovolemic shock which can follow their abrupt removal. The caveat is that no one—you, EMT-basic, or

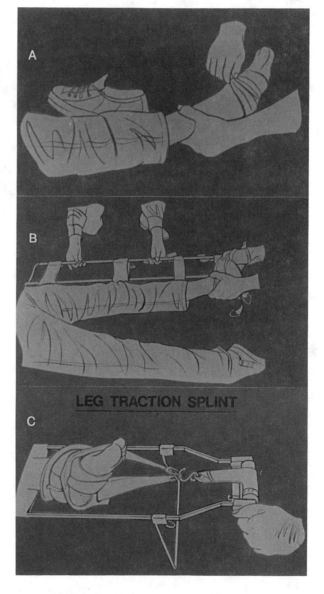

Figure 21–5. Application of a Hare traction splint for immobilization of a femur fracture. (A) In-line traction on the limb is applied by grasping the ankle. (B) An ankle hitch is applied and thereafter used to maintain the traction. The splint is placed under the limb and the proximal end (half-ring) pressed firmly against the ischial tuberosity. (C) The ankle hitch is then fastened to the distal end of the splint and the windlass turned to provide further traction as needed. Restoration of blood flow and/or relief of pain and muscle spasm are desired end points. Finally, the straps are adjusted to support and to secure the limb to the splint, and neurovascular status is again reassessed. (From the American College of Surgeons Committee on Trauma, Subcommittee on Advanced Trauma Life Support, Instructor Manual slides, 1982, with permission.)

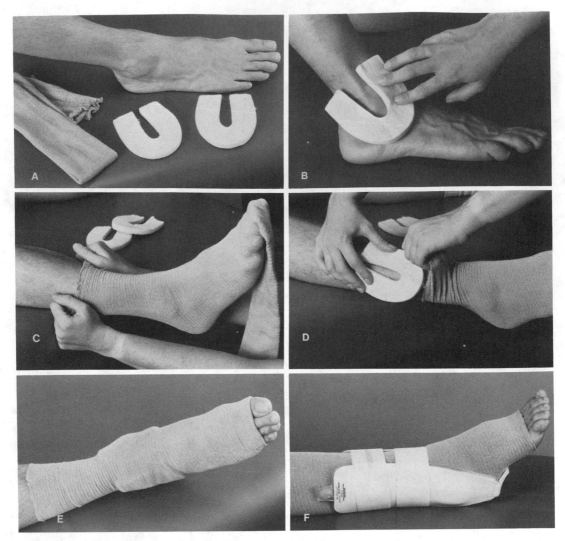

Figure 21–6. Application of a compression wrap for an acute ankle injury. (A) An elastic wrap, preferably elasticized stockinette, and two horseshoe-shaped pads are used. The pads can be fashioned from ABDs. (B) The pads are placed so as to fill in the hollows around the malleoli. (C–E) Stockinette is then applied over the padding. (F) If ambulation is to be permitted, a stirrup-type splint is then applied over the compression wrap. (From Garrick and Webb,[3] with permission.)

chief of surgery—be allowed to deflate the MAST pants until all the lines are in and either the vital signs have been stabilized or the patient is in the operating room. When MAST pants are deflated outside the operating room, first the abdominal part, then one limb, then the other are gradually deflated while the vital signs are continually monitored.

Rigid or semirigid splints generally provide the best immobilization of a limb. The important factor is that they be adequately padded. Of the several types, my favorite is the Jones' compression splint or "cotton cast" (Fig. 21–4). Although not usually applicable at the scene, it is especially useful for long interfacility transport (e.g., from ski resort emergency room to urban hospital). It provides good comfort, uniform compression with little risk of neurovascular or cutaneous compromise, and excellent immobilization.

Traction splints are special types of rigid splints. They are particularly useful for femur fractures, which are usually associated with considerable muscle spasm. Traction is provided via an ankle hitch; and countertraction, by pressure against the ischial tuberosity (Fig. 21–5). Thus, ankle or pelvic injuries may limit their usefulness. However, these ubiquitous devices make pretty good splints for most lower limb injuries, whether or not traction is required. They can be used, for example, with a lot, a little, or no traction, for splinting femur, tibia-fibula, and knee fractures, respectively.

The initial treatment of most acute, uncomplicated musculoskeletal injuries will include rest, ice, compression, and elevation (RICE). (Obviously, the RICE mnemonic does not apply in cases complicated by hypothermia, cold-induced tissue injury, or open wounds). Depending on the severity of injury, "rest" may be either relative (i.e., simple avoidance of pain-producing activity) or absolute (i.e., immobilization of the injured part). With lower limb injuries, rest also usually implies using crutches for ambulation. When immobilization is not required, non-weight-bearing crutch ambulation is advanced to partial weight-bearing ambulation with heel-to-toe gait as tolerated. "Ice" implies application of crushed ice for 20 minutes at least once every 4 waking hours. It can and should be applied over any compression wraps, splints, casts, and the like. Ice treatment is continued until the swelling stabilizes. Most immobilizers do not provide adequate compression, so "compression" usually means application of a separate compression wrap. Typically, this consists of felt or similar padding around bony prominences held in place by a snug elastic wrap or elasticized stockinette (Fig. 21–6). "Elevation" implies keeping the injured part at or above heart level (or at least waist level) at all times that the athlete is not actively using the part (e.g., for ambulation or exercise). Both compression and elevation are continued until all swelling is resolved. At first, elevation may be intuitive, as the athlete soon realizes the injured part hurts more when it is dependent. Later, however, the athlete may have to be reminded to keep it elevated conscientiously.

Adequate compression and immobilization for acute knee injuries can usually be achieved as follows (see Fig. 21–6). ABD pads or a horseshoe-shaped felt pad is placed just above and on either side of the patella.

An elastic wrap or, preferably, elasticized stockinette is then applied over the padding. The wrap should extend from below the calf to midthigh. A knee immobilizer is then applied over the compression wrap. The immobilizer should have stiff medial, lateral, and posterior stays. It may be necessary to bend the posterior stays or to put some padding behind the knee so that the knee can be held in a position of comfort; that is, 20 to 30° of flexion.

A final important aspect of initial assessment and management is the disposition. As a general rule, an orthopedic surgeon should be involved in the management of all musculoskeletal injuries for which the diagnosis or preferred treatment is uncertain, as well as those for which surgery is clearly required.

Referral on an *emergent* basis is indicated for fractures or dislocations complicated by neurovascular impairment. Referral on an *urgent* basis is generally indicated for unreduced dislocations, penetrating joint wounds, open or structurally significant fractures, grade III strains, and mechanical disruption of normal joint function (e.g., locked meniscal tears). With the possible exception of lateral ankle sprains, referral is also indicated whenever severe ligamentous injuries (grade III sprains) are suspected and cannot be ruled out.

SUMMARY

The scope of this chapter is limited to winter sports injuries that require emergent or urgent care. The objective is to provide the reader with an efficient, prioritized plan for carrying out the initial assessment and management of such injuries.

Adapted from the American College of Surgeons' Committee on Trauma, my recommended approach to the severely or multiply injured athlete comprises a primary survey, resuscitation, a secondary survey, and definitive care. Treatment priorities for both multiple system injuries and extremity injuries are emphasized, with particular attention in each case to the prevention of further injury. Key diagnostic, treatment, and referral decisions to be made by the primary physician and the pitfalls to be avoided are also pointed out. I strongly recommend the American College of Surgeons' Advanced Trauma Life Support Course for Physicians to all physicians who are in positions to care for severely injured athletes.

REFERENCES

1. Caroline, NL: Emergency Care in the Streets, ed 2. Little Brown, & Co, Boston, 1983.
2. Casey, MJ: Renal trauma. Mil Med 129:136–142, 1964.
3. Garrick, JG and Webb, DR: Sports Trauma: An Algorithmic Approach to Common Problems. WB Saunders, Philadelphia (in press).
4. Oh, S: Cervical injury from skiing. Int J Sports Med 5:268–271.
5. Rogers, WA: Fractures and dislocations of the cervical spine. J Bone Joint Surg 39A:341–376, 1957.
6. Shields, CL, Jr, Fox, JM, Shannon, E, and Stauffer, E: Cervical cord injuries in sports. Phys Sportsmed 6:71–76, 1978.
7. Subcommittee on Advanced Trauma Life Support (ATLS) of the American College of Surgeons (ACS) Committee on Trauma: Advanced Trauma Life Support Course: Instructor Manual. American College of Surgeons, Chicago, 1984.
8. Tator, CH and Edmonds, VE: National survey of spinal injuries in hockey players. Can Med Assoc J 130:875–880, 1984.
9. Tator, CH, Ekong, CE, Rowde, DW, and Schwarz, ML: Spinal injuries due to hockey. Can J Neurol Sci 11:34–41, 1984.
10. Torg, JS (ed): Athletic Injuries to the Head, Neck, and Face. Lea & Febiger, Philadelphia, 1982.
11. Wales, LR, Knopp, RK, and Morishima, MS: Recommendations for evaluation of the acutely injured cervical spine: A clinical radiologic algorithm. Ann Emerg Med 9:422–428, 1980.
12. Williams, CF, Berstein, TW, and Jelenko, C: Essentiality of the lateral cervical spine radiograph. Ann Emerg Med 10:198–204, 1981.

CHAPTER 22

Head Injuries in Winter Sports

JAMES B. McQUILLEN, M.D.

Serious head injuries are unusual in winter sports. Between 1983 and 1984, only 1 head fracture and 44 head contusions were reported from all of the venues operated by the Olympic Regional Development Authority at Lake Placid.[2] The fracture occurred at the Mount Van Hoevenberg Bobsled and Luge Complex and was not associated with severe concussion or neurologic signs. The bobsled and luge complex also reported 11 head contusions. Twenty-four head contusions occurred at the Whiteface Mountain Alpine Ski Center; five head contusions occurred at the Lake Placid Olympic Arena, and two were reported each at the Intervale Ski Jump and the Mount Van Hoevenberg Cross-Country Skiing Complex. None of these contusions was considered to be critical or severe.

Yet for all winter sports—skiing, skating, and sliding—the risk of severe head injuries is ever present (see Chapters 1, 29, 32, 35, 36, 39, and 41). This chapter looks to the Vermont skiing experience to discover that head injuries were a common denominator for the fatal accidents that occurred. The circumstances of these accidents are examined to determine the underlying factors that led to the fatal injuries. Then, major syndromes and complications of head injuries are discussed with an eye to defining those factors that may be managed to prevent fatal outcomes.

THE VERMONT EXPERIENCE

The State of Vermont considers itself the "skiing capital of the East." As such, skiing injuries, especially lethal injuries, assume immense importance and are carefully investigated. During seven Vermont ski seasons (1979 to 1986) representing 24.2 million skier days, 16 skiing fatalities were logged by the State Medical Examiner's Office.[6]

The leading cause of skiing death is craniocerebral trauma. Other winter sports share similar injuries, but Alpine skiing remains the prototype winter sport and, with increased speed, has introduced new clinical and pathologic syndromes never before recognized. Fourteen of the 16 cases were documented by complete autopsy.

Because the death of any person "from violence or by casualty or as a result of an injury" in Vermont must be reported by law to a regional medical examiner, it is unlikely that any cases of skiing fatality were omitted in this study. Autopsy may be ordered by the State's Attorney or the Chief Medical Examiner. Therefore, all accidental ski deaths must be certified by the medical examiner system.

Of the 16 deaths, 15 were secondary to craniocerebral trauma. Fifteen of the 16 accidents were witnessed, and the common denominator for all was that the skier was out of control. Death occurred at the scene in three instances, and in the emergency room or within one-half hour of arrival at a hospital in seven other cases; in all other fatal cases involving survival more than 30 minutes after hospital admission, the patients died of edema and herniation. Skull fractures were present in 13 of the 16 cases, and occipital skull fractures were by far the most common.

Fourteen of the 16 deaths occurred because of a collision between the skier and a stationary object, usually a tree. Two of the 16 deaths were secondary to falls. Ability was not a significant factor, as equal numbers were found in beginners and experts. The difficulty of the trails did not appear significant: in two cases the trail exceeded the skier's competence, in six the skier appeared to be on an adequate and appropriate slope for level of ability, and in seven cases the skier's competence exceeded the difficulty of the trail. Alcohol was not an important factor. Blood alcohol was determined in 13 cases. It was absent in 12 of these cases, and a minimal level was present in the other case. It did appear that fatigue was an important factor, and excessive speed was the lethal factor.

DISCUSSION

Skull Fractures

Fractures of the anterior aspect of the skull were unusual among the Vermont skiing fatalities, and when they did occur, anterior fracture occurred only with associated basal skull fractures. Basal and occipital skull fractures were by far the most common and frequently occurred as an isolated fracture. The frequency of occipital and basal skull fractures is explained by the lack of protective reflexes when the human body is falling backward. Reflexes for self-defense are aimed at protecting the anterior aspect of the skull. For that reason, the latter type of skull fracture was infrequent. The lethal nature of the skull fracture is explained by the tendency of a blow to the occiput to cause contrecoup lesions. The concept of coup and contrecoup brain injury has long been accepted as established fact. When one critically examines the results of multiple skull injuries, however, it becomes apparent that a coup delivered to the frontal part of the skull infrequently produces a significant contrecoup lesion in the occipital lobes; whereas a coup lesion produced in the occiput produces a severe and significant contusion on the orbital surface of the frontal lobes and the tips of the temporal lobes. This is explained by the fact that cerebral contusions tend to occur where the bony skull has the firmest grip upon the brain.[7]

Subdural Hematoma

Subdural hematomas were noted in seven cases. In only one case was the subdural hematoma of clinical significance,[4] exceeding 100 ml. Epidural hematoma was an unusual event, occurring in only one case. Two cases of subarachnoid hemorrhage were noted. Both of these were associated with subdural hematoma. Only a single intraparenchymal hemorrhage was seen.

Other Lesions

Pontine medullary lacerations were noted in two cases. This is not an uncommon lesion in motor vehicle accidents when there is hyperextension of the chin on impact,[3] but when pontine medullary lacerations are seen in a nonvehicular accident, they attest to the skier's speed at the time of impact.

Diffuse Axonal Injury

For over 150 years, it has been suspected that rapid rotational forces producing a shear effect in the brain could tear axons. These lesions produce a clinical syndrome of immediate neurologic deficit at the time of impact, and if survival occurs, it is in an akinetic, mute, or vegetative state.[1] None of the skiers involved in this report survived sufficiently long to develop histologic evidence of this syndrome (eosinophilic rounded retraction balls within the white matter of the brain); however, the gross lesions characteristic of this syndrome were noted (tearing of the corpus collosum and contusion of the mesenocephalic tegmentum), and it was these gross lesions that indicated the diagnosis despite the rapidity of demise.

Malignant Cerebral Edema

There is a syndrome termed "malignant cerebral edema," which is seen in children. This syndrome is characterized by sudden neurologic deterioration following cranial trauma, which is associated with rapid bilateral swelling of the brain and usually unassociated with a neurosurgical lesion.[5] The basic pathophysiology appears to be vasodilatation and initial hyperemia with redistribution of blood from the subarachnoid and pial vessels into the parenchyma of the brain. Similar rapid brain swelling may be seen in young adults, and here it may be unilateral.

An example of "malignant cerebral edema" was demonstrated in an 18-year-old downhill racer on the Italian World Cup team. During the previous month, he had won his first downhill race in World Cup competition. On the day of his collapse while racing at Lake Placid, he was severely jarred as he struck a mogul. He did not fall at the time of impact; however, as he was approaching the finishing line, for no apparent reason he fell and slid across the line. He stood and watched the continuation of the race for several minutes, and then he complained of dizziness and collapsed. A team physician reached him almost immediately and found fixed, dilated pupils, deep coma, and shallow respirations. A computerized tomographic (CT) scan revealed massive swelling of the left cerebral hemisphere. He remained in a chronic vegetative state until his death. It was subsequently discovered that 2 weeks prior to his sudden collapse he had fallen on the slopes, sustaining a "minor" head injury.

The possibility that sequential injuries may lead to sudden brain swelling, as occurred in this skier, was reinforced by the demise of a 19-year-old college football player. Five days prior to his collapse he was involved in a fist fight, during which he received a blow to the head and briefly lost consciousness. He noted headaches for the ensuing 3 days. By the fourth day, he was well enough to play football. Following a running play in which he was involved as a blocker, he walked from the field and collapsed, despite accounts of no unusual head trauma. Examination immediately after his collapse revealed fixed, dilated pupils, deep coma, and ataxic respirations. A CT scan performed within 30 minutes of collapse revealed extensive swelling of the right hemisphere with marked midline shift. Despite all efforts, he died 4 days following his collapse. Neuropathologic examination revealed marked cerebral edema with herniation. There was also a right frontal lobe contusion, which histologically proved consistent with the date of his concussion. It was hypothesized that the sudden brain swelling was secondary to sequential trauma that had created mild cerebral swelling and diminished intracranial compliance. It appears that by causing vasomotor paralysis, sequential trauma can produce self-sustained increased intracranial pressure with diminished intracranial compliance, so that even minor trauma can lead to sudden, catastrophic brain swelling.

CONCLUSIONS

In the vast majority of serious head injuries from skiing accidents described, medical therapy was not possible; and in those few in which it was possible, it was ineffective. If craniocerebral trauma is to be prevented, medical efforts should be aimed at the major risk factor: loss of control secondary to fatigue and excessive speed.

A second important consideration is the

prevention of sequential craniocerebral trauma with rapid brain swelling that may follow a too hasty return to sporting participation following a concussion. From our experience we recommend discontinuation of skiing, and other sports in which head trauma is risked, for at least 3 weeks following a concussion to avoid the peril of minor sequential trauma leading to "malignant cerebral edema."

The high speeds generated in winter sports and the liability to falls and impacts pose the risk of head injuries for both competitive and recreational participants. The insights gained by examining factors that probably contributed to the lethal outcomes of the cases described should help coaches and participants as they plan their training, competitive, and recreational activities.

REFERENCES

1. Adams, JH, Mitchell, DE, and Graham, DI: Diffuse brain damage of immediate impact type. Brain 100:489–502, 1977.
2. Dick, B, Hornet, J, and Pazienza, J: Sports Injuries at Lake Placid: 1983–1985, A Descriptive Study. Albany Medical College Department of Family Practice, Albany, NY, 1986.
3. Lindenberg, R and Freytag, E: Brain stem lesions characteristic of traumatic hyperextension of the head. Arch Pathol 90:509–515, 1970.
4. McLaurin, RL and Tutor, FT: Acute subdural hematoma. Review of ninety cases. J Neurosurg 18:61–67, 1961.
5. McQuillen, JB, McQuillen, EN, and Morrow, P: Trauma, sport, and malignant cerebral edema. Am J Forens Med Pathol 9(1): 12–15, 1988.
6. Morrow, P: Unpublished data, 1987.
7. Young, HA and Schmidek, HH: Complications accompanying occipital skull fractures. J Trauma 22:914–920, 1982.

CHAPTER 23

Eye Injuries in Winter Sports

MICHAEL EASTERBROOK, M.D.

Recent studies in the United States indicate that over 10 percent of more than 35,000 eye injuries per year resulted from trauma sustained during sports or recreational activities.[2] The adoption of specific safety measures, such as the strict enforcement of game regulations and the constant use of standardized protective equipment (see Chapter 29), has been associated with significant reductions in the number and incidence of eye injuries sustained in North American ice hockey.[7,10]

Although proper adherence to the rules and the appropriate use of protective equipment are capable of preventing most sports-related eye injuries in the contact sports and those which use a projectile,[2,4,5,8,9] the activities involved in the majority of winter sports have not lent themselves thus far to the application of these measures. Eye injuries are uncommon in cross-country skiing and the noncontact skating sports, whereas eye and periorbital trauma as the result of sliding and Alpine skiing accidents are ever present concerns for athletes and those who render their immediate care.[3,6] Fortunately, even in these winter sports the occurrence of eye injuries is infrequent.[10] Between 1983 and 1985, only 3 to 4 percent of injuries reported during training and competition from the Mount Van Hoevenburg bobsled and luge venue and the Whiteface Mountain Alpine skiing facility at Lake Placid were to the eye.[3] However, when eye injuries do occur in sporting events, the outcome can be most tragic. Serious competitors are generally young people, who may be confronted with a long life

195

of impaired vision when disabling eye injuries are sustained.[2]

This chapter looks at experiences gained from frequent consultations for eye injuries sustained during ice hockey training and competition, to discuss management and to develop guidelines for the primary health care provider regarding trauma to the face and periorbital tissues (also see Chapter 21). Prompt and appropriate referral to ophthalmologic care may well help save the eye of an injured athlete.[1]

ASSESSMENT OF THE ATHLETE AFTER ACUTE TRAUMA TO THE EYE

A simple history and examination on the ski slopes or in the skating rink can define the patient who should have immediate ophthalmologic evaluation and management. The following cases and discussion are presented to illustrate several points of history and eye examination that will help to define the injured player who needs referral to an ophthalmologist, in contrast to the player who may be treated conservatively and returned to competition.

HISTORY

Case 1 _____

This 29-year-old hockey player was high sticked by a defenseman as he skated for the puck (Fig. 23–1). He had no loss of vision, no photophobia, and no diplopia. Cold compresses were used to reduce the swelling, and he was able to return to action the following night.

Foreign-Body Sensation

Patients who complain of a foreign-body sensation when the eyelid blinks may have a corneal abrasion produced by a stick, a ball, or a puck, or they may have a small foreign body under the upper lid. Most ophthalmologists have a Desmarre retractor to evert the upper lid (Fig. 23–2); however, a simple paper clip may be bent in such a way (Fig. 23–3) that the eyelid can be inverted (Fig. 23–4), revealing the upper tarsus for visual inspection with a flashlight (Fig. 23–5). Examination of the cornea may reveal lack of

the normal clear light reflex. Fluorescein staining and a cobalt-blue filter readily demonstrate a small corneal abrasion, but if a foreign-body sensation persists with a normal everted upper eyelid, the irregular surface of a corneal abrasion can be recognized on the slope or on the rink with a simple penlight (Fig. 23–6).

Case 2 _____

This National Hockey League defenseman was struck in the eye with a stick (Fig. 23–7). He stated that he went completely blind before his vision began to return.

Blurring of Vision

Because of a history of vision loss, this hockey player had ophthalmologic evaluation. His pupil was dilated using mydriatic drops, and a retinal detachment was found (Fig. 23–8). The retinal detachment was successfully repaired, and the player went on to resume his professional career.

PHYSICAL EXAMINATION

Examination of the Eyelid Margin

Eyelid margin lacerations (Fig. 23–9) such as those caused by a hockey stick injury may produce notching (Fig. 23–10) of the lid unless the edges are very carefully sutured together to prevent entropion or ectropion of the lid margin. Any eyelid laceration involving the canaliculus (Fig. 23–11) is of particular concern. These patients must be referred for examination under anesthesia for careful localization and microscopic suturing of the cut ends of the canaliculus (see Chapter 21).

Examination of the Subconjunctiva

Small subconjunctival hemorrhages (Fig. 23–12) are of little consequence if the patient has had no vision loss and no symptoms of photophobia, and if examination shows a normal pupil. Such hemorrhages will usually clear in a few days. Even players with extensive subconjunctival hemorrhages (Fig. 23–13) but no history of significant vision loss and no photophobia can be returned to the

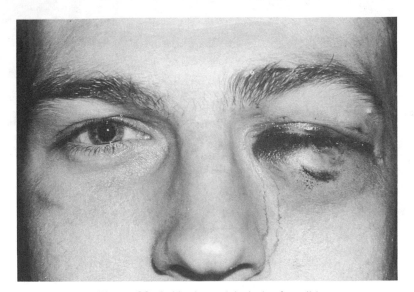

Figure 23–1. Hockey stick slash of eyelid.

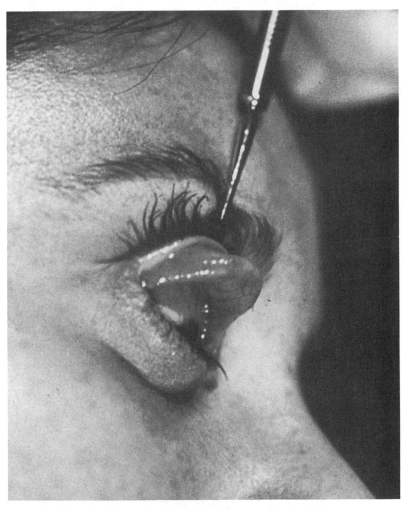

Figure 23–2. Desmarre retractor everting lid.

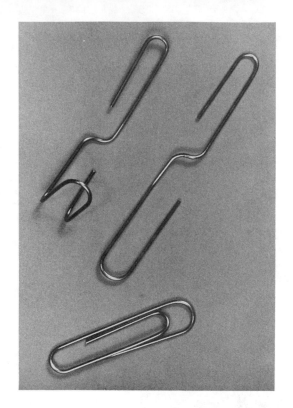

Figure 23–3. Paper clip bent to act as lid retractor.

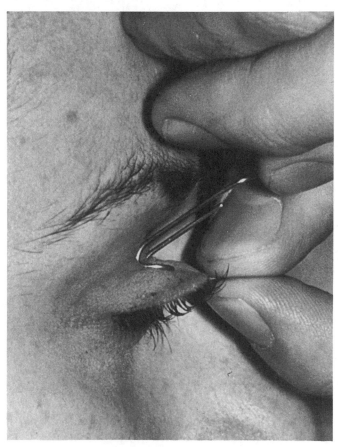

Figure 23–4. Applying bent paper clip.

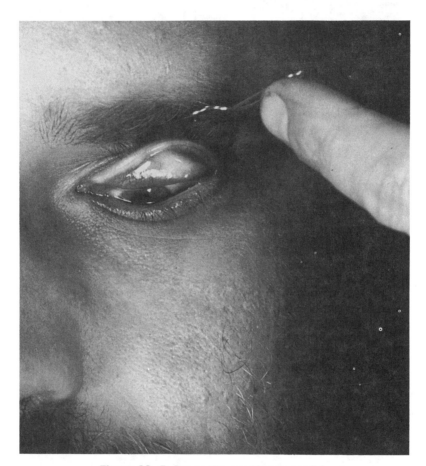

Figure 23–5. Paper clip everting upper lid.

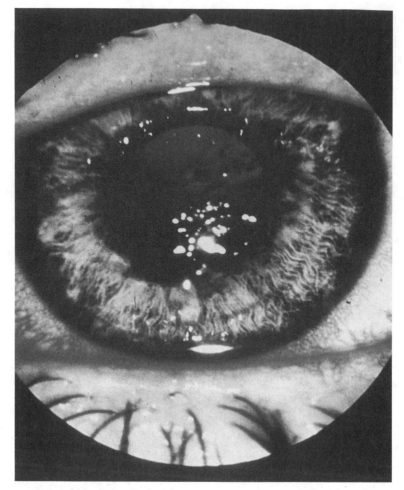

Figure 23–6. Irregular corneal reflex without fluorescein.

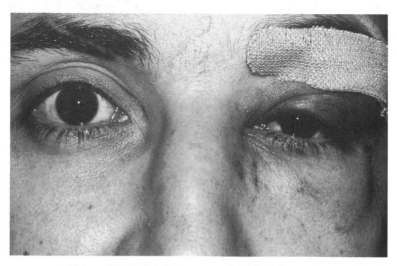

Figure 23–7. Ocular trauma to NHL defenseman.

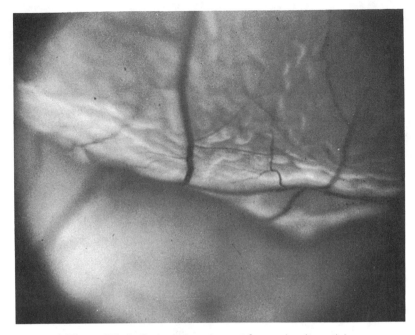

Figure 23–8. Retinal detachment from a hockey stick.

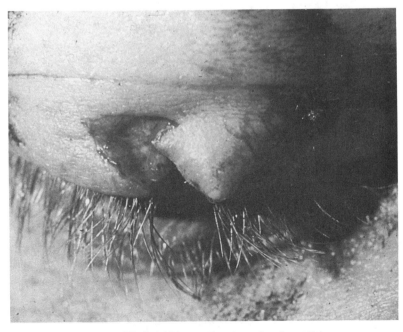

Figure 23–9. Lid laceration by a hockey stick.

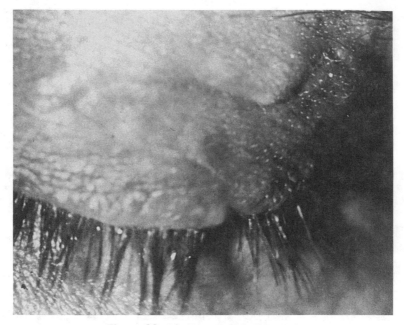

Figure 23–10. Preventable lid notch.

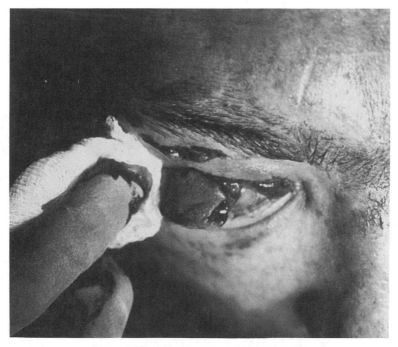

Figure 23–11. Laceration of canaliculus.

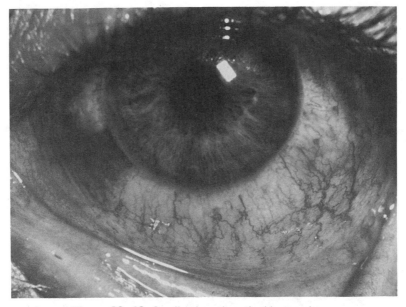

Figure 23–12. Small subconjunctival hemorrhage.

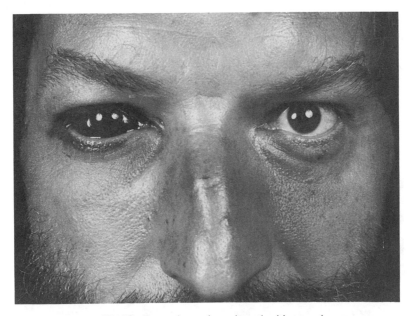

Figure 23–13. Extensive subconjunctival hemorrhage.

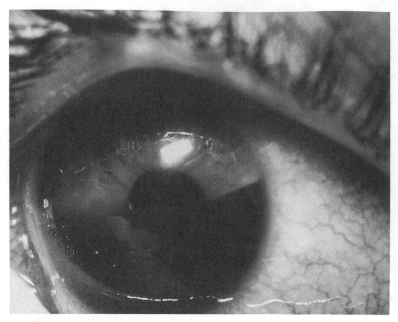

Figure 23–14. Classic hyphema—the most common reason for hospital admission.

field, although the hemorrhage may take several weeks to clear.

Examination of the Anterior Chamber

Classical hyphema (Fig. 23–14) caused by a contusion that results in tearing of the iris vessels and bleeding into the aqueous fluid of the anterior chamber appears only some hours following injury, after the patient has remained still, so that by gravity the blood has settled out to form a clear layer. These patients should be referred for ophthalmologic evaluation and will often require hos-

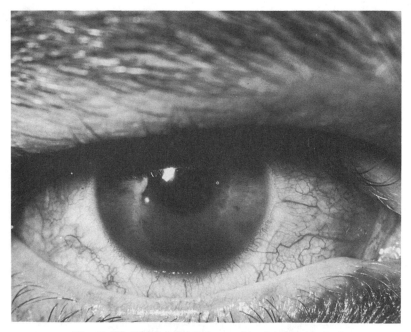

Figure 23–15. Small hyphema: Iris detail is blurred.

pitalization for prevention and management of further hemorrhage and acute glaucoma. Clouding of the anterior chamber immediately following eye injury is a common manifestation of bleeding into the anterior chamber (Fig. 23–15). If iris details are not clear on examination, a microscopic hyphema should be suspected, and the patient should be referred for slit-lamp examination.

Examination of the Pupil

Case 3 _____

This National Hockey League goal tender was struck through the eye opening in the mask by his own defenseman's stick. The astute team plastic surgeon noticed a slightly irregular pupil (Fig. 23–16) and referred the player for a slit-lamp examination. A microscopic hyphema was found, and the patient was hospitalized for 7 days. The hyphema did not rebleed and the patient continued his hockey career.

_____

The importance of carefully visualizing the pupil following an eye injury cannot be overstressed. Examination of an irregular pupil and cornea with a penlight can reveal corneal lacerations with a small iris prolapse (Fig. 23–17), which will necessitate ophthalmologic referral for slit-lamp examination and immediate surgical repair.

Examination of the Retina

Patients who present with immediate blurring of vision after an eye injury may demonstrate a retinal hemorrhage.

Case 4 _____

An eye injury that resulted in a macular hemorrhage (Fig. 23–18) ended this excellent player's National Hockey League career.

_____

All patients who sustain significant blunt trauma to the eye should have their pupil dilated for ophthalmoscopic examination.

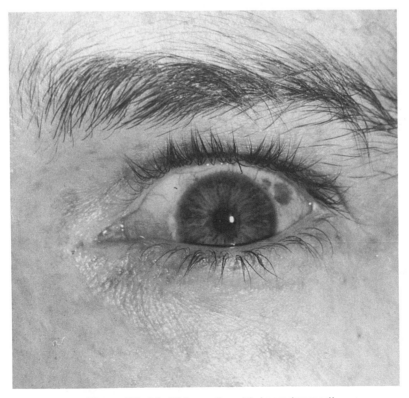

Figure 23–16. NHL goalie with irregular pupil.

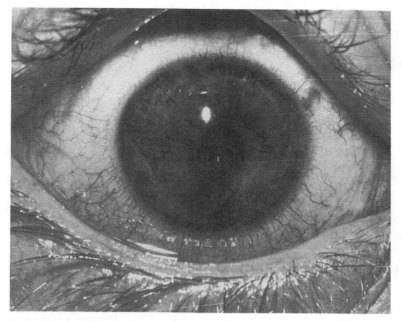

Figure 23–17. Irregular pupil from iris prolapse through corneal laceration.

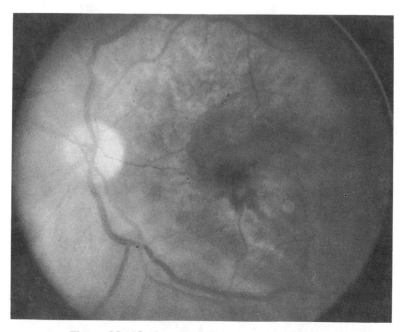

Figure 23–18. Career-ending macular hemorrhage.

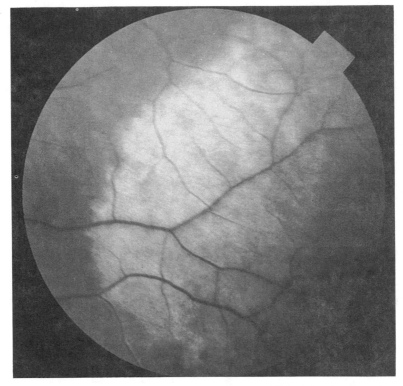

Figure 23–19. Retinal edema in Toronto NHL defenseman.

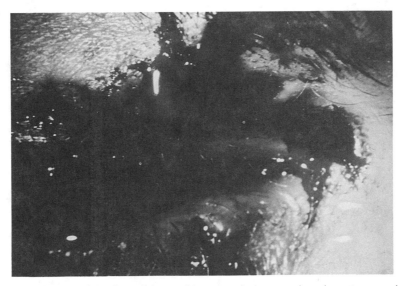

Figure 23–20. Eyelid laceration from injury with streetwear nonpolycarbonate prescription glasses.

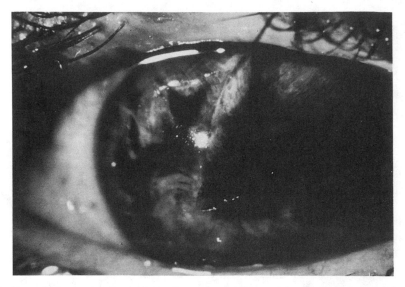

Figure 23–21. Corneal laceration and iris prolapse from injury with streetwear nonpolycarbonate prescription glasses.

Case 5

This National Hockey League defenseman, who had previously sustained a lid laceration and hyphema, developed retinal edema (Fig. 23–19) following a blow from a hockey stick. These retinal changes were transient and resolved in 10 days.

THE ATHLETE MOST AT RISK OF EYE INJURY

Case 6

This athlete, who was wearing hardened glass prescription lenses when he was struck, sustained lacerations to his eyelid (Fig. 23–20) and cornea (Fig. 23–21). Al-

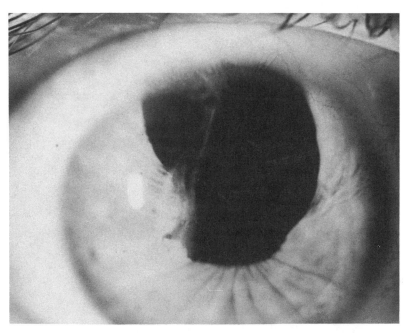

Figure 23–22. Corneal scar from broken prescription glasses.

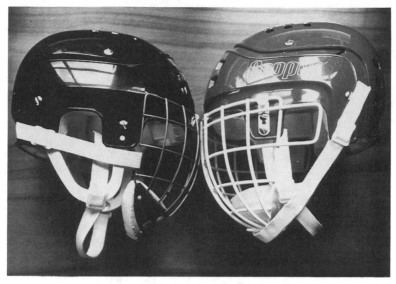

Figure 23–23. Wire eye protectors for hockey.

though the corneal laceration was success-fully repaired, the patient required a full-sec-tor iridotomy. Subsequent sequelae included photophobia, a corneal scar (Fig. 23–22), and best corrected vision of 20/100.

CONCLUSIONS

The lessons taught by the foregoing dis-cussion of hockey injuries should be applied to the initial examination of all athletes who sustain direct or indirect trauma to the eye on

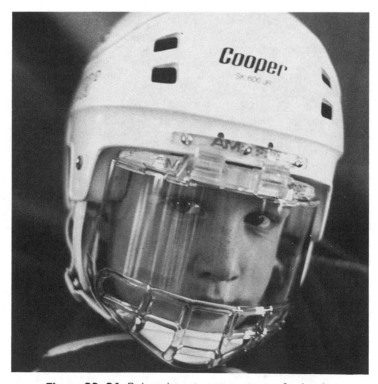

Figure 23–24. Polycarbonate eye protector for hockey.

Table 23–1. FACE MASKS APPROVED
FOR ICE HOCKEY PLAY, 1988

Canada*	United States†
St. Lawrence	St. Lawrence
Cooper Canada	Cooper Canada
Karlu Titan Canada	Karlu Titan Canada
Sports Maska (CCM)	Sports Maska (CCM)
1 Tech	1 Tech
—	Protec In.

*Canadian Standards Association
†Hockey Equipment Council

ski slopes or in the ice rink. A history of blurred vision, light sensitivity, diplopia, or loss of vision necessitates immediate referral for ophthalmologic evaluation.

Careful examination of the eyelid margin, the subconjunctiva, the cornea, the anterior chamber, the pupil, and the posterior pole with a flashlight and an ophthalmoscope should permit the physician attending an injured athlete to diagnose significant ocular trauma and to decide whether the athlete should be referred for ophthalmologic management or returned to play.

Finally, work by Dr. T. J. Pashby[7] in Canada and Paul F. Vinger[9] in the United States has significantly reduced and virtually eliminated eye injuries among organized amateur hockey players through emphasis on the strict enforcement of regulations and the use of protective face and head gear. Eyeguards approved for amateur hockey in Canada (Figs. 23–23, 23–24) have been designed to withstand 350 pounds of force over the eyes and mouth by a static test and 20 foot-pounds by kinetic testing. Table 23–1 lists the eyeguards that are currently approved for hockey play by the Canadian Standards Association and the Hockey Equipment Council in the United States.

Extrapolation of this experience to other sports that put the eyes at risk of trauma bespeaks the importance of adequate and appropriate protective equipment to prevent serious ocular injuries.[9] Whether their play is recreational or competitive, all athletes who must use prescription lenses for vision correction to participate in these sports should wear polycarbonate safety lenses mounted in industrial frames with sideshields or injection-molded eye protectors that include their prescription. Streetware eyeglasses and contact lenses offer no protection and may pose additional hazard for eye laceration if struck with sufficient force.

Adherence to these recommendations should go far toward the prevention of eye injuries and elimination of visual impairment for those who participate in winter sports.

REFERENCES

1. Antoki, S, Labelle, P, and Dumas, J: Retinal detachment following hockey injuries. Can Med Assoc J 117:245–246, 1977.
2. Bell, JB: Eye trauma in sports: A preventable epidemic. JAMA 246:156, 1981.
3. Dick, B, Hornet, J, and Pazienza, J: Sports Injuries at Lake Placid: 1983–1985. A descriptive study. Department of Family Practice, Albany Medical School, Albany, NY, 1986.
4. Easterbrook, M: Eye injuries in racquet sports: A continuing problem. Can Med Assoc J 123:268–269, 1980.
5. Easterbrook, M: Eye protection in racquet sports: An update. The Physician and Sportsmedicine 15:180–186, 1987.
6. Hart, GG: Final report, frequency of visits by ICD-9 diagnostic code. Medical Report of the XIII Winter Olympic Games. Lake Placid Olympic Organizing Committee Medical Services, Lake Placid, NY, 1980.
7. Pashby, TJ: Eye injuries in Canadian hockey. Phase II. Can Med Assoc J 117:670–677, 1977.
8. Vinger, PF: Ocular injuries in hockey. Arch Ophthalmol 94:74–76, 1976.
9. Vinger, PF: Sports-related eye injury. A preventable problem. Surv Ophthalmol 25:47–51, 1980.
10. Vinger, PF: The incidence of eye injuries in sports. Int Ophthalmol Clin 21:21–46, 1981.

CHAPTER 24

Maxillofacial Injuries in Winter Sports

LESTER M. CRAMER, D.M.D., M.D.

The high speeds, difficult technical maneuvers, and potential for collision involved in many of the winter sports predispose participants to facial injury. In evaluating and treating the face, one must especially consider the cosmetic aspect of the visage; the airway, especially with regard to the breathing function and its relation to endurance; and the preservation of teeth, which can be so easily lost.

PRESEASON EXAMINATIONS

The preseason history and physical examination of athletes should include determination of visual adequacy, airway patencies, bilateral hearing capability, presence and security of the teeth and their occlusion. No one team doctor can make all these necessary observations accurately. The general screening examination should be augmented by specialists who can elucidate abnormalities in the area of visual and internal nasal anatomy.

Although visual screening programs administered by paraprofessionals can be organized, complete eye examinations are preferable to screening examinations only. Eye examinations ideally should include five parameters: (1) dynamic visual acuity, (2) depth perception, (3) stereopsis, (4) fusion, and (5) refraction. Based on these results, the need for further testing will be determined by the examiner. This ideal is attainable if each team will avail themselves of local volunteers with expertise in sports vision from the fields of optometry, opticianry, and ophthalmology.

The standardization of any screening program is difficult but critical, and logistics for the follow-up of positive findings must be built into the program. About 25 to 30 percent of those examined will be found to have some pathology that must be further managed. The National Association for Sports Vision in Harrisburg, Pennsylvania can assist in locating volunteer sports vision specialists and in designing either a complete examination system or a screening program. The development of this baseline for all athletes will be most helpful in dealing with those who subsequently become injured. It can also be the basis around which a vision training program can be developed to enhance performance skills (see Chapter 10).

Nasal screening examinations often detect the presence of deviated nasal septums, which if uncorrected may hinder the endurance of athletes. In these cases, a rather minor surgical correction by a plastic surgeon or otorhinolaryngologist could change the athlete's whole career.

Dental consultation should be obtained for evaluation of the teeth and jaws to rule out tooth or jaw pathology and to construct the mouth guards needed in contact sports.

PROTECTIVE EQUIPMENT

Safety measures have been determined by the governing bodies of amateur sports, and league/team officials mandate protection for professional athletes. Each sport has its own unique protective requirements according to its techniques, amount of body contact, and the missiles and speeds involved. This protection may involve the use of helmets and face protectors. Some athletes object to the use of such protective equipment. They complain that it is more difficult to see or that their movements are constrained when wearing helmets or facial shields. With modern equipment, these complaints usually are not valid. These feelings can be overcome even in established veteran competitors, who will take time to become accustomed to them. Although some older competitors may need psychologic counseling to help them become accustomed to head gear, younger players who grow up with this equipment

often state that they feel undressed if they play without the protection. It is proven that facial injuries can be nearly abolished, and the severity of injuries that do occur can be markedly decreased by the use of proper shields, helmets, and mouthpieces. Athletes and their coaches and trainers should see to it that the mandated protective equipment is worn at all times, including practice (see Chapter 29). Furthermore, officials and manufacturers should continue to search for improvements in protective equipment so that good devices are being constantly made better.

SOFT TISSUE INJURIES

The most common soft tissue injuries of the face are contusions, hematomas, abrasions, and lacerations. Contusions and hematomas should be treated with ice and rest, although occasionally a large hematoma may require drainage. Large or deep abrasions should be anesthetized so that they may be adequately cleaned. Removal of all embedded substances must be accomplished. This can be done best by scrubbing the injured area with a brush, by excising or picking out foreign material with a scalpel, or by washing out the injury with a pulsating irrigator. Any retained foreign material in the deeper layers of the dermis or in the subcutaneous tissues may leave a "tattoo mark," which is particularly objectionable on the face. Careful application of dressings is an art that should be perfected by persons caring for injured athletes. On the face, dressings must be designed to protect the eyes, ears, and nose; provide for drainage; and, above all, stay in place. The inner lining must not be an impervious one, which would impede drainage. For lacerations, a lightly greased hydrophilic single layer of gauze should be used next to the wound. Abrasions are best covered with a semipermeable membrane. For the first 24 to 48 hours, inner dressings should be covered with a lightly compressing dressing, which serves to decrease both pain and swelling. This can be done best with polyester batting next to the lining dressing, because it is soft, compressible, and nonwettable.

The use of antibiotics is controversial and should be decided on an individual case-to-case basis. For small lacerations, abrasions, or contusions, antibiotics are obviously not necessary. If the area or volume of injury increases, or if there is a puncture, short courses of high-dose antibiotics are indicated. Antibiotics are also indicated when there is questionable viability, or if a deeper structure such as a sinus or nasal-lacrimal duct is also involved. Topical antibiotics are helpful in treating small abrasions and may be placed on the suture lines of wounds that will not be or cannot be dressed (e.g., the free border of the lip) and in areas that are left exposed after the first several days of dressings.

Facial lacerations will present a variety of differing problems, depending on the severity of the trauma. If the laceration is a simple, straightforward cut, proper anesthesia followed by good cleansing and layer-to-layer coaptation of tissues will suffice. This can be accomplished under aseptic conditions at the athletic site or in any suitably clean place. However, if the laceration is markedly contused, jagged, complex, or stellate, or if it involves either deeper structures or special surface areas, then the wound is best cared for in a facility designed for surgical procedures. The operating area may be an office, clinic, emergency room, or an operating room, depending on the situation. In many cases, local anesthesia may suffice, but in others general anesthesia will be needed. Good lighting, adequate instrumentation, and good assistance will give the best chance for an excellent result.

Complex lacerations require mature surgical judgment and meticulous technique. Debridement techniques that are applied to injuries elsewhere on the body may need modification when one deals with facial injuries. Many times, elsewhere on the body, small pieces of tissue that are of borderline viability are discarded, but on the face they should be preserved because they may be just the piece that will help preserve critical architecture, and on the face they may well survive because there they have a richer vasculature. The very act of "squaring up the edges," which is taught because it is mechanically correct, may be just the wrong thing to do in any specific area where survival of that tissue will preserve a small but vital anatomic structure. Thus, the treatment of these complex lacerations is best done by an experienced plastic surgeon. Although

secondary plastic surgical revisions may be done when needed, primary local preservations are usually preferable when they are indeed possible.

Eyelids and Periorbita

Whenever there is trauma to the periorbital region, fractures must be considered, and a thorough examination of the globe must be performed. Injury to the conjunctiva, sclera, lens, globe, retina, or bone should be discovered and managed accordingly by the appropriate medical or bone specialist.

Deep lacerations of the eyelid rim should be debrided carefully under $\times 4.5$ loupe magnification. Careful layered suturing must approximate the gray line, the white line, the sclera, and the tarsus. Direct, secure, accurate suturing has replaced the need for the outmoded halving and stepping. With correct deep alignment, the skin closure will easily follow. If structures are missing because of the injury, small free grafts should be done, using the nasal septum as the source for cartilage to replace tarsus, and either the retroauricular or supraclavicular areas to replace the thin color-matching skin. The buccal mucosa is a prime source for replacement of missing conjunctiva.

Medial lid lacerations may sever the canaliculi draining the tears. Immediate repair of lower canaliculi should always be done. The ducts are easy to identify with modest ($\times 4.5$) magnification. Lacrimal duct probes are used to dilate the punctum as well as the cut end of the ducts. Any special obturator rod may be inserted from punctum to the inferior nasal meatus to splint the ducts, and then the cut ends are repaired using 8-0 suture technique.

The medial canthal ligaments are rarely severed in an isolated soft tissue injury. Their disruption usually is part of fractures in this region and will be discussed later. Conversely, although not a common occurrence, laceration of the lateral canthal ligament is possible when there is no fracture. Awareness is the key, because repair of canthal lacerations at the time of initial injury is not difficult. However, if they are allowed to heal in an abnormal position, later repair is difficult. At the acute injury, the ligament is either cut in midligament or detached from the bony orbit. If cut in midligament, the repair is straightforward suturing with nonabsorbable suture. If the ligament has been severed at the orbital rim, it is necessary to drill a hole through the bone for secure reattachment.

The eyebrows are frequently lacerated, occasionally avulsed. The important factors are the alignment of the superior and inferior margins. If this is done accurately, the eyebrow will appear much better than if any stepping is allowed. If the lacerations are jagged, undermined, or very irregular, it is particularly important that they should not be trimmed or squared. Every possible shred should be saved and pieced together. Even though this may seem like a jigsaw-puzzle arrangement and the blood supply may be precarious, gentle handling and the use of very fine 6-0 or 7-0 suture material will probably result in survival of the eyebrow and give a more reasonable appearance than if the pieces had been debrided. If a portion of eyebrow has been avulsed, a very thin split-thickness graft should be used to provide early coverage. This thin graft will then have maximum contracture later, and after several months it may be small enough and have pulled the hair into good enough position so that only an excision and closure, rather than a full reconstruction, will be necessary. If this has not been successful, the brow must be modified by either local flap rotations, free hair grafts, or an island pedicle scalp flap.

Lips and Mouths

Three common errors must be avoided when repairing the lips. They are as follows:

1. Be sure not to leave hematoma.
2. Be sure not to misalign the vermilion.
3. Be sure not to leave free muscle unapposed.

The use of a headlight and $\times 3.5$ loupe magnification will help avoid these common errors, because the lip is deceptively thick, especially when swollen. Commonly, lip lacerations are through and through, and frequently the bleeding from the cut labial arteries is profuse. Judicious use of injectable and topical epinephrine plus basic hemostatic coagulation and ligation will allow visualization so that good wound toilet and accurate approximations can be accomplished. Awareness of the vermilion geography is critical, because accurate alignment of the mucovermilion border and cutaneovermilion borders are necessary to give correct appearance to the lip. This is an especially neat way to prevent errors as one approaches the oral commissures. Layer-by-layer closures are critical, particularly when one is dealing with the two layers of the orbicularis oris muscle.

Intraoral lacerations are frequently badly handled. Accurately approximating them to preserve the labial and buccal gutters is very important. This frequently requires a good assistant to align the surface while the surgeon performs approximation. In the cheek area of the mouth, the parotid duct orifice must be preserved. Likewise, in the floor of the mouth, the submaxillary duct and orifice must be recognized, and preserved or repaired if necessary. The old-time practice of letting major tongue lacerations heal by themselves is no longer acceptable. Unless it is a very small laceration in a child, the necessary suturing of muscles and mucosa should always be accomplished, even if it necessitates general anesthesia. In the athlete, this will ensure earlier eating for nourishment and earlier return to practice and competition.

Nose

Formidable hemorrhage frequently thwarts the repair efforts of soft tissue injuries of the nose unless these injuries are promptly and efficiently handled. Topical cocaine-epinephrine intranasal packing augmented by local anesthetic solutions containing epinephrine will help control bleeding to the point that the necessary coagulation or ligatures can be provided. Closure without first securing hemostases in this area particularly predisposes to bothersome or destructive hematomas and to inaccurate repairs. Septal hematomas can lead to secondary perforations or saddle-nose defects. Nasal hematomas are also highly susceptible to infection.

Accurate replacement of and repair of intranasal mucosa are essential to the future function and appearance of the nose and are not difficult when proper instrumentation, light, and assistance are used. Only after the mucosa has been accurately closed should the external nose be reassembled. This assemblage is best done in layers, using absorbable sutures in the cartilage and perichondrium and in the many tiny muscles. Accurate alignment should be accomplished using as few sutures as possible but as many as necessary. These cartilaginous and muscular repairs are supported by either external splints within the nose (i.e., packing or magnetic devices) and/or external supports suspended from head caps, wires, or lead plates.

Great care must be expended around the nostril, to align the specialized intranasal skin as well as the alar cartilages. In addition, the very difficult skin foldings at the rims must be carefully sutured; small errors can lead to notches that are difficult to correct later. Prevention here is very important; a few accurately placed 7-0 nylon sutures will obviate the need for a secondary reconstructive procedure that may not be successful.

Ears

Following injuries to the ear, the external auditory canal must be carefully inspected after proper cleansing to be certain that the bleeding is coming from external sources and that the tympanic membrane is intact. If the skin of the canal is disrupted, it usually can be reassembled with no or very few sutures and held in proper position with light packing. When the pinna is injured, it can be nicely reassembled with a few very fine absorbable sutures in the cartilage and perichondrium. Sutures in the cartilage should be placed so as to avoid the rim notches. These internal sutures are critical, but again they should be kept to a minimum. Accuracy in the cartilage alignment helps insure a cosmetically pleasing ear structure. The entire repair is then bolstered by a carefully molded, soft, slightly compressive dressing to support the cartilage and to discourage bleeding. Hematomas are poorly tolerated by the ear, so prevention is a key to good results. Small drains should be placed and the dressing changed early. Drains should be removed on either day one or day two, and any hematomas that have occurred should be evacuated.

Hematomas in nonlacerated ears are not commonly seen in winter sports. However, if one is encountered, it must be promptly drained by aspiration or incision. The injured ear should be reexamined daily, and these procedures must be repeated, if needed, to prevent accumulation. Failure to do so can lead to a cauliflower ear.

Cheeks

All deep cheek lacerations sever one or more of the mimetic muscles. These are often larger than expected, easy to repair, and frequently overlooked. They should be identified and carefully reapproximated with 4-0 absorbable sutures whenever encountered, so that functional results of facial animation are optimum.

Also at risk but not frequently severed in cheek lacerations is the parotid duct. In any major cheek injury, the parotid duct should always be demonstrated to verify its integrity. If it is cut, it should be promptly anastomosed with either 7-0 or 8-0 nylon over a polyethylene stent that is led out through the buccal mucosal orifice.

Severed facial nerve branches are best repaired during the primary operation because the scarring from wound healing makes them difficult to find later. The deformity of a paralyzed face can be devastating, whereas a primary interfascicular microneurorrhaphy can result in 100 percent return of function. Therefore, it is critical for an experienced microsurgeon to be part of the repair team.

FACIAL FRACTURES

The diagnosis of an acute facial fracture should never be missed. Even nondisplaced fractures are readily discerned. Clinical examination, conventional x-ray examinations, and, when indicated, coronal computerized tomography (CT) scans should be 100 percent accurate in the diagnosis and lead to full therapeutic success in every case. Thus, it behooves us to be sure that the clues to diagnosis are well enough known so that all these correct diagnoses can be made. This is critical for obtaining good results following facial fractures, because secondary treatment after healing in a malaligned position is so much more difficult, and the outcomes are frequently less satisfactory.

Nose

The nasal bone is the most frequently fractured facial bone in sporting accidents. Injuries may result in simple depressed fractures that are obvious to diagnose and straightforward to elevate into position. However, thorough intranasal and radiographic evaluation must be done to avoid missing septal fractures or hematomata. If these are seen, early prompt reduction and fixation with special forceps can be readily accomplished with proper anesthesia. If swelling has intervened, it is usually best to wait a few days to carry out definitive treatment after much of the swelling has subsided.

Occasionally, severe trauma to the interorbital area will cause a widened and depressed nasal bridge, telecanthus, and rounded palpebral openings. This nasoethmoidal severe fracture needs prompt open reduction of the bones and reapproximation of the canthal ligaments to the bones, and occasionally requires a supplemental bone graft and exterior wires or lead plates for support.

Zygoma

The arch of the zygoma lies between the orbit and the ear, where it serves to support the cheek. When the zygoma is fractured in an isolated fashion, it will be depressed, and this is clinically obvious. Such fractures can be demonstrated by a submentovertex x-ray view. After zygomatic fractures, mandibular motions may be impeded by the decreased size of the infratemporal space, which encroaches upon the coronoid process and the temporalis and internal pterygoid muscles. Surgical reduction under local or general anesthesia is done via a low lateral scalp incision behind the temporal hairline.

The most common zygomatic fracture, the tripod fracture, separates the bone through the suture lines that join the zygoma to the frontal bone, the temporal bone, and the maxilla. The disjuncted zygoma is displaced downward and backward to give the following clinical signs: flattened cheek, palpable step of infraorbital rim, anesthesia in the distribution of the infraorbital nerve (ala nasi, upper lip, medial 3½ upper teeth on the ipsilateral side), horizontal diplopia, fluid level of blood in maxillary sinus, bloody nose from the sinus leaking into the nose, lateral subconjunctival hemorrhage, and antimongoloid palpebral displacement downward of the lateral canthal ligament. A Waters' x-ray view is diagnostic; and a coronal CT x-ray examination is the state-of-the-art method for diagnosing precise fragment size and localization, as well as for determining the exact status of the floor of the orbit—for the orbital floor can be badly fractured and still not be clinically apparent.

However, orbital floor fractures are usually obvious. The most common signs are vertical diplopia and lowering of the globe. These signs may be masked by hematoma and edema, and the trapping of the globe may be difficult to ascertain if the orbital floor is extremely comminuted. Enophthalmos may not be apparent for these reasons and may become apparent only after the edema recedes, the fat atrophies, and the scar tissue contracts. To prevent this, the specific diagnosis is best corroborated by coronal CT scan. If orbital floor fracture is found, prompt surgery is indicated.

Surgical reduction and fixation of the zygoma is done under general anesthesia. The incisions should be small and placed in the camouflage areas beneath the eyebrow and subciliary. Usually, these two incisions can allow for total bone exposure and orbital floor correction. Small wires or plates are used for the fixation; bone, Teflon, or silicone pieces are used to replace the orbital floor after the muscles and fat have been freed and replaced into the orbit. Occasionally, supplementary incisions may be needed in the mucobuccal sulcus to allow the placement of intra-antral balloons to help support the orbital floor. Another supplemental incision that is sometimes needed to reduce these fractures, especially in difficult cases when interposed tissues cannot be otherwise exposed, can be either in the temporal scalp or directly on the cheek. Hospitalization is short, usually only 1 day. Systemic antibiotics are used for a few days, and decongestants are prescribed for a few weeks. The return to competition is prompt if there is no residual diplopia.

Maxilla

The maxilla characteristically fractures in one of three places, as originally documented and classified by LeFort. LeFort I, a horizontal detachment of the palate and alveolar ridges of the maxilla, is the most common maxillary fracture, and the easiest to treat. LeFort II is a pyramidal detachment of the central portion of the face, consisting of the medial portion of the maxillae, the medial half of both antra, the medial half of both infraorbital rims and orbital floors, and the nasal bones. LeFort III, the most serious fracture occurring from severe trauma, includes a LeFort II fracture in continuity with bilateral zygoma fractures. It is this fracture that is frequently associated with other problems such as airway obstruction, intracranial obstruction, intracranial concussion, cervical spine fracture, laryngeal injury, and cerebral spinal fluid leakage.

Clinical diagnosis of maxillary fractures is made by noting pain and extensive swelling over the mid face, often accompanied by malocclusion of the teeth and distortions of the face, including a dish-face appearance. Telecanthus, infraorbital anesthesia, and diplopia may be associated with fractures of the maxilla. Clinical observations correlated with the radiologic findings on both standard views and the use of both computerized axial tomography (CAT) and coronal CT scans will guide the way to correct treatment. Arch bars are applied to the maxillary and mandibular teeth, and appropriate incisions (frequently a bicoronal incision) are made. Following reduction, fixation is accomplished with wires, screws, or plates. Intermaxillary fixation is continued for 4 to 7 weeks. Three months is a short recuperative period for this injury. It must be emphasized that this is most difficult surgery that is frequently done in very sick people. Fortunately, maxillary fractures rarely result from athletic injury, particularly since the advent of protective devices.

Mandible

The mandible is the second most commonly fractured facial bone. It rarely breaks in one place only. This is probably because of its peculiar bent-U-shape and inherent bone weaknesses secondary to the placement of teeth of differing shape and size. Particularly weak areas are found in the parasymphyseal area just medial to the canine tooth, in the area of the third molar region near the angle, and also at the base of the neck of the mandibular condyle. Various

combinations of these three weak areas result in the common fracture combinations, which usually occur in a contracoup arrangement; that is, on opposite sides of the midline. The incidence of these commonly occurring fracture pairs are as follows:

1. Parasymphyseal-condylar neck
2. Parasymphyseal-angle
3. Condylar neck-condylar neck
4. Parasymphyseal-parasymphyseal
5. Angle-condylar neck
6. Angle-angle

Clinical examination following mandibular fractures will reveal malocclusion, pain, palpable defects along the lower border of the mandible or within the mouth, and ecchymoses in the floor of the mouth. X-ray examinations will delineate these fractures, and treatment can be guided by the direction and stability of the reduced fracture and by whether total stability can be achieved by external fixation. Most fractures can be treated by means of closed manual or elastic traction reduction and external fixation, using arch bars on the maxillary and mandibular teeth to maintain the reduction. Following reduction and fixation of mandibular fractures, it is necessary to maintain the teeth in occlusion for 4 to 6 weeks. If adequate closed reduction cannot be achieved, then open reduction from either the intraoral or cervical approach is used. The bones are reduced, and then internal fixation is achieved by wires, screws, or plates. Until recently, this would always require augmentation by maintaining the teeth in occlusion with intermaxillary wires for 4 weeks. In the past few years, the development of compression techniques has allowed such firm fixation of stable fractures that intermaxillary fixation has not been necessary. These newer techniques will allow an athlete to return to training within 10 to 14 days and to compete in noncontact sports by 1 month.

SUMMARY

Preseason physical examinations of winter athletes should include good evaluation of vision, airway, hearing, and occlusion to establish baselines and to pick up preexisting pathology that may be treated. Thereby, serious facial injuries are largely preventable during most winter sporting endeavors. When facial trauma does occur, prompt diagnosis and treatment are mandatory to give the optimum cosmetic and functional results. Return to training can occur quickly, except for the most severe injuries. Although further research is needed to design the ideal protective equipment, currently available helmets, shields, and mouth guards are quite effective.

REFERENCES

1. Converse, JM: Surgical Treatment of Facial Injuries, ed. 3. Williams & Wilkins, Baltimore, 1974.
2. Dingman, RO and Converse, JM: Reconstructive Plastic Surgery, ed 2, vol II. WB Saunders, Philadelphia, 1977.
3. Schulz, RC: Facial Injuries. Year Book Publishers, Chicago, IL, 1970.
4. Soll, DB: Management of Complications in Ophthalmic Plastic Surgery. Aesculapius Publishing, Birmingham, AL, 1977.
5. Vinger, PF: Sports eye injuries: A preventable disease. Am Acad Ophthalmol 88:108–113, 1981.

PART IV

Skating

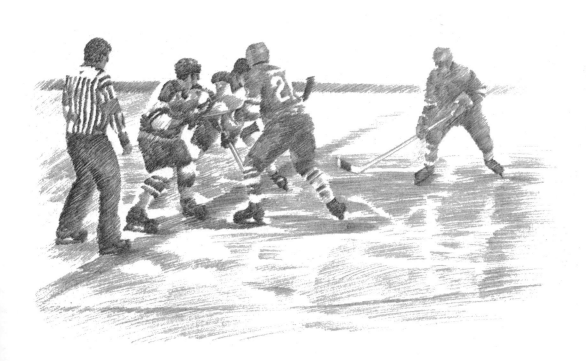

CHAPTER 25

The Physiology of Speed Skating

CARL FOSTER, Ph.D

NANCY N. THOMPSON, M.S.

Speed skating is an important international sport in which the United States has periodically enjoyed great competitive success. Speed skating may be characterized as an energy-demand sport in which the primary determinant of success is the ability to move the skater from point A to point B in the shortest possible time. In terms of average speed, skating is somewhat comparable to bicycling equivalent distances without the assistance of a pack. Speeds of over 900 meters per minute (35 mph) are routinely attained during sprint competition. In this chapter, we will review studies of the physiology of speed skating that have been performed both in our laboratory and elsewhere. We hope that they will provide a perspective for understanding the sport and for allowing individual skaters to achieve improved performances.

HISTORICAL PERSPECTIVE

Although speed skaters have been studied for some time, the first systematic report in English was the monograph of Ekblom and associates.[14] In this study of elite Swedish skaters, a variety of acute responses to exercise were described. These skaters were mostly specialists in the long distances, including recent World and Olympic medalists in the 10,000-meter event. These athletes were characterized by having high values for maximal oxygen consumption (VO_{2max}) and were not characterized as being particularly strong. Geijsel[22] studied Dutch marathon speed skaters and observed that the ability to tolerate a heavy but probably submaximal load on the cycle ergometer was predictive of success in long-distance (40-km) races.

Our early studies (1979 to 1980) with the United States Speed Skating team indicated that contrary to the findings of Ekblom and colleagues[14] and Giejsel,[22] skaters had only modestly elevated values for $\dot{V}O_{2max}$ in l/min and very ordinary values (averaging 63 ml/kg) for $\dot{V}O_{2max}$ normalized for body weight.[29] The values attained in our laboratory in 1980 were considerably improved over similar values attained by Maksud and colleagues[31] prior to the 1968 Olympiad. Even ultrasuccessful all-around skaters such as Eric Heiden of the United States (5.3 l/min) (unpublished data from our laboratory) and Hein Vergeer of the Netherlands (5.1 l/min)[26] do not have particularly remarkable values for $\dot{V}O_{2max}$. Companion studies of body composition indicated that skaters were not particularly large relative to athletes in general, with an average body weight of only about 75 kg for the elite male skaters. Skaters are comparatively lean in relation to other athletes. Body composition values of approximately 8 percent fat are typical. There seemed to be a marked segregation of elite and developmental skaters, particularly with regard to the elite skaters having greater lean body weight (LBW).[32] Female speed skaters are also comparatively lean, averaging about 17 percent fat,[33] a level that is markedly

lower than the percent body fat of nonathletic women (see Chapter 6).

ACUTE RESPONSES TO EXERCISE

During speed skating, maximal cardiovascular demands (as reflected by heart rate) are attained in all events ranging from 500 to 10,000 meters (Fig. 25–1). The heart rate at any given absolute $\dot{V}O_2$ is higher during skating or simulated skating on the slideboard (see Chapter 2) than during cycle ergometry. However, when the heart rate is normalized to the percent of the ergometer specific $\dot{V}O_{2max}$, the heart rate/$\dot{V}O_2$ relationship is fundamentally the same during skating as during cycling (Fig. 25–2).

Pulmonary ventilation (V_E) during speed skating apparently increases more or less in concert with $\dot{V}O_2$.

Accordingly, V_{Emax} during speed skating is often lower than during cycle ergometry or during running (Fig. 25–3). Studies in our laboratory, using a slideboard rather than on-ice conditions, suggest that $V_E/\dot{V}O_2$ may be slightly higher during skating than during cycling at the same $\dot{V}O_2$.

AEROBIC POWER

Several authors have evaluated $\dot{V}O_{2max}$ during skating. As indicated earlier, skaters do not have particularly large $\dot{V}O_{2max}$ values, compared with other athletes, regardless of whether $\dot{V}O_2$ is expressed as l/min or ml/kg. Only Ekblom and colleagues[14] have found

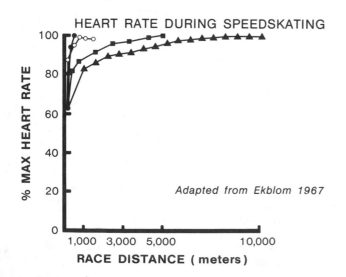

Figure 25–1. Schematic representation of heart rate response during speed-skating competitions of various durations, expressed as a percent of the maximal heart rate observed in the laboratory during cycle ergometry. (Adapted from the data of Ekblom and colleagues.[14])

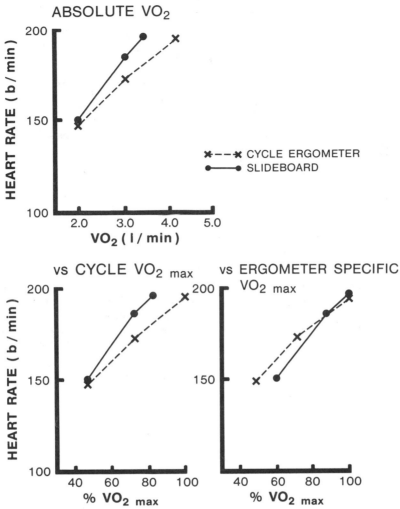

Figure 25–2. Heart rate response during cycle ergometry and during simulated skating on a slideboard. The data are from the author's laboratory and are presented relative to absolute $\dot{V}O_2$ and to relative $\dot{V}O_2$ on cycle ergometer and slideboard.

values consistently above 70 ml/kg in elite male skaters. In general, $\dot{V}O_{2max}$ during skating or simulated skating averages 85 to 90 percent of that attained during either running or cycle ergometry (Fig. 25–4). $\dot{V}O_{2max}$ during roller skating, a common training activity, is typically somewhat higher than during ice speed skating,[11] probably because the higher preextension knee angle during roller skating allows for enhanced blood flow to the legs.[10] There is generally a step-down in $\dot{V}O_{2max}$ from better skaters to less accomplished skaters and from male to female skaters. Uniquely, elite female skaters from the United States do not seem to have a higher $\dot{V}O_{2max}$ than their developmental

counterparts. This, together with the comparatively low value for $\dot{V}O_{2max}$ among speed skaters, suggests that aerobic power output per se, and particularly $\dot{V}O_{2max}$ in ml/kg, may not be as important during speed skating as it is, for example, in running or Nordic skiing.

Studies conducted in our laboratory have suggested that performance at either 500 or 1500 meters in speed skating is generally well correlated to $\dot{V}O_{2max}$ (l/min).[17] However, the similar correlation when performance is expressed relative to LBW suggests that overall body size and gross power output may be more important than $\dot{V}O_{2max}$ per se (Fig. 25–5). This is particularly true when one consid-

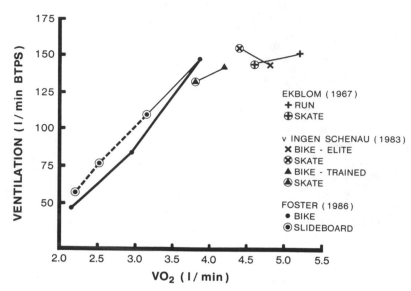

Figure 25–3. Pulmonary ventilation during cycle ergometry and during either speed skating or simulated skating on the slideboard. Maximal on-ice data from Ekblom and others[14] and van Ingen Schenau and colleagues,[38] suggest that V_E is reduced during skating in proportion to the reduced $\dot{V}O_2$. Data from the author's laboratory support this observation but also suggest that $V_E/\dot{V}O_2$ during submaximal skating may be slightly elevated over cycle ergometry.

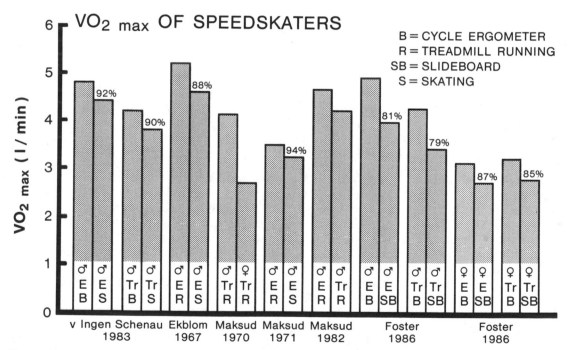

Figure 25–4. $\dot{V}O_{2max}$ data obtained on speed skaters from several laboratories during cycle ergometry (B), treadmill running (R), skating (S), or on the slideboard (SB). Percentages above skating or slideboard data indicate the relative $\dot{V}O_{2max}$ in the same group of athletes to data obtained during either running or cycle ergometry.

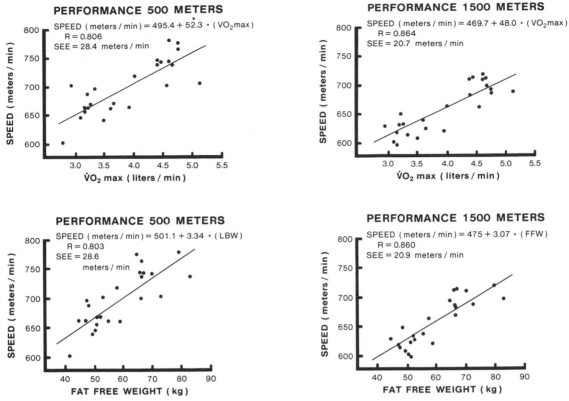

Figure 25–5. Relationship of $\dot{V}O_{2max}$ during cycle ergometry and lean body weight to performance in 500- and 1500-meter skating events. All laboratory data for this study were collected within a week of competition, and all races occurred on the same evening for all athletes under nearly ideal ice and weather conditions.

ers the comparatively small opportunity for aerobic metabolism during the 37- to 45-second duration 500 meter event. Van Ingen Schenau and de Groot[37] observed a very high power output to $\dot{V}O_{2max}$ ratio in elite female skaters when compared with similarly trained male skaters. They suggested that this improved performance ratio may allow competitors with fairly low values for $\dot{V}O_{2max}$ to be competitive. Geijsel[22] observed that the ability to tolerate a very high power output of 5 watts/kg was well related to marathon skating performance, and that improved skating within the season of training and competition was associated with increases in work time on the ergometer. This suggests that the ability to maintain homeostasis at workloads approximating or even exceeding $\dot{V}O_{2max}$ may be central to speed skating performance. We have found that $\dot{V}O_{2max}$ measured during slideboard exercise is somewhat more highly correlated with

skating performance than is $\dot{V}O_{2max}$ during cycle ergometry. This, of course, is reasonable considering the known importance of the specificity of muscular work (Fig. 25–6).

The lack of relationship between $\dot{V}O_{2max}$ in ml/kg with speed skating performance undoubtedly reflects the way resistance is provided to the skater. In running, the center of gravity must be lifted to allow propulsion. Using appropriate skating technique, the center of gravity is moved side to side but is never lifted.[36] Accordingly, body weight probably represents a fairly small resistance factor. However, the crouched posture of the speed skater (which requires great muscular endurance of the gluteal and quadricipital muscle groups) allows even large skaters to achieve a fairly small frontal area. The ability of large skaters to achieve an aerodynamic profile suggests that $\dot{V}O_{2max}$ relative to the average frontal area projected is the appropriate method of expressing $\dot{V}O_{2max}$. However,

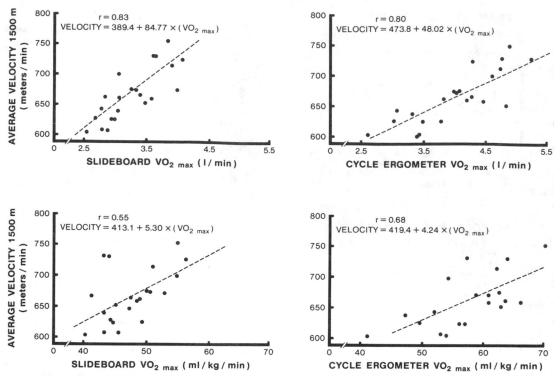

Figure 25–6. Comparative relationship between $\dot{V}O_{2max}$ measured on cycle ergometer or slideboard and skating performance at 500 and 1500 meters. Expression of $\dot{V}O_{2max}$ in l/min results in a better correlation with performance regardless of the type of ergometer used.

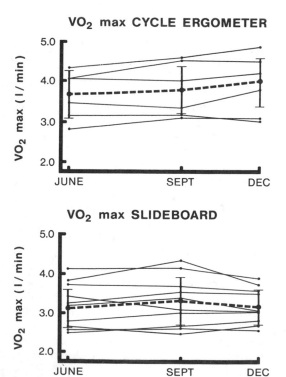

Figure 25–7. Serial changes in $\dot{V}O_{2max}$ measured on cycle ergometer and slideboard in the same athletes over the course of the dry-land and early on-ice training period. There were no significant changes noted for either ergometer.

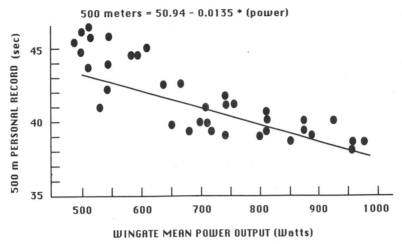

Figure 25–8. Relationship of anaerobic power output observed during the Wingate cycle ergometer test to personal best performance at 500 meters.

no researcher has yet published this correlative study.

We have found in a number of studies that $\dot{V}O_{2max}$ is a very stable value in speed skaters,[16,19] as it is in other athletes.[8] Despite the intensity of training over long periods of time, this variable, whether measured during treadmill running, cycle ergometry, or on the slideboard, does not seem to change very much over time (Fig. 25–7). Workers in the

Netherlands, however, have noted substantial variation in $\dot{V}O_{2max}$ throughout the year, with peak values observed during the winter competitive period.[27]

ANAEROBIC POWER

Because of the relative brevity of metric style speed skating events, the contribution of anaerobic power output cannot be mini-

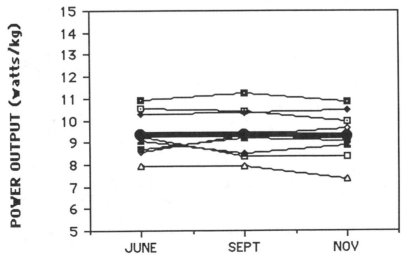

Figure 25–9. Serial changes in anaerobic power output observed during the Wingate test at various times during the training year corresponding to early (June) and late (September) dry-land training and after 6 to 8 weeks of on-ice training (November). Data are expressed as the average power output observed over the standard 30-second duration of the test.

mized. In the Netherlands, Giejsel and colleagues[21] have found that anaerobic muscular performance, as measured during the Wingate cycle ergometer test, correlates more highly with skating performance than does $\dot{V}O_{2max}$. These results are similar to the good correspondence between exercise tolerance at 5 watts/kg and performance noted by Geijsel[22] and the correspondence between average power output in 3 minutes and performance noted by van Ingen Schenau and de Groot.[37] We also have found that the power output during the Wingate test is well correlated with personal best performances over 500 meters (Fig. 25–8). Like $\dot{V}O_{2max}$, anaerobic muscular performance is a remarkably stable measure across a period of time of at least months (Fig. 25–9).[34] It also appears to be primarily related to lean body mass.[1] Interestingly, within this data (see Fig. 25–8) are individual points that do not fall closely along the line of identity. We have found several skaters who are markedly faster than would be predicted by their anaerobic power output. These individuals are, almost without exception, very accomplished at the tech-

nically demanding sport of indoor speed skating and, by visual observation, are thought to have good "technique." Other skaters who skate slower than would be expected on the basis of anaerobic power output are unique in that they, also almost without exception, have obvious technical flaws. These data suggest that skill elements in speed skating may be of considerable importance.

ENDURANCE TIME ON THE CYCLE ERGOMETER

Geijsel[22] noted that the endurance time on the cycle ergometer at a workload of 4 watts/kg changed more or less in concert with skating performance in Dutch marathon skaters. Recent data from our laboratory have shown remarkable improvement on this test during the summer dry-land training period in American metric style skaters (Fig. 25–10). Given that we have failed to observe changes in either $\dot{V}O_{2max}$ (see Fig. 25–7) or anaerobic power (see Fig. 25–9) during comparable periods of time, these results suggest the utility

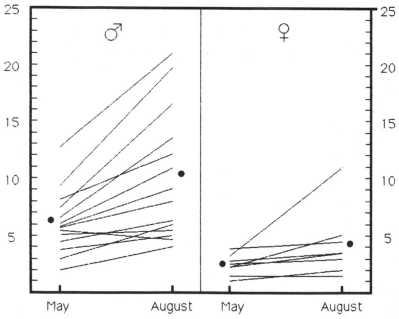

Figure 25–10. Serial changes in endurance time on the cycle ergometer at a workload of 5 watts/kg. During this test the rpm was restricted to 60 rpm. Only 2 of 22 skaters failed to improve on this test. Data were collected in cooperation with Dr. Ann Snyder of the University of Wisconsin, Milwaukee.

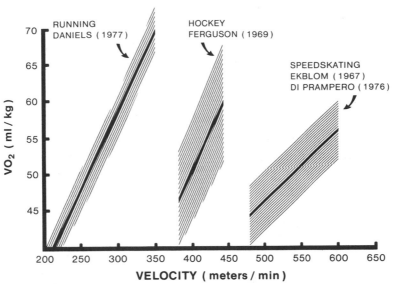

Figure 25–11. Schematic representation between pace of running or skating and $\dot{V}O_2$. For skating the curve is generally right shifted and widened, indicating a greater intrinsic variability in the aerobic demands of skating than that of running. For speed skating the curve is right shifted relative to hockey skating, reflecting the reduced drag attributable to different clothing and posture.

of this simple but demanding test in evaluating changes in basic fitness in speed skaters. The aerobic requirement of riding at 5 watts/kg is about 65 ml/kg. The range of performance times observed in our laboratory is consistent with a workload requiring approximately the $\dot{V}O_{2max}$.[28] The rather low endurance times and small improvements observed in female skaters suggest that 5 watts/kg may be too heavy a workload for practical use. Using the logic that $\dot{V}O_{2max}$ in female skaters is about 88 percent of that in males,[33] a workload of 4.3 watts/kg would seem to be appropriate.

SKATING ECONOMY

In many sports—notably running and swimming—differences in economy (the relative oxygen uptake at a given speed) seem to explain differences in performance beyond that explainable by $\dot{V}O_{2max}$. Although there are limited data on the energy costs of speed skating, the two available studies by Di-Prampero and associates[13] and Ekblom and colleagues,[14] suggest that there is a notable degree of variation in the energy cost of speed skating. If one combines the results with energy cost data obtained during skating in hockey players,[15] and compares these results to those obtained with equally elite runners,[7] the great variability in the energy cost of skating is apparent (Fig. 25–11). These data further suggest the importance of skill elements within the continuum of variables contributing to speed skating performance. However, the importance of changing aerodynamics attributable to towing Douglas bags or to postexercise oxygen consumption measurements has limited previous studies of the energy cost of speed skating to ranges of speeds that are far below those employed by contemporary skaters. Likewise, if one assumes that athletic events requiring less than 10 to 15 minutes are completed at work rates in excess of $\dot{V}O_{2max}$,[28] then even the longest event usually skated by contemporary speed skaters (10,000 meters) is likely to require an energy output approximating $\dot{V}O_{2max}$. For this reason, measurement of $\dot{V}O_2$ during skating at competitively representative speeds may not be very meaningful.

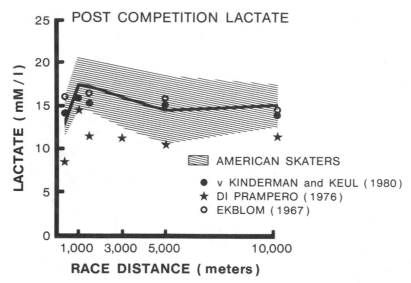

Figure 25–12. Postcompetition blood lactate concentrations obtained following speed skating competitions by the authors (shaded area is mean ±1 standard deviation). The data from von Kinderman and Keul[39] and Ekblom and others[14] agree well with our data. The data from DiPrampero and co-workers[13] were originally presented as delta lactate from a nonspecified resting value. In this figure we have added 1mM/l to the delta lactates reported by DiPrampero and associates.

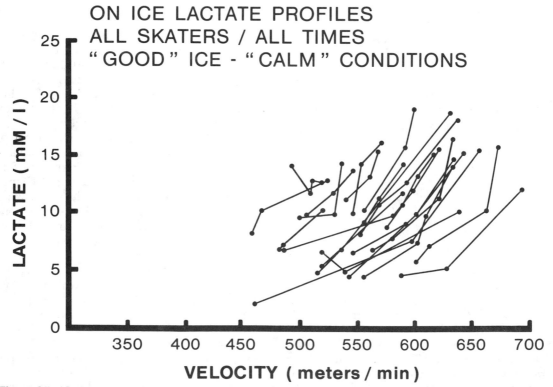

Figure 25–13. Relationship of skating speed to plasma lactate accumulation. Each trial represents skating 1500 meters at a steady pace. Fingertip blood samples were collected 2 minutes postexercise for each trial. Data were collected in cooperation with Drs. Peter van Handle and Jackie Puhl of the USOC-OTC.

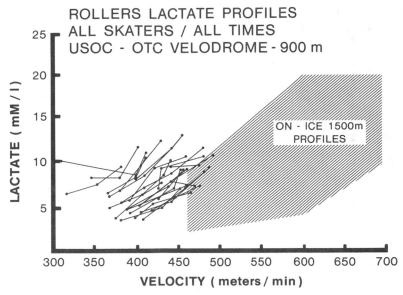

Figure 25–14. Plasma lactate responses in relation to velocity during roller skating. These studies were conducted at the USOC-OTC (elevation 2000 meters) and are compared with responses during speed skating at the Olympic Rink In West Allis, WI (elevation 100 meters) (shaded area). The data were collected in cooperation with Dr. Jackie Puhl of the USOC-OTC.

LACTATE METABOLISM

Skating is a very high-intensity sport. Three of the five international distances for men in metric-style speed skating are completed in less than 2 minutes, and the longest event is completed in less than 15 minutes, corresponding to running performances of no more than 5000 meters. Accordingly, peak postcompetition lactate levels in speed skaters are typically fairly high. In Figure 25–12, we present values that we have observed with American skaters, together with results presented by other investigators. We have found that peak postexercise lactate levels are highest in the 1000 and 1500 meter events (1 minute 15 seconds to 2 minutes), with slight reductions at shorter and longer distances. Values averaging 17 mM/l are quite common, and values as high as 24 mM/l have been observed. Peak postexercise lactates in speed skaters are, however, lower than those observed by von Kinderman and Keul[39] in runners and fairly comparable to those obtained in swimmers. Whether this means that speed skating is less anaerobic than sprint running or whether the comparatively large isometric component of speed skating prevents blood lactate from

being an accurate reflection of disturbances in intramuscular pH remains to be resolved.

In an attempt to develop a method of evaluation suitable for supramaximal exertion, we have, in cooperation with Drs. Peter van Handel and Jackie Puhl of the United States Olympic Committee–Olympic Training Center (USOC–OTC), performed lactate profiles for members of the United States Speed Skating Team (Fig. 25–13). From these profiles we can note several things: (1) As the speed of skating increases, lactate begins to accumulate in the familiar curvilinear fashion. (2) Only rarely is the plasma lactate level in speed skaters as low as the 4 mM/l value, which seems to be a point of reference for runners and cyclists.[24] From our experience, it appears that as soon as the skater assumes the characteristic sitting posture, a blood lactate concentration of 5 to 7 mM/l is virtually assured. (3) These data also indicate a tremendous variability in the velocity-lactate relationship. Some of this is clearly related to conditioning differences among these athletes. However, if one considers the individual athletes contributing to this particular profile, there are strong suggestions that skaters with relatively good technique may have a right-shifted curve and skaters with

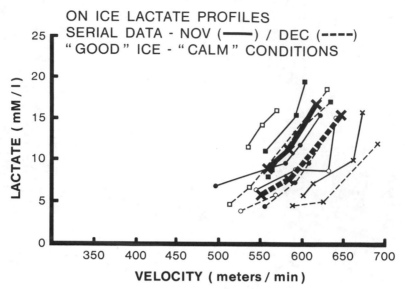

Figure 25–15. Serial lactate profiles collected in five skaters during the early on-ice training period during November and just prior to international selection trials in December. Each trial represents skating 1500 meters at a steady pace. Fingertip blood samples were collected 2 minutes postexercise for each trial. Data were collected in cooperation with Drs. Peter van Handle and Jackie Puhl of the USOC-OTC.

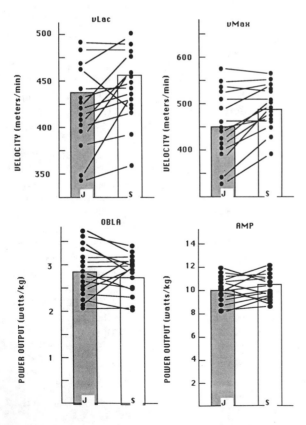

Figure 25–16. Changes in the velocity of skating associated with a blood lactate concentration of 10 mM (vLac) and in maximal velocity for 1500 meters on an indoor short-track course (vMax) during the summer training period. Also shown is the lack of change in fitness-related variables OBLA and AMP during this period of time.

relatively poor technique may have curves that are left shifted. These responses seem to occur over and above differences that we can account for by differences in fitness.

Lactate profiles during roller skating are presented in Figure 25–14. These data were collected at the USOC–OTC in Colorado Springs (elevation 2000 m) in cooperation with Dr. Puhl. They are compared with the phantom of the speed-lactate relationship observed in West Allis, Wisconsin (elevation 100 m) during speed skating with good wind and ice conditions. Ignoring differences attributable to altitude, the relative speed differences between roller and ice skating are consistent with the data of de Boer,[10] who observed that maximal roller skating for 4 to 5 minutes was performed at about 82 percent of the speed of ice skating for a comparable time. The curve for roller skaters displays many of the same characteristics as those for ice skaters; that is, the curvilinear character

of the relationship, the high minimum values, and the marked individual variability. The importance of skill differences is supported by serial lactate profile data that we have collected (Fig. 25–15). In this case, lactate profiles were first obtained in November after approximately 4 weeks of on-ice training, and in December after another 6 weeks of on-ice training (see Chapter 2). There is a rightward shift in the lactate profile, which is not obviously related to either ice conditions or conditioning status, suggesting improved economy.

Subsequently we[20] have studied lactate accumulation, maximal skating performance, and physiologic responses during cycle ergometry before and after experimental alterations in the summer dry-land training program. During the summer the skaters included two to three on-ice workouts on an indoor short course, with particular emphasis on technique. The velocity at which blood

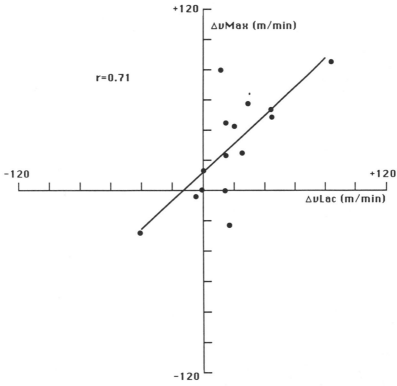

Figure 25–17. Comparison of changes in vLac and vMax during the course of the summer training period. During this period of time the skaters performed selected technical drills on ice two to three times weekly. Large positive changes in both variables were usually noted in slower and/or less experienced skaters, suggesting the need for continued on-ice training much longer than typically practiced by contemporary skaters.

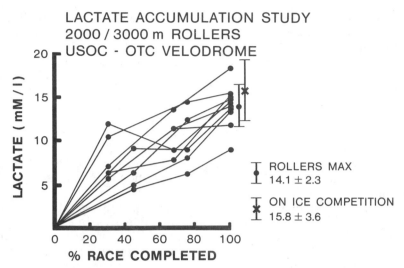

Figure 25–18. Pattern of lactate accumulation during simulated competition on roller skates. Intermediate distance values were obtained on a separate day by having the athlete skate at the same pace as observed during competition and stop after a predetermined intermediate distance. Data were collected in cooperation with Dr. Jackie Puhl of the USOC-OTC.

lactate levels rose to 10 mM (vLac) increased significantly, as did the maximal average velocity for 1500 meters (vMax). These changes were particularly evident in slower and/or less experienced skaters. During this period there were no changes in either the cycle ergometer power output at a lactate concentration of 4 mM (OBLA) or in the maximal power output during the Wingate test (AMP) (Fig. 25–16). Changes in vMax were well correlated (r = 0.71) with changes in vLac (Fig. 25–17), but not with changes in either OBLA (r = 0.22) or AMP (r = 0.06). However, because changes in vLac were not significantly correlated with changes in OBLA (r = 0.02), we feel that the improved vLac and vMax are attributable to improved technique rather than to differences in lactate metabolism.

During simulated competition on roller skates,[6] we have noted a progressive and essentially linear increase in blood lactate during the course of the event. In these studies, skaters performed maximal efforts at 2000 and 3000 meters, corresponding timewise to 3000 and 5000 meters on ice. On separate occasions they skated at the same pace but stopped after 35 to 40 percent and 75 percent of the total distance had been completed. Lactate sampled in this manner provided an index of what occurred during competition without the necessity for interrupting the competitive effort (Fig. 25–18). Some of the individual data, in which the athletes demonstrated fairly minor nonuniformities in pacing, suggest that lactate may accumulate very rapidly during the early part of the race. This may account for the profound decrement in average speed observed during competitive speed skating races in the 1000 and 1500 meter events (Fig. 25–19). This pace decrement, particularly with the supporting lactate data, suggests that the pace pattern in the middle distance skating events needs to be reconsidered. Although there may be tactical and emotional advantages to be gained from starting at a high velocity, the combination of reduced power output and deteriorating technique act to slow the skater greatly. (The last 400 meters in a 1500 meter race is often similar to the same athlete's average velocity in 3000- to 5000-meter races.)

During our early studies with American skaters, we found that peak postexercise lactate levels were comparatively low ($\approx$ 8 mM/l).[19] Because these values were so far below those reported by Ekblom and associates[14] and DiPrampero and colleagues,[13] we were concerned as to their potential significance. Analysis of skaters' training programs and dietary habits suggested to us that they were subject to chronic glycogen depletion, such as that often seen in athletes

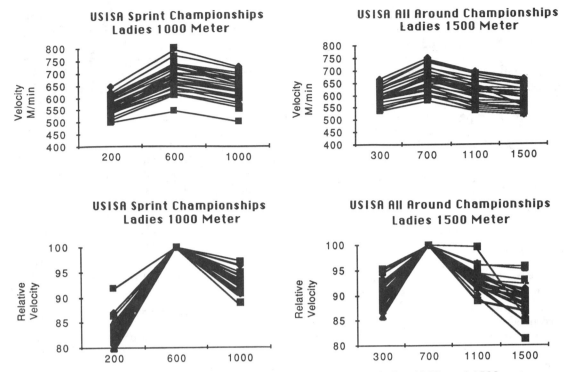

Figure 25–19. Relative velocity pattern of American speed skaters during 1000- and 1500-meter competitions. The data are expressed in both absolute velocity and normalized to the highest full-lap velocity. Note the substantial decrease in velocity during the latter half of both events.

undergoing severe training.[4] This observation led us to experiment with the use of carbohydrate supplements. In these studies, we observed that the appropriate use of a carbohydrate supplement beverage following training could effectively increase the percentage of carbohydrate in the diet without adversely affecting the overall nutrient intake.[18] It was associated with favorable subjective responses during subsequent workouts, enhanced work performance in the laboratory, and higher postexercise lactate levels. Our subsequent experience over the last 4 years with the United States National Team is that these commercially available carbohydrate supplements form an important adjunct to facilitating recovery from training. Although it may be argued that appropriate dietary selections could effect the same end, we have thus far been unsuccessful in achieving satisfactory levels of carbohydrate intake without the use of supplements.

There is some evidence that muscle glycogen resynthesis may be facilitated in the immediate postexercise period. This has led to suggestions that easily digestible liquid foods rich in carbohydrate should be consumed in the warming hut within minutes of finishing training or competition.[3]

MUSCLE METABOLISM

Although the percutaneous muscle biopsy procedure has minimal risks, we have been unwilling to assume even the minimal risk of performing what are essentially descriptive studies. The few data available come mostly from work with elite competitive cyclists who also happened to be speed skaters, and these suggest that fiber composition is very mixed and probably averages near the average for the population as a whole. Skaters tend to self-select into sprinters (500, 1000 meters), all-arounders (500, 1500, 3000, 5000 for ladies and 500, 1500, 5000, 10000 for men), and marathon specialists (5000 meters to 40 km). This suggests that there may be some selection along the lines of fiber composition similar to that noted for runners.[5] Documentation for this is lacking, however.

Green[23] has evaluated the muscle glycogen depletion pattern during continuous and interval skating in hockey players. During continuous skating for 1 hour at 60 percent of $\dot{V}O_{2max}$, most of the glycogen depletion occurred in the type 1 or slow-twitch muscle fibers. There was limited glycogen depletion in the type 2 fibers. Studies conducted during high-intensity intermittent exercise (10 $\times$ 1 minute at 120 percent of $\dot{V}O_{2max}$) indicated a profound degree of total glycogen depletion, with particular depletion in the type 2 or fast-twitch muscle fibers. These findings were consistent with the general knowledge of glycogen depletion rate and pattern during cycle ergometer exercise. Given that the intensity of both training and competition for most metric-style speed skaters has some similarity to the high-intensity exercise pattern used by Green,[23] it is probably reasonable to assume that speed skating induces rapid glycogen depletion from both type 1 and type 2 muscle fibers. Thus, even relatively brief training sessions and/or races may be associated with a profound need to restore muscle glycogen. This suggestion is consistent with our observation that skaters have great difficulty in performing training that requires prolonged "sitting" in the skating position without evidence of glycogen depletion.

This is some evidence that speed skating—at least at marathon distances—may be associated with muscle damage as evidenced by substantial release of muscle enzymes.[25] The longer metric-style races are also usually associated with persistent muscular soreness, which might suggest muscle damage, although biochemical or histochemical documentation is lacking. However, the association between severe exertion and muscle damage is well documented, and one must presume that the problems of frequent muscular overuse are as meaningful for speed skaters as for other athletes.[2]

MUSCULAR STRENGTH

The rather awkward crouched posture adopted by contemporary speed skaters puts a particular strain on the gluteal and quadricipital muscle groups. Ekblom and associates,[14] however, noted that speed skaters were not particularly strong during leg ex-

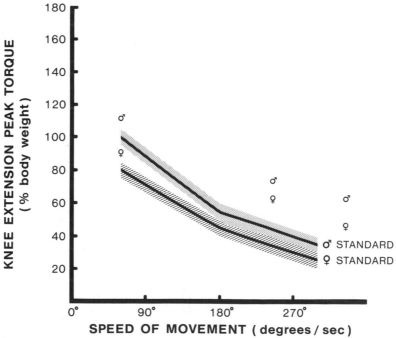

Figure 25–20. Relative peak torque in relation to velocity of male and female skaters during isokinetic knee extension compared with normative data suggested by Davies.[9]

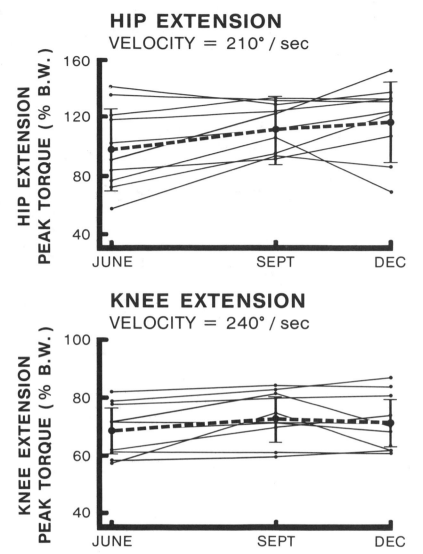

Figure 25–21. Changes in the relative peak torque of the hip and knee extensors in speed skaters (7 male, 4 female) during the course of dry-land and early on-ice training.

tension activities and observed that skaters who were better sprinters seemed to be somewhat stronger than distance-oriented skaters. Certainly, the pattern of power output during the skating stroke[11,12] would favor individuals capable of generating very large muscular forces at high rates of limb extension.

Our experience with the American speed skating team has been that speed skaters are very strong compared with ordinary individuals (Fig. 25–20). We have found also that peak torque of both hip and knee extensors (Fig. 25–21) increases subsequent to training.

During weight training, American skaters typically perform sets of 5 squats with 2 to 2½ times body weight by the end of the summer dry-land training period. This is particularly remarkable considering the very deep position favored for this exercise. It is generally accepted from biomechanical studies that skating performance is related to skating posture, specifically the preextension knee angle.[35] Studies in our laboratory have suggested that skating posture improves throughout the preparatory period (Fig. 25–22). These data also suggest an overall parallelism between changes in strength of the

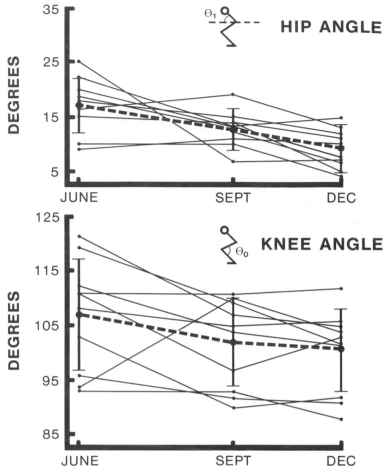

Figure 25–22. Changes in skating posture, defined as preextension knee angle (θ_0) and hip angle (θ_1) during maximal slideboard exercise during the preparatory period for skating. Decreasing values for θ_0 and θ_1 are generally regarded as indicative of improved fitness for competition.

hip and knee extensors and changes in skating posture. These changes seem to allow the skaters to sustain a more favorable posture, at least during slideboard exercise, as the training program progresses.[16]

It may be argued that peak torque of the hip and knee extensors, which usually occurs midway through the range of motion, is an inappropriate measure of muscular strength in speed skaters. Torque at the angles of hip and knee flexion typical of the gliding phase of the stroke may be a more meaningful index of strength for skaters. This is particularly likely because of the high rates of hip and knee extension in speed skating and the lack of contribution of terminal hip and knee extension forces to the skating stroke.[11]

SUMMARY

In summary, speed skating is an important international sport that despite a relatively small base of participants has been the focus of notable success by American athletes during several Olympic winter games. The sport is typically populated by rather small, muscular athletes who do exceedingly well in anaerobic and strength-type activities. Contrary to early reports from Scandinavia, which focused on long-distance specialists, contemporary all-around speed skaters are probably more similar to the 200- to 800-meter runner of intermediate hurdler than they are to the 10,000-meter runner (which represents the dominant model in sports physiology). We have noted a pattern in which more successful skaters give evidence of better skill as opposed to only better physiology. The rather striking variability in the limited data regarding the energy costs of speed skating and the data that we have collected on lactate metabolism during skating suggest that components of neuromuscular skill may be of considerable significance. Certainly future research into the physiology of speed skating must address this issue rather than follow a model that assumes that conditioning is of central importance. Lastly, it appears that strength-related variables are of particular importance to speed skaters. More intensive inquiry into this as yet poorly understood area is clearly indicated.

ACKNOWLEDGMENTS

Research in our laboratory has been supported by grants from the Sport Sciences Division of the U.S. Olympic Committee and from Ross Laboratories, Columbus, OH. Several other individuals have made substantive contributions to our efforts with the U.S. Speed Skating team. They include Paul Abler, PT; Kurt Alt, PT; Paul Bodenback, ATC; Ann Brophy, PT; M. Jayne Conway, MS; Kurt Kuettel, BS; Kathy Lemberger, MS; and W. Drew Palin, MD; as well as coaches Mike Crowe, Dan Immerfal, Dianne Holum, Susan Sandvig, and Nancy Swider-Peltz. Of course, the patience and understanding of the athletes with our often inept inquiries were a necessary prerequisite for these studies. Our fondest hope is that they are beginning to reap the rewards of their patience.

REFERENCES

1. Abler, P, Foster, C, Thompson, NN, Crowe, M, Alt, K, Brophy, A, and Palin, WD: Determinants of anaerobic muscular performance. Medicine and Science in Sports and Exercise 18:51 (Abstracts), 1986.
2. Armstrong, RB: Muscle damage and endurance events. Sports Medicine 3:370–381, 1986.
3. Brouns, F, Saris, WHM, and ten Hoor, F: Nutritional factors influencing physical performance. In Rispens, P and Lamberts, R (eds): Physiological, Biomechanical and Technical Aspects of Speed Skating. Private Press, Gronigen, The Netherlands, 1985, pp 112–133.
4. Costill, DL, Bowers, R, Branham, G, and Sparks, K: Muscle glycogen utilization during prolonged exercise on successive days. J Appl Physiol 31:834–838, 1971.
5. Costill, DL, Daniels, J, Evans, W, Fink, W, Krahenbuhl, G, and Saltin, B: Skeletal muscle enzymes and fiber composition in male and female track athletes. J Appl Physiol 40:149–154, 1976.
6. Crowe, M, Foster, C, Thompson, NN, Phul, J, Baldwin, C and Katz, A: Blood lactate and perceptual responses during simulated competition. Medicine and Science in Sports and Exercise 18:59 (Abstract), 1986.
7. Daniels, J, Scardina, N, Hayes, J, and Foley, P: Elite and subelite female middle and long distance runners. In Landers, DM (ed): Sport and Elite Performers. Human Kinetics, Champaign, IL, 1986, pp 57–72.
8. Daniels, J, Yarbrough, R, and Foster, C: Changes in $\dot{V}O_2$ and running performance with training. Eur J Appl Physiol 39:249–254, 1978.
9. Davies, GJ: A Compendium of Isokinetics in Clinical Usage: Workshop and Clinical Notes. S & S, LaCrosse, WI, 1984.
10. de Boer, RW: Training and Technique in Speed Skating. Free University Press, Amsterdam, The Netherlands, 1986.
11. de Boer, RW, van Ingen Schenau, GJ, and de Groot, G: Specificity of training in speed skating. In Rispens, P and Lamberts, R (eds): Physiological, Biomechanical and Technical Aspects of Speed Skating. Private Press, Groningen, The Netherlands, 1985, pp 49–59.
12. de Groot, G, van Ingen Schenau, GJ, de Boer, RW: Evaluation of speed skating capacity on the basis of tests. In Rispens, P and Lamberts, R (eds): Physiological, Biomechanical and Technical Aspects of Speed Skating. Private Press, Gronigen, The Netherlands, 1985, pp 39–48.
13. DiPrampero, PE, Cortil, G, Mogoni, P, and Saibene, F: Energy cost of speed skating and efficiency of work against air resistance. J Appl Physiol 40:584–591, 1976.
14. Ekblom, B, Hermansen, L, and Saltin, B: Hastighetsakinng pa Skridsko: Idrottsfysiologi rapport nr 5. Trygg-Hansa, Stockholm, 1967.
15. Ferguson, RJ, Marcotte, GG, and Montpetit, RR: A maximal oxygen uptake test during ice skating. Medicine and Science in Sports 1:207–211, 1969.
16. Foster, C, Abler, P, Brophy, A, Crowe, M, Holum, D, Lemberger, K, Thompson, N, and Palin, D: Serial changes in aerobic power, skating posture and strength in elite speed skaters. AAHPERD Abstracts, 1986.
17. Foster, C, Holum, D, Lemberger, K, Pollock, ML, and Pels, AE: Laboratory correlates of speed skating performance. Medicine and Science in Sports and Exercise 17:269 (Abstract), 1985.
18. Foster, C, Meyer, L, and Hare, J: Nutritional support in the elite athlete. AAHPERD Abstracts, 1984.
19. Foster, C, Pollock ML, Farrell, PA, Maksud, MG, Anhom, J, and Hare, J: Training responses of speed skaters during a competitive season. Res Q Exerc Sport 53:243–246, 1982.
20. Foster, C, Thompson, N, Crowe, M, Conway, MJ, Kuettel, K, Sandvig, S, and Swider, N: Effectiveness in speed skating. Medicine and Science in Sports and Exercise 19:104 (Abstract), 1987.
21. Giejsel, J, Bomhoff, G, van Velzen, J, de Groot, G, and van Ingen Schenau, GJ: Bicycle ergometry and

speedskating performance. Int J Sports Med 5:241–245, 1984.

22. Geijsel, JSM: Training and testing in marathon speed skating. J Sports Medicine Physical Fit 19:277–284, 1979.

23. Green, HJ: Glycogen depletion patterns during continuous and intermittent ice skating. Medicine and Science in Sports 10:183–187, 1978.

24. Jacobs, I: Blood lactate: Implications for training and sports performance. Sports Medicine 3:10–25, 1986.

25. Janssen, GME: Skating and muscular overuse. In Rispens, P and Lamberts, R (eds): Physiological, Biomechanical and Technical Aspects of Speed Skating. Private Press, Gronigen, The Netherlands, 1985, pp 88–93.

26. Lamberts, R and Rispens, P: Aerobic power in speed skating. In Rispens, P and Lamberts, R (eds): Physiological, Biomechanical and Technical Aspects of Speed Skating. Private Press, Gronigen, The Netherlands, 1985, pp 13–20.

27. Lamberts, R and Rispens, P: Determinations of Anaerobic threshold in athletes. In Rispens, P and Lamberts, R (eds): Physiological, Biomechanical and Technical Aspects of Speed Skating. Private Press, Gronigen, The Netherlands, 1985, pp 21–38.

28. Leger, L, Mercier, D, and Gauvin, L: The relationship between % $\dot{V}O_2$ and running performance time. In Landers, DM (ed): Sport and Elite Performers. Human Kinetics, Champaign, IL, 1986, pp 113–120.

29. Maksud, MG, Farrell, PA, Foster, C, Pollock, ML, Hare, J, Anholm, J, and Schmidt, DH: Maximal $\dot{V}O_2$, ventilation and heart rate of Olympic speed skating candidates. Journal of Sports Medicine and Physical Fitness 22:217–223, 1982.

30. Maksud, MG, Hamilton, LH, and Balke, B: Physiological respones of a male Olympic speed skater—Terry McDermott. Medicine and Science in Sports 3:107–109, 1971.

31. Maksud, MG, Wiley, RL, Hamilton, LH, and Lockhart, B: Maximal $\dot{V}O_2$, ventilation and heart rate of Olympic speed skating candidates. J Appl Physiol 29:186–190, 1970.

32. Pollock, ML, Foster, C, Anholm, J, Hare, J, Farrell, P, and Maksud, M: Body composition of Olympic speed skating candidates. Res Q Exerc Sport 53:150–155, 1982.

33. Pollock, ML, Pels, AE, Foster, C, and Holum, D: Comparison of male and female speed skating candidates. In Landers, DN (ed): Sport and Elite Performers. Human Kinetics, Champaign, IL, 1986, pp 143–152.

34. Thompson, NN, Foster, C, Crowe, M, Rogowski, B, and Kaplan, K: Serial responses of anaerobic muscular performance in competitive athletes. Med Sci Sports Exerc 18:51 (Abstract), 1986.

35. van Ingen Schenau, GJ and Bakker, K: A biomechanical model of speedskating. Journal of Human Movement Studies 6:1–18, 1980.

36. van Ingen Schenau, GJ, de Boer, RW, and de Groot, G: Mechanical aspects of speed skating. In Rispens, P and Lamberts, R (eds): Physiological, Biomechanical and Technical Aspects of Speed Skating. Private Press, Gronigen, The Netherlands, 1985, pp 72–87.

37. van Ingen Schenau, GJ, and de Groot, G: Differences in oxygen consumption and external power output between male and female speed skaters during supramaximal cycling. Eur J Appl Physiol 51:337–345, 1983.

38. van Ingen Schenau, GJ, de Groot, G, and Hollander, AP: Some technical, physiological and anthropometrical aspects of speed skating. Eur J Appl Physiol 50:343–354, 1983.

39. von Kinderman, W and Keul, J: Anaerobic supply of energy in high speed skating. Deutsche Zeitschrift fur Sportsmedizin 5:142–147, 1980.

CHAPTER 26

Biomechanics of Skating

NANCY L. GREER, Ph.D.

BIOMECHANICS OF SPEED SKATING
BIOMECHANICS OF ICE HOCKEY
CONCLUSIONS

In both speed skating and ice hockey, an important component of performance is the ability to skate fast. In speed skating, the skater with the fastest start, straightaway, and turn techniques will win the race. In hockey, the faster player has an advantage in getting to the puck, creating unbalanced offensive situations, and being more effective defensively.

Coaches and researchers associated with these sports have independently attempted to determine the mechanical components of skating technique that contribute to faster performance. In each sport, initial research efforts were primarily descriptive and relied on stopwatches and measures made from tracings produced on new ice surfaces. Currently, high-speed film and electronic measurement and recording devices are being used to study and to quantify performance.

In this chapter, research relevant to the question of improving skating speed is outlined, and findings focusing on similarities between the sports of ice hockey and speed skating are summarized.

BIOMECHANICS OF SPEED SKATING

Early research efforts in speed skating concentrated on velocity changes during the course of the race or within an individual stroke. In 1980, a mathematical model was developed by van Ingen Schenau and Bakker[11] to describe the skating technique in mechanical terms. The work done during hip and knee extension resulted in an increase in velocity and, therefore, kinetic energy of the

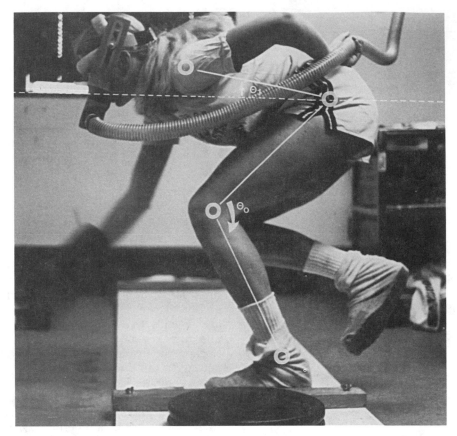

Figure 26–1. Combined biomechanical-physiologic study of a speed skater during simulated skating on the slideboard. Preextension knee (θ_0) and hip (θ_1) angles are measured directly from stop-action video tapes.

center of gravity. The increase in kinetic energy represented the external work per stroke. Combining this term with the stroke frequency provided a measure of the total external usable power. Their model of speed also included resistance to movement that was attributable to air and ice frictional losses.

To evaluate the model, top male skaters were filmed during the 500-, 1500-, 5000-, and 10,000-meter races at the 1978 World Championships.[11] A kinematic analysis of the data indicated that the trunk angle, measured relative to the horizontal, was greater (more upright) during the 500-meter race as compared with the longer events. As the length of the race increased, the thigh angle increased, indicating that the thigh was held more vertically during the longer events. Possible explanations for these findings were the difference in lever arms at the knee and

hip as well as the ability of the larger muscle groups to withstand the effects of fatigue over longer time intervals. See Figures 26–1 and 26–2 for examples of how joint angles are measured and then reduced to stick figures.[11]

Independent values for external power were determined using pre-extension knee angle (the angle between the thigh and shank just before push-off), body length, and stroke frequency. When the two power values were compared, the agreement was considered excellent, especially in light of the many assumptions made. From this finding, it was suggested that for top skaters, the skating movement is determined primarily by the pre-extension knee angle, stroke frequency, and air and ice friction. When the actual amount of work per stroke was measured and compared with that predicted by the pre-extension knee angle, it was determined that skaters increase their external work output at higher velocities by an increase in stroke frequency. Using a corrected model, the speed in 52 of 53 races could be predicted within an absolute error of 5 percent. This indicated that approximately 95 percent of the performance of these elite male skaters could be explained by the extension of the knee and hip joints, the stroke frequency, and the air and ice friction.

Subsequent studies were directed at validating the model for other groups of skaters. "Top" and "sub-top" skaters were compared during a 3000-meter race.[12] The sub-top group was found to fit the previously described model as well as the elite group, indicating that the variables identified for the top skaters were also important for the sub-top group. Specific differences between the two groups were observed in the position of the trunk (the elite skaters maintaining a more horizontal position), the pre-extension knee angle (with smaller values observed for the elite skaters), and the stroke frequency (which showed a higher value for the top skaters). The combined effect of these measures was a higher external power among the top skaters.

Trained and elite skaters have also been studied during a 1500 meter event.[4] Differences in performance levels were attributed to increased work per stroke in the elite skaters. Overall, the elite skaters skated at a faster speed, had greater power and more work per stroke, and displayed a shorter push-off phase.

Performances of male and female elite skaters have also been compared.[14] Previous research had indicated that during cycling, female skaters were capable of delivering the same external power relative to body weight as the male skaters.[16] The authors consequently hypothesized that differences in skating performance between male and female skaters were due to differences in technique or frictional losses. The greatest difference between the two groups was observed for the pre-extension knee angle, with females showing a larger value. A greater thigh angle, measured relative to the horizontal plane, accounted for most of the difference. Trunk position did not differ significantly between the two groups. Lower external power values were found for the female skaters at all distances. Because the stroke frequency values were similar for men and women, this was attributed primarily to lower work per stroke, as related to the pre-extension knee angle.

The combined influence of anthropometric, physiologic, and technical factors has also been considered.[16] Fourteen sub-elite skaters and five elite skaters were evaluated in a series of on-ice and off-ice performance tests. Anthropometric measurements and estimations of lean body mass were included in the test battery. The results indicated that the elite skaters had shorter thighs and longer shank values relative to the sub-elite group. This configuration generally should be to the skater's advantage as lower muscle forces would be required by the extensors of the hip and knee. A significant difference in pre-extension knee angle was also observed. The difference was primarily a result of a greater thigh angle relative to the horizontal plane. Inability to maintain the thigh and, therefore, knee angles was hypothesized to be due to the larger muscle forces required. It was also speculated that achieving a lower body position would require greater use of the anaerobic energy systems. Differences in speed

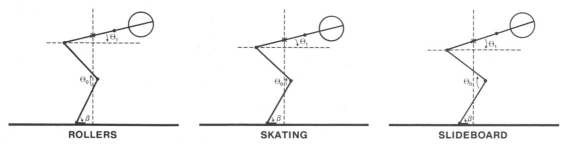

Figure 26–2. *Reduced data showing skating position for the same speed skater during speed skating, roller skating, and simulated skating on the slideboard.*

and external work were attributed to differences in both external work per stroke and stroke frequency. Elite skaters were able to increase stroke frequency to compensate for a decrease in work per stroke.

The ability of female elite skaters to control their speed has also been investigated.[15] This question encompassed two distinct areas: (1) the variables related to performance differences among skaters at similar levels and (2) the ability to regulate speed at different distances. In regard to different distances, it was observed that skaters controlled their speed by varying the stroke frequency. The amount of work per stroke did not differ greatly despite the difference in power output. A ratio that compared stroke frequency on the curved sections to stroke frequency on the straight sections increased as the distance of the race increased. The difference was attributed to a greater decrease in the straight section frequency as compared with the curved section frequency. In an attempt to differentiate performances of similarly skilled skaters, several new variables were introduced into the study. These included the maximum knee extension angle, maximum knee extension velocity, effectiveness of the push-off, the gain in potential energy during the glide phase (reflected in the difference in knee angles prior to push-off and at the time of weight transfer), and the difference in initial and final knee angles associated with the push-off phase. Performance scores of velocity and external power were positively correlated with the angle of the support leg at the time of weight transfer and with the variables describing the change in potential energy and the effectiveness of the push-off. The performance values were not correlated with the maximum angular velocity of the knee, perhaps because the skate is lifted from the ice prior to full extension of the knee.

More recently, attention has been directed to the study of forces in speed skating.[18] Push-off forces were measured using skates instrumented with strain gauge elements between the shoe and the skate blade. When skating on the straight portion of the track, an increase in force was evident near the end of the stroke. An increase in velocity was not accompanied by an increase in force. When skating the curve, a peak in the force curve was not observed. The difference in the patterns was attributed to the lack of rotation from the lateral to the medial portion of the skate when skating the curved portion of the track.

Force data have also been combined with kinematic information in order to examine the moments of force and the associated power values at the hip, knee, and ankle.[2] Muscle activity patterns and muscle contraction velocities were also recorded. Based on the results from two well-trained skaters, it was concluded that the knee-extension phase could be characterized as a "catapult-like" action. The gluteus maximus and vastus medialis muscles were considered to be largely responsible for the power output during the push-off phase.

Mechanical aspects associated with skating the curves have also received attention recently. Performances of elite and trained male skaters have been compared.[2] Elite skaters had shorter stroke times and greater push-off angles than did the trained group. The result was a greater work per stroke that contributed to greater values for speed and power in the elite group.

Utilizing the geometry of the speed skating oval, a mathematical model of the power output in skating the curves was developed.[3] A study of 16 elite female skaters resulted in differences of about 3 percent between measured power and predicted power. Much of this more recent work has been summarized by van Ingen Schenau.[13]

Other research related to improving performance in speed skating has focused on body position and starting techniques. Wind tunnels have been used to investigate the effects of skaters' body build and posture on the drag coefficient.[6,10] The use of a constant drag coefficient value for all subjects has been shown to be inaccurate. The skin suits worn by present-day skaters cause less drag than older, woolen suits. Shielding, or skating close behind another skater, reduced the drag by 16 percent when the skaters were 2 meters apart and 23 percent when the distance was 1 meter. When the effects of skating with and against the wind were considered, it was recommended that skaters attempt to maintain a constant power and allow the speed to fluctuate slightly, as opposed to skating at a constant speed.

A three-dimensional analysis of starting techniques in the women's 1000-meter event has indicated that both the starting positions and initial movements vary even among elite skaters.[9] Additional research is required before a complete understanding of a "best" start may be achieved.

BIOMECHANICS OF ICE HOCKEY

The ability to accelerate quickly from a stationary or "gliding" position has been recognized as an important element of ice hockey performance. Lariviere[19] investigated the relationships between velocity, length of stride from the rear skate to front skate at the time of take-off, angle of forward inclination of the leg at take-off, and angle of propulsion between the blade and the direction of motion. It was concluded that a greater velocity was associated with a larger angle of propulsion, a smaller angle of forward lean, and a greater stride length.

Page[25] also studied the technical components associated with greater velocity. The characteristics of skaters with higher velocity values were

1. longer strides
2. wider strides with greater width between strides
3. greater abduction of the leg
4. quicker return of the skate to the ice
5. quicker set of the inside edge
6. quicker extension of the knee
7. greater flexion of the knee prior to push-off
8. greater forward lean of the trunk and legs

Increased skating velocity has been observed to be positively correlated with stride rate and negatively correlated with single-support and double-support times.[21] Three skating velocities were studied. It was found that skaters' stride lengths did not significantly relate to their velocities, and at slow and medium speeds the skaters were subjectively observed to assume more upright postures and have longer glide phases.

Marino and Weese[23] studied the patterns of acceleration and deceleration during a skating stride. Three phases were identified: glide during single support, propulsion during single support, and propulsion during double support. A period of deceleration was observed during the initial stages of single support. Acceleration began approximately halfway through the single-support phase and was maintained through the end of double support. Concurrent with the start of the acceleration phase were an external rotation of the thigh and an initiation of extension of the hip and knee. They concluded that during the recovery phase, the foot should be brought back close to the ice to maintain balance and to complete the single-support phase quickly.

The statistical method of multiple regression has been used to explore the relationship of various parameters describing technique to acceleration ability.[20] Beginning from a stationary start, the following factors were all found to contribute significantly to the prediction of the average acceleration over a 20-foot interval: a high stride rate, forward lean of the trunk, placement of the recovery foot under the body, and a low angle of the leg at take-off of the propulsive leg. Similar parameters were identified in the prediction of time to skate 6 meters.[22] The subjects analyzed in this study represented a wide range of skating ability.

To determine whether the regression equation for prediction of acceleration would apply to elite skaters, participants in the 1983 National Sports Festival were studied.[7] Predicted values derived from this equation were not significantly different from measured values, thereby indicating that the model was appropriate for elite skaters. To evaluate the effects of changes in technique on performance, the values for trunk flexion and leg angle were altered, and a new predicted acceleration was derived. Changing the trunk angle produced only a small change in the acceleration value, whereas changing the leg angle by 9 degrees improved the predicted acceleration from 3.51 m/s^2 to 4.04 m/s^2.

The question remained whether a more appropriate equation could be produced for the elite skaters. A stepwise regression program was used to develop a new regression model. Statistically, the model was not as strong as Marino's.[20] However, similarities between the two equations were apparent. In each case, either stride rate or single- and double-support times, which sum to the reciprocal of stride rate, were significant predictors. This agrees with previous findings,[23,25] which advocated the quick return of the skate to the ice, quick set of the inside edge, and quick extension of the knee and hip to produce greater velocity. Both models also emphasized a small angle at the trunk and take-off leg. A low body position would be advantageous in putting the skater in a position to exert force in a horizontal direction and thus benefit from a greater ground reaction force in the direction of the desired movement.

Changes in skating technique as a player fatigues have been evaluated.[8] An endurance test has been developed that requires the player to skate 6 lengths of the ice in an all-out effort. To study the effects of fatigue, the first four strides of the second, fourth, and sixth lengths were filmed. These films were then analyzed to determine stride rate, single-support time, double-support time, non-support time, and angular position data for the trunk, hip, knee, and leg. Time to skate each length was recorded using photocells.

Performance times were found to be significantly slower between the second and sixth lengths. Stride rate decreased significantly, and the support times increased significantly as the skater completed the test. Knee angle at the time the propulsive foot left the ice and the trunk, knee, and leg angles at the time when the recovery foot returned to the ice all were significantly changed over the course of the test. The direction of the changes was such that the trunk was placed in a position of greater forward lean and the leg was in a more vertical position with less flexion at the knee as the skater fatigued. Thus, the skater was unable to maintain a low posture relative to the ice. When comparisons were made between the three lengths evaluated, the change in knee angle was greatest between the second and fourth lengths, whereas the change in trunk angle was greatest between lengths four and six. This pattern of changes would appear to reflect fatigue of the quadriceps followed by fatigue of the hip extensors and other lower back muscle groups.

Hockey researchers have also attempted to determine the most effective starting techniques. Three basic techniques may be used to initiate movement from a stationary position: (1) the front start, (2) the crossover start, and (3) the thrust-and-glide start. In the front start, the player begins facing in the direction of movement with the feet perpendicular to the imaginary starting line. For the crossover

start, the player stands sideways, with the feet parallel to the starting line, and initiates the forward movement with the rear foot crossing over the front foot. The thrust-and-glide start begins from a sideways position. The front foot is then turned out to point in the direction of movement while the back foot pushes off.

Jones[17] studied university-level varsity and junior varsity hockey players. In this group, faster skating times, velocities, and accelerations—measured at 30 feet and 60 feet from the starting line—were recorded when the front start was used.

Performance over the first 20 feet was recorded by Naud and Holt.[24] High-speed film and timing devices were used. The thrust-and-glide start was found to be faster for the Bantam, Junior "B," and college-level hockey athletes, but no significant difference was observed for professional players. Biomechanically, the thrust-and-glide technique allowed the rear leg to make the initial thrust with the skate at a 90° angle to the direction of movement. The center of gravity began to move forward immediately; whereas in the crossover technique, the center of gravity was vertically elevated for a short period of time.

Roy[26] compared the ground reaction forces produced by the three starting methods. Using a force platform embedded in a synthetic ice surface, it was found that the vertical impulse was highest using the crossover technique, whereas the lateral impulse was greatest using the front start. The fore-aft component impulse was similar for each of the starting styles.

CONCLUSIONS

The results of research efforts in speed skating and ice hockey show several similarities. In both sports, faster skaters are characterized by lower body positions. Elite speed skaters were found to have a more horizontal trunk position and lower pre-extension knee angle. Faster hockey skaters have been shown to have greater forward lean of the trunk and propulsion leg. Greater flexion of the knee prior to push-off was also observed. These parameters have also been reported to change as the skater becomes slower because of fatigue. The advantage of a lower body position would appear to be related to the ability to increase the horizontal component of the ground reaction force associated with skating thrust.

Stroke frequency in both speed skating and ice hockey has also been found to be related to performance. Assuming that a low body position can be maintained to maximize the effectiveness of the stroke, the skater who can execute more propulsions has the advantage.

Recent directions for research include some areas of interest common to both sports. These are analyses of starting techniques and performance in skating the curved sections of the speed skating track or executing hockey crossovers and control turns. Through continued research efforts in both sports, improvements in performance and training may be expected.

REFERENCES

1. Boer, RW de, Cabri, J, Vaes, W, Clarijs, JP, Hollander, AP, de Groot, G, and van Ingen Schenau, GJ: Moments of force, power, and muscle coordination in speed-skating. Int J Sport Med 8:371–378, 1987.
2. Boer, RW de, Ettema, GJC, van Gorkum, H, de Groot, G, and van Ingen Schenau, GJ: Biomechanical aspects of push-off techniques in speed skating the curves. Int J Sport Biom 3:69–79, 1987.
3. Boer, RW de, Ettema, GJC, van Gorkum, H, de Groot, G, and van Ingen Schenau, GJ: A geometrical model of speed skating the curves. J Biomechanics 21:445–450, 1988.
4. Boer, RW de, Schermerhorn, P, Gademan, J, de Groot, G, and van Ingen Schenau, GJ: Characteristic stroke mechanics of elite and trained male speed skaters. In J Sport Biom 2:175–185, 1986.
5. Dillman, CJ, Stockholm, AJ, and Greer, NL: Movement and velocity patterns of ice hockey players during a game. Paper presented at the Second International Symposium on Biomechanics in Sports, Colorado Springs, CO, January 1984.
6. Di Prampero, PE, Cortili, G, Mognoni, P, and Saibene, F: Energy cost of speed skating and efficiency of work against air resistance. J Appl Physiol 40:584–591, 1976.
7. Greer, NL and Dillman, CJ: The influence of biomechanical factors upon the acceleration capabilities of elite ice hockey players. Paper presented at the Second International Symposium on Biomechanics in Sports, Colorado Springs, CO, January 1984.
8. Greer, NL, Dillman, CJ, and Blatherwick, J: A biomechanical evaluation of changes in skating technique with fatigue. In Thorton-Trump, A (ed): Proceedings of the Third Biannual Conference of the Canadian Society for Biomechanics. Winnipeg, 1984, pp 67–68.
9. Hartfel, M, Swigart, J, Erdman, AG, Stoner, LJ, Greer, N, Sandvig, S, and Foster, C: A kinematic analysis of sprint starts of females in speed skating. Int J Sport Biom (submitted).
10. Ingen Schenau, GJ van: The influence of air friction in speed skating. J Biomechanics 15:449–458, 1982.
11. Ingen Schenau, GJ van and Bakker, K: A biomechanical model of speed skating. J Human Movement Studies 6:1–18, 1980.
12. Ingen Schenau, GJ van and Bakker, K: A mathematical model of speed skating. In Morecki, A, Fidelus, K, Kedzior, K, and Wit, A (eds): Biomechanics VII-B. University Park Press, Baltimore, 1981, pp 492–497.
13. Ingen Schenau, GJ van, de Boer, RW, and de Groot, G: On the technique of speed skating. Int J Sport Biom 3:419–431, 1987.
14. Ingen Schenau, GJ van and de Groot, G: On the origin of differences in performance level between elite male and female speed skaters. Human Movement Science 2:151–159, 1983.
15. Ingen Schenau, GJ van, de Groot, G, and de Boer, RW: The control of speed in elite female speed skaters. J Biomechanics 18:91–96, 1985.
16. Ingen Schenau, GJ van, de Groot, G, and Hollander, AP: Some technical, physiological, and anthropometrical aspects of speed skating. Eur J Appl Physiol 50:343–354, 1983.
17. Jones, BE: Comparison of ice skating starting styles used in ice hockey. Unpublished master's thesis. The University of British Columbia, 1969.
18. Koning, J de, de Boer, RW, de Groot, G, and van Ingen Schenau, GJ: Push-off force in speed skating. Int J Sport Biom 3:103–109, 1987.
19. Lariviere, G: Relationship between skating velocity and length of stride, angle of forward inclination, and angle of propulsion. Unpublished master's thesis, University of Oregon, 1968.
20. Marino, GW: Multiple regression models of the mechanics of the acceleration phase of ice skating. Unpublished doctoral thesis, University of Illinois, 1975.
21. Marino, GW: Kinematics of ice skating at different velocities. Res Q 48:93–97, 1977.
22. Marino, GW: Selected mechanical factors associated with acceleration in ice skating. Res Q Exer Sport 54:234–238, 1983.
23. Marino, GW and Weese, R: A kinematic analysis of the ice skating stride. In Terauds, J and Gros, H (eds): Science in Skiing, Skating, and Hockey. Academic, Delmar, CA, 1979, pp. 65–74.
24. Naud, RL and Holt, LE: A comparison of selected hockey skating starts. Can J Appl Sports Sci 4:8–10, 1979.
25. Page, P: Biomechanics of forward skating in ice hockey. Unpublished master's thesis, Dalhousie University, 1975.
26. Roy, B: Biomechanical features of different starting positions and skating strides in ice hockey. In Asmussen, E and Jorgensen, K (eds): Biomechanics VI-B. University Park Press, Baltimore, 1978, pp 137–141.

CHAPTER 27

Medical Aspects of Speed Skating

MICHAEL P. WOODS, M.D.

This chapter presents the medical aspects of speed skating from the viewpoint of a competitive skater who is also a physician. Experience with training and skating at all levels of competition has permitted me to focus on several areas of medicine and sports science that hold particular importance for the skaters, their coaches, and their health care providers.

INJURIES

It is interesting to note that while most sports-governing bodies concerned with the Olympic sports are desperately scrambling to find adequate liability insurance coverage, speed skating has had little or no difficulty in obtaining such coverage. Since its inception, the United States International Speed Skating Association has had no suits filed in regard to medical liability. The reason for this is that, by nature, the sport is relatively injury free. The speed skating motion provides little stress to bones and joints; training for the sport involves heavy strength work on the quadriceps, adductor, and lower back muscle groups, which in itself helps provide protection to the lower back and knee joints. Competition is on a "one skater at a time" time-trial basis, so falls are relatively infrequent. When falls do occur, they are usually cushioned by snow or a long slide before significant impact is made. Thus, orthopedic injury directly related to the action of the sport is rare. When acute orthopedic injuries do occur, they are usually related to dry-land training.

However, acute lacerations of the calcaneus tendon incurred from the return skate during the start have been reported, and falls that are improperly cushioned can result in severe deceleration injuries to almost any bone or joint. This is especially true of indoor and/or pack-style racing, which is not currently recognized as an Olympic sport. Hockey rink boards make poor deceleration cushions. Because short-track skating was a demonstration sport in the 1988 XV Winter Olympic Games at Calgary and will be a full part of the program in the 1992 Winter Olympic Games, the overall injury picture for skaters may be changing. Chronic orthopedic injuries do occur in relation to the skate boot, secondary to dry-land training and secondary to inadequate flexibility training in a sport that requires severe flexion, particularly of the lower back. The process of dry-land training covers a great realm of activities, including running; power and endurance weightlifting; bicycle riding and racing; roller skating at high speeds; slideboarding; and a long compendium of various jumps, squats, and duckwalks—all of which are aimed at strengthening the lower back and thigh muscles, especially the quadriceps group. It is beyond the scope of this chapter to cover the many and various orthopedic problems that can occur secondary to participating in such a wide range of athletic activities, but the most troublesome and common off-season injuries to speed skaters include low back and knee pain from weightlifting; joint pain, muscle pulls, and tendinitis from running and cycling; and, not necessarily the least, bumps and contusions from bicycle accidents.

It should be mentioned here that back pain also can be caused by the skater's position, which includes forward flexion and right lateral flexion and rotation of the spine at the lower back. This is especially marked when the skater is turning the corners. Prevention is better than cure for these chronic back problems. The use of sand bags placed on the lower back rather than barbells for squats has been suggested as a solution to weightlifting back injuries, and proper flexibility exercises seem to be effective in the prevention

of inflection injuries caused by chronic "position" problems of the skater. Flexibility training is also important in the prevention of restrictive injuries to muscle and tendon groups that are involved in the skating motion.

Boot-related injuries are centered about three areas of the foot. The peroneus longus and brevis tendons may be pinched between the skate counter, which is a hard shell that fits snugly around the heel of the foot, and the lateral malleolus, resulting in tendinitis (see also Chapter 28). Calluses and tendinitis can form on the foot extensors, which traverse an area that may be constricted when the boot is tightened. A similar area of possible callus formation and tendinitis is the Achilles tendon, which may rub at the point where the rear top of the boot ends. Finally, the cuneiform-first metatarsal bones and joint may form callus secondary to pressure and rubbing. This also is an area where the boot laces are very tight. Solutions to these various boot-related problems are preventive in nature and include proper padding, properly fitted skates, and careful tightening of the skates. It is hoped that, in the future, boots will be designed with comfort as well as performance in mind. In the case of such injuries during the competitive season, padding must be used to transfer pressure away from the injury site. These injuries may be severe enough to hamper performance and should be tended to immediately upon detection.

The start in sprint events is an extremely violent, although coordinated, movement that includes maximum speed in return of the skate to a position at one's center of gravity. This motion can result in two types of injuries. The first type of injury that may be incurred at the start of a sprint involves lacerations and stab wounds should the skate blade be guided too far medially, thus hitting the opposite leg before it is set down. The second start-related injury is strain to the adductor muscle group. In managing these lacerations, it is important to bear in mind the possibility of tendon damage, particularly damage to the calcaneus tendon. Rest and appropriate ice treatment for 24 hours followed by heat and whirlpool applications are standard therapy for these adductor strains. Proper warm-up, especially in very cold weather, may help prevent this common injury.

ENVIRONMENTAL PROBLEMS

Speed skating is a winter sport, and training is conducted on an open surface, where exposure to high winds is common. Wind chill is enhanced by the skating speeds, which reach close to 35 miles per hour. Additionally, for aerodynamic and flexibility reasons, clothing is sparse at best. Elite skaters train outside daily, no matter what unpleasant conditions the weather may hold. In Milwaukee, that can include $-15°F$ $(-26.1°C)$ temperatures with wind chill as low as $-70°F$ $(-56.7°C)$. There are three direct cold-related problems that the speed skating community faces: frostbite, hypothermia, and cold-induced bronchospasm and bronchitis.

For the speed skaters, frostbite commonly occurs on the toes, hands, nose tip, and occasionally the eye. In male skaters, the penis is an organ that is painfully at risk! During distance races, the left hand is particularly vulnerable because it is held on the back without movement throughout the race. Usually these cases are superficial and will heal without specific treatment; however, sloughing of skin can occur, particularly with inexperienced athletes. Initial treatment of frostbite[3] is warming of the area in 40 to 44°F (4.4 to 6.7°C) water. Exercising the part, massaging it, or subjecting it to high temperatures should be avoided. The erroneous practice of rubbing the part in the snow will increase pain and edema. If frostbite is moderately severe, analgesics may be required during the warming period. Vesicles, bullae, and eschars should be left alone (see Chapter 18). Although antibiotics, tetanus antitoxin, and regional sympathectomy may be necessary in the most severe cases of frostbite, there have been no cases from the United States Speed Skating Team that required such radical treatment. However, even small frostbite injuries may leave parts permanently hypersensitive to cold. The best treatment of frostbite is prevention. Proper clothing and covering, use of mittens rather than gloves, utilization of face masks and skate covers, and rewarming at frequent intervals

in bitter cold are simple measures for the prevention of frostbite.

Life- or health-threatening hypothermia is not a serious problem in speed skating, because of the level of exercise during training, the clothing that is worn, and the relatively short periods of time that are spent outside during competition. However, race performance is definitely affected by extreme cold. At the molecular level, enzymes involved in muscular function work poorly at extremes of temperature, and as suspected, most American speed skating records have been set at above-freezing temperatures on refrigerated ice surfaces. The only currently available means of keeping muscle temperature adequate are extra clothing, which proves restrictive, and surface-heating substances, which are inadequate. The effect of cold on performance and protection from cold in elite speed skating are potential areas of research that sorely need examining.

A syndrome fairly common to speed skaters following the highly anaerobic events (1000, 1500, and 3000 meters) consists of severe postcompetition bronchitis with cough and excess production of sputum. This can last up to 2 days following a race. Some athletes appear to be more prone to developing these symptoms than others. These symptoms seem directly related to decreasing temperature and decreasing humidity and appear to occur only when maximum air flow is involved in the race; they are rarely a problem after races of 5,000 or 10,000 meters, in which aerobic capacities play a larger role. Although wearing a mask provides humidity and heat to inhaled air, this decreases air flow and decreases elimination of carbon dioxide, both of which will be detrimental to performance. Mucolytic agents may be of some value in treating this syndrome.

DIET

Recent research on the diets of speed skaters displayed eating habits that should be improved.[1] Measurements in 1983 indicated that members of the United States Speed Skating Team ate a high-fat and relatively low-carbohydrate diet. Foster and colleagues[1] concluded from their study that increasing the carbohydrate percentage in the diet resulted in better glycogen storage and less chronic glycogen depletion during very heavy training in the late off-ice season, during August and September (see Chapters 2 and 4). Carbohydrate was increased in the diets of athletes both by adding short-chain carbohydrate supplements and by dietary counseling. Caloric consumption in these athletes may exceed 5000 calories per day, and dietary counseling and supplements may help improve performance. This, too, is an area that is fertile for research.

SEASONAL ILLNESSES

Speed skaters, as all winter athletes, are subject to common winter illnesses. These include colds, flu syndrome, mononucleosis, rhinorrhea, and exercise-induced asthma (see Chapters 14, 15, and 19). Therapy for these illnesses is usually symptomatic, except in the case of exercise-induced asthma.

Exercise-induced asthma can be triggered not only by exercise but also by emotional upset and low temperatures. Competitive speed skating accentuates all three of these triggering mechanisms. Treatment can include one or more of the following medications: (1) aminophylline or its derivatives; (2) β_2 adrenergic agonists, including isoetharine, metaproterenol, terbutaline, and albuterol—all of which act by bronchodilation; and (3) steroids, which probably act by decreasing mucosal edema and by preventing bronchoconstrictor release. Cromolyn sodium, which is only of value as preventative treatment, acts by decreasing the release of bronchoconstrictors from mast cells. Aminophylline and the beta stimulators act through inhibition of cAMP breakdown or by stimulation of cAMP release. As such, all have some β_1 activity to varying extent; that is, they are myocardial stimulants. The types and dosages of these drugs, which may be used while competing in International Olympic Committee sanctioned events, are limited (see Chapter 12). Currently, cromolyn, aminophylline, theophylline, beclomethasone, and nasalide (a steroid anti-inflammatory nose spray for rhinitis) are all legal within certain dose ranges (see Chapter 19). However, the drug and dosage list changes from year to year. If athletes involved in national or international competition need these medications, valuable advice can be found at the United States Olympic Committee (USOC) Headquarters, 1750 E. Boulder St., Colorado Springs, CO. A letter should be written to the USOC Head of Sports Medicine, including the following:

1. The names and addresses of the athlete and providing physician;
2. The sport that is involved;
3. The diagnosis of the illness being treated;
4. The medicine of choice for that illness;
5. The dosage and frequency of the medicine being used.

In return, an identification card will be sent by the USOC to the athlete, which will allow him or her to compete at a national level. In addition, a letter from the athlete's doctor should also be included if competition is at an international level. Athletes and their physicians also can obtain information from the USOC drug control hotline (1-800-233-0393).

PSYCHOLOGY AND SPEED SKATING

There are several contributions to high stress levels in the elite speed skater's life. The time invested in the sport is huge. When one considers travel time, time spent with equipment, and time for extra sleeping and showering, these factors can easily mount to an 8 to 10 hour per day time investment into the sport, even though actual training may directly require only 2 to 5 hours per day. The money invested in the sport is also high. Equipment, travel, and living away from home for a significant part of the year, often in Europe, quickly mounts both in terms of monetary costs above a normal budget and in terms of the opportunity costs of time lost from normal employment. Furthermore, in the sport of speed skating, there is little or no financial reward unless the competitor is among the very best in the world. Because of these time and financial investments, speed skaters frequently are forced to limit to a minimum the physical, intellectual, and social activities outside of their sport. Finally, the technical factors of speed skating are such that hard work in the sport is not always a guarantee of success. The number of important speed skating competitions is limited to those that are trials for the World Championships or Olympic Games and the championships themselves. Poor performance for whatever reason in even a single race can negate years of physical, psychologic, financial, social, and time-consuming efforts.

Studies with candidates for the United States Speed Skating Team have shown that large fluctuations in mood state are associated with poorer performance.[2] It appears that those who consistently win have fewer mood swings, tend to channel anxiety to their advantage, and seem to psychologically peak at the time of competition. Properly dealing with the psychologic pressures of speed skating can mean the difference between success and failure. Although controlled studies of speed skaters are not yet available, relaxation therapy, biofeedback, coping strategy and visualization therapy may be of considerable value to these athletes (see Chapter 8). During the past 6 years, three of America's top women speed skaters, each having won medals in either World Championships or the Olympics, have retired from elite skating before their full potential was met. This was primarily because of their unwillingness to cope with the pressure or to commit the time felt necessary to ready themselves for major competition.

Speed skating shares with other winter sports—and in some ways exaggerates—certain problems of financial, educational, and lifestyle sacrifices. A concerted effort to develop programs that require less time by the provision of more facilities than are currently available, and to promote scholarships, meaningful employment, and readily available counseling, should certainly help improve the social, economic, and psychologic well-being of speed skaters.

It seems unfair to limit this discussion to only the negative psychologic impact of speed skating. Obviously there are benefits from planning, working toward and achieving one's goals, winning, and also learning to deal with losses. These benefits help develop the achievement skills needed to cope with the stresses of life beyond speed skating.

Further research and the use of already available methods of psychologic support should be aimed at better protecting the psychologic health of speed skating athletes while preparing them for competition and life as they find it.

TRAVEL AND THE CIRCADIAN RHYTHM

World Cup, World Championship, and Olympic competitions in speed skating occur in all parts of the world. As such, skaters are subjected to flights to countries as far away as Australia, Korea, China, and Japan. Travel across more than six time zones has been associated with deterioration of subsequent athletic performance. It appears that flights going east are more disruptive than those going west. Athletic performance is best between 1200 and 2100 hours and is poorest between 0300 and 0600. Obviously, traveling will result in disruptions of the normal day-to-day rhythm of activity and performance.[4] It is suggested that travel plans allow for at least 6 to 10 days of adjustment of destination, especially if the travel is over more than five or six time zones. Presetting sleeping and waking times while the athlete is still at home does not appear to be of value; however, adjusting activity times may help in improving performance earlier. Furthermore, the athlete should direct his or her activities and sleeping and waking times to appropriate local time on the first day of arrival at the new time zone.

OVERTRAINING

The causes, symptoms, and results of overtraining are not easily understood. The term "overtraining" itself still is ill defined (see Chapter 9). A slew of psychologic, autonomic, physical, dietary, and fluid and electrolyte related theories have come forth on this topic. Suffice it to say here that overtraining indeed does occur in speed skaters. Overtraining is an especially frequent problem in young inexperienced athletes who have suddenly increased their training load. The problem appears to be worst in sports that combine technique with the necessity for long hours of endurance and strength training. Speed skating is a good example of this type of sport. Symptoms of overtraining include a consistent decrease in performance level in competitive events when no other explanation for the poor performance can be found; thus it is a diagnosis of exclusion. True physiologic overtraining is not easily treatable and may take months of recovery time. If, during a period of overtraining, technical changes are made in hope of improved performance and these changes are detrimental to effectiveness, careers can be ruined.

Physicians may see overtrained athletes in their offices. Unfortunately, by the time the problem comes to medical attention, there is no treatment for the truly overtrained athlete except rest. Rest patterns appear to be as important as training patterns in the prevention of this syndrome, and the build-up to world-class training programs should occur over years, not weeks. Very gradual increases in the training load are as important as a "feeling" for when oneself or one's athlete is on the verge of being overtrained.

Overtraining needs more precise definitions, and various causes—physiologic as well as psychologic—need to be found and defined. This is an area of sports science that deserves ongoing research with elite class athletes as well as developing athletes.

CONCLUSIONS

Noteworthy common threads throughout this discussion of the medical aspects of speed skating are the importance of preparation and prevention. In virtually every aspect discussed, knowledge is currently available to help speed skating athletes avoid or at least minimize some of the most significant health problems that can adversely affect their training and performance.

However, there continue to be gaps in our knowledge and understanding of many of these problems, which for the benefit of future skaters may be closed through further research in medicine, technology, and the sports sciences.

REFERENCES

1. Foster, C, Hare, J, Meyer, L: Practical demonstrations of nutritional support in elite athletes. AAHPERD Abstracts 1984.
2. Gutmann, M, Pollock, M, Foster, C, Schmidt, D: Training stress in olympic speedskating: A psychological perspective. The Physician and Sportsmedicine 12:45–57, 1984.
3. Lapp, NL, and Juergens, JL: Frostbite. Mayo Clinic Proceedings 40:932–948, 1965.
4. Winget, C, DeRoshia, C, Holly, D: Circadian rhythm and athletic performance. Medicine and Science in Sports and Exercise 17:498–516, 1985.

CHAPTER 28

Overuse Injuries in Figure Skating

LESTER M. CRAMER, D.M.D., M.D.

CRAIG H. McQUEEN, M.D.

The very nature of competitive figure skating maneuvers (Table 28–1), the unreasonable training schedule and rink conditions (Table 28–2), and the outmoded design of the skate (Table 28–3) mark the elite competitor as easy prey for overuse syndromes. Add to these factors the perceived and probably actual need to be thin, the incredible psychologic stresses being placed on adolescents, and the exercise-induced amenorrhea in female skaters with its potential for attendant osteoporosis (see Chapter 6), and it becomes even more understandable that one or another of the overuse syndromes is a part of nearly every skater's life. Further complicating the problem is the fact that figure skating is not a team sport. Not only is it not a team sport, but there is a very pervasive private, nearly secretive, aspect associated with the endeavor. Many coaches and athletes selfishly guard their techniques and training methods not only from other competitors but also from the national governing boards. Frequently the skater does not have access to sports medicine personnel who have experience in the diagnosis, treatment, and rehabilitation of injuries peculiar to the sport.

There have been very few studies concerning the incidence of figure skating injuries. These studies have involved relatively small groups, but they have shown similar patterns (Table 28–4). Most injuries have been to the back and lower extremity (Table 28–5). These problems are growing as the intrica-

Table 28–1. MANEUVERS PREDISPOSING TO OVERUSE INJURIES

I. The need to be on deep edges, especially inside edges
II. Position requirements:
   A. Hyperlordotic back
   B. Extended knee and pointed toe, free leg
   C. Extended knee, spinning
   D. Flexed knee, spinning
   E. Abducted hip, camel spin
   F. Stroking positions
   G. Hyperflexed ankle, spinning
III. Jumps
   A. Use of picks puts pressures on ankle, foot, toes, knee.
   B. Speed, height, and revolutions make both good landings and poor landings stressful.
IV. Skating programs are maximally aerobic. Anaerobic bursts are frequently superimposed. Fine psychomotor skills must be maintained when skater is maximally fatigued.

cies of more revolution jumps dominate the drive to succeed, and poorly supportive boots with insecurely attached blades are inadequate to combat the rotational and impaction forces that are generated.

The modern care of athletes still must emphasize good history taking and careful physical examinations, augmented with a knowledge of the specific requirements and hazards that characterize the sport (Tables 28–6 and 28–7). Differentiation of the several pain syndromes will frequently require special studies, such as bone scans, computerized tomography (CT) scans, laminograms, and magnetic resonance imaging (MRI), which have helped make precise diagnosis the hallmark of modern sports medicine. Be-

Table 28–2. THE UNREASONABLE TRAINING SCHEDULE AND CONDITIONS

1. Yearly: season not defined, train 11–11½ months
2. Daily: 5–6 hours on ice, 1–3 hours off ice
3. Weekly: 6–7 days
4. Rinks: cold; seldom have space for any off-ice maneuvers
5. No time to warm up and to warm down

cause of the youthful ages of figure skating athletes, the sports physician must be most cautious in the use of x-ray examination, particularly during evaluation of the back and the hip.

Principles of treatment are also changing. Long periods of rest are no longer the basis of treatment programs. Current philosophy embraces short-term immobilization; manipulation and massage; modalities such as ultrasound, transcutaneous electrical neuromuscular stimulation (TENS), electrical stimulation, and deep icing; short-term systemic steroids or other nonsteroidal anti-inflammatory medications; early mobilization; and vigorous rehabilitation of the cardiovascular, neuromuscular, and psychologic systems.

THE BACK

The back is one of the more commonly injured regions in figure skaters. However, the diagnostic complexities of back pain are so extensive that they cannot be fully covered here. Suffice it to say that the back is very heavily stressed by impactional and torsional forces that subject it to at least multiple microtraumas, if not macrotraumas, during each skating day. These traumas are cumulative throughout life. X-ray examination in these young people must be carefully selected and performed, and sophisticated interpretation is often necessary. The differential diagnosis and treatment of the back pain can be so difficult that early referral to a competent orthopedist or chiropractor should always be considered. The proper resolution of back problems can be critical to the skater's career.

Dr. Lyle Micheli[9] has felt that tight lumbar dorsal fascia and low back inflexibility are common problems in skaters, and that these problems combined with tight hamstrings can lead to chronic low back pain. Preventive off-ice flexibility programs combined with abdominal and back resistive exercises are helpful in eliminating most low back complaints. However, if back pain persists in spite of conservative management, a bone scan may be necessary. Bone scans can be helpful in determining whether there is a stress fracture of the pars interarticularis, which occurs in skaters.

Table 28–3. PROBLEMS CAUSED BY
THE SKATE*

1. Too heavy
2. Too rigid
3. Poor malleolar support and configuration
4. Leather tongues bind, crack, and irritate
5. Tight lacing, irregularly spaced
6. Sole irregular and becomes rigid with blade attached
7. Arch support poor
8. Toe support insufficient or inaccurate
9. Heel countersupport inaccurate
10. Superior heel folds over
11. Shock absorption weak or absent
12. Boot-blade assemblage unreliable
13. Laminated heels separate or crack
14. Blade radii generic

*Many of these can be prevented by wearing of custom boots.

THE GROIN

The painful groin, or so-called groin strain, is common in figure skaters because of the following predisposing causes: (1) imbalance between the low extremity adductors and the gluteus medius, (2) forcible stroking push-off adducting the thigh, (3) forcible external rotation of the abducted leg (e.g., slipping off a landing edge), and (4) forcible abduction of the thigh (e.g., the straddling injury from doing splits, either in the air or on the ice).

The differential diagnosis will be between tendinitis of the iliopsoas, rectus femoris, or gracilis and partial avulsion of the adductor origin from the pelvis. The torn adductor origin will have tenderness on the subcutaneous edge of the pubic ramus, and pain will be increased by passive abduction of the thigh or forced active abduction. Groin pain from iliopsoas tendinitis is also increased by

Table 28–4. ANATOMIC INCIDENCE
OF OVERUSE SYNDROMES

1. Back	16%
2. Hip, groin, thigh	5%
3. Knee	18%
4. Leg	15%
5. Ankle	30%
6. Foot	16%

Adapted from Garrick.[5]

abduction, but in addition, it will be increased by both extension and external rotation, and also the lesser trochanter will be tender. The role of the gluteus medius is important because it becomes so overdeveloped in figure skaters from camel spins that it may overwhelm an unbalanced adductor system. In addition, the gluteus medius itself may become inflamed. Chronic tendinitis of the gluteus medius at its attachment to the trochanter will cause increasing pain with active abduction of the hip but not with passive range of motion examination.

The treatment of groin strain is ice, rest, massage, nonsteroidal anti-inflammatory drugs, and hip spica wrapping with the thigh flexed and externally rotated. Crutches, cane, and avoidance of stair climbing are advised. Later treatment consists of heat, ultrasound, diathermy, isometrics, and therapeutic stretching.

Prevention of groin strain is very important, and we now know from studying skaters that proper flexibility and strengthening are necessary requirements to help prevent groin strain. Skaters should be on a regular exercise program using eccentric and concentric contractures of the adductor muscles and also the abductor muscles of the hip. They should also be on a regular stretching regimen. This will really help prevent most of the groin strains. Also, it will enhance the stroking ability of skaters who have to do a lot of stroking.

THE KNEE

The painful swollen knee is the single most significant problem occurring in skaters. The most common cause of sore knees is chronic patellar tendinitis (CPT), the "jumper's knee" syndrome that is seen in many sports. Differentiation from the spectrum of acute and chronic knee injuries is mandatory and may be complex. Orthopedic examination, frequently supplemented by x-ray examination, aspiration, and arthroscopy, should be done promptly because many knee injuries may require early surgery. It is critical not to miss the diagnosis of a torn meniscus or anterior cruciate ligament, osteochondral fracture, or disruption of the medial or lateral collateral ligament. When these conditions are ruled out and the location of the pain and swelling are extra-articular, the

Table 28–5. CLASSIFICATION OF TYPES OF FIGURE SKATING INJURIES

1. Fracture and dislocation	11.6%
2. Sprain	8.3%
3. Contusion	11.1%
4. Strain	15.7%
5. Inflammation	19.8%
6. Overuse	19.4%
7. Degeneration	1.2%
8. Impingement	2.1%

Numbers 4–8 are overuse syndromes totaling 58.2% of problems seen.

Adapted from Garrick.[5]

specific tendinitis or bursitis diagnosis should be made and the correct treatment and rehabilitation instituted. Prevention should be part of the regimen for all skaters, but it is especially important in those with predisposing factors that may lead to knee problems. These factors are a wide pelvis, found frequently in female skaters and occasionally in males, an increased Q angle ("knock" knees or valgus), a high-riding patella (patella alta), tight Achilles tendons, pronated feet with lowered arches, tight hamstring muscles, and weak quadriceps, perihip, or gastrosoleus muscle complexes. Recent testing of elite skaters has shown a direct correlation between quadriceps inflexibility and symptoms of jumper's knee and Osgood-Schlatter's disease. When skaters are placed on a proper flexibility program that they do on a regular basis they can increase their flexibility and help overcome these overload symptoms at the knee. Hamstring and quadriceps strengthening are also important.

The specific stresses placed on the knee must be understood intelligently to approach the diagnosis and treatment of knee problems. These stresses are more than can be enumerated succinctly, but as one analyzes some of the common stresses of figure skating on the knee, one wonders how the knee survives as well as it does.

1. Jump take-off: The weight-bearing flexed knee suddenly must be snapped into full extension. In toe-assisted jumps, the non-weight-bearing flexed knee receives a shock from its toe and then goes into full extension.

2. Jump landing: As the full weight re-

Table 28–6. COMMON OVERUSE SYNDROMES IN ELITE FIGURE SKATERS

Site	Most Common Problems	Principal Differential Diagnoses
Back	Tight lumbodorsal fascia	Spondylolysis Rotational strains S-I joint subluxations
Groin	Adductor tears	Iliopsoas tendinitis
Knee	Chronic patellar tendinitis	Chondromalacia patellae Patellar subluxation Osgood-Schlatter's disease Patellofemoral stress syndrome
Leg	Shin-splints	Anterior compartment syndrome Posterior tibial tendinitis Tibial stress fracture
Anterior and lateral ankle	Ankle impingement Bursitis Tendinitis	Anterior tarsal tunnel syndrome Peroneal subluxation Ligament sprains or tears
Postankle and hindfoot	Achilles tendinitis Plantar fascitis	Posterior tunnel syndromes Calcaneal pathologies Retrocalcaneal bursitis
Midfoot	Tarsotarsal subluxations Tarsometatarsal subluxations	
Forefoot	Soft tissue irritations Reverse turf toe Metatarsal stress fracture	

Table 28–7. ANATOMIC PROBLEMS CONTRIBUTING TO FIGURE SKATERS' OVERUSE SYNDROMES

I. General anatomic problems
  A. Scoliosis
  B. Increased Q angle
  C. Poor track of quadriceps mechanism
  D. Pronated feet
  E. Cavus feet
  F. Tibia varus
  G. Tibia valgus
  H. Talus varus
  I. Talus valgus
II. Specific defects seen in the figure skating athlete
  A. Tight lumbodorsal fascia
  B. Weak hamstring muscles
  C. Tight quadriceps muscles
  D. Short Achilles tendons
  E. Weak upper body musculature
  F. Overdeveloped gluteus medius

turns suddenly from airborne to the ground, full axial loading is superimposed on the derotational forces being applied to a flexed knee.

3. Spinning:

a. Upright "scratch" spin: The knees are forcibly locked in full extension.

b. Camel spin: Full weight is borne by one knee locked in extension with the hip in full extension and external rotation.

c. Sit spin: Full weight is borne by one knee in a semiflexed position with the hip semiflexed and externally rotated.

4. Stroking: The flexed knees are each on a different skate edge, and the thighs are forcibly rotated against the hip in one direction with the knee in the opposite direction while each extremity rotates opposite to the other.

5. In figures: The positions leading to stress are numerous. One example is the use of a strong inside skate edge to execute a loop with the knee flexed. One knee bears the full weight, pressing firmly against the tibia in internal rotation, with the hip markedly externally rotated.

Jumper's Knee

Severe chronic patellar tendinitis (CPT) or "jumper's knee" is a common problem that should be largely preventable. Presently, about 15 percent of figure skaters are afflicted with CPT. Predisposing anatomic and biomechanic factors that contribute to CPT have already been mentioned above. The pain and swelling of CPT are located at the distal patellar tip 85 percent of the time. About 15 percent have a variant CPT (chronic quadriceps tendinitis) and will exhibit these symptoms just above the patella. The patient with CPT will complain of pain with exercise, which subsides with rest. A feeling of weakness or "giving way" is often described. This is aggravated by using the stairs, especially by going downstairs.

Clinical examination of CPT should include the entire lower back and both lower extremities, including the feet, to determine the strengths, flexibilities, and lengths of the hip and gluteal musculature as well as the hamstrings, quadriceps, and gastrosoleus muscles. Frequently, it is found that the hip and gluteal muscles are weak, the hamstrings are tight, and the quadriceps are both weak and tight. The Achilles tendon is short, the foot is pronated, the tibia is internally rotated, the patella tracks laterally, and the Q angle is increased. Range of motion will be normal except that it is limited by pain at the end of the extension. With the hip extended, there will be limited knee flexion because of the contracted extensor mechanism. Palpating the exact location of pain and tenderness is facilitated by extending the knee and gently manipulating the patella distally to locate the tenderness under the inferior (sometimes the superior) pole of the patella. With CPT there is no joint effusion and no joint line tenderness. The tip sign is positive. This is tenderness of the inferior pole of the patella elicited by "tipping" the apex of the patella anteriorly by the application of pressure on the superior aspect; then the area just beneath the patella can be more readily palpated. Assessment of the patellar alignment frequently will show that it is high riding (patella alta) and that it is tracking laterally. This is frequently either because the vastus medialis obliquus is weak or because a pronated foot with flattened arch has turned the tibia inward against the fixed femur. Therefore the patella is pulled upward and laterally by the quadriceps muscles, as they try to stabilize the knee.

The differential diagnosis of CPT includes the following:

1. Poor patellar tracking
   a. Subluxation
   b. Dislocation
   c. Chondromalacia patellae
2. Patellofemoral stress syndrome
3. Osgood-Schlatter's disease
4. Bursitis

A four-phase classification[1] is helpful in determining treatment:

Phase 1: Pain only after workout.
Phase 2: Pain during workout, can participate.
Phase 3: Pain during and after workout, interferes with participation.
Phase 4: Tendon disruption.

The treatment of phases 1 and 2 consists of three parts:

1. Proper warm-up and warm-down
2. Therapy modalities
3. Rehabilitative techniques

Most skaters warm up insufficiently because of the constraints of their schedules. Free-style skating sessions are short and immediately follow the figure sessions. It would be desirable to schedule a 5- to 10-minute warm-up period between figures and free styles and to allow 5 or 10 minutes after the free-style session for warm-down, using the time efficiently, particularly for slow stretching of the hips, thighs, gastrosoleus complexes, and Achilles tendons. The best therapeutic modalities for CPT are immediate icing, intermittent hot packs followed by ice packs or iced galvanic whirlpool. Isometric muscle strengthening is employed, and then after a few weeks—when the pain has decreased—this is supplemented by a resistive program of strengthening designed for use at home. A carefully designed stretching program for hip flexors, adductors, and abductors is begun early and supplemented by stretching of both the Achilles tendons and the hamstrings. As the pain subsides, stretching of the quadriceps and gastrosoleus complex is added. During the work-up, a simple but specific patellar-restraining brace should be fashioned. This consists of a felt pad or strap across the superior pole of the patella to help prevent it from riding up and laterally.

If these methods fail and phase 3 is entered so that the patient cannot skate because of pain, complete rest is indicated for many weeks. If this is unsuccessful, then a special operation for jumper's knee can be undertaken. This is done by preparing the patient for a general anesthetic, but using local anesthetic on the skin over the distal patellar pole before the patient is put to sleep. Then, while the patient is still awake, an incision is made, and the maximal area of tenderness of the distal patellar tip is found, using palpation and also a small needle. This is because the tear of the tendon in jumper's knee is on the undersurface of the patellar tendon. If the tendon is repaired and the granulation tissue from the tear is removed, the symptoms of jumper's knee will abate. It must be emphasized that this is a last-ditch effort, and that all efforts should be made to manage this conservatively with proper flexibility and strengthening exercises.

In addition to tracking problems and chondromalacia, the three most common problems in the differential diagnosis of CPT are bursitis, Osgood-Schlatter's disease, and the patellofemoral joint stress syndromes. The various bursae around the knee may be inflamed. Their specific location away from the patellar tendon aids in the diagnosis. Acute prepatellar bursitis, resulting from direct trauma to the knee, presents with well-localized subcutaneous swelling, so that the diagnosis is apparent. Treatment is ice packs, compression, aseptic aspiration if extensive, and early return to on-ice training with a knee support. The deep retropatellar bursa has not been studied adequately in figure skaters. It probably becomes inflamed in some skaters and should be considered in the differential diagnosis of knee pain, particularly if there has been a previous history of Osgood-Schlatter's disease. Swellings of the lateral bursae are rare.

Patellofemoral joint stress syndrome is the most common internal derangement in figure skating. The repeated stresses in deceleration maneuvers cause injuries to this joint. The clinician treating jumper's knee must always remain alert to the possibility of patellofemoral joint stress syndrome with subluxation. If there is actual instability with "giving way," full orthopedic work-up is indicated. Patellofemoral joint stress syndrome with or without associated osteochondral fracture and torn medial or lateral meniscus or the ACL must be considered. Patellofemoral tracking problems are directly related to weakness of the vastus medialis obliquus (VMO) structure. As one of the first stages of treatment for chondromalacia of the patella and/or lateral patellar compression syndrome, exercises should be undertaken to strengthen the vastus medialis obliquus. This is most safely done with straight leg raising exercises with resistance at the ankle. Also, short arc quad exercises can be done with the goal in mind of strengthening the VMO muscle. If patients with patellofemoral tracking problems and lateral patellar compression syndrome are allowed to exercise with a full bent knee at 90°, particularly against resistance, they will often worsen their patellofemoral symptoms. Dr. Ben Kibler[7] of Lexington did a large study on jumping of athletes in which they strengthened selectively the hamstring musculature. This seemed also to be very helpful in the prevention of anterior knee pain and overload syndromes at the knee. Thus rehabilitation of the hamstring muscles is also very important.

THE LEG

The knee, ankle, and foot cause frequent clinical problems in figure skaters, whereas the leg has not been involved as much as one would expect. In the running sports, excessive pronation and poor absorption of the impact shock lead to posteromedial leg and ankle pain. In skating, with its great impacts in descent from the height of jumps and frequent rotational movements, it would seem that shin-splints and other leg problems would be common, but, indeed, now they are uncommon. However, for the skaters of the 1970s, shin-splints were a major problem.

Pathologic leg conditions that may afflict figure skaters are

1. Shin-splints, medial tibial syndrome (MTS)
2. Stress fractures, primarily tibial, occasionally fibular
3. Compartment syndromes
4. Posterior tibial tendinitis

Shin-Splints

Posteromedial shin pain can be a continuum of pathology running the gamut from medial tibial syndrome (MTS) "shin-splints" to stress fractures. In MTS the pain and tenderness are along the distal medial tibia, involving the posteromedial compartment and the long flexors to the foot, and extending down to the medial ankle. The patient will usually have both short Achilles tendons and pronated feet with heel eversion, tibia vara, subtalar varus, and forefoot supination. Well-localized tenderness will cover a 9- to 16-cm^2 area approximately 6 to 8 cm above the medial malleolus at the origin of the posterior tibialis tendon. Myositis and low-grade periostitis are present. The patient will be able to "exercise through" the pain, which is an important differentiation point, because a patient with a chronic compartment syndrome may have no pain at rest but develop increasing pain with exercise, and the patient with a stress fracture or posterior tibial tendinitis will have resting pain that is increased by exercise. If periostitis is a significant part of the MTS, it can progress and the symptoms will worsen.

Compartment Syndromes

Before settling on a clinical and radiologic diagnosis of shin-splints, it is important to be certain that no more severe pathology is present. To this end, a chronic anterior compartment syndrome may be ruled out by the history, but it may be necessary to perform a stress wick test, measuring intracompartmental pressure by means of an indwelling catheter with the knee at work.[8] Radioisotope bone scans, CT scans, or MRI scans are frequently necessary; they can be diagnostic when the conventional x-ray examinations have been normal. Physical examination is the best way to rule out posterior tibial tendinitis. Palpating the tendon down to its insertion on the talus, one will frequently encounter exquisite pain and tenderness over a prominent or accessory navicular bone. Because rest is part of the treatment for posterior tibial tendinitis and exercise is allowed in the treatment for shin-splints, the differentiation is important; rupture of the posterior tibial tendon is a distinct possibility that must be avoided.

In differentiating MTS from anterior compartment syndrome, it should be noted that the latter includes the following findings: (1) tenderness over the anterior compartment, (2) decreased sensation between the first and second toes, (3) increased pain on foot dorsiflexion, and (4) increased pressure demonstrated by a stress wick test.[8] However, an exercise-induced anterior compartment syndrome may cause pain only, and pressures would be elevated only after exercise.

The treatment for MTS involves the use of

1. Icing before and after exercising
2. Nonsteroidal anti-inflammatory drugs
3. Preexercise stretching
4. Proper warm-up
5. Special exercises to strengthen posterior tibial muscle
6. Modalities to relieve pain
   a. Massage
   b. Ice, whirlpool
   c. Ultrasound
   d. Spray and stretch
7. Special support
   a. Correct taping to support the arch
   b. Orthoses placed in both shoes and skates—these should prevent pronation, supply padding, support the arch, cushion shock, and prevent overuse of the posterior tibial tendon
8. Leg warmers

Stretching before workout should concentrate on the Achilles tendon and the posterior tibial tendon, and should be done for 30 seconds, with two repetitions for each leg. They are best accomplished by either wall pushes with the knees locked, wall pushes with the knees bent, or stair stretches.

Special stretching exercises include (1) sitting on the floor with the legs in front and maximally dorsiflexing to stretch the Achilles tendon, (2) doing the same maneuver with maximal plantar flexion, (3) rotating both medially and laterally with the foot plantar flexed, and (4) stretching and strengthening all extensors.

Stress Fractures

If a stress fracture has occurred, the area should be protected with a functional splint for 3 to 4 weeks. Activity should be decreased, flotation hydrotherapy will be helpful, and stretching should be instituted after the first week of functional splinting.

Posterior Tibial Tendinitis

Posterior tibial tendinitis is not a common diagnosis, but when made, it has grave importance because of the possibility of tendon rupture. Rest is mandatory. This should be augmented with icing and nonsteroidal anti-inflammatory drugs. Orthoses with a medial heel wedge for support are used. Whirlpool and ultrasound may be helpful. A non-weight-bearing, short leg cast with the foot in inversion is placed for an additional 2 weeks. After cast removal, specific strength and flexibility programs are instituted.

THE ANTERIOR AND LATERAL ANKLE

The most common overuse syndromes of the anterior and lateral ankle in figure skaters are

1. Impingements
2. Bursitis
3. Tendinitis
4. Sprains and tears of ligaments
5. Neuropathy; tarsal tunnel syndromes
6. Peroneal tendon subluxation

Dislocations, Fractures, and Impingements

All significant anterior and lateral ankle injuries should be x-rayed to exclude fracture or dislocation. If stable ankle injuries are found, they should be treated promptly to control edema. Minimal but protective support should be provided. Physical therapy should begin with early manipulation and proprioceptive rehabilitation maneuvers. When ankle injuries are unstable or if there is denervation of the posterior tibial nerve or peroneal nerve, casting or surgery may be necessary as determined by clinical, radiographic, and arthroscopic examinations.

Bursitis and Tendinitis

Pain and swelling of the anterior, medial, or lateral ankle often reflect either bursitis or tendinitis of the flexor hallucis longus, anterior tibialis, posterior tibialis, extensor hallucis longus, or extensor digitorum longus muscle tendons. These are caused or enhanced by the constant irritation of anterior leg bending with stroking and landing against the unyielding and frequently poorly padded skate tongue with tightly laced skate boots. Although these injuries are not necessarily serious medical problems, they can be extremely painful and bothersome to skating athletes and do impede their performances. Bursitis and tendinitis must be differentiated from more serious pathology, namely, the anterior impingement syndrome and the anterior tarsal tunnel syndrome.

The pain and swelling that reflect the irritational tenosynovitis of the anterior or posterior tibialis tendons medially and the extensor hallucis longus or extensor digitorum longus tendons anteriorly must be differentiated from inflammation of the bursae that overlie the medial and lateral malleoli. Pain and swelling anterolaterally may reflect either peroneal tenosynovitis or subluxation. Posterior tibialis tenosynovitis is not common but is very important to rule out because it can lead to tendon rupture. To reiterate, the posterior tibialis tendon runs behind the medial malleolus, where pain and tenderness with tenosynovitis are increased with resisted supination and passive pronation. However, anterior tibialis tenosynovitis pain and tenderness are usually localized to the tendon at the extensor retinaculum in front of the medial malleolus and stops at the navicular-metatarsal-cuneiform insertion. Tenosynovitis of the anterior tibialis is more readily responsive to treatment with rest, ice, ultrasound, and nonsteroidal anti-inflammatory drugs than posterior tibialis tenosynovitis.

Flexor hallucis longus tenosynovitis is not common among figure skaters but must be considered when there is swelling and pain behind the medial malleolus in the "picking" foot. The fibro-osseous tunnel of the flexor hallicus longus going posterior and lateral to the malleolus may become stenotic, thereby limiting great toe passive extension or even flexion of the great toe at the metatarsalphalangeal joint. Direct anterior ankle swelling and tenderness occur in figure skaters with great frequency, because of either bursitis or tenosynovitis of the extensor hallucis longus or extensor digitorum longus. These conditions must be differentiated from, although they may be accompanied by, an anterior impingement syndrome (AIS). The pain from tenosynovitis and bursitis is more superficial than that from AIS and can be outlined in the anatomy of the tendon or the bursa. The pain of AIS will be more diffuse, because it is related to the thickened synovium, and it is directly associated with both active and passive ankle motions. The trauma is usually on the landing foot because of tibiotalar compression resulting from acute flexion during landing. X-ray views may show talar or tibial spurs. Occasionally, a CT scan or an MRI may be indicated, and ankle arthroscopy must be done to confirm the diagnosis.

Sprains and Tears

Sprains and tears of the ankle ligaments are not common injuries in competitive figure skaters. When they do occur in these athletes, they are usually the result of off-ice activity.

Anterior Tarsal Tunnel Syndrome

Anterior tarsal tunnel syndrome (ATTS) is caused by compression of the deep peroneal nerve by the extensor retinaculum at the talonavicular joint on the dorsum of the foot. The extensor retinaculum tightens during plantar flexion and during dorsiflexion of the toes. Nerve involvement causes aching and tightness where the anterior ankle meets the dorsum of the foot. There will be hypesthesia in the first web space in the distribution of the deep peroneal nerve and a Tinel's sign over the nerve just lateral to the dorsalis pedis pulse. As the disease progresses, there may be atrophy of the extensor digitorum brevis. Although this is an unusual syndrome, it is necessary to be aware of it in the differential diagnosis of anterior ankle pain. Tight shoes or boots or a midtarsal osteophyte may be a contributing cause. Conservative therapy of rest and boot loosening may suffice. If these measures fail, this is one of the few situations in managing skating athletes in which we advocate steroid injections. However, in the long run, surgery may be the only effective treatment.

Peroneal Tendon Subluxation

Lateral ankle pain and swellings are not common in figure skaters. The three entities that occur that can cause these symptoms are fibular stress fracture, peroneal tenosynovitis, and peroneal tendon subluxation.

Chronic peroneal tendon subluxation (PTS) occurs in the "picking" foot when it is inverted. The subluxation can be demonstrated by asking the patient to evert and to dorsiflex the foot. The retinaculum may be torn, or there may be an avulsion fracture of the lateral ridge of the distal fibula. The tenderness and swelling are posterior to the fibula and superior to the ankle.

Treatment of PTS is controversial, but certainly a trial of conservative management is indicated. Compression taping over a felt pad reinforced with a splint may suffice, or a well-molded cast that places gentle pressure on the peroneal tendons may be needed. If conservative management is unsuccessful, surgical reconstruction must be considered.

Stress fractures of the fibula usually involve the distal third of the bone about 5 to 6 cm above the lateral malleolus. Lateral ankle pain is a common first symptom. Differentiation must be made mainly from peroneal tendinitis, which is rather uncommon. With fibular stress fracture there will be pain and swelling along the peroneal tendons, and the pain is increased by eversion of the foot. X-ray examinations, bone scans, and CT scans or MRI are necessary for the differential diagnosis. The treatment is rest, heel cord and ankle stretching, and muscle-strengthening exercises. If there is pain on full weight bearing, cast immobilization and crutches may be needed for approximately 4 weeks.

THE POSTERIOR ANKLE AND HEEL

The most common posterior ankle and heel problems in figure skaters are

1. Achilles tendinitis and paratendinitis
2. Plantar fascitis

These problems must be differentiated from a variety of unusual entities:

1. Calcaneal stress fracture
2. Tarsal tunnel syndrome
3. Posterior ankle impingement
4. Calcaneal spurs
5. Calcaneal apophysitis
6. Calcaneal periostitis

There are a number of other causes of painful heels. Among them are bruises and hematomas, superficial irritations leading to fissured heels, mosaic verrucae, blisters, macerations, and calluses. Bursitis of the Achilles tendon leading to pump bump is unusual in skaters.

Achilles Tendinitis

Achilles tendinitis (AT) is common in skaters because of the plantar flexed position mandated by the skate, the manner of push-off or stroking, and the amount of energy absorption that is accepted by the hindfoot when both stroking and landing. Irritational pressures from the boot then compound the problem.

The pathology is either microtears in the tendon itself, which are more common at the distal insertion on the calcaneal tuberosity, or inflammation of the paratenon, which usually occurs more proximally at the musculoskeletal junction. These injuries may occur singly, but they usually occur together and are clinically indistinguishable. About 70 percent of patients with AT have pronated feet, and 90 percent have a valgus heel, accompanied by forefoot varus and tibia vara. The pain of AT is usually at the insertion of the tendon just distal to the calcaneal tuberosity. The pain then continues proximally for several centimeters. Pain is increased by motion with examination or when a physical activity begins but may decrease as the activity continues. Examination will usually show foot pronation, valgus heel position, and decreased active and passive dorsiflexion. Similar pain and tenderness can be seen with bursitis. However, with bursitis, swelling can be demonstrated either in front of the Achilles tendon or behind the calcaneus by applying pressure medially and laterally anterior to the tendon just above its insertion. This is an important differentiation because steroid injections into the bursa may clear symptoms quickly, whereas steroid injections of Achilles tendinitis are definitely contraindicated.

The treatment program for AT is aimed at relieving pain and inflammation, strengthening weak muscles, stretching tight structures, and correcting biomechanical problems. Ice, ultrasound, iontophoresis, and later heat and diathermy are helpful. A 3- to 6-week course of nonsteroidal anti-inflammatory drugs also can help alleviate symptoms. The clinical examination will reveal which muscle groups need stretching. Frequently it is any or all of the following: the musculature and fascia of the back, the hip adductors, the iliotibial band, the hamstrings, the quadriceps, the gastrocnemius, the soleus, the Achilles tendon, and the plantar fascia. Particularly, the gastrosoleus complex, the Achilles tendon, and the plantar fascia should be viewed as a single linkage system. The gastrosoleus complex restrains the forward motion of the tibia to stabilize the leg and to mediate the rate of extension and flexion of the ankle and knee, making it an important mechanism for shock absorption. It is critical that calf stretching be emphasized. It should be noted that the gastrosoleus complex stretches more effectively if the tibialis anterior muscle has been isometrically exercised prior to calf stretching. Calf stretching should be done for 30 seconds, four repetitions, four times a day. Calf stretching is best accomplished by standing at arm's length from a wall with the feet together and flat on the floor. The knees should be extended. Then with the elbows bent, the patient leans forward to place the forearms against the wall with the back and lower extremities straight. Every few days the patient should move a little farther away from the wall. These exercises should then be repeated with the knees flexed. Calf and ankle stretches are especially important to do before and after each workout and before and after warm-up sessions because the position in the boot causes plantar flexion, which must be overcome.

Strength training by use of isometrics with surgical tubing, free weights, or resistive machines is important. Determinations should be made regarding which muscles are weak, and specific exercises should then be designed to strengthen them. Usually, the gastrosoleus complex, the vastus medialis obliquus, and the hamstrings need the most concerted effort. Orthotics can be extremely helpful (see Chapter 7). Medial support and heel posting can prevent pronation on push-off and control the valgus heel position. A heel lift in both shoe and boot also can help decrease pain. For some skaters with AT, a 2-week period in a non-weight-bearing cast may be necessary to relieve pain. If casting is done, electrical stimulation of the lower extremity musculature should be used to limit muscle atrophy. Some skaters will require surgical intervention, but this should not be undertaken until at least 6 months or more of conservative treatment. Rupture of the Achilles tendon is always a threat that can be a career-ending event.

Tendo Achillis Bursitis

Tendo achillis bursitis, or "pump bump," is seen in the bursa between the skin and the Achilles tendon. It becomes inflamed in persons with a prominent superior calcaneal tuberosity who use footwear with closely fitting heel counters. A characteristic swelling occurs on the posterolateral aspect of the heel directly beneath the position of the boot heel counter. The bony prominence can be palpated there, and superficial swellings are found between the Achilles tendon and the skin. Treatment consists initially of ice and exercise, and later heat and a brief period of rest. To diminish pressure against the pump bump, a heel counter with a cutout in the cup is used.

Posterior ankle impingement of the tibia on the talus and calcaneus is important to differentiate from pump bump. With posterior ankle impingement, diffuse pain and synovial thickening can mimic Achilles tendinitis. It is present in the "picking" foot and common when the skater is overworking to perfect a new toe jump or to gain reliability on an already mastered jump, particularly the triple lutz. Manipulative maneuvers are important in the management of posterior ankle impingement as well as the symptomatic use of ice, ultrasound, iontophoresis and galvanic whirlpool. Arthroscopy may be needed for diagnosis if the symptoms do not subside.

Plantar Fascitis

The pain of plantar fascitis (PF) develops insidiously and is most marked at the medial tubercle of the calcaneus. It may radiate along the longitudinal arch and also into the fascial insertion on the plantar aspect of the calcaneus. Examination may reveal painful nodularity along the medial border of the fascia. The pain of PF worsens upon arising from bed in the morning and decreases during the day. At the beginning of skating, pain from PF decreases, but it increases and may become intolerable by the end of the workout. Tenderness is found at the medial calcaneal tubercle and may extend proximally along the course of the medial calcaneal nerve, longitudinally along the arch, and on the plantar aspect of the interior calcaneus, where a spur may be palpated and can be seen on x-ray examination. Passive dorsiflexion of the foot or great toe will increase pain. The foot may be either pronated or cavus, but the Achilles tendon is always short, and the calcaneus is in a flexed position.

Differentiation of PF must be made particularly from the posterior tarsal tunnel syndrome, which is caused by entrapment of the medial or lateral plantar nerves. In the posterior tarsal tunnel syndrome, the pain is usually burning in character and there is no tenderness over the plantar fascia, but a positive Tinel's sign is found behind and below the medial malleolus. Intrinsic muscle weakness is a late sign. X-ray examinations may be used to rule out calcaneal stress fractures in many cases, but some may need bone scan, CT scan, or MRI. Apophysitis and spurs can likewise be ruled out with these scanning studies. An S-1 radiculopathy could also cause this pain pattern, but no local tenderness on stretch is found with radiculopathy, and other characteristic signs will be found during the neurologic examination.

Most cases of PF will subside with conservative care. All cases need rest, ice massage alternating with heat, nonsteroidal anti-inflammatory drugs, and orthotics. Stretching is primarily for the cavus foot; the pronated foot must not be stretched unless the Achilles tendon is extremely short. The cavus foot can be rested by an adhesive strapping and an arch support. It will also benefit from stretching of the gastrosoleus complex and Achilles tendon and from plantar fascia stretching with a rolling pin. The molded arch support should have a cutout to relieve pressure. Separate supports should be made for the skate boot and for street shoes. Because the pronated foot has already overstretched the plantar fascia during weight bearing, there is an insufficiency of the bony and ligamentous tissues. Therefore, stretching should be confined to the short Achilles tendon and the gastrosoleus complex. The plantar fascia should *not* be stretched; it must be strengthened by isometric dorsiflexion and posterior tibial action, and it should be supported with medial longitudinal arch supports and taping. Occasionally, a cast is the only way to relieve the pain of PF. A heel pad of Sorbuthane helps some patients, but a plastic heel cup (TULI) is usually more effective because it seems to gather the fatty tissues of the heel together to provide better cushioning. Steroid injections remain controversial. We consider steroid injections for PF to be potentially dangerous because they may lead to rupture of the fascia.

Patients who do not respond to these conservative regimens for PF may need surgery to release the fascial origin, resect the degenerative areas, decompress and reroute the medial calcaneal nerve, and remove any bone spur impinging on the nerve to the abductor digiti quinti muscle.

If a diagnosis of tarsal tunnel syndrome has been made, treatment consists of ice, nonsteroidal anti-inflammatory drugs, and accurate steroid injections directly into the tunnel. An orthotic to control pronation and to correct heel valgus is also helpful (see Chapter 7). If the signs persist, surgical decompression is a successful maneuver and does not keep the patient too immobile after the first 2 weeks following surgery.

Skin calluses, fissures, verrucae, blisters, and maceration from the heel pad are usually quite obvious and can be accurately diagnosed by inspection. Good hygiene is necessary for the skate boot, the shoe, and the foot. Calluses can be kept thin by soaking and filing. A customized cutout orthosis may be able to correct the callus by distributing the forces correctly. Fissures can be treated by collagen injection. Verrucae may best be handled by laser ablation. Blisters can be prevented by the use of petrolatum in areas known to be susceptible; if they occur, they should be aspirated aseptically with a tiny needle, leaving the skin intact for protection. All of these conditions can benefit from a heel cup or better fitting boots.

THE MIDFOOT

The midfoot is an extremely important complex to the skater, but it is also a poorly understood, often a painful, region. The pain may occur across the entire midfoot or may be isolated to the lateral or the medial tarso-metartarsal joints. Patients may report an acute "popping" followed by pain, or they may have chronic "popping" and subluxing of the joints and tendons. The foot position in the boot, plantar flexion with the toes gripping the sole in extreme plantar flexion, is mainly compensated during skating by the forward position of the tibia on the talus with the knee flexed. However, when the skate is removed and the upright position for walking is assumed, the bones respond by assuming stressed positions, especially in a person with alignment predisposition. Some people feel that there are some displacements, such as talus anterior cuneiform, superior navicular, superior cuboid lateral, cuboid medial, and calcaneus medial. However, it has not been documented—at least not orthopedically—that manipulation of these is of any benefit. Therefore, supporting the foot in the proper boot seems to be the most important and helpful prevention of midfoot problems in skaters.

THE FOREFOOT

Irritated lesions of the skin are more common around the toes and the plantar surfaces of the distal metatarsals. Calluses, athlete's foot, hard and soft corns, blisters, and ingrown toenails are prone to occur because of the toe box and sole conformations of the skate boot. These are nagging problems that can become secondarily infected. They are best dealt with by cleanliness, protectors, fungicides, orthoses, collagen injections, and laser or conventional surgery as specifically indicated.

Reverse Turf Toe

The act of "picking" during toe jumps requires hyper-plantar-flexion of the foot and toes. The proximal phalanx of the great toe absorbs the greatest amount of this force, which is transmitted to the first metatarsal joint. This joint is therefore susceptible to acute or subacute sesamoiditis and traumatic arthritis. Occasionally, there will be small avulsion fractures on the dorsum of the proximal portion of the most proximal phalanx. Appropriate x-ray examinations must be taken for diagnosis. Treatment will be avoidance of the offending maneuver, gentle manipulation, compression dressing, elevation, ice, ultrasound, whirlpool, taping, padding, and nonsteroidal anti-inflammatory drugs.

Metatarsal Neuroma

Metatarsal neuroma must always be considered in the differential diagnosis of forefoot pain. Although metatarsal neuromas are uncommon in most young people, they may occur in the elite skater because of the stresses placed on this area by constant plantar flexion gripping action of the toes in the boot. When decreased sensation in the distribution of a digital nerve to the toes is associated with distally radiating knifelike or electricity-like metatarsal pain, which can be elicited by squeezing the appropriate interspace, a diagnosis of metatarsal neuroma must be entertained. Most commonly these neuromas occur on the most lateral branch of the medial plantar nerve between the third and fourth metatarsal bones. Steroid injections may alleviate the signs and allow the skater to complete the competitive season. The only cure for metatarsal neuromas may be surgical, but the skater must understand that at least a 2-month period of rest will be necessary postoperatively.

Metatarsal Stress Fractures

Metatarsal stress fractures are not uncommon and are easily overlooked. A high index of suspicion must be kept in mind when dealing with forefoot pain, and prompt x-ray examination is needed. Metatarsal stress fractures may not be visible during the first examination, so if the pain persists, reexamination by x-ray supplemented by bone scan or CT scan may be necessary to establish this diagnosis. Treatment consists of a walking cast and reduced activity.

CONCLUSION

The lower extremity overuse syndromes appear to be inevitable in figure skating because of the demands of the sport. However, we should strive to minimize their occurrence and severity by accurate physical examination to determine anatomic predisposition and modification of equipment and training activities. Once we have determined an anatomic predisposition to stress injury, we can write a prescription for special flexibility and strengthening programs, technique modifications, on-ice and off-ice orthoses, or special modification of the skating boots. The use of corticosteroids in treating these syndromes needs special mention. Systemic steroids on a long-term basis are definitely contraindicated. Although short-time high-dose corticosteroids may occasionally be helpful in extremely painful situations, we consider even short-term use of corticosteroids to be contraindicated in young skaters because of the potential biochemical and psychologic hazards of these drugs. The local injection of corticosteroids should rarely be used because it masks diagnosis and can lead to tendon rupture. However, selective use and placement of local corticosteroids at certain injection sites can have a place in the treatment of bursitis and nerve entrapments.

The figure skating season now encompasses 11 or more months of the year, and the portion of this season that is devoted to competitive preparation may involve as many as 6 hours of skating and 3 hours of conditioning each day. The competitive figure skater is further vulnerable to incredible psychologic stresses (see Chapters 8 and 11). Recognition of these factors and close observation to spot overuse and overtraining syndromes (see Chapter 9) in the earliest stages will allow intervention to prevent detrimental outcomes. Education of the coach, athlete, and family by sports science professionals will be the most fruitful way to deal with these problems.

It has now been well shown through serial studies of figure skaters that they benefit from regular flexibility and strength training. However, these should be monitored, and the skaters need to be trained in the proper ways.

As a basic rule, we can state the following regarding flexibility training: Flexibility should be done on a daily basis. It should be a static type of stretching with a slow, gradual stretch of the muscle, and this should be done for all the major muscle groups of the lower extremities, including the hamstrings, the quadriceps, the calf, and adductor and abductor muscles. Also, low back flexibility should be stressed, and even upper extremity flexibility is important in the pairs and dance skaters. Therefore, on a daily basis, flexibility should be worked on and is best done as an off-ice activity.

Strength training, on the other hand, needs to be done at least three times weekly and should be done at a facility where various types of weight equipment can be used and programs can be followed. Programs have been designed for figure skaters using free weights, and universal and Nautilus equipment. If proper resistive training is understood by the skater, then such programs can be of some benefit. The skaters should be instructed and should learn programs where they use a combination of eccentric and concentric contractions of the muscle, and they also should understand plyometrics in the function of jumping with the lower extremities. It has also been observed in figure skaters that upper extremity strength is very necessary for successful jumping, for two reasons: (1) the upper extremities help in take-off, and (2) during the rotational phase of a triple jump, the arms have to be held in against centrifugal force in order to maintain the rotation. As soon as the arms begin to unfold, then the skater will check out of the jump and the jump is finished. Therefore, in the later part of a program when a skater wants to do a triple jump, upper extremity strength becomes critical.

There are some important definitions that should be given now so that people such as coaches and skaters can understand the type of strength training that is necessary. An eccentric contraction is that type of contraction that occurs when the muscle is working as it lengthens. This happens when the muscle works as a shock absorber, as does the calf muscle when the skater lands. This is done by slowly lowering weight while the muscle is lengthening. A concentric contraction is a contraction that occurs when the muscle is shortening, and this is the most familiar type of strength training, in which work is done with the muscle becoming shorter and larger as the resistance is undertaken. Plyometrics is a special type of training and is defined as the use of an eccentric contraction immediately followed by a concentric contraction. Energy developed in a forceful eccentric contraction is important in contributing to a more forceful concentric contraction. Michael Stone and Dennis Wilson[10] state that eccentric and plyometric training are necessary to enhance elastic energy and to maximize the muscles' capability for typical movements. Proper training, instruction, and understanding of the way muscles work are important for the figure skater's maximal performance. It is important that each individual skater be examined carefully, and then, that a specific program of weight and flexibility training be outlined for them. As a basic program, however, all skaters should be on a daily flexibility program and a 3-days-a-week strength-training program in order to maximize their performance and to help prevent injuries. We feel that if this is continued on a regular basis, it can improve skaters' ability to endure the overload work schedules that many of them must follow.

REFERENCES

1. Boland, AL: Soft tissue injuries of the knee. In Nicholas, JA and Hershman, EB (eds): The Lower Extremity and Spine in Sports Medicine. CV Mosby, St. Louis, 1986, pp 983–1012.
2. Bradley, M: Survey of injuries in competitive figure skaters during 1985. Personal communication, 1985.
3. Brown, EW and McKeag, DB: Training, experience and medical history of pairs skaters. The Physician and Sportsmedicine 15:100–114, 1987.
4. Cramer, LM, McQueen, C, Silby, H, and Smith, AD: Data from USFSA Junior Elite Sports Camps, 1986–1988, in preparation.
5. Garrick, J: The character of the patient population in a sports medicine facility. The Physician and Sportsmedicine 13:73–76, 1985.
6. Huffman, D: The causes and prevention of injuries. Skating Magazine, January 1985.
7. Kibler, B: AAOS poster publication, 1987.
8. Matsen, FF: Compartmental Syndromes. Grune & Stratton, New York, 1980.
9. Smith, AD and Micheli, LJ: Injuries in competitive figure skaters. The Physician and Sportsmedicine 9:1036–1047, 1982.
10. Stone, M and Wilson, D: Resistive training and selected effects. Med Clin North Am 69(1):109–122, 1985.

CHAPTER 29

Ice Hockey Injuries

JAMES V. MOGAN, M.D.

MECHANICS
INJURIES
PREVENTION
SUMMARY

Ice skating was introduced in Holland around the year 1400. Since then it has evolved into four main areas, namely, recreational skating, speed skating, figure skating, and ice hockey. The sport of ice hockey, as we know it today, began as a combination of ice skating and field hockey. The term hockey most likely derives from the old French *hoquet*, meaning shepherd's staff.

The first known ice hockey competition took place on Christmas Day, 1855, in Kingston, Ontario, when the Royal Canadian Rifles, after having cleared snow from the harbor ice, played a game on the ice using field hockey sticks, a lacrosse ball, and ice skates strapped to their boots. The formal organization of hockey took place in the late 1800s. The first organized, or sanctioned, hockey game occurred in Montreal in 1879. Written rules came about, and in 1890 the Ontario Hockey Association, the parent of all hockey organizations, was formed in Toronto, and the game rapidly spread across Canada and eventually into the United States.

The governing body of hockey in the United States is the Amateur Hockey Association of the United States (AHAUS). It was founded in 1937. Since then it has undergone a phenomenal growth and today includes approximately 11,500 teams with over 200,000 participants.

Unfortunately, as the popularity of the game increased, so did the number of injuries. This is attributed not only to an increase in participants but also to refinements in both the game and the equipment. As the game has evolved, speed and size have been emphasized, and collisions have become more devastating. Sticks are now carried higher, the slap shot has been introduced, and defensemen have begun to drop down to block shots. It also should be pointed out that North American hockey is basically a violent game, in contrast to European-style hockey, in which speed, skills, and play making are emphasized. Fist fights are commonplace in the top echelons of American professional hockey, which does not set a good example for young amateur participants.

Increasing rates of certain injuries have been noted by governing bodies during recent years, and amateur organizations have responded with rules changes that have led to decreases in a number of these injuries. A good example is the decrease in severe eye injuries, which has followed the institution of rules requiring face protectors in amateur hockey. Unfortunately, the National Hockey League has not followed suit and is currently dealing with an increase in severe eye injuries.

MECHANICS

The forces and velocities created by skating are significant. Although the ice surface may appear large, measuring approximately 200×85 feet, it is relatively small to contain the speeds at which the players are skating and at which the puck is traveling. Forward skating speeds have been measured at 35 mph and backward skating speeds at 17 mph.[2] Bobby Hull (former National Hockey League star) has slapped a puck at 117 mph. The skating push-off force of a hockey player has pounds and vertical twisting forces that can reach 40 to 80 inch pounds. With these speeds and forces, it is easy to understand not only the frequency but also the severity of ice hockey injuries.

Hockey injuries result from impact, and impact is a result of mass and speed. There are basically two types of impact: (1) low-mass, high-velocity (i.e., puck or stick), and (2) high-mass, low-velocity (i.e., body or boards). The injuries produced by each type of impact are quite different. The former tend to cause contusions or lacerations; whereas the latter result in fractures and ligamentous damage.[2] The severity of an injury caused by impact can be dramatically decreased if the impact force is absorbed as much as possible and distributed over a larger area. This is the main principle involved in protective equipment.

Finally, although there are serious knee and ankle injuries, there are not as many per player as in many other contact sports, in spite of the speeds and forces involved. This has been attributed to three factors: (1) there is less friction between the foot and playing surface, (2) the player's center of gravity is usually well past the weight-bearing knee when full extension is obtained, and (3) hockey is usually not a jumping sport.

INJURIES

One of the main problems in reviewing the literature is that there is no one accepted definition of a hockey injury. Therefore, statistics from study to study are difficult to compare. For example, the National Hockey League definition of an injury is an event that causes a player to miss action in a game situation. Another study lists injury as any physical abnormality resulting from direct or indirect trauma that causes pain, disability, or other signs of tissue damage. Still another study defines injury as any problem that leads to consultation with a physician or results in a missed practice or game. In spite of these limitations, useful information about hockey injuries can be obtained from the literature.

Over the past 10 to 15 years, certain trends have been noted. One, unfortunately, has been the marked increase in severe spinal cord injuries. Between 1948 and 1973, at two spinal cord injuries centers in Ontario, there were no reported spinal injuries due to hockey. Between 1976 and 1983, 42 spinal injuries were reported. This alarming increase led to a study of these injuries.[3] This study found that a blow to the head from a push or check into the boards was the most common antecedent event. Most of the players had been struck from behind with the unexpected check, which did not allow the player to tense his muscles to resist the impact. The injury, therefore, was due to axial loading plus flexion. No adverse effect or vulnerability to neck injury was attributed to helmet use. The conclusions were that new rules against checking from behind should be instituted, and indeed, they have been in amateur leagues. It also was suggested that an educational program should be directed toward the players to make them aware of this potentially catastrophic injury and how it may be prevented through an increased emphasis on neck muscle conditioning programs.

Another significant event over the past 20 years has been the impact of the helmet and facial protectors in reducing eye and facial trauma. As severe facial and blinding eye injuries increased in the early 1970s, amateur hockey ruling bodies took steps to lower the players' sticks. A movement also developed to require head, face, and eye protection. With improvement in the technology of face masks and eye protectors, amateur bodies began to require their use. As a result, there has been a sharp decline in the number of severe injuries. It has been estimated that through the use of these devices 1.2 million players have averted a projected 70,000 eye and facial injuries per year, at an annual savings to society of over 10 million dollars in medical expenses.[4] The discussion of various types of protectors (e.g., wire mesh, polycarbonates, and so forth) is beyond the scope of this paper. It should be mentioned, however, that if a wire mesh is used, the holes should be small enough not to allow the penetration of the hockey stick; this is not always the case (Fig. 29–1).

Recent studies of hockey injuries reveal that there is a slight decrease in the incidence of injuries as the season progresses. Factors having no bearing on the occurrence of hockey injuries are whether the team won or lost and whether they played on home ice. Injuries are fewest in the first period of play,

and the lowest number take place in the neutral zone. Forwards have the highest incidence of injuries (52 percent), followed by defensemen (31 percent), and goalies (7 percent). With regard to puck control, the lowest incidence of injuries is away from the puck, and the highest incidence occurs when controlling or fighting for the puck.

Overall, the major cause of hockey injuries is body contact. Penalties are associated with 26 percent of injuries.[1] Most injuries are soft tissue (88 percent), and most are minor (86 percent). Soft tissue injuries include contusions, strains, sprains, and lacerations. Anatomic location of injuries has changed, with earlier studies showing that the head and face were most frequently injured. Since the advent of helmet and face protectors, head and facial injuries have dropped remarkably. The lower extremity is more frequently injured than the upper extremity and the trunk. As the levels of hockey play progress from pre-high-school to professional ranks, the incidence rate of injuries increases dramatically from 1 per 100 hours of play by the young amateurs to 1 per 7 hours of play at the highest level.[2]

One by-product of the rules requiring the use of head and face protectors in amateur hockey is that players now tend to hold their sticks higher because faces are protected. When the collegiate players then arrive in the professional ranks, they seem to have an increased tendency toward high sticking, and this may be contributing to the rash of injuries being seen in professional play.

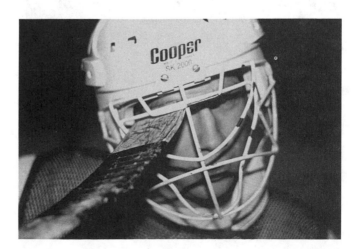

Figure 29–1. Inadequate mask allowing the stick to penetrate.

PREVENTION

The prevention of hockey injuries, or at least a significant decrease in their frequency, certainly is a worthwhile goal. There are four main modalities that can be used to achieve this goal: (1) equipment improvement, (2) training, (3) player education, and (4) better rules and enforcement.

Regarding equipment, the space age has arrived. Felt and fiber pads, one-piece ash sticks, and leather tube skates—once so popular—are now obsolete. New foams, plastics, nylons, and fiberglass are used to make equipment lighter and stronger. In 1982, the Toronto Maple Leafs spent $1,500.00 per man on equipment. The benefits of helmets and face masks have already been mentioned. Shoulder pads that are double cantilevered appear to offer more protection than those that are single cantilevered (Fig. 29–2). Newer elbow pads incorporate more forearm

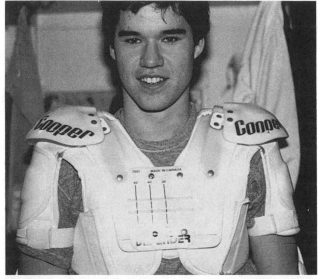

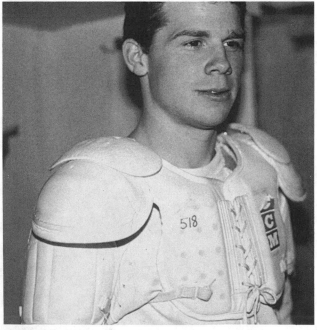

Figure 29–2. *Top,* Single cantilevered shoulder pads. *Bottom,* Double cantilevered shoulder pads.

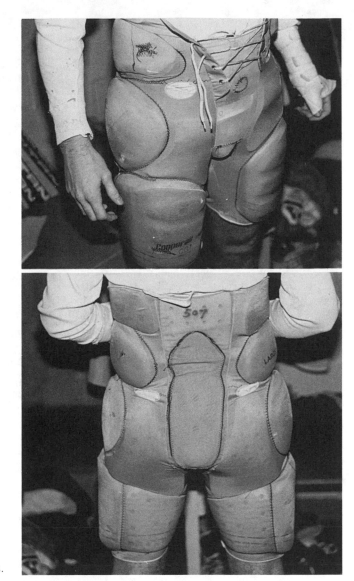

Figure 29–3. New girdle garments.

protection and are better fitting so that they do not slip off the bony prominences. Improved hockey gloves offer adequate protection to hand and fingers, but not necessarily to the wrist. New girdle garments have been designed that fit well and do not slip during turning maneuvers. These offer improved protection for not only the thigh and hip but also for the lower abdomen and chest wall (Fig. 29–3). The new plastic skate boots seem to provide much better ankle protection and support when compared with the leather boots. Finally, custom-fitting orthoplast splints can be fashioned by therapists to pro-

tect minor injuries and to allow quicker return to action.

In regard to conditioning and training, much has been learned in the past 20 years. Despite the anaerobic nature of hockey, a greater emphasis has begun to be placed on aerobic conditioning, because good aerobic capacity provides the basis for endurance and fast recovery. Added emphasis has been placed on strength training, both during the season and in the off season. Overall conditioning has been found to drop off if strength training is not continued during the season. Because fatigue is a season-long problem and tired players are much more predisposed to injury, there should be a reevaluation of the integration of practice and training sessions with games. The frequency and scheduling of games have to be a factor in this equation. Because hockey requires both skill and endurance, drills should be arranged so that skill-learning activities are practiced before endurance activities. Unless this sequence is followed, players are often already fatigued when they attempt drills designed to improve their skills.[1]

Players should understand the principles behind their training. They should be aware of the factors that lead to injuries, and they should know how injuries can be prevented. Recognizing that most severe spinal injuries are caused by checking from behind and that a training program to strengthen neck muscles might help prevent this injury should strongly motivate hockey players to train in this manner and to try to avoid the kind of contact that could be crippling for life.

Finally, rules need to be improved and enforced. More severe penalties for high sticking and other flagrant rules infractions are necessary. Steps should be taken to eliminate fighting in professional hockey. Players at all levels should be required to wear helmets and face protectors.

SUMMARY

Hockey is an exciting, action-filled sport. As players become larger and faster and improve their skills, sports scientists are encouraged to continue study of the physiology, biomechanics, and injury patterns that are special to this game. This knowledge will provide essential data to hockey governing bodies that will help them develop appropriate regulations for the protection of both the players and the sport.

REFERENCES

1. A Round Table: Hockey: Optimizing performance and safety. The Physician and Sports Medicine 11, 12:73–83, 1983.
2. Sutherland, GW: Fire on ice. Am J Sports Med 4:264–269, 1976.
3. Tator, CH, Ekong, CEU, Rowed, DW, Schwartz, ML, Edmonds, VE, and Cooper, PW: Can J Neuro Sci 11:34–41, 1984.
4. Vinger, PF: Sports eye injuries, a preventable disease. Am Acad Ophthalmol 88:108–113, 1981.

PART V

Skiing and Sliding

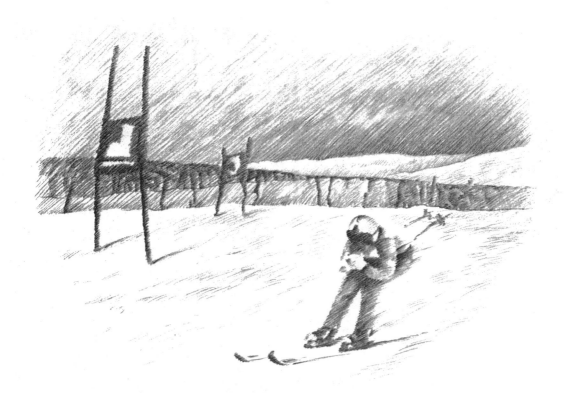

CHAPTER 30

Physiology of Cross-Country Skiing

JOHN M. KELLY, D.P.E.

Although cross-country skiing has existed for centuries, it has been given limited scientific study. On-snow studies have been difficult to control because inconsistent climatic conditions make it hard to obtain reliable physiologic data. Furthermore, the logistics of data collection are complicated as a result of severe climatic conditions. Finally, it has been difficult to mimic the skiing motion in the laboratory. The recent advent of the skating technique has further complicated study of Nordic skiers.

As a consequence of these difficulties, much that has been written about the physiology of skiing has been adapted from research in related activities. For example, because distance running and skiing have much in common, studies involving runners are often used as the basis for ski training. Additionally, many skiing studies are difficult to interpret because methodology varies greatly from laboratory to laboratory. Evaluation of arm and combined arm and leg exercises provides an example of problems associated with interpreting data. Few authors precisely describe the arm exercise protocol used in their studies, thus causing confusion when they attempt to compare the results with other studies.

This chapter is not intended to be a comprehensive review of the physiology of cross-country skiing. There is little value in repeating what can be obtained from a host of other publications.[3,14] Rather, it is my purpose to discuss some aspects of Nordic skiing that have received limited attention in the literature.

COMPARING NORDIC SKIERS TO RUNNERS

The first factor to consider when studying cross-country skiing is the physical structure of the skier. Cross-country skiing requires intensive development of the upper body as well as the legs, and this provides the major physical distinction between runners and skiers. The middle- to long-distance runner typically has a highly trained lower body and an undertrained upper body. In an unpublished study from our laboratory, Grogan[6] studied the response of seven highly trained runners to arm, leg, and combined maximal exercise. The runners' arm $\dot{V}O_{2max}$ was only 60 percent of their leg (running) $\dot{V}O_{2max}$. According to Sharkey,[14] highly trained skiers can be expected to perform arm exercise approximating 85 percent of their leg $\dot{V}O_{2max}$. In another related study, Street[17] found that when runners were required to perform combined arm and leg work, their $\dot{V}O_{2max}$ decreased by 6 percent, compared with leg work alone. Because maximum cardiac output remains unchanged or increases slightly with leg or combined work,[5] a plausible explanation for the reduced $\dot{V}O_{2max}$ is that the runner's arms received a disproportionately large amount of the cardiac output, thereby limiting blood flow to the legs.

In addition to having greater upper body endurance and strength, cross-country skiers tend also to be larger than runners. Male and female world class distance runners commonly weigh an average of 130 and 110 pounds, respectively. Although there is great variability in weights of skiers, averages are around 160 pounds for men and 130 pounds for women. Because there is little difference in body fat percentage between runners and skiers,[9,11,14] the major difference between them is that the skier has a greater fat-free mass. The advantage for skiers in having greater fat-free mass appears to be twofold. First, a greater muscle mass provides the potential for greater power, which is a more important aspect of cross-country skiing than of distance running. In this respect it would be fair to compare skiing more to bicycling than to running. Both sports demand frequent surges in energy expenditure, whereas running involves a relatively even disbursement of energy. The second advantage to the larger body mass is an enhanced ski-snow interface, allowing for greater glide as the weight increases (see Chapter 31). Bergh[3] points out that a very large skier (220 lb) can compete in international competition with a $\dot{V}O_{2max}$ of 70 ml kg^{-1} min^{-1}, but a smaller skier (130 lb) might require a $\dot{V}O_{2max}$ of 90 ml kg^{-1} min^{-1} to be equally successful.

As in all sports that rely heavily upon endurance, a highly developed oxygen transport system is a prerequisite for elite status in cross-country skiing. Top skiers usually have maximal oxygen uptakes in excess of 80 and 70 ml kg^{-1} min^{-1} for men and women, respectively.[3] Astrand and Rodahl[1] indicate that cross-country skiers have recorded the highest values for $\dot{V}O_{2max}$ ever measured in humans: 94 and 75 ml kg^{-1} min^{-1} for men and women, respectively. Interestingly, the same authors have observed that data collected on the best Scandinavian skiers have not changed during the period between 1955 and 1985. This suggests that improved performances over the past generation are attributable to other, more subtle, physiologic factors or to improved technique and equipment.

COMPARISONS OF UPPER AND LOWER BODY WORK

The study of arm, leg, and combined arm and leg work in Nordic skiing research has attracted considerable scientific attention. Because Nordic skiing places great emphasis on muscle contraction of the upper and lower body, much information can be learned from these investigations.

Well-documented studies have shown only slight increases in the maximal oxygen consumption ($\dot{V}O_{2max}$) of elite athletes during simultaneous leg and arm work when compared with leg work during uphill treadmill running.[1,9,12,13] However, other studies have shown that individuals with poorly trained upper bodies often experience a decrease in $\dot{V}O_{2max}$ with combined arm and leg exercise, and one investigator reported slightly greater combined $\dot{V}O_{2max}$ responses (2 percent) in skiers with well-conditioned upper bodies.[7]

The apparent reason why $\dot{V}O_{2max}$ is not increased with greater muscle involvement is that maximal cardiac output is not increased by the greater muscle demands, because leg work involves enough muscle to elicit maximal cardiac output. Therefore, beyond a critical mass of active muscle involvement, as in running, each muscle group must compete for its share of the blood flow. In other words, each muscle group has less perfusion than if it performed alone. In athletes with poorly trained arms, the upper body may demand more blood than it can use efficiently, while the legs are deprived of available oxygen.[12] This results in early fatigue owing to the inefficient distribution of blood. Interestingly, Secher and associates[12] suggest that during these periods of uneconomical blood distribution, the arms may disproportionately release more lactate than the legs, thereby contributing to premature fatigue.

During combined work, fatigue occurs early when the upper extremities are required to carry too much of the load. In conditioned nonathletes, the maximal arm load does not exceed more than 30 percent of the total work;[4] for untrained individuals, this critical arm load percentage would be considerably less than 30 percent. However, in well-trained athletes, this percentage may be closer to 40 percent.

Having the capability of distributing the work more evenly between the musculature of the upper and lower body is a distinct advantage for the cross-country skier. Even though the $\dot{V}O_{2max}$ remains about the same, more work can be accomplished during combined work than with leg work alone. Astrand and Rodahl[1] report that one of their subjects could tolerate a power output of 350 watts for 3 minutes with leg exercise but was able to continue exercising for 6 minutes when the effort was distributed between the legs and arms. Similar results have been observed by other investigators.[9,13] These researchers found that the perceived exertion of their subjects at equivalent power outputs was lower during combined work than with leg exercise alone. Additionally, it was found that the ventilatory threshold was significantly delayed during combined arm and leg ergometery.[9,10]

As an explanation for the increased work time, Astrand and Saltin[2] proposed that even though blood lactate concentrations were similar during leg and combined exercise, a higher leg muscle lactate concentration existed during the leg exercise. The elevated muscle lactate concentration during maximal leg work presumably reflected a higher relative load and lower pH in the working muscles, and this contributed to early fatigue. Street[17] offered another reason for increased power output during combined work. He theorized that some of the muscles active in balance and stabilization during leg work contribute to the power output during combined exercise.

In summary, it may be concluded that the length of time that a given power output can be maintained at the same oxygen uptake is related to the fraction of total muscle mass that is involved in the exercise. From a practical point of view, this means skiing efficiency will increase as work is more evenly distributed throughout the body.

STRENGTH TRAINING

The improvement of endurance through strength training without affecting $\dot{V}O_{2max}$ is an interesting but poorly understood phenomenon. Prior to recent research, it was commonly assumed that muscular endurance was dependent exclusively upon oxygen uptake and that increased oxygen delivery was essential for improvements in endurance. It also was believed that strength training would be of little value in endurance sports because of its inability to improve $\dot{V}O_{2max}$. Recently, several investigations have forced reevaluation of these assumptions. Hixon and Rosenkoetter[8] studied the effects of a 10-week strength program on $\dot{V}O_{2max}$ and on bicycle and treadmill endurance times. Although only a 4 percent increase in bicycle $\dot{V}O_{2max}$ was observed, a 47 percent increase in performance time was realized. Grogan[6] found similar results when he trained a group of seven quality runners ($\dot{V}O_{2max}$ mean: 68.0 ml kg^{-1} min^{-1}) in a 10-week upper body conditioning program. Initially, the runners' arm $\dot{V}O_{2max}$, determined on a weighted pulley system,[9] was 60 percent of their leg and combined $\dot{V}O_{2max}$ values (Fig. 30–1). Following an intensive upper body training program, in addition to maintaining normal running mileage, arm $\dot{V}O_{2max}$ increased by 8 percent in these subjects, although no gains were made in leg or combined arm-leg $\dot{V}O_{2max}$. Apparently a plateau was reached in the ability of these athletes to transport oxygen to the working muscles.

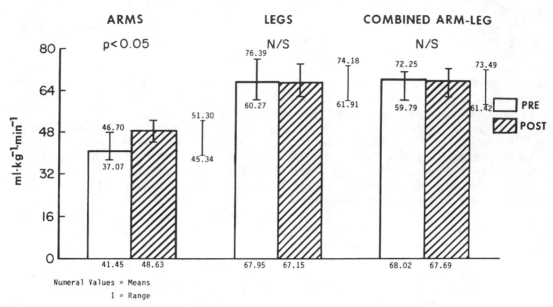

Figure 30–1. Changes in combined arm and leg $\dot{V}O_{2max}$ as a result of upper body training.

Even with a better-conditioned upper body, they were unable to increase their $\dot{V}O_{2max}$.

These observations support the contention that the oxygen transport system is the limiting link in one's ability to consume oxygen. Despite only modest improvement in $\dot{V}O_{2max}$ (8 percent in the arms), exercise time to exhaustion showed gains of 25 percent for the arms and 12 percent for the combined arm-leg tests. Additionally, a mean increase of 400 percent was observed on the roller board, which is a device frequently used by skiers for upper body training and served as one of the training devices in Grogan's study. An untrained control group failed to make improvements in any of the studied variables.

Although precise reasons for the gains in endurance times that resulted from strength training are unknown, Hixon and Rosenkoetter[8] speculate that greater muscle size, increased amounts of adenosine triphosphate (ATP) in the muscles, and enhanced motor unit recruitment patterns may be at least partially responsible. Further investigations regarding this phenomenon will be required to understand the mechanisms behind these increases in endurance; from a

practical point it appears that programs emphasizing strength and muscular endurance may be extremely beneficial to skiers, even though little or no improvement may be realized in $\dot{V}O_{2max}$. Finally, it is important to recognize that the strength-training program employed in Grogan's study emphasized muscular endurance as well as strength training, and that many of the exercises were specific to skiing (i.e., they employed muscle groups in fashions similar to skiing). These concepts are supported by Bergh,[3] who maintains that strength and endurance training are important considerations for skiers but that they need to be specific to skiing and should emphasize the endurance component. Bergh also feels that light resistance (10 to 30 percent of maximum) be employed because heavy resistance training is of little value to skiers.

BLOOD DISTRIBUTION

It is well established that the volume of blood leaving the heart per minute (i.e., the cardiac output [$\dot{Q}$]) is the major determinant of $\dot{V}O_{2max}$. However, given the same $\dot{Q}$ and $\dot{V}O_{2max}$, two individuals may differ substantially in their endurance times for a specific event. In addition to pumping large quantities of blood, the athlete must be able to effectively orchestrate the blood distribution. Because $\dot{Q}$ is finite and all of the working muscles are competing for their share of $\dot{Q}$, even small inadequacies in blood distribution may have profound effects upon performance. For example, if a skier calls upon greater arm involvement than can be effectively supported, blood flow will be directed from the legs to the arms.[5,12] Thus, valuable oxygen essentially will be wasted, contributing to early fatigue. A well-conditioned upper body can effectively use a greater percentage of the $\dot{Q}$ without compromising performance. It appears that consistent training is essential in developing the delicate control of blood flow required for optimal performance. In skiing this not only suggests the need for upper body training but also the need for combined arm and leg training in the same neuromuscular patterns as the sport demands. Although there is little available scientific evidence to substantiate this hypothesis, some investigators have offered circumstantial support.[4,10,12,16] Thus, it would seem that an important effect of task-specific training occurs in the peripheral circulation by a more economic distribution of blood flow.[5] These assumptions may be interpreted as an endorsement for training programs to include activities that require coordinated arm and leg work, such as roller skiing and roller blading.

This distribution of $\dot{Q}$ and work to the upper and lower body may help explain why Nordic skiers are able to compete at high intensities on successive days. It is interesting to compare skiers who are able to compete in 30- to 60-kilometer races on successive weekends with runners who must space several months between events of this length. The full explanation is unknown, but several speculations can be offered: By distributing the work over a larger muscle mass, no single muscle group, such as the lower extremities, is required to carry the full burden. It is possible that elite skiers may distribute only 70 percent of their work to the lower body. This will result in more economic recruitment of motor units, conservation of glycogen, increased fat metabolism, and delayed onset of lactic acid accumulation. Further-

more, because of the smooth, atraumatic pattern of skiing as compared with running, one may anticipate less tissue strain. Sherman and others[15] speculate that the trauma associated with running may delay muscle glycogen resynthesis. A comparison of the effect of running and skiing on glycogen repletion would be an interesting study.

SPORT-SPECIFIC TESTS

Several authorities have recommended tests that are sport-specific when evaluating athletes.[7] Stromme and colleagues[18] found that skiers achieved 2.9 and 3.1 percent higher $\dot{V}O_{2max}$ values when skiing uphill, as opposed to running, for women and men, respectively. On the contrary, others found no differences in $\dot{V}O_{2max}$ values attained through ski walking and running.[9,17] These small differences apparently result from the training and experience of the athletes.

The development of sport-specific laboratory tests for skiing has posed some problems for the scientist because ergometers that closely simulate the actions of skiing are nonexistent. Consequently, most laboratories have studied skiers using treadmills or bicycles. According to Street,[17] the treadmill is an adequate device for testing average skiers. However, these methods may not adequately assess elite skiers with well-trained upper bodies.

Perhaps a good place to begin in sport-specific ski testing would be the development of a standardized technique for assessing arm exercise. The literature has been very confusing in this respect, as it is nearly impossible to compare the results obtained from different experimental procedures. For example, unpublished data from our laboratory showed a significant difference in the $\dot{V}O_{2max}$ of 14 skiers using different protocols to assess upper body endurance. Using a prototype arm ergometer developed by Street, arm endurance was measured with three protocols and compared with data from an uphill treadmill test and an arm-cranking test. The ski ergometer required the subjects to pull on straps attached to a calibrated resistance with a diagonal poling motion at 120 strokes per minute. The resistance was increased each minute until exhaustion. In the standing unrestricted test, the subjects as-

Table 30–1. THE COMPARISON OF
METABOLIC DATA USING FIVE MAXIMAL
PROTOCOLS, N = 14

Method	$\dot{V}O_2$ L min^{-1}	HR	$\dot{V}E$ L min^{-1} STPD	R
Running	4.496	192	126.8	1.23
	(.465)	(11)	(10.4)	(.04)
Arm (standing unrestricted)	3.500	181	108.3	1.04
	(.472)	(10)	(20.4)	(.03)
Arm (standing restricted)	2.838	172	99.1	1.09
	(.471)	(16)	(25.6)	(.06)
Arm (sitting)	2.944	173	99.0	1.11
	(.490)	(11)	(20.9)	(.05)
Arm (cranking)	2.721	170	85.2	1.19
	(.457)	(12)	(19.5)	(.07)

Values are means, with standard deviation in parentheses.
R = respiratory exchange ratio
From Johnson, DA: Master's thesis. St. Cloud, MN, St. Cloud State University, 1987.

sumed a standing position and were not restricted in the motion they applied. The standing restricted test limited the motion of the upper body by requiring the subject to keep the sternum in constant contact with a rigid support. In the sitting test, the subjects were strapped in a chair with their legs doubled back under the chair. The arm-cranking test used a Monarch ergometer adapted for arm work and required the subject in a sitting position to maintain 56 revolutions per minute with an increase of 0.5 kilopond each minute until exhaustion. $\dot{V}O_{2max}$ values ranged from 4.496 to 2.721 liters min^{-1} for running and arm cranking, respectively (Table 30–1). When the four arm tests were compared with the running test, $\dot{V}O_{2max}$ varied from 61 percent for arm cranking to 78 percent for the standing unrestricted test. This range in variability makes it impossible to interpret data collected when employing different exercise protocols. For example, Sharkey[14] concluded that the arm $\dot{V}O_{2max}$ in untrained individuals seldom exceeds 70 percent of the leg $\dot{V}O_{2max}$; whereas trained skiers can achieve 85 percent of the leg value. One can see the problems associated with this generalization when the arm protocol is not specified. Obviously, by using an unrestricted protocol, the athlete is able to utilize a greater portion of his or her total muscle mass. When permitted, athletes will use the great muscles of their backs and even their legs to achieve the highest obtainable score.

CONCLUSION

This chapter has discussed several of the more important concepts and problems related to physiologic research in cross-country Nordic skiing. In this scope it is impossible to cover all of the physiologic concerns related to the sport. It is suggested that cross-country skiing has much in common with other endurance sports, but there is also much that is unique. Development of the skier's oxygen transport system to its greatest capacity is of paramount importance. This requires training of the central cardiovascular system and training of the individual muscle groups to improve peripheral blood flow and the oxidative and anaerobic machinery. The central adaptations to training may be viewed as common to all endurance sports, but the peripheral changes remain specific to cross-country skiing.

As yet, there have been few scientific contributions to the sport of cross-country skiing because of the difficult nature of the sport and limited technology. Presently this wonderful sport has caught the eye of the scientist. The exciting and demanding nature of cross-country skiing makes it a very attractive model for the researcher. New and adapted technology—along with the cooperative efforts of enthusiastic athletes, coaches, and researchers—provides much promise for expanding our knowledge of this sport in the near future.

REFERENCES

1. Astrand, PO and Rodahl, K: Textbook of Work Physiology Physiological Bases of Exercise, ed 3. McGraw-Hill, New York, 1986, pp 661–665.
2. Astrand, PO and Saltin, B: Maximal oxygen uptake and heart rate in various types of muscular activity. J Appl Physiol 16:977–981, 1961.
3. Bergh, U: Physiology of Cross-Country Ski Racing. Human Kinetics, Champaign, IL, 1982.
4. Bergh, U, Kanstrup, IL, and Ekblom, B: Maximal oxygen uptake during exercise with various combinations of arm and leg work. J Appl Physiol 41:191–196, 1976.
5. Clausen, JP: Effect of physical training on cardiovascular adjustments to exercise in man. Physiological Reviews 57:779–815, 1977.
6. Grogan, J: Master's thesis. St. Cloud, MN, St. Cloud State University, 1987.
7. Hermansen, L: Oxygen transport during exercise in human subjects. Acta Physiologica Scandinavica (Suppl. 399): 19–36, 1973.
8. Hixon, RD, Rosenkoetter, MA, and Brown, MM: Strength training effects on aerobic power and short term endurance. Med Sci Sports Exerc 12:336–339, 1980.
9. Millerhagen, JO, Kelly, JM, and Murphy, RJ: A study of combined arm and leg exercise with application to nordic skiing. Can J Appl Sports Sci 8:92–97, 1983.
10. Reybrouck, T, Heigenhauser, GF, and Faulkner, JA: Limitations to maximum oxygen uptake in arm, leg, and combined arm-leg ergometery. J Appl Physiol 38:774–779, 1975.
11. Rusko, H, Havu, M, and Karvinen, E: Aerobic performance capacity in athletes. Euro J Appl Physiol 38:151–159, 1978.
12. Secher, NH, Clausen, JP, Klausen, K, Noer, I, and Trap-Jensen, J: Central and regional circulatory effects of adding arm exercise to leg exercise. Acta Physiologica Scandinavica 100:288–297, 1977.
13. Secher, NH, Ruberg-Larsen, N, Binhorst, RA, and Ponde-Petersen, F: Maximal oxygen uptake during arm cranking and combined arm plus leg exercise. J Appl Physiol 36:515–518, 1974.
14. Sharkey, BJ: Training for Cross-Country Ski Racing. Human Kinetics, Champaign, IL, 1984.
15. Sherman, W, Costill, DL, Fink, WJ, Haggerman, FC, Armstrong, LE, and Murray, TF: Effect of a 42.2 km footrace and subsequent rest or exercise on muscle glycogen and enzymes. Journal of Applied Physiological Respiratory Environmental Exercise Physiology 55:1219–1224, 1983.
16. Stamford, BA, Weltman, A, and Fulco, C: Anaerobic threshold and cardiovascular responses during one versus-two-legged cycling. Res Q 49:351–362, 1978.
17. Street, GM: Maximal Cardiorespiratory Responses and Vertical Power Outputs Associated With Combined and Leg Exercise in Highly Trained Athletes. Master's thesis, St Cloud State University, 1983.
18. Stromme, SB, Ingjer, F, and Meen, HD: Assessment of maximal aerobic power in specifically trained athletes. Journal of Applied Physiological Respiratory Environmental Exercise Physiology 42:833–837, 1977.

CHAPTER 31

Biomechanics of Cross-Country Skiing

GLENN M. STREET, Ph.D.

International cross-country ski racing is currently passing through a very exciting period in its history. In just 5 years, from 1977 to 1982, the sport completely shifted from its classic skiing techniques to a new, radically different style of skiiing called skating.[26] The change was so swift and sweeping that the official governing body of international ski racing, Federation Internationale de Ski (FIS), felt compelled to establish rules to control the growth of the skating techniques. The first rules banned skating in the last 200 meters of all races, the first 100 meters of mass start relay races, and all tag zones in relays.[22] As a further step, the FIS ruled that half of the 1985–1986 and 1986–1987 World Cup races would be classified as "classic races" (skating prohibited) and the other half as "open races" (skating permitted).

Prior to the skating revolution, a limited number of biomechanical studies on the classic techniques were published in scientific journals. However, because of (1) the excitement over skating, (2) the increasing number of biomechanists with interests in cross-country skiing, and (3) the availablity of new research funds from the Scientific Committee of the United States Olympic Committee (USOC), the number of biomechanical studies being conducted on cross-country skiing is gradually increasing. Because the published biomechanical data are sparse, this chapter will focus on a theoretic discussion of the forces that act on a skier to both propel and to resist his or her forward progress and how these forces are related to skiing performance.

SKIING TECHNIQUES

For those readers with a limited knowledge of skiing techniques, three classic and three skating techniques will be described briefly. The three classic techniques are the diagonal stride, double pole, and kick-double pole. The three skating techniques are the marathon skate, V2 skate, and V1 skate.

Classic Techniques

All of the classic techniques have one thing in common: They all involve skiing in a set of parallel tracks. Prior to a classic race the course is machine groomed, which results in a hard, compressed trail with two parallel tracks routed into the snow, one track for each ski. Except for sharp corners, steep uphill sections, or challenging downhill runs, the skis always remain in the prepared tracks.

Two of the classic techniques, diagonal stride and kick-double pole, rely entirely on friction between the ski and snow to generate a kicking force. Adequate friction is obtained by the application of a "sticky" kick wax to the middle third of the base of the ski. During a kick in the diagonal stride or kick-double pole, the ski is brought to a complete stop and is driven against the snow so that the kick wax, which is under high pressure, grips the snow.

Diagonal Stride

The diagonal stride was the mainstay of cross-country skiing for all skiers until the skating revolution in the early 1980s, and it remains the dominant technique for most of the nonracing ski community. The diagonal stride can be considered an extension of walking because the basic movements of the limbs are the same in both activities. The major difference between walking and the diagonal stride is that in skiing the arms are actively involved in propulsion as opposed to passively swinging, as is observed during walking. "Diagonal" in the name "diagonal stride" refers to the fact that the opposite arm and leg act together.[5]

The general movement pattern of a skier performing the diagonal stride is illustrated in Figure 31–1a. A half cycle of the diagonal stride, as viewed from the side, is shown in six sequential frames. The half cycle begins in frame 1, with the thighs of the skier together, and ends with frame 6, when the thighs are together again. Frame 1 marks the beginning of the kick phase as the skier prepares to plant the right ski against the snow and drive forward. From frame 1 to frame 2 the skier thrusts forward with the right leg and left arm. The skier then glides on the left ski (frames 2 to 4), while the right pole is swung forward in preparation for pole plant (frame 4) and the right kick leg is extended backward. From frames 4 to 6 the skier poles with the right pole to aid in maintaining glide speed. During this pole phase the thighs move back together as the skier readies for the next kick with the opposite leg, thus beginning the second half of the cycle.

The diagonal stride is used extensively during most classic races and is most commonly employed on moderate to steep uphills (greater than 4°). The technique is also employed with some regularity on relatively flat sections of a course.

Double Pole

The double pole is the least complex of the classic techniques and is the only style of skiing, classic or skating, that relies entirely on the arms and trunk for propulsion. A full cycle of the double pole technique is illustrated in Figure 31–1b, beginning with planting of both poles (frame 1). The skier then poles with both arms (frames 1 to 3), followed by a glide phase (frames 4 to 5), during which the arms and trunk recover in preparation for the next pole plant.

The double pole technique is most frequently used at high skiing speeds, faster than typical diagonal stride and kick-double pole speeds, but slower than speeds at which a skier might assume an aerodynamic tuck position. Within a certain range of relatively high skiing speeds, it is considerably easier to maintain an effective double pole technique than it is a diagonal stride or kick-double pole technique. The technique is used most frequently on downhills but is also used on level or slight uphill sections under fast track conditions, such as ice-covered trails.

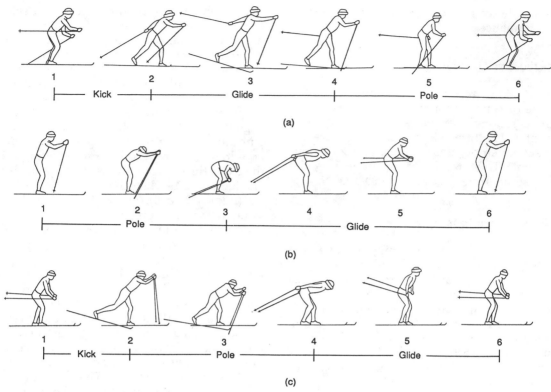

Figure 31–1. General movement pattern for (a) the classic or diagonal stride, (b) for the double pole technique, and (c) for the kick-double pole technique.

Kick-Double Pole

The kick-double pole is a slight variation of the double pole because of the addition of a single kick. A half cycle of the kick-double pole is shown in Figure 31–1c, beginning with the skier in a position in which the thighs are together immediately preceding a kick. The skier drives forward by kicking with the right leg (frames 1 to 2), while both arms swing forward simultaneously in preparation for a synchronized planting of the poles. The skier plants both poles in the snow and double poles (frames 2 to 4) as the kick leg is swung forward. A glide period follows during which the skier recovers to the original body position (frames 4 to 6). Immediately following frame 6, the second half of the cycle begins as the skier initiates the next kick with the same or the opposite leg. The more highly skilled skiers typically alternate legs on successive kicks so that each leg is given adequate time for recovery.

As a general rule, the kick-double pole technique is used at speeds between the normally slower pace of the diagonal stride and the faster pace of the double-pole. Terrains that are frequently conducive to the kick-double pole are mild uphill and downhill slopes ($\pm 5°$ from horizontal).

Skating Techniques

Among the unique aspects of the skating techniques are that (1) at least one ski is angled obliquely to the resultant direction of travel, (2) the skis never stop moving over the snow, even during the kick, (3) kick wax is not used, only a glide or alpine wax, and (4) the skier skis on a flat, hard-packed trail. The net effect of the many differences between the skating and classic techniques is that skating is a considerably faster method of skiing. In an analysis of finish times of Olympic medal winners and World Cup performers from 1964 to 1985, an abrupt rise ($\sim$

15 to 23 percent) in the average race pace was noted with the advent of skating.[25]

Marathon Skate

The marathon skate is considered the original style that started the skating revolution. Its use began in the mid 1970s when a Finnish skier, Paul Siitonen, employed it in marathon length (Worldloppet) races.[24] The Worldloppet skiers in the late 1970s were the first to use the marathon skate technique throughout entire races. However, it was not until 1982 that an American skier, Bill Koch, popularized the technique in the shorter races of the World Cup Circuit.[22]

A side view of a cycle of the marathon skate is shown in Figure 31–2a. Beginning with frame 1, the skier has the left ski positioned in the prepared track; the left ski will remain in the track throughout the cycle. The right ski is out of its track and placed at a

slight angle across the track (frame 1). With the right ski angled outward and both poles planted, the skier simultaneously double poles and drives the right ski out to the side (frames 1 to 4) for forward thrust. The weight of the skier is transferred back to the left ski to mark the beginning of the glide phase. During the glide phase (frames 4 to 6), the arms and right leg are swung forward, which places the skier back to the starting body position. The skier is now in position to repeat the cycle. The cycle is normally repeated with the same leg until it tires, at which time the roles of the legs are switched.

Currently, the marathon skate is used sparingly because the newer skating techniques, such as the V1 and V2, are proving to be faster. The marathon skate will occasionally be used on a tracked downhill section (instead of the double-pole technique), after the skier comes out of the tuck position. A good example of where the marathon

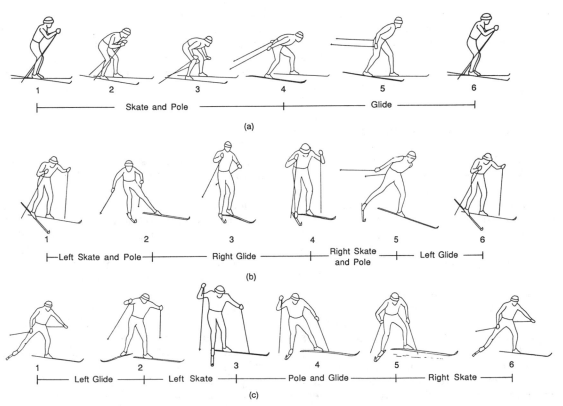

Figure 31–2. General movement patterns in the recently evolved ski-skating techniques, including (a) the marathon skate, (b) the V2 skate, and (c) the V1 skate.

skate might be used is at the end of a steep downhill section when the speed of the skier begins to decrease. Upon slowing down, the skier, who is still in the prepared tracks, will rise from the tuck position and begin marathon skating. As speed decreases further, the skier typically switches to one of the V skate techniques.

V2 Skate

The V2 skate is performed on a wide, unrouted, machine-prepared trail. Both skis are angled out, and the skier skates from side to side in a manner similar to ice skating, only with the addition of a double-poling action with each kick. The skier glides diagonally on one ski before edging the ski and simultaneously kicking and double poling off the ski and stepping onto the opposite ski. This marks half of the cycle. The new skate ski then glides diagonally before it and the poles are used to thrust the skier out over the original ski. This set of symmetrical side-to-side movements represents one complete cycle. The "V" in the term "V2" describes the pattern the skis make in the snow. The "2" indicates that the skier is double poling twice during one complete cycle.

A complete cycle of the V2 skate is shown in Figure 31–2b. The skier begins by double poling and kicking with the left ski and stepping onto the right ski (frames 1 to 2). The skier then glides on the right ski (frames 2 to 4) before thrusting with the same ski and both poles back onto the left ski (frames 4 to 5). The cycle ends as the skier glides on the left ski (frames 5 to 6) to the starting body position (frame 1 = frame 6).

During the 1986 to 1987 ski season, the V2 skate technique was used sparingly by cross-country skiers in the World Cup Circuit; V1 was the dominant style. However, just the opposite situation existed with biathlon (cross-country skiing and riflery). The biathletes in 1986 to 1987 World Championship events chose the V2 technique over the V1. In some respects, it seems unreasonable that two independent groups of elite skiers selected two different skating techniques for competition. One would assume that both groups would have, through hours of experimentation and training with the different techniques, gravitated toward the same, and presumably more economical, skating style.

There are several differences between the two sports, however, that may partially explain this difference in technique selection. In biathlon, a rifle is strapped to the back of the skier. Any twisting or side-to-side acceleration of the trunk is undesirable because both of these factors would tend to cause the rifle to move on the skier's back. The V2 technique may help minimize this problem by decreasing the number of times the skier moves from side to side. Unpublished data from a comparative study of the V2 and V1 techniques[19] have shown that the number of cycles per minute is less for the V2 (33) than for the V1 (50). This means that a skier moves from side to side only 66 times in a minute (two steps per cycle) in the V2 versus 100 times in the V1.

An additional factor that may contribute to this discrepancy of technique selection is the type of pace that the two groups maintain during a race; biathlon is more intermittent in nature because of the periods of shooting. These "rest" periods may permit the biathletes to ski with greater intensity, thereby allowing them to ski uphills using the V2 technique. The current thought among most skiers is that the V2 is difficult to perform economically at slow speeds. Consequently, if the V2 is used on moderate to steep uphills, where skiing speeds are normally slow, the skier is forced to increase skiing intensity.

V1 Skate

The V1 skate, as its name implies, involves skating with both legs. The "1" indicates that the arms double pole once during a complete cycle; double poling occurs on every other kick. The synchronization of the double pole with respect to the legs' actions is different in the two techniques. In the V1 skate, the skier double poles during the glide phase of the skate ski. In the V2 skate, the skier double poles during the kick.

A complete cycle of the V1 skate is depicted in Figure 31–2c. The cycle begins with the skier gliding on the left ski in frame 1. As the skier glides (frames 1 to 2), the arms and right ski are swung forward in preparation for pole plant and a weight shift to the opposite (right) ski. The skier then thrusts off the left ski and steps onto the right ski (frames 2 to 3) and begins the right glide phase (frames 3 to 5). During this glide phase, the skier double poles in order to maintain speed. Toward the end of the glide phase, the skier thrusts off the right skate ski (frames 5 to 6) and steps back onto the left ski, marking the end of one complete cycle.

The V1 skate was used more extensively than any of the other skating techniques in open races during the 1986 to 1987 cross-country World Cup season. The V1 skate is used on terrains ranging from slight downhills to relatively steep uphills. One factor that might partially account for the use of V1 over V2 is that the arms and torso have a slightly longer (~ 23 percent) recovery period. Recovery time between pole phases are approximately 0.78 s for the V1, but only 0.63 s for the V2.[20] In addition, skiers generally find it less difficult to maintain balance with the V1 technique because of the shorter periods of time spent on each glide ski.

FORCES DURING SKIING

A typical starting point in most sport biomechanics research is describing movement patterns of athletes and their equipment. This area of study is referred to as kinematics and has become one of the more powerful tools in biomechanical research, allowing biomechanists to quantify movements of an athlete with great detail. A number of kinematic studies have been conducted and published on the diagonal stride technique in cross-country skiing. They include investigations on (1) the length and frequency of the stride;[8–10,15,18] (2) durations of the various phases within the stride, such as the glide, pole, and kick phases;[8,9,12,18,27] and (3) angles of select joints of the body at particular points within a stride.[8,12,15,27] Fewer kinematic studies have been conducted on the other classic techniques and are thought to be unpublished. Because skating is relatively new, limited kinematic work has been completed on this technique, and the research is still unpublished.

Although kinematics provides the biomechanist, coach, and skier with a better understanding of a skiing style, a more thorough understanding of a technique is obtained only when the forces that cause these movements are studied. This area of study is known as kinetics. Although kinetic studies offer the biomechanist a clearer picture of the sport, they are conducted less frequently because of the sophisticated and expensive equipment needed to measure the forces. Three kinetic studies on cross-country skiing are known to have been published, and all are on the classic techniques.[7,11,14] All three investigations measured the poling and kicking forces during the diagonal stride and double pole techniques.

There are four external forces that govern the movement of a skier (Fig. 31–3). One of these forces, snow drag, always acts to slow the skier down. Another, ground reaction

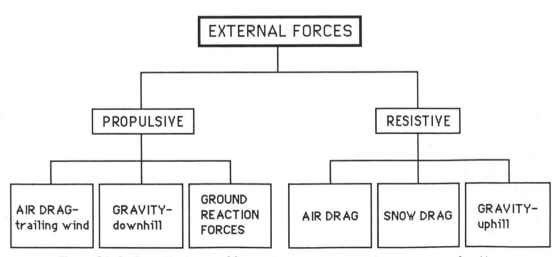

Figure 31–3. Overall scheme of forces that act to govern the movement of a skier.

force, always propels the skier forward. In this chapter, only the reaction forces to poling and kicking will be treated as ground reaction forces. Snow drag could be considered a ground reaction force but will be considered as a separate type of force. The other two external forces, air drag and gravitation, can either speed up or slow down the skier. All four of these external forces will be defined and discussed briefly in the subsequent sections, followed by the final section, which evaluates the relative importance of each resistive force under different conditions.

All estimated forces, mechanical power outputs, and skiing speeds in this chapter were computed for a 75-kg, 178-cm male skier with a maximal oxygen uptake of 80 $ml\cdot kg^{-1}\cdot min^{-1}$ and a maximal sustainable mechanical power output of 380 watts. The mechanical power output was predicted from a reasonable estimate of the skier's maximal sustainable rate of oxygen consumption for a 10 30-km race: 90 percent of maximum.[1] Prediction of mechanical power output from oxygen consumption was made from bicycle ergometry data.[1]

Air Drag

Air drag is a force that normally acts to slow a skier down and is a result of air molecules hitting the skier. At impact, the air molecules apply a net force on the skier. If the molecules hit the back of the skier, the net force acts to propel the skier forward. In the opposite case, the molecules strike the front of the skier and tend to slow him or her down.

Air drag is a function of four factors: (1) air density, (2) frontal area, (3) coefficient of drag, and (4) flow velocity. Air drag is directly proportional to three (frontal area, coefficient of drag, and air density) of the four factors, which means that if one of these doubles, with everything else held constant, air drag doubles. However, with flow velocity, air drag is related exponentially: air drag is proportional to the square of flow velocity. When flow velocity is doubled, air drag increases fourfold. Consequently, flow velocity has a greater influence on air drag than the other three factors, and its importance increases at faster skiing speeds.

These relationships are summarized in the following formula for air drag. All estimates of air drag presented in this chapter were calculated with the following formula and indicated constants. The constants are average values from several sources.[13,16,17,28]

$$air\ drag = \frac{1}{2}\cdot \rho \cdot A \cdot C_d \cdot v^2$$

where: ρ = air density = $1.25\ kg\cdot m^{-3}$
  A = projected frontal area of skier (0.9 m^2 standing position, 0.5 m^2 tuck position; male skier)
  C_d = coefficient of drag (0.9)
  v = flow velocity ($m\cdot s^{-1}$)

Flow Velocity

Flow velocity is the velocity of the air molecules with respect to the skier. It can be thought of as the average impact velocity of the air molecules. There are three possible types of flow velocities: (1) positive flow velocity: air molecules move toward and strike the front of the skier; (2) zero flow velocity: the air molecules do not strike the skier because the skier and air molecules have the same velocities; and (3) negative flow velocity: the air molecules hit the back of the skier. In the first case, which is the most common situation in skiing, the air molecules act to slow the skier down. In the second case of zero flow velocity, the air molecules have no effect on propulsion. In the final situation, in which a sufficiently strong trailing wind causes the air molecules to hit the back of the skier, air drag acts to *propel* the skier.

The effect of flow velocity on air drag is illustrated in Figure 31–4. Air drag was estimated for the previously mentioned male skier across a range of flow velocities from 0 to 11 $m\cdot s^{-1}$ for the standing and aerodynamic tuck positions. In the absence of wind, the flow velocities in Figure 31–4 can be considered to be equal to skiing speeds. Under this condition, the indicated ranges of flow velocities for uphill, level, and downhill skiing are valid. Flow velocity, and consequently air drag, are lowest for uphill skiing. In the standing position, peak air drag during uphill skiing is estimated to be only 8 Newtons (1 Newton [N] = 0.23 pounds). It is approximatley half this for the tuck position. Even across the flow velocities that are typi-

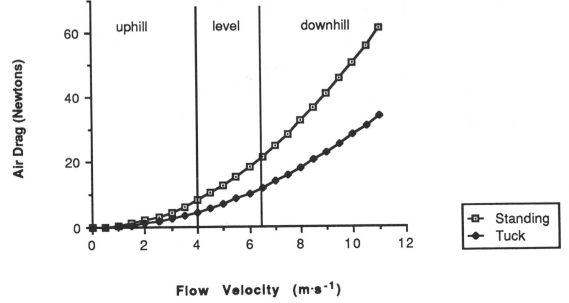

Figure 31–4. Relationship of the rate of air movement past the skier's body (flow velocity) to the amount of drag exerted by the air on the skier. The importance of a favorable aerodynamic position is obvious at the higher flow velocities.

cal of level terrain skiing, peak air drag approaches only 22 N. It is not until the higher flow velocities of downhills that air drag becomes sizable. Estimated air drags at flow velocities of 9 and 11 m·s^{-1} are 41 and 61 N in the standing position, and 23 and 34 N in the tuck position.

As just discussed, the magnitude of air drag is normally relatively small (0 to 34 N) in cross-country skiing because of the typically low flow velocities (0 to 9 m·s^{-1}). However, on steep downhill runs or when facing a strong head wind, air drag can become a major source of resistance. A head wind is a wind that directly opposes a skier. The practical significance of a head wind is that it results in an increase in mechanical power output and rate of energy expenditure for a given skiing speed. Consequently, when faced with a head wind, a skier normally decreases the pace of skiing so that a relatively constant mechanical power output is maintained.

Figure 31–5 illustrates the effect of various head winds on a skier's speed for level skiing. The skier's maximal sustainable mechanical power output against air and snow drag was assumed to be 380 watts. At this constant power output, the skiing speeds across the range of head winds were estimated with the following formula:

$$P = (F_1 + F_2) \cdot v_s$$

where: P = total power output of air and snow drag (380 watts)
F$_1$ = air drag
F$_2$ = snow drag
v$_s$ = skiing speed

Air drag (F$_1$) was calculated using the previously defined formula and constants for a male skier skiing in an erect position. Snow drag (F$_2$) was estimated using the snow drag formula that is defined in a subsequent section. The coefficient of snow drag used was 0.08.

It is apparent from Figure 31–5 that when skiing across level terrain, a head wind has a sizable effect on the speed that a skier can maintain. When there is no head wind, the skier is able to ski at approximately 5.5 m·s^{-1}. With a mild head wind of 1.5 m·s^{-1} (3 mph), the estimated maximal sustainable skiing speed decreases by 8 percent to 5.08 m·s^{-1}. With more stiff head winds of 3 and 6 m·s^{-1} the skier is forced to slow down to

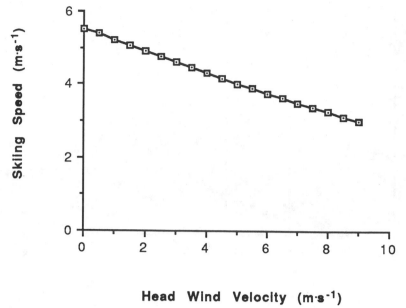

Figure 31–5. Overall effect of changes in head wind velocity to the maximal sustainable skiing speed at a constant power output.

estimated speeds of 4.6 and 3.8 m·s^{-1}: 16 and 32 percent reductions, respectively.

Although not commonly practiced, in certain situations drafting can play an important role in cross-country skiing by partially shielding trailing skiers from the wind and reducing air drag. In a study of bicyclists, Kyle[16] found sizable reductions in air drag (27 to 47 percent) for riders who rode in the slipstream. The reductions were largest when the spacing between cyclists was small. In an upright position and with a spacing of 3.5 m between cyclists, which is a reasonable spacing for skiers, the reduction in air drag was approximately 30 percent. The reductions in air drag were relatively constant across the test speeds of 6.7 to 15.6 m·s^{-1}. A 30 percent reduction of air drag in skiing on the level at 5.5 m·s^{-1} with no head wind would result in approximately a 6 percent reduction in total mechanical power output. At the same speed of skiing but with a head wind of 4.5 m·s^{-1}, the total power output savings for the trailing skiers is estimated to be about 14 percent.

The available evidence on aerodynamics of human movement and the preceding estimations of power output savings suggest that a skier can significantly reduce the energy cost of skiing by staying in the slipstream of another racer. The greatest advantage is realized when flow velocity is large and air drag is the major component of the net resistive force. These conditions exist under many circumstances and include (1) skiing any uphill into a stiff head wind and (2) skiing on the level or downhill, with or without a head wind, particularly when the snow conditions are fast (minimal snow drag).

Projected Frontal Area

Projected frontal area refers to the maximal coronal planar area of a skier. Frontal areas vary with body type and posture of the skier. Irrespective of the size of a skier, air drag can be decreased by about half by going from a standing to a tuck position; frontal area is about half as large in the tucked position. This percentage reduction in air drag is true across all flow velocities and becomes increasingly important at higher flow velocities, as shown in Figure 31–4.

Coefficient of Drag

The coefficient of drag is a measure of the air resistance of a particular geometric shape. It takes into account the roughness of surfaces and shape of the object. The coefficient of drag can be lowered slightly through the use of special fabrics or faring devices. Such changes have resulted in 1 to 3 percent reductions in total air drag in alpine skiing. During the past several years, cross-country ski racers and racing suit manufacturers have begun paying more attention to these details. Tight-fitting, one-piece suits have now replaced the older, looser-fitting suits and knickers. More recently, stretch suits that include an integral hood appear to be increasing in popularity among international racers in certain countries. Although the energy savings of clothing modifications may be relatively small, it is still to the skier's advantage to employ the most aerodynamic clothing and equipment that are currently available.

Air Density

Air drag is proportional to the density of the air: the more dense the air, the greater the air drag. Air density is affected differently by three factors: (1) temperature, (2) humidity, and (3) barometric pressure. Air density increases at colder temperatures. Air is about 4 percent more dense at −10°C (14°F) than at 0°C (32°F).[29] As the humidity increases, air density decreases. Humid air is less dense because water molecules have lower molecular weights than air molecules. The changes in air density as a result of humidity are normally quite small—less than 1 percent.[6] Lastly, as air pressure increases, air density also increases. Air pressure normally does not change more than about 3 to 4 percent from day to day at any given altitude. Barometric pressure is dependent not only on climatic changes but also on altitude (see Chapter 42); the higher the site of the race, the lower the barometric pressure. Consequently, denser air conditions are present on dry, frigid, and clear (high-pressure) days. Less dense air conditions are associated with warm, moist, low-pressure weather systems. With everything else being equal, air drag will be 3 to 6 percent less on a warm (0°C [32°F]), moist day than on a cold (−10°C [14°F]), dry day.

Snow Drag

Snow drag is the resistance the snow offers to a gliding ski. It always acts opposite to the direction of travel and, therefore, is a retarding force for the skier. Snow drag is a complex phenomenon becuase of the large number of factors that influence it. This is a direct result of the variable nature of snow and the multitude of ski designs. For the purpose of the present general discussion, snow drag will be simplified and considered to be reasonably estimated by the following equation:

$$\text{snow drag} = N \cdot \mu_{sd}$$

where: N = normal force beneath the ski
μ_{sd} = snow drag coefficient

Normal force is the component of the reaction force of the snow against the ski that is perpendicular (90°) to the ski bottom. During skiing the normal force continually fluctuates between 0 and 1.5 to 2.5 times body weight.[11,14] In the case where a skier skis across flat terrain, the average value of the fluctuating normal force will be slightly lower than body weight. The average normal force is less than body weight because of the contribution the ski pole reaction force makes to the net positive vertical impulse. In level skiing, the net negative vertical impulse that is due to the weight of the skier (gravitation) must equal, in magnitude, the sum of the positive vertical impulses of the reaction forces beneath the poles and skis, because the net vertical acceleration of the skier is zero. The more extensively the poles are used, the greater the reduction in average normal force beneath the ski, which results in a proportional drop in snow drag. The skiers and ski techniques that generate large poling forces benefit from this principle. Vertical force-time curves presented by Ekström[11] on the diagonal stride were used to approximate the average normal force beneath the ski (97 percent of body weight).

As on the level terrain, the poling forces act to decrease the average normal force beneath the skis on uphills and downhills. In addition, in the case of the diagonal stride and kick-double pole techniques, there is further reduction in the normal force, which becomes more pronounced with increasing steepness. If skiing speed is constant up a uniform slope, the average normal force will decrease as a function of the cosine of the angle of the hill (normal force = cosine of the hill angle-body weight). At hill angles of 5°, 10°, 15°, and 20°, the normal force is reduced further by 0.5, 1.5, 3.5, and 6.0 percent. Reductions in the normal force are detrimental to a skier performing the diagonal stride or kick-double pole technique on uphills. A drop in the normal force results in a proportional drop in the propulsive component of the kicking force. This is one of the factors that is responsible for the increased incidence of slippage on uphills. On downhills, however, the additional decrease in normal force is advantageous, because it will reduce snow drag.

The snow drag coefficient (μ_{sd}) is the ratio of snow drag to the normal force. Researchers[2,21] have reported μ_{sd} values ranging from 0.07 to 0.20. As μ_{sd} increases, snow drag increases. In general, μ_{sd} is lowest when air temperature is −5 to 0° C (23 to 32° F) and highest at the coldest temperatures. Although the evidence is sketchy,[2,23] it suggests that for a given snow condition, μ_{sd} is relatively constant across the speeds that are typical for cross-country skiing. However, at extremely slow speeds, less than 0.05 m·s⁻¹, μ_{sd} increases rapidly toward the static coefficient of friction (μ_s) of the wax.

Results from studies on sliding over ice and snow[2,3,21] and friction of ice and snow[3,23] indicate that snow drag is a result of two separate forces: (1) friction and (2) snow compression and displacement. Original studies on sliding over ice and snow[2,21] used procedures that resulted in the measurement of the combined effect of friction and snow compression. These investigators pulled a skier, or a sled with ski runners (sledge), over the snow and measured sliding resistance (snow drag). Their reported values for μ_{sd} were 0.07 to 0.20.

The second group of studies[3,23] isolated friction through the use of a stationary test device. Shimbo[23] used a disk coated with ski wax that was spun on prepacked snow. Because the device was not going through loose snow, the effects of snow compression and displacement were virtually eliminated. The resistive forces (friction) measured in these studies were considerably smaller than those measured in the sliding experiments. The kinetic coefficients of friction (μ_k) on ice and snow reported by Bowden[3] and Shimbo[23] ranged from 0.03 to 0.07. The coefficients of friction (μ_k) and snow drag (μ_{sd}) are mathematically similar values. On average, coefficients were three times larger in the snow drag (sliding) studies than those reported in the studies on friction (0.12 versus 0.04).

Bowden[3] identified snow compression and displacement as being responsible for the higher coefficients in the sliding studies. From the data, it appears that friction accounts for approximately one third of total snow drag, with snow compression and displacement accounting for the remaining two thirds.

Friction

When one solid body is slid over another there is a resistance to the motion, called friction. Friction (F) is a function of the normal force (N) and a kinetic coefficient of friction (μ_k): $F = N \cdot \mu_k$.

The coefficient of friction (μ_k) for two solid objects is largest when the sliding surfaces are perfectly dry. As soon as a layer of fluid is introduced between the objects, μ_k drops dramatically. The thickness of the lubricating layer and the size of the surface asperities (microscopic surface irregularities) determine the extent of the drop in μ_k. When the lubricating layer is relatively thin, many of the asperities from opposing surfaces make direct contact during sliding. As the lubricating layer thickens, fewer asperities make contact, until a thick enough layer is reached so that no direct contact is made and μ_k reaches its minimal value. In this situation, the resistance to motion arises solely from the viscosity of the lubricant.[4]

In cross-country skiing, a water layer is formed beneath the ski as a result of melting due to frictional heat.[3] Melting due to pressure beneath the ski is not a factor. To lower the melting point of snow just 1 degree, from 0 to −1° C (32 to 30.2° F), a 75-kg skier would have to exert a force of approximatley 11 times body weight to the ski (assumptions: surface area of ski = 0.0810 m², and even pressure distribution). Because of the water layer, the coefficients of friction on snow and ice are quite small: μ_k = 0.02 to 0.07.[2,23] The water layer is thickest under warm conditions and gradually thins as the temperature drops. It is hypothesized that a thick water layer minimizes the number of snow crystals that make direct contact with the wax, thereby minimizing friction.[3] As the water layer thins under colder conditions, the wax comes into direct contact with more of the sharp snow crystals and the coefficient of friction increases twofold to threefold: μ_k = 0.02 at 0° C (32° F) and 0.05 at −20° C

($-4°$ F).[23] Because of these phenomena, cold temperatures provide the skier with superior traction, which is needed to perform the classic techniques, but increased resistance to gliding becomes a problem. In the midrange temperatures, adequate traction is achieved and glide resistance is moderately small. With still warmer temperatures, up to $0°$ C ($32°$ F), glide resistance is optimal, but traction for the diagonal stride and kick-double-pole techniques is compromised. Skiers are forced to use tacky klister waxes during warmer conditions to achieve adequate traction.

Snow Compression and Displacement

When a ski glides over the snow, it compresses and displaces the snow. This compression and displacement are a result of a force that the ski applies to the snow. The snow exerts an equal and opposite reaction force to the ski. One component of the reaction force, which is oriented opposite to the direction the skier is traveling, acts to slow the skier down. It is this component that contributes to snow drag.

The size of the reaction force that exists because of snow compression and displacement is a function of numerous factors, including (1) condition of the ski trail, (2) force applied to the ski by the skier, and (3) pressure profile beneath the ski. The harder the snow, the less it will compress and displace, and hence the ski will experience a smaller retarding force. An icy track would compress and displace the least and therefore would offer low resistance, whereas a loosely packed snow or a cold crystalline snow would offer the greatest resistance. The mechanized ski trail grooming equipment that is currently in use plays an important role in reducing snow drag by firmly packing the snow.

For a given snow condition, the harder the skier drives the ski into the snow, the greater the snow compression and displacement will be, thereby raising snow drag. Another factor to affect snow compression and displacement is ski design. Some skis ("klister") are intentionally designed to be stiff and to have high pressures beneath the tip and tails of the ski.[11] However, because these characteristics are detrimental in soft, crystalline snows, klister skis are generally used only on very hard packed or icy trails where

snow compression and displacement are minimal.

Gravitation

The earth attracts other objects to its center. This attractive force is called gravitation and is what gives an object its weight. In skiing, gravitation plays an important role on the hills. A component of body weight assists a skier on downhills but hinders the skier on uphills. On level sections, body weight has no direct effect on the forward progress of a skier. Recall that gravitation (body weight) acts downward. Consequently, on the level, body weight does not have a component that acts parallel to the direction the skier travels. A parallel component would tend to speed up or to slow down the skier, depending on its orientation. Figure 31–6 illustrates the effect of gravitation on a 75-kg skier for hill angles ranging from 0 to $20°$.

On downhills, a component of body weight acts to propel the skier down the hill (propulsive component of gravitation = skier weight · sine [hill angle]); the steeper the downhill, the larger the propulsive component. The same components of body weight act to retard the motion of the skier on uphills. The magnitudes of the resistive components of body weight are equal to the propulsive components for the same hill angles, only opposite in direction and function. Consequently, Figure 31–6 can be used to determine the magnitudes of both the resistive and propulsive forces that are due to gravity for given uphill or downhill slopes.

On uphills, gravitation is normally the dominant resistive force. Even on a slight uphill, the resistive component of body weight is sizable. Typical uphills in skiing range from 1 to $15°$, and occasionally up to $20°$. On a $5°$ uphill, the resistive component of gravitation is 9 percent of body weight, which for a 75-kg skier results in a retarding force of 64 N. At an angle of $10°$, the force becomes 17 percent of body weight, or 128 N. On an even steeper hill of $20°$, the force becomes extremely large: 34 percent of body weight (250 N).

Ground Reaction Forces

The propulsive forces in level and uphill skiing are a direct result of muscular forces

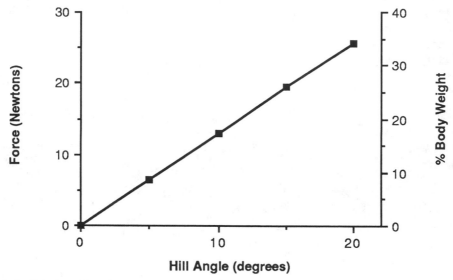

Figure 31–6. Relationship of the steepness of the skiing hill to the force (percent of the skier body weight) directed down the hill.

generated by the skier. During the kicking and poling actions, large forces are transferred through the skis and poles to the snow. Peak kicking and poling forces in the diagonal stride are 1.5 to 2.5 and 0.3 to 0.4 times body weight, respectively.[11,14] The ground, in turn, resists the ski and pole (and consequently the skier) with equal and opposite forces. The tangential components (parallel to the snow's surface) of these reaction forces are responsible for propelling the skier forward. The peak magitudes of these propulsive components in the diagonal stride are less than 25 percent and 10 percent of body weight at the ski and pole, respectively.[14]

The propulsive components of the ground reaction forces at the ski are distinctly different for the two styles of skiing: classic and skating. In the diagonal stride and kick-double pole techniques, the propulsive component is due to static friction between the ski and snow. However, in skating, the ski is always moving, even during the kick. Consequently, the skier does not rely on static friction for traction. Instead, a step is formed in the snow by edging of the ski. The gliding ski is driven against this step and a large reaction force is generated, a component of which is propulsive. The reaction force is oriented normal to the bottom of the ski. Because the ski is edged and angled obliquely

to the direction of the skier's travel, the reaction force has three components that are oriented (1) normal to the ski trail, (2) side to side, and (3) in the direction of travel. The functions of the three components are to support the skier's weight and to propel the skier laterally and forward.

During the kick phase in the classic techniques, the ski is brought to a complete stop and the kick wax is pressed against the snow for traction. The higher the static coefficient of friction (μ_s) of the kick wax, the better the traction. With the incorrect kick wax (too low a μ_s), the skier is unable to generate large propulsive forces with the legs and must rely more heavily on the arms and trunk for propulsion. Many classic races are won on selection of the correct kick wax.

Another factor that affects traction in the diagonal stride and kick-double pole techniques is the pressure profile under the ski. If the pressures are high beneath the tips and tails that are coated with glide wax, and low beneath the midsection that is coated with kick wax, traction will be poor (the resultant μ_s will be small). This situation is common when a skier chooses a ski with a stiff camber or when the skier becomes tired and generates smaller kicking forces. When an excessively stiff pair of skis is used or a weak kicking force is generated, the pressure profile of the ski will exhibit large pressures under the tip and tail, and low pressure under the midsection.[11] However, when a large kicking force (1.5 to 2.5 times body weight) is applied to the ski, the pressure is greatest under the kick wax, which results in good traction (large resultant μ_s).

A third factor that affects traction in the classic techniques is the angle at which the skier orients the kicking force. On a level section, a 90° angle represents a vertical kicking force and an angle of 80° corresponds to a force tilted 10° from the vertical plane. If the kicking force is directed at an angle close to the vertical plane, the ski will have adequate traction to prevent slipping. However, as the kicking force is directed more horizontally, the ski will eventually slip because of the low μ_s values that are typical in skiing (0.12 to 0.24). The estimated critical leg thrust angles for impending slipping of the ski are shown in Figure 31–7. It is interesting to note in Figure 31–7 that because of the relatively poor traction (low μ_s values) that is inherent in skiing, the leg thrust force can only, at best, be oriented approximately 14° from the vertical plane before slipping will occur. This constraint is a major factor that is responsible for causing the time of leg thrust in the diagonal stride and kick-double pole techniques to be brief (less than 270 ms).[14] Traction is lost shortly after the kick is initiated as the leg begins to extend backwards.

RESISTIVE FORCES: THE BIG PICTURE

The four external forces that govern the forward progress of a skier were discussed in the previous sections, with theoretic and experimental approximations of each force. In this section, the approximate magnitudes of the three resistive forces (air drag, snow drag, and gravitation) will be compared under various conditions to illustrate the relative importance of each force.

Estimated magnitudes of the three resistive forces are shown in Figures 31–8 and 31–9 for downhill, level, and uphill grades. In the figures, each resistive force is represented by a layer. The height of the layer is proportional to the magnitude of the resistive force. For example, in Figure 31–9c the resistive force due to gravity on a 20° uphill is approximately 250 N (340 − 90 = 250). The snow drag is about 65 N (90 − 25 = 65), and air drag is 25 N (25 − 0 = 25). Viewing the same graph at a slope of 0°, resistance due to gravity equals 0 N, snow drag equals 57 N, and air drag is 56 N.

The magnitudes of the resistive forces in all six parts of the figures were estimated for

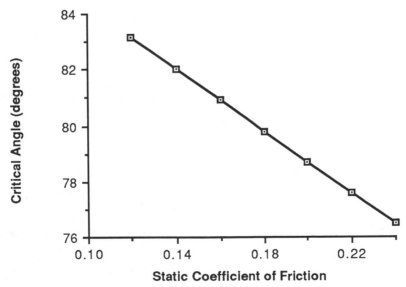

Figure 31–7. Relationship of the static coefficient of friction (the degree to which the pushing foot adheres to the snow surface) to the critical angle (the greatest forward angle at which effective forward propulsion can be achieved).

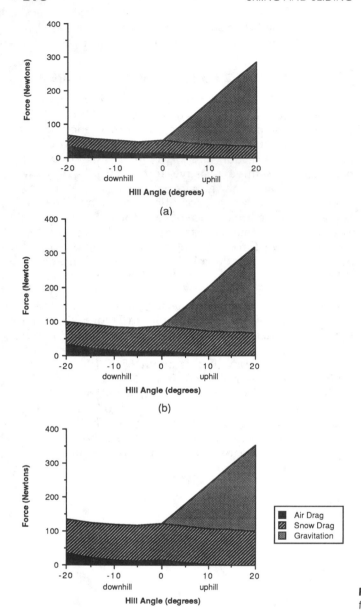

Figure 31–8. The effect of different coefficients of snow drag on the overall summated resistive forces.

a 75-kg skier using the formulas discussed earlier in the chapter. Air drag was calculated using estimated skiing speeds of 0.5, 1.5, 2.5, 4, 5.5, 6.5, 7.5, 9.5, and 11.5 m·s^{-1} for the hill angles of −20°, −15°, −10°, −5°, 0°, 5°, 10°, 15°, and 20°. Speed estimates were obtained from unpublished kinematic and timing data, experiments,[8–10,12,28] and predictive equations.[13] A tuck position (frontal area = 0.5 m^2) was assumed for the −20 to −5° downhills, and a standing position (frontal area = 0.9 m^2) for the remaining angles. Snow drag was calculated with snow drag coefficients of 0.05, 0.10, and 0.15 for Figures 31–8a, b, and c, respectively, and 0.08 for Figures 31–9a to c. A head wind of 0 m·s^{-1} was used in Figures 31–8a to c, and head winds of 0, 2.5, and 5 m·s^{-1}, for Figure 31–9a, b, and c, respectively.

The general pattern of the resistive forces in skiing, as can be observed across Figures 31–8 and 31–9, is that gravitation has no resistive effect on downhills or level sections. On uphills, however, gravitation becomes extremely important; here it is the major contributor to total resistance on uphills steeper than 5°. Consequently, on uphill terrain, gravitation is the dominant resistive force.

Snow drag is normally the next largest contributor to total resistance. On typical downhills of −10 to −1°, snow drag accounts for approximately 56 to 99 percent of the total resistance (Figures 31–8 and 31–9).

On extremely steep downhills (−20 to −11°), snow drag becomes a little less important as the speed of the skier increases and air drag becomes an important contributor to resistance.

The effects of different coefficients of snow drag (μ_{sd} = 0.05 to 0.15) are illustrated in Figure 31–8a to c. If the μ_{sd} of 0.05 accurately represents the resistance of an icy track and 0.15 a slow condition, a comparison of Figure 31–8a with 31–8c clearly demonstrates

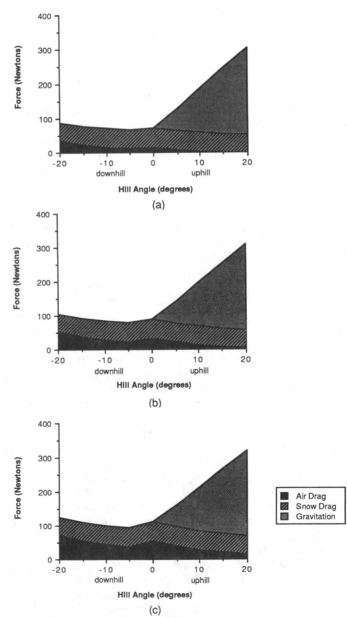

Figure 31–9. The effect of different levels of air drag on the overall summated resistive forces.

that a skier must contend with dramatically different snow drag forces. Snow drag increases from 51 to 122 N with the 0.1 increase (0.05 to 0.15) in μ_{sd} on level terrain.

Air drag, under most skiing conditions, is the smallest of the three resistive forces. On uphills, air drag is usually minimal, even with a substantial head wind. Air drag normally contributes less than 3 percent to the total resistance on uphills steeper than 5°. Even with a stiff head wind of 5 m·s^{-1}, air drag on a 5° uphill increases to only 25 percent of the total resistance (Figure 31–9c). The effect of air drag increases considerably on downhills, particularly when the skier is in a standing position. Recall that air resistance is approximately twice as large in the erect position for any given flow velocity.

A head wind has a fairly sizable effect on increasing the relative contribution of air drag. Without a head wind, air drag accounts for 17 percent of the total resistance on a 5° downhill (Figure 31–9a), but with head winds of 2.5 and 5.0 m·s^{-1}, air drag accounts for 29 and 40 percent respectively (Figures 31–9b,c).

A reduction of any one of the three resistive forces is advantageous to the skier, allowing the skier to maintain a faster skiing pace. The skier has no control over some of the factors that determine the size of the resistive forces, such as the weather, snow conditions, and angle of the uphill. However, many of the factors may be manipulated by the skier to cause reductions in all three of the retarding forces, several of which are subsequently discussed here.

In the case of gravitation, the variable with the most influence (angle of the uphill) is unchangeable. Other factors that the skier does have some control over are equipment and body weight. Any reduction in the system weight (skier and equipment) results in improved performance. Consequently, gains can be made by selecting the lightest equipment available. Although the savings are marginal because of the relatively small contribution ($\sim$ 3 percent) to total system weight, they are differences that can be meaningful to the international racers who finish seconds or fractions of seconds apart. More sizable gains can be made if the skier loses excess body fat. To illustrate, if a 75-kg male skier with 15 percent body fat dropped to 10 percent body fat, the resistive effect of

gravitation would substantially decrease by approximately 5.6 percent.

Factors that affect snow drag and that the skier has some control over include poling forces, ski base preparation, and ski selection. As previously discussed, lower snow drag is expected when larger poling forces are generated. It might be hypothesized that the potential is quite large for substantial reductions in snow drag, based on the accomplishments of arm-trained athletes, such as wheelchair competitors, rowers, and kayakers, and the relatively low to moderate arm training of many cross-country skiers.

Considerable attention is paid to ski base preparation and waxing. The savings in snow drag from these practices are probably important for particular types of snow conditions (greater than 0° C [32° F]). However, for many snow conditions (−8 to 0° C [17.6 to 32° F]), the gains are probably disproportionately small for the amount of time spent preparing and waxing ski bases. Many waxes work well when air temperature is between approximately −8 and 0° C (17.6 and 32° F).

In trying to reduce air drag, the skier can wear aerodynamic clothing and equipment and expect small reductions (1 to 3 percent) in air drag. More importantly, as previously discussed, larger potential exists for reductions in air drag and energy consumption by drafting approximately 3.5 m behind another skier. Although drafting in cross-country skiing is currently an uncommon practice, its potential as an aid to performance seems promising, particularly when skiers are faced with stiff head winds.

CONCLUDING REMARKS

The biomechanics of Nordic skiing is a field of study that is still in its infancy. As was evident from the overview presented in this chapter, considerable experimental kinematic and kinetic research is needed before reasonable predictive models for skiing performance can be developed. Such models will eventually allow biomechanists to identify the more important factors that govern skiing performance.

ACKNOWLEDGMENTS

Appreciation is extended to Brenda Palmgren and Nancy Street for their assistance in the art work and to Virginia Fortney, E. C. (Ned) Frederick, Jill McNitt-Gray, Richard Nelson, Gerry Smith, and Nancy Street for their editorial comments.

REFERENCES

1. Åstrand, PO and Rodahl, K: Textbook of Work Physiology: Physiological Bases of Exercise. Mc-Graw-Hill, New York, 1977.
2. Bowden, FP: Friction on snow and ice. Proceedings of the Royal Society of London 217(A):462–478, 1953.
3. Bowden, FP and Hughes, TP: The mechanism of sliding on ice and snow. Proceedings of the Royal Society of London 172(A):280–298, 1939.
4. Bowden, FP and Tabor, D: The Friction and Lubrication of Solids. Oxford University Press, London, 1964.
5. Brady, MM: Nordic Touring and Cross Country Skiing. Port City Press, New York, 1972.
6. Brancazio, PJ: Sport Science: Physical Laws and Optimum Performance. Simon & Schuster, New York, 1984.
7. Dal Monte, A, Fucci, S, Leonardi, LM, and Trozzi, V: An evaluation of the diagonal stride technique, in cross-country skiing. In Matsui H and Kobayashi K (eds): Biomechanics VIII-B. Human Kinetics, Champaign, IL, 1983.
8. Dillman, CJ and Dufek, JS: Cross-country skiing: A comparative analysis between roller and on-snow skiing. Ski Coach 6:4–8, 1983.
9. Dillman, CJ, India, DM, and Martin, PE: Biomechanical determinations of effective cross-country skiing techniques. Journal of the United States Ski Coaches Association 2:38–42, 1979.
10. Dillman, CJ and Martin, PE: Biomechanics of cross-country skiing. Ski Patrol Magazine, Fall 1984, pp 20–23.
11. Ekström, HE: Force interplay in cross-country skiing. Scandinavian Journal of Sports Science 3:69–76, 1981.
12. Gagnon, M: A kinematic analysis of the alternate stride in cross-country skiing. In Morecki A, Fidelus K, Kedzior K, and Wit, A (eds): Biomechanics VII-B. Polish Scientific Publishers, Warszawa, Poland, 1981.
13. Gros, HJ: Basic mechanics and aerodynamics applied to skiing. In Terauds J, Gros H (eds): Science in Skiing, Skating and Hockey. Academic Publishers, New York, 1979.
14. Komi, PV: Ground reaction forces in cross-country skiing. In Winter D, Norman R, Wells R, Hayes K, and Patla A (eds): Biomechanics IX-B. Human Kinetics, Champaign, IL, 1985.
15. Komi, PV, Norman, RW, and Caldwell, G: Horizontal velocity changes of world-class skiers using the diagonal techniques. In Komi, PV (ed): Exercise and Sport Biology. Human Kinetics, Champaign, IL, 1982, pp 166–175.
16. Kyle, CR: Reduction of wind resistance and power output of racing cyclists and runners travelling in groups. Ergonomics 22(4):387–397, 1979.
17. Leino, MA, Spring, E, and Suominen, H: Methods for the simultaneous determination of air resistance to a skier and the coefficient of friction of his skis on the snow. Wear 86:101–104, 1983.
18. Marino, WG, Tetley, B, and Gervais, P: A technique profile of the diagonal stride patterns of highly skilled female cross-country skiers. In Nadeau, CH, Holliwell, WR, Newell, KM, and Roberts, GC, (eds): Psychology of Motor Behavior and Sport. Human Kinetics, Champaign, IL, 1980, pp 614–621.
19. McNitt-Gray, J, Street GM, and Nelson, RC: Temporal analysis of skating technique. Unpublished manuscript, Penn State University, Biomechanics Laboratory, 1986.
20. Nelson, RC, McNitt-Gray, J, and Smith, G: Biomechanical analysis of the skating technique in cross country skiing: Final report. Unpublished manuscript, Penn State University, Biomechanics Laboratory, 1986.
21. Outwater, JO: On the friction of skis. Medicine and Science in Sports, 4:231–234, 1970.
22. Robbins, P: The inside edge: Controversy and competition. Cross Country Skier November 1984, pp 32–34.
23. Shimbo, M: Friction on snow of ski soles, unwaxed and waxed. In The Society of Ski Science (ed): Scientific Study of Skiing in Japan. Hitachi, Tokyo, 1971, pp 99–112.
24. Stevens, S: Skating the Worldloppet. Cross Country Skier November 1984, pp 34–36.
25. Street, GM, McNitt-Gray, J, and Nelson, RC: Timing study: World cup cross country ski race. Unpublished manuscript, Penn State Unviersity, Biomechanics Laboratory, 1985.
26. Tabor, J: Face to face, Bill Koch. Ultrasport Magazine November 1985, pp 14–21.
27. Waser, J: Filmanalyse biomechanisher parameter beim skilanglauf. In Fetz, F (ed): Biomechanik des schilaufs. Inn-Verlang, Innsbruck, 1977, pp 54–66.
28. Watanabe, K and Ohtsuki, T: The effect of posture on the running speed of skiing. Ergonomics 21:987–998, 1978.
29. Weast, RC and Astle, MJ: CRC Handbook of Chemistry and Physics. CRC Press, Boca Raton, FL, 1980.

SUPPLEMENTAL SOURCES

Ekström, HE: A technical method developing the mechanical function of cross-country skiing. Journal of the United States Ski Coaches Association 3:23–31, 1979.

Ekström, H: Future developments in cross-country skiing equipment. In Johnson, RJ and Mote, CD Jr (eds): Skiing Trauma and Safety: Fifth International Symposium. American Society for Testing and Materials, Philadelphia, 1985, pp 433–441.

Pierce, J, Pope, M, Johnson, R, and Punia, D: Force analysis in cross-country skiing. J Biomechanics 16:290 (Abstract), 1983.

CHAPTER 32

Cross-Country Ski Injuries

ROBERT J. JOHNSON, M.D.

STEPHEN J. INCAVO, M.D.

Cross-country skiing is an ideal recreational sport. It can be enjoyed by individuals of all age groups and levels of fitness. It involves cardiovascular endurance, and exercises nearly all of the musculoskeletal system. It is relatively inexpensive and does not require highly specialized areas. It is relatively safe, and most importantly, it is an enjoyable winter sport.

This chapter deals with some of the more common cross-country ski injuries and relates them to the biomechanics of the sport and the equipment that is used.

TECHNIQUES AND MUSCLE STRESSES

Cross-country skiing techniques can be divided into three categories: diagonal stride, double poling, and skating (Figs. 32–1 to 32–3).[2] In recent years, the skating technique has gained in popularity owing to the increased speed athletes are able to achieve with this method (see Chapter 31). The approximate speeds that are obtainable with the various cross-country skiing techiques are diagonal stride, 6 meters per second; double poling, 6 to 7 meters per second; and double poling with skating, 8 to 9 meters per second.

Whatever technique is used, great demands are placed on the thrusting muscles. Hip extensors, knee flexors, and ankle plantarflexors are all susceptible to overuse injuries. Skating additionally involves the hip adductors and external rotators. Consider-

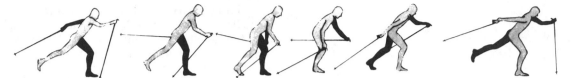

Figure 32–1. Diagonal stride technique. (From Ekstrom, H,[2] with permission.)

able compressive and shearing forces acting on the lumbar disks can occur during cross-country skiing. Back extensors and abdominal muscles also are subjected to high demands.

EQUIPMENT

Fiberglass cross-country skis have virtually replaced the older wooden skis because of the lighter weight, increased speed, less waxing, and improved friction characteristics of the more modern skis. One drawback with fiberglass skis is that they have a high breaking strength, which may result unfavorably in the transmission of increased energy to the lower extremity. Whereas older, wooden, skis would break under high strain, fiberglass skis may not break in adverse circumstances, but, instead, a lower extremity ligament may be torn or a bone may be fractured.

Cross-country ski bindings serve to fix the forward tip of the ski boot while leaving the heel free to elevate off the ski. Heel fixation is variable, depending on the heel plate, which can be a simple serrated plate, a ridged heel plate with a grooved boot heel, or a peg and locator (Figs. 32–4 to 32–6). Improved heel fixation affords better ski control during turning, especially on downhill terrains, but this carries an increased risk of injury to the lower extremity during a twisting fall if the skier's weight cannot be removed from the heel. In general, cross-country skis have minimal side cut and no metal edges, which means less control than Alpine equipment on downhill terrain.

Ski boots should be flexible to allow both free forefoot and ankle motion. If downhill skiing with a fixed heel binding is to be performed, the ski boots should have a stiffer ankle. To afford better control while going downhill with cross-country skis, several devices, termed convertible mountaineering devices, have been designed that have the ability to lock the heel down or to free it for regular cross-country techniques. As a general rule, these devices have not met the safety standards of modern Alpine bindings.

INJURIES

Cross-country skiing has traditionally been considered a low-risk sport, but severe injuries are reported.[1,6] Fiberglass skis and well-packed ski tracks have led to increased skiing speeds. Snow plowing with cross-country skis to control speed can be difficult, because the ski edges do not afford enough resistance. Also, skiers—especially those at the top level, who train several hours daily—are at risk for overuse injuries.

In controlled, prospective studies, the Al-

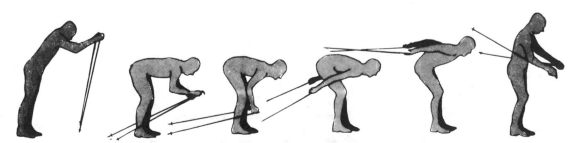

Figure 32–2. Double poling technique. (From Ekstrom, H,[2] with permission.)

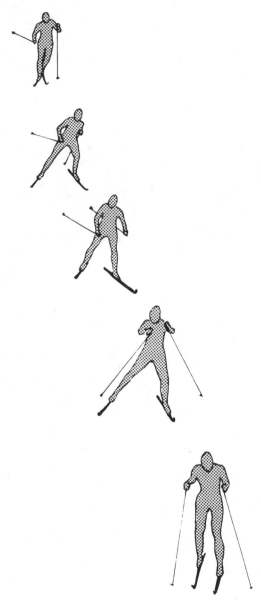

Figure 32–3. Double poling with skating technique. (From Ekstrom, H,[2] with permission.)

pine skiing injury rate has been reported at approximately 3 per 1000 skier days.[5] Estimated rates of cross-country skiing injuries from Europe varied from 0.2 to 0.5 per 1000 skier days.[3,9] A controlled prospective study of cross-country ski injuries in northern Vermont was carried out over two seasons, 1979 to 1981. The combined injury rate was found to be 0.7 per 1000 skier days.[1] This may be due in part to the fact that skiers in Vermont are less skilled than their European counterparts. Ten to 20 percent of cross-country skiers can be classified as active skiers, but the majority are "ski walkers."

The reporting of cross-country injuries suffers from many factors and probably underestimates the true incidence of injury.[3] Cross-country ski facilities generally lack organized medical personnel. In addition, much of cross-country skiing is done on unpatrolled terrain, and thus injuries that are sustained may not be reported. Moreover, many minor injuries, especially overuse injuries, go unreported. Notwithstanding these shortcomings, the cross-country ski injuries that were observed in a prospective study at five northern Vermont ski touring centers are listed in Table 32–1.[1] Table 32–2 lists the causes of accidents and injuries in the same study. Some interesting findings of this study were that (1) ski lessons did not reduce the likelihood of injury; (2) a background in Alpine skiing appeared to reduce the risk of injury, (3) a trend toward increased lower extremity injuries from torque transmission occurred when heel plates of the ridge and groove design were used, and (4) almost all injuries (88 percent) occurred on downhill terrain. These findings have been confirmed by other investigators.[6–8]

Shoulder dislocations and acromioclavicular separations as well as injury to the ulnar collateral ligament of the thumb meta-

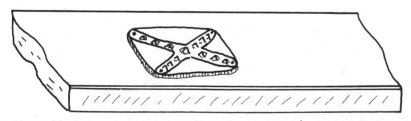

Figure 32–4. Serrated heel plate. (From Boyle, J et al,[1] with permission.)

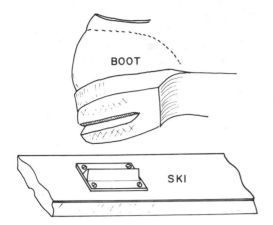

Figure 32–5. Ridged heel plate with a grooved boot heel. (From Boyle, J et al,[1] with permission.)

carpal phalangeal joint (skier's thumb) are common upper extremity injuries seen in cross-country skiing. Lower extremity injuries that occur in both Alpine and cross-country skiing include knee ligament injuries and tibial and fibular fractures.

By its very nature, cross-country skiing lends itself to overuse injuries, including muscular strains, tendinitis, and stress fractures. Some of the more common injuries include rotator cuff tendinitis; tendinitis of the posterior part of the deltoid; triceps tendinitis; lateral epicondylitis; muscular strain of the hip extensors, flexors, and adductors; and iliotibial band syndrome. These conditions often begin during the nonskiing season, when they are associated with distance running, which is frequently used by cross-

Table 32–1. CROSS-COUNTRY SKI INJURIES FOR 1979–1980 AND 1980–1981 SEASONS (49 INJURIES IN 43 PATIENTS)

Upper Extremity (40.8%)	
Thumb sprains	6
Shoulder dislocations	3
Shoulder contusions	3
Colles' fracture	2
Finger sprains (PIP)	2
Elbow contusions	2
Elbow fracture-dislocation	1
Hand contusions	1
	20
Lower Extremity (48.9%)	
Knee contusions	4
Ankle sprains	3
Hip contusions	2
Knee ligament total disruptions (MCL and ACL)*	2
Knee ligament partial ruptures	2
Leg contusions	2
Subtrochanteric femur fracture*	1
Patellar tendon open rupture*	1
Tibia and fibula fracture	1
Ankle fracture	1
Patellar subluxation	1
Hamstring strain	1
Knee laceration	1
Knee abrasion	1
Hip, massive subcutaneous hematoma*	1
	24
Head, Face, and Trunk (10.2%)	
Fracture of sacrum	1
Concussion	1
Mandible fracture*	1
Skull contusion	1
Ear laceration	1
	5

*Required surgery

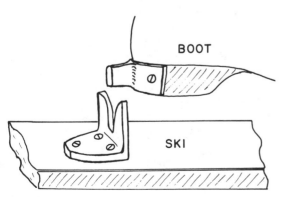

Figure 32–6. Locator heel plate with a peg on boot heel. (From Boyle, J et al,[1] with permission.)

country skiers for conditioning. The hallmark of treatment for these conditions is resting the injured structure until local pain and tenderness disappear. For the serious athlete, however, resting need not be equated with complete cessation of activity. Rather, it may mean a change in technique or modification of activity level. This may be supplemented with immobilization of the injured extremity. Nonsteroidal anti-inflammatory drugs may hasten the recovery as well as ice in the acute phase and heat after

Table 32–2. CAUSES OF THE ACCIDENTS
AND INJURIES

Cause of Accident		Cause of Injury	
Loss of edge control	15	Impact with snow surface	21
Caught ski tip	10	Impact with object*	10
Struck bare spot	3	Twisted body part	8
Deliberate fall	3	Impact with ski pole	3
Caught edge	3	Impact with another person	1
Slipped while standing	3		43
Broke through crust	2		
Miscellaneous	4		
	43		

*Tree, rock, pole, etc.

the acute phase has subsided. Resumption of activity should be gradual, and pain and tenderness should be used as markers for activity tolerance. During recovery, stretching and strengthening of the injured area will help prevent recurrence.

Stress fractures can be considered a special subset of overuse injuries. Repeated loading can fatigue bone, and a crack can develop. If repeated loading continues, this crack may progress to a complete fracture. The hallmark of a stress fracture is localized pain and tenderness. Generally these heal with resting of the extremity; however, tibial stress fractures may be an exception to this rule. Reported sites of stress fractures in cross-country skiers include the humerus, the calcaneus, and the metatarsals.

Foot and ankle problems occur not infrequently and are in part due to the cross-country ski boot, which does not protect the ankle as effectively as an Alpine ski boot. These injuries include lateral ankle ligamentous sprains, dislocation of the peroneal tendons, partial tears of the Achilles tendon, and ankle fractures. Chronic Achilles tendinitis with localized bursitis (retrocalcaneal or superficial Achilles bursa) may also occur. Plantar fasciitis and Morton's neuroma also can be seen in cross-country skiers.

Low back pain is more common in cross-country skiers than in nonskiers.[4] This seems to occur especially if cross-country skiing was done during the adolescent growth spurt. In the kick phase of the diagonal stride technique, repetitive hyperextension motions occur. In double poling, recurrent flexion and extension motions are used. Consid-

erable compressive and shear forces act on the disk with these movements. The etiology of low back pain in cross-country skiers may be fatigue fractures of the pars interarticularis or inflammation of the paraspinal muscle insertions around the spinous processes.

Spine trauma is not very common in cross-country skiing.[4] However, a seated fall or collision may produce a lumbar compression fracture. These usually are stable injuries and require only symptomatic treatment. Cervical spine injuries have been observed after falls from telemark turning.

SUMMARY

Enjoyment is only one of the many benefits of cross-country skiing. It is a relatively safe sport that can be performed at varying degrees of expertise. Cardiovascular fitness can be improved, and the musculoskeletal system can benefit from cross-country skiing. Recent developments in cross-country equipment and facilities, while contributing to the pleasure of this sport, have also increased the velocity of the skier. In the future, therefore, more serious injuries similar to those seen in Alpine skiing may become more prevalent. Presently, the most common injuries seen in cross-country skiers come from overuse. Fortunately, most of these can be prevented, and those that do occur are relatively easy to treat.

REFERENCES

1. Boyle, J, Johnson, R, Pope, M, et al: Cross country skiing injuries. In Johnson, R and Mote, C (eds):

Skiing Trauma and Safety: Fifth International Symposium. American Society for Testing and Materials, Philadelphia, 1985, pp 411–422.

2. Ekstrom, H: Future developments in cross country skiing. In Johnson, R and Mote, C (eds): Skiing Trauma and Safety: Fifth Internitonal Symposium. American Society for Testing and Materials, Philadelphia, 1985, pp 433–441.

3. Eriksson, E: Ski injuries in Sweden: A one year survey. Orthop Clin North Am 7:3–9, 1976.

4. Frymoyer, J, Pope, M, and Kristiansen, T: Skiing and spinal trauma. Clin Sports Med 1:309–318, 1982.

5. Johnson, R, Ettlinger, C, Campbell, R and Pope, M: Trends in skiing injuries. Analysis of a six year study (1972–1978). Am J Sports Med 8:106–113, 1980.

6. Lyons, J and Porter, R: Cross country skiing: A benign sport. JAMA 239:334–335, 1978.

7. Shealy, J: A comparison of downhill and cross-country skiing injuries. In Johnson, R and Mote, C (eds): Skiing Trauma and Safety: Fifth International Symposium. American Society for Testing Materials, Philadelphia, 1985, pp 423–432.

8. Shealy, J, Geyer, L, and Hayden, R: Epidemiology of ski injuries: An investigation of the effect of method of skill acquisition and release bindings used on accident rates (Industrial Engineering Research Report). State University of New York, Buffalo, 1973.

9. Westten, N: Injuries in long distance cross country and downhill skiing. Ortho Clin North Am 7:1–2, 1976.

CHAPTER 33

Physiology of Ski Jumping

KENNETH J. HARKINS, M.S.

The sport of ski jumping provides us with an opportunity to satisfy one of mankind's most persistent dreams, namely to fly through the air like birds. Flights by ski jumpers have steadily increased in length. In the 1930s, Sepp Bradl of Austria became the first man to exceed 100 meters in a ski jump. More commonly in that era, flight lengths in the major competitions were in the 40- to 50-meter range. Now the flights from ski-flying hills are approaching 200 meters. Distances of 100 to 110 meters are quite common in international competition and, in fact, necessary if a jumper expects to do well.

Ski jumpers enter the air at speeds of up to 115 kilometers per hour and land at speeds measured to be much higher than that. For these flights, the jumper relies only on relatively simple equipment and himself or herself. Success or failure on a given jump is most often determined by how the jumper meets the physiologic and biomechanical requirements for a perfectly performed ski jump.

THE SKI JUMP

In international competition today, the most common jump sizes are 70 meters and 90 meters. These jumps allow for flight lengths of up to 90 meters and up to 120 meters respectively. In addition, there are six ski-flying hills (120 meters) in the world, and it is in these jumps that flights of close to 200 meters are achieved. To help understand the physiologic requirements for the sport, a short review of the parts of the ski-jump hill

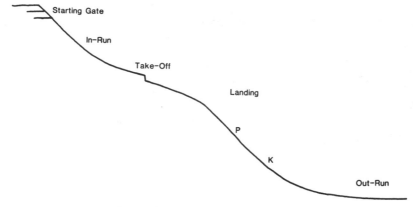

Figure 33–1. The ski jump in profile.

and its relation to the jump is appropriate (also see Chapters 34 and 36) (Fig. 33–1).

The Starting Gate

The starting gate is at the top part of the jump where the jumper enters onto the inrun (Fig. 33–2). Modern ski jumps have numerous starting gates to allow for appropriate speed selection. Frequently the jumper must enter the inrun from a start that is set off to the side. This requires a quick turn into the tracks, which are at the center of the inrun. In recent years jumpers have even had to use starting points that are below the existing starting gates. This can make starting somewhat difficult because of the steepness of the inrun. Inrun grades are usually between 35 and 40°. The movement in jump construction has been to install bar starts, which allow the jumper to start at the center of the inrun at various heights.

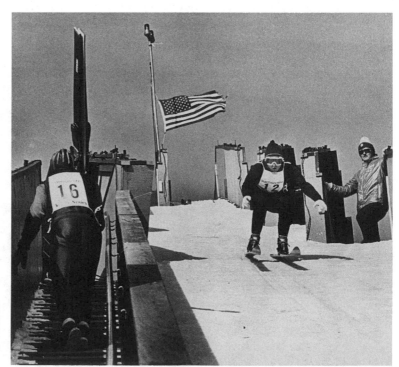

Figure 33–2. A jumper turns into the track at the top of the inrun of a ski-flying hill. (Photo: Charles Curtis, *Duluth News Tribune and Herald.*)

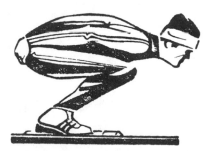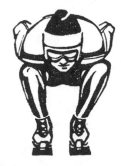

Figure 33–3. A schematic representation of the inrun position from the side and from the front.

The Inrun

The inrun includes the long, steep, straight portion of the jump and the transition curve that leads to the take-off. It is in the inrun that the jumper builds up the speed for flight. In the inrun the jumper assumes the "inrun position." This is usually a low, tuck-type position with the arms held along the jumper's sides to minimize wind drag (Fig. 33–3). This position must also allow the jumper to be in good balance and position for take-off.

The Take-off

The takeoff is a straight section at the end of the inrun. It usually is at an angle of 8 to 12° below the horizontal plane. It can be as long as 20 meters or as short as 4 meters. It is here that the jumper performs the "take-off movement." This is a very quick, powerful movement from the crouched inrun position to the stretched-out flight position. The movement takes from 0.2 to 0.5 seconds and must be executed with power, perfect timing, and in an aerodynamically correct manner.

Flight

The time that the jumper is in the air over the landing hill is the flight. Optimal angles for the body and skis in flight have been determined and generally described; the jumper's body is approximately parallel with the skis with a slight bend at the waist, and the arms are held along the sides (Fig. 33–4).

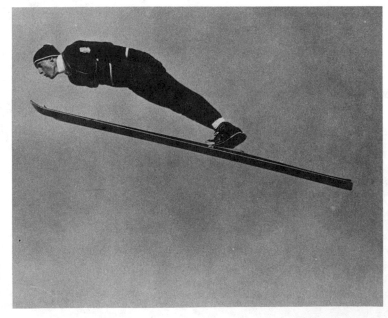

Figure 33–4. Man in flight. (Photograph courtesy of Dick Ferris, *Iron Mountain News*, Michigan.)

This position is not unlike the cross-sectional profile of an airplane wing. Every good jumper has experienced the unique lifting sensation that a well-positioned body and skis in flight can give.

The Landing

The landing area is well defined to be between the P (normal point) and the K (critical point) in the landing hill (see Fig. 33–1). This is the steepest (between 37 and 42°) and therefore the safest area to land. The distance between the take-off and the P point is the determinant of the ski-jump size. For example, if that distance is 70 meters, then that is considered a 70-meter ski jump. Beyond the critical point, the landing hill begins to flatten, and flights ending in this area could result in excessive landing forces, which can be dangerous to the jumper. The jumper lands with one leg in front of the other. Both knees bend to absorb the force. This is called a "Telemark" landing.

The Outrun

This is the area where the landing hill flattens out and the jumper decelerates and is able to come to a stop.

PHYSIOLOGIC REQUIREMENTS FOR SKI JUMPING

Although ski jumping is unquestionably a sport that heavily involves biomechanics and aerodynamics, there are physiologic factors that also are very important in determining whether an individual will be successful as a ski jumper.

The inrun position requires the jumper have adequate range of motion in the hip, knee, and ankle joints to allow him to sit in a position that has the least amount of wind resistance. This position must be such that the angles at those joints are appropriate for performing the take-off movement in a biomechanically proper manner. It is also important that the jumper can be relaxed and well balanced in the inrun position, for safety as well as performance reasons. Flexibility of the muscles around the hip, knee, and ankle joints is therefore a priority.

The take-off is the determining factor for success in ski jumping. The goal of the take-off is to come as quickly as possible out into the flying position in the highest possible flight curve with the least amount of air resistance.[18] Muscular power is the major requirement in the take-off. In a comparison of top junior athletes in Finland, the ski jumpers were the group with the highest values for muscular power, as well as for maximum isometric leg force.[15] Kornexl[13] studied top jumpers from six nations in a muscular power test and found that the jumpers were significantly more powerful than a group of sport university students. Furthermore, among the jumpers, he found a positive relationship between performance in the power test and length of jumps in a series of four jumps in 70-meter and 90-meter ski jumps. Force platform analysis of the take-off movement of one of the world's best jumpers showed that this jumper developed full vertical force within 0.1 seconds of beginning the movement, whereas less successful jumpers required 0.2 seconds.[18] Obviously muscular power is an important attribute for a ski jumper.

It is important to recognize, however, that if the jumper executes the take-off movement in a manner that is not biomechanically proper (see Chapter 34) (e.g., if the jumper presents too much wind resistance), the jump cannot be successful, regardless of how much force the jumper applies. The take-off represents a fine balance between maximum force generation and proper biomechanics.

It is in the landing that the jumper needs the most strength. The landing force is directly related to the angle of fall onto the landing. It has been calculated that at a fall angle of 8° to the landing hill with the speed of 90 kilometers per hour, an 80-kilogram jumper experiences a force of 630 kilograms at the landing instant.[14] This force is primarily absorbed eccentrically by the extensor muscle groups of the knee and hip joints. Abdominal and back muscles are also involved for stabilization because of the magnitude of the force at the landing movement.

CARDIOVASCULAR FITNESS IN SKI JUMPERS

It is evident that a high level of cardiovascular fitness is not necessary to perform one single ski jump. However, a jumper may jump many times consecutively during a training day. Imhof[10] used telemetry to monitor heart rates in a group of nine international class jumpers during training and found that heart rates ranged from a low of 126 beats per minute at 90 seconds prior to the start, to a high of 155 beats per minute at 15 seconds after landing. Heart rates during the ascent to the top ranged from 140 to 147 beats per minute. The tachycardia in ski jumpers had two components: emotional tachycardia while standing at the top of the jump waiting to start, and exertional tachycardia during the climb to the top. The metabolic cost of the climb up a ski jump was calculated to be 2.0 liters $O_2 \times min^{-1}$ or 28.5 ml $O_2 \times$ kilogram $\times min^{-1}$ in a 70-kilogram skier. This implies that a reasonable level of cardiovascular fitness is important for a ski jumper. Astrand,[2] Arstila and Rusko,[1] and Rusko and colleagues[16] have all reported values for maximum oxygen consumption in groups of ski jumpers at 60 ml $O_2 \times$ kilogram $\times min^{-1}$ or above. This level of fitness is necessary not only for training at the ski jump but also for the dry-land or off-snow training in preparation for the sport.

TRAINING

Training for ski jumping falls into two categories: (1) training for the techniques of the sport, and (2) training to improve physiologic capabilities of the individual.

Training for Technique

Although it is not the purpose of this chapter to discuss ski-jumping technique training from a biomechanical perspective, it is important to recognize that proper technique development is essential for top-level performance in the sport. Optimally, this is accomplished by extensive ski-jump training on snow. However, this would limit training time to the winter months, which is an unacceptable situation for world class athletes. Therefore, alternatives have been developed. Ski jumps are used in the snowless months by covering the landing area and outrun with plastic mats, and equipping the inrun with a refrigerated rail (e.g., Frost Rail by Porkka of Lahti, Finland) or a plastic rail or plastic mats. This affords excellent training that is very similar to jumping on snow. The refrigerated rail type of inrun compares more closely with snow; however, this is quite expensive.

Jumpers now are able to spend the majority of their training time on the ski jumps. The national team members in Finland jump approximately 1200 times per year, and because of the availability of summer jumping hills, they seldom go more than 10 days to 2 weeks throughout the year without actually being engaged in ski jumping.[19]

In the United States there are five sites for summer ski jumping, and only one of those has a refrigerated rail inrun (Ely, Minnesota). American jumpers do not jump as much in the snowless months as their European counterparts, but continued development and improvement of domestic facilities may help remedy this discrepancy.

Training for Physical Performance

Muscular power for the takeoff is the most important physiologic characteristic for the ski jumper. Muscular strength is also important for holding a proper inrun position in the transition curve from the inrun to the take-off and for absorbing the forces of landing. The focal point of dry-land ski-jumping training should be the development of power and strength to optimal levels in the appropriate muscles. Lower in priority, but certainly not ignored, is training for flexibility and neuromuscular coordination. Cardiovascular endurance training is not usually a major part of the training program, but as noted above, a certain level of cardiovascular fitness appears to be important.

Muscular Power Training

It is a basic physiologic property that stretching an activated muscle results in greater work and power output during the shortening phase of contraction.[8] A concentric contraction preceded by eccentric contraction is superior in power output to concentric contraction alone. This has been shown by difference in jumping heights[11] and in ground reaction forces and calculated mechanical power in jumping.[3] Power output during a jump in which countermovement is allowed exceeds the power output of a static jump by up to 81 percent.[5] Rate of stretch in the countermovement phase and eccentric force are directly related to performance in the concentric phase, whereas the time between eccentric and concentric contractions (coupling time) is inversely related.[5] This means that a short, quick countermovement is most effective for improving force production in the ensuing concentric contraction. Potentiation of muscle performance is most likely the combined result of the utilization of elastic energy in the muscle and the activation of alpha motor neurons via the stretch reflex.[3,5,6]

In the ski jump, the jumper actually utilizes this physiologic property of muscle by starting the take-off movement with a quick, short countermovement. Muscles are also prestretched by the centripetal force placed on them as the jumper rides through the transition curve to the take-off. Jumpers also utilize these physiologic principles in their training by an emphasis on jumping-type exercises. It has been shown that eccentric training is more effective than concentric training in muscle tension development,[12] and jumping-type training can be considered eccentric training. This has been called plyometric training;[7] however, the ski jumpers prefer to call this training "general speed" or "special speed" training.

General speed training in the form of repeated jumps should be done up to 20 times in succession. These jumps are usually done from the inrun position, but other positions also may be used. Special speed training can be accomplished with very few jumps, usually not more than five, and many times just a single jump. Drop jumps are also practiced. Here the ski jumper drops off a platform of up to 90 centimeters in height. Drop jumps are done with an immediate jump upon landing, or just by absorption of the dropping force with no jump at all upon landing. Body weight alone can be used in this training, or light weights can be added to increase the resistance. Sometimes elastic cords are applied to give a less-than-body-weight effect. These are the predominant types of training used by top-level ski jumpers, who are among the best of all international class athletes in utilizing the elastic energy potential of their extensor leg muscles.[4]

The use of heavy resistance weight training in ski jumping has been deemphasized, probably because the speed of contraction during heavy resistance training is not fast enough and the coupling time is not short enough to enhance the utilization of stored elastic energy.[9] Also, it has been shown by Tesch and associates[17] that heavy resistance training has a negative effect on some contractile enzyme activities, especially in those subjects who experienced pronounced muscular hypertrophy.

In most training regimens, flexibility, coordination, and cardiovascular fitness are dealt with during the warm-up and cooldown portions of jump-training sessions, and special sessions can be designed specifically for these purposes.

CONCLUSION

Ski jumpers fly farther than ever before, and they are doing this with lower take-off speeds and, therefore, with a decreased likelihood of dangerous falls. These are very attractive developments that have happened as a result of several factors. Great emphasis has been given to ski-jump design, which must adhere to strict guidelines; consequently ski jumps are safer and better. Skis are wider and fly better than earlier models, boots are more stable, and aerodynamically correct protective head gear is used by virtually all jumpers. Because summer ski jumping has become common, jumpers are able to train extensively on ski jumps, and this is certainly a reason for much of the positive change that has been seen in the sport. Just as important is the fact that ski jumpers have learned to train effectively, and in almost all cases they are well prepared physiologically for the performance demands in the sport.

REFERENCES

1. Arstila, A and Rusco, H: Fitness Profiles of Elite Finnish Athletes. Research Report Number 10, Department of Biology of Physical Activity, University of Jyvaskyla, Finland, 1976.
2. Astrand, P and Rodahl, K: Textbook of Work Physiology. McGraw-Hill, New York, 1977.
3. Bosco, C and Komi, PV: Potentiation of the mechanical behavior of the human skeletal muscle through prestretching. Acta Physiologica Scandinavica 106:467–472, 1979.
4. Bosco, C and Komi, PV: Muscle Elasticity in Athletes. In Komi, PV (ed): Exercise and Sport Biology, Vol 12, Human Kinetics, Champaign, IL, 1982.
5. Bosco, C, Komi, PV and Ito, A: Prestretch potentiation of human skeletal muscle during ballistic movement. Acta Physiologica Scandinavica 111:135–140, 1981.
6. Bosco, C, Viiatasalo, JT, Komi, PV, Luhtanen, P:

Combined effect of elastic energy and myoelectrical potentiation during the stretch-shortening cycle phase. Acta Physiologica Scandinavica 114:557–565, 1982.

7. Brooks, GA and Fahey, TD: Exercise Physiology: Human Bioenergetics and its Applications. John Wiley & Sons, New York, 1984.

8. Cavagna, GA, Saibene, FP, and Margaria, R: Effect of negative work on the amount of positive work performed by an isolated muscle. J Appl Physiol 20:157–158, 1965.

9. Hakkinen, K and Komi, PV: Alterations of mechanical characteristics of human skeletal muscle during strength training. Eur J Appl Physiol 50:161–172, 1983.

10. Imhof, PR, Blatter, K, Fuccella, LM, and Turri, M: Beta-blockade and emotional tachycardia; radio-telemetric investigations in ski jumpers. J Appl Physiol 27:366–369, 1969.

11. Komi, PV and Bosco, C: Utilization of stored elastic energy in leg extensor muscles by men and women. Med Sci Sports 10:261–265, 1978.

12. Komi, PV and Buskirk, ER: Effect of eccentric and concentric muscle conditioning on tension and electrical activity of human muscle. Ergonomics 15:417–434, 1972.

13. Kornexl, E: Zum speziellen Sportmotorischen Eigenschafts niveau des Skispringers. Liebesubungen. Liebeserzienhung 27:74–80, 1973.

14. Monsen, JH, Mork, I, and Rimeslatten, E: C-Kurs Hopp. Norges Skiforbund, Oslo, 1974.

15. Rusko, H, Arstila, A, and Hirsimaki, Y: Aerobic and Anaerobic Performance Capacity of Junior Athletes. Unpublished presentation, FIS-Skilauf Kongress, Vuokatti, Finland, 1976.

16. Rusko, H, Havu, M, and Karvinen, E: Aerobic Performance Capacity in Athletes. Research Report Number 9, Department of Biology of Physical Activity, University of Jyvaskyla, Finland, 1976.

17. Tesch, PA, Hakkinen, K, and Komi, PV: The effect of strength training and de-training on various enzyme activities. Medicine and Science in Sports and Exercise 17:245, 1985.

18. Thyness, P and Monsen, JH: Ski Hopp. Norges Skiforbund, Trondheim, 1972.

19. Windsperger, G: Personal communication, 1986.

CHAPTER 34

Biomechanics of Ski Jumping

KEVIN R. CAMPBELL, Ph.D

INRUN
TAKE-OFF
FLIGHT
SUMMARY

Biomechanical analysis of ski jumping dates back to 1927, when R. Strauman presented a detailed mechanical analysis based on wind-tunnel experiments.[4] Since that time, many European and Japanese researchers have contributed to the evolution of the modern techniques employed by ski jumpers. The following analysis draws upon these studies as well as on the results of research conducted in the United States.

Often ski jumping is divided into separate phases for analysis. Because of the continuous nature of the jump, it is difficult to isolate these phases, as what often happens during one part of the jump greatly influences the rest of the performance. However, by making such divisions, we may identify the objectives of each phase and study the proper means of meeting these objectives. This article presents an analysis of ski jumping by examining proper inrun, take-off, and flight techniques.

INRUN

The goal of the ski jumper during the approach is to maximize velocity. As the ski jumper stands at the top of the jump, he or she possesses a large amont of potential energy. Moving down the inrun, this potential energy is changed to kinetic energy, which is reflected by velocity. During this change from potential to kinetic energy, there is an energy loss caused by various forces acting on the jumper-ski system.

Figure 34–1 illustrates the proper inrun position and the external forces acting on the

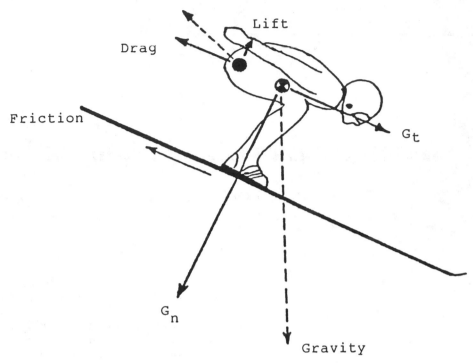

Figure 34–1. Proper inrun position.

jumper-ski system. The gravitational force can be separated into a component parallel to the track, called the tangential component of gravity (G_t), and a component perpendicular to the ramp surface, called the normal component of the gravitational force (G_n).

The friciton force is determined by normal gravitational force (G_n) and the coefficient of friction (μ_k), which reflects the nature of the contacting surfaces, ski and snow, and the resistance to movement between them. To reduce friction, the ski jumper must place himself or herself on the skis such that the skis lie flat on the snow, increasing the area of contact.

The force that creates the speed of the jumper-ski system is the G_t (see Fig. 34–1). As the mass of the ski jumper increases, G_t increases also. At the same time, friction increases because of an increased G_n, and the frontal area of the skier increases, causing an increase in air resistance. Sports scientists have found that the mass, or weight, of a skier is not the main factor on which the speed of straight descent depends. It has been found that velocity is most sensitive to aerodynamic forces, or air resistance, during a straight descent on skis.[3] In Figure 34–1,

the aerodynamic forces, lift and drag, are shown acting at the center of pressure as they affect the skier on the inrun. The drag force is the force acting in the direction opposite to the motion of the jumper, and the lift force is the force acting perpendicular to the direction of motion. To minimize the effects of these forces, the jumper must minimize frontal surface area and be in a position that does not create much turbulence. The proper position is illustrated in Figure 34–1. Wind tunnel tests and mathematical studies have demonstrated that the back should be flat and parallel to the skis, with the feet 4 to 6 inches apart and the legs upright. The arms are positioned back along the trunk, parallel to the skis. Small change in arm position may cause drag differences up to 20 percent. This is especially important in the last 25 meters of the approach when velocity is above 20 m/s.

During the transition, friction force is increased because of the effect of centrifugal forces, and the rate of speed increase is drastically reduced. The centrifugal force also tends to push the skier into the track and to cause the skier to sit back more. This must be resisted, because any movement back will place the skier in an unfavorable position for jumping and will decrease the effectiveness of the take-off movement.

TAKE-OFF

In modern ski jumping, the take-off has the most significant effect on the length of flight. Sports researchers have often disagreed on the purposes of the take-off and how this movement should be performed. Questions have arisen as to whether the take-off movement should be performed in an upward or outward direction and whether vertical velocity created in the take-off movement is at all related to distance jumped. Recent studies have begun to answer these questions. It can be stated that the objectives of the take-off are (1) to give the jumper-ski system a maximum normal (vertical) velocity, (2) to produce a favorable body position at the jump's edge, and (3) to provide an initial turning moment or angular momentum for the forward rotation of the body over the skis immediately after take-off. This should be accomplished without significantly decreasing the tangential velocity.

Results of a biomechanical study of the take-off at the 1979 pre-Olympic games (70-meter competition) at Lake Placid found that the following performance variables measured during the take-off phase were related to distance jumped: position of the center of gravity relative to the base of support, angle of the lower leg, normal acceleration and velocity, take-off angle, and angular velocity at the hip and knee joints. Furthermore, a comparative analysis examined the results of the top nine highly skilled performers as compared with the results for less skilled jumpers. It was found that generally the problems encountered during take-off can be considered as existing in two areas. The first area deals with the positioning of the skier during the movement, and the second problem considers the input from the skier in the jumping motion, such as timing, rate, and strength of movement.

The results from research at Lake Placid have indicated that the position of the center of gravity of the skier with respect to the ankle or base of support during take-off is related to distance jumped.[2] The position of the center of gravity is described by the distance(s) (Fig. 34–2) along the track surface as measured from the perpendicular projection of the ankle joint to the projection of the center of gravity. In general, at the initiation of the take-off or thrusting movement, the center of gravity is located slightly behind the ankle. However, the smaller this distance is, the better the performance.

Figure 34–2 illustrates the positions characteristic of a highly skilled jumper and of a less skilled ski jumper, respectively, just after the initiation of the upward thrust. The highly skilled jumper has positioned the center of gravity more forward than the less skilled skier. Note that the less skilled skier's center of gravity is still behind the ankle, whereas the highly skilled skier has moved the center of gravity in front of the base of support. This more favorable forward position is directly related to the lower leg angle. Decreasing this angle places the center of gravity in a more forward position, whereas increasing the lower leg angle moves the center of gravity back.

In Figure 34–3 it can be seen that the highly skilled ski jumper maintained the small lower leg angle throughout the take-off and continued to demonstrate a more forward position at the instant of take-off. The more skilled skier also demonstrates a greater trunk angle relative to the air flow. A study by Strauman[5] suggested that immediately after take-off the trunk should be positioned at an angle of 28° with the air flow for the most aerodynamically efficient preflight position. It was also indicated that a range from 20 to 40° was acceptable. The top nine finishers at the 1979 pre-Olympic games demonstrated an average angle of 22° immediately after take-off, whereas the less skilled competitors demonstrated a trunk angle of 17.5° with respect to air flow. Based on Strauman's recommendations, the top jumpers are not in the optimal position, but they are within the allowable limits. The less skilled competitors are below the allowable range and not in an efficient preflight position. However, this low trunk position is necessary during preflight to compensate for the lack of a forward position of the center of gravity. To explain this, it is necessary to examine the force acting on the ski jumper and the turning moment developed at take-off.

The turning moment (or amont of rotation) created by the jumping force can be determined by multiplying the magnitude or size

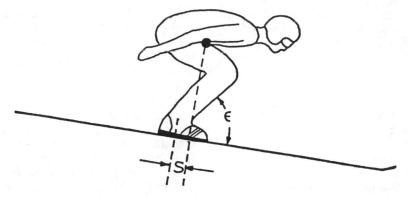

A. Highly Skilled Ski Jumper

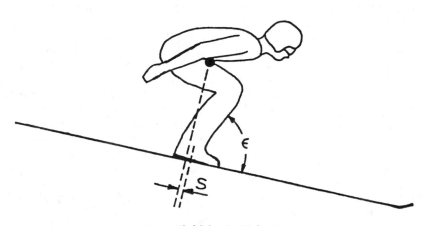

B. Skilled Ski Jumper

Figure 34–2. Position at the initiation of the thrust.

of the force by the perpendicular distance from the force to the axis of rotation. This distance is referred to as the moment arm. To calculate the turning moment created at take-off, one needs to know the axis of rotation, the length of the moment arm, and the magnitude of the force. In the jumper-ski system, the center of gravity can be considered as the axis of rotation. The distance from the ankle to the center of gravity reflects the length of the moment arm for the perpendicular force created during the extension, which acts through the feet of the ski jumper. Assuming

equal strength of extension (or force) for the highly skilled and skilled jumpers (it will be seen later that the highly skilled jumpers generally create a larger force), the more forward position of the center of gravity as exhibited by the highly skilled skier will create a greater moment arm and therefore a greater turning moment.

It was also found that the highly skilled ski jumpers are moving their centers of gravity forward with respect to the ankle at a higher rate than the skilled jumpers. This fact, in conjunction with the increased turning moment, allows the highly skilled skier to open the trunk more to the air earlier and to use the surface to create lift. Lift and drag forces are related to the size of the surface area exposed to the air flow. The low trunk position of the skilled skier at take-off (see Fig. 34–3) exposes only a small surface area to the air flow, resulting in small lift and drag forces. The larger trunk angle, as demonstrated by the highly skilled jumper, exposes more sur-

face area to the air, therefore creating larger lift and drag forces.

The lift and drag forces created by the trunk cause a backward turning moment about the center of gravity. The skier who opens the trunk to the air to create lift is also slowing the rotation forward, whereas the ski jumper who keeps the trunk down and minimizes the lift forces will slow the rotation forward.

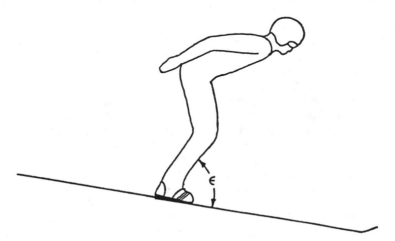

A. Highly Skilled Ski Jumper

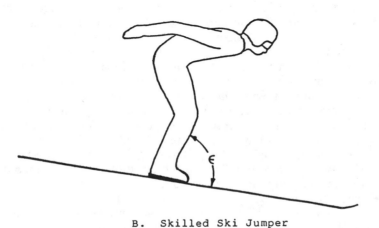

B. Skilled Ski Jumper

Figure 34–3. Position at take-off.

The ski jumper who does not demonstrate a strong forward position of the center of gravity at the take-off must minimize the backward turning moment created by the resultant lift and drag forces acting on the trunk. If these forces are not kept small, the skier will not be able to move into the strong forward-leaning flight position. The more skilled skier who is moving forward at a higher rate and generates a larger turning moment, because of the position of the center of gravity and a stronger movement, is able to use the trunk to create lift early and still move into the favorable forward-leaning flight position. In a sense, the ability to create a large forward turning moment during the take-off dictates the amount of lift that can be generated by the trunk surface during the preflight and still allow the jumper to move forward into a favorable flight position.

The second area to be considered relative to take-off deals with the input from the skier. This area includes strength and rate of movement as well as the sequencing and timing of the extension. The ability of a ski jumper to generate a velocity normal or perpendicular to the ramp is related to distance jumped. During the Lake Placid study[2] the average maximum vertical velocity for the top nine finishers in the 70-meter jump was found to be 2.32 meters per second (2.30 m/s at take-off.), whereas the average maximum normal velocity for the less skilled ski jumpers was 2.13 meters per second (2.12 m/s at take-off). This represents a significant difference, which was reflected in the distance jumped (82.6 meters versus 73.9 meters).

Normal (vertical) velocity is related to the ability to generate force in the direction perpendicular to the ramp. Newton's second law states that force equals mass times acceleration. It can been seen that if mass does not vary significantly between jumpers, then acceleration in the normal direction will reflect the force exerted in that direction. The top nine finishers at the 1979 pre-Olympic games 70-meter competition demonstrated an average maximum acceleration of 8.98 meters/sec/sec. The average maximum acceleration for the less skilled competitors was 6.76 meters/sec/sec, indicating a smaller normal force.[2]

The jumping motion is caused by exten-sion at the ankle, knee, and hip joints. In raising the center of gravity from a low position, the contribution from extension of the ankle joint represents approximately 10 percent of the total change in height, and extension about the knee and hip reflect approximately 65 percent and 25 percent, respectively, of the total elevation. Therefore, it can be seen that the ability to extend the knee is a primary factor in jumping and also that extension about the hip contributes significantly to the ability to raise the center of gravity.

The results from the Lake Placid study indicated that the top finishers demonstrated significantly higher angular velocities (the rate of increase in the angle) about the knee and hip joints during the take-off movement.

The angular acceleration, or rate of change of the angular velocity, is also important. The ability to generate large angular velocities rapidly allows the skier to stay in the inrun position longer and to maintain speed along the track. Less skilled skiers generally take more time to change maximum angular velocity during the take-off. This slower movement exposes more surface area to the air flow over a longer period of time and results in a slightly lower velocity along the track and a significantly lower vertical velocity at take-off. For highly skilled skiers, the maxima for the angular velocities have been shown to coincide with take-off. The less skilled jumper normally reaches maximum velocities just after take-off, indicating late execution of the movement.

Finally, the extension should continue after take-off. If this motion is completed before take-off, a greater surface area is exposed to the air flow and there is a resultant decrease in velocity. The final extension after take-off also helps raise the ski tips as the jumper prepares for the flight phase.

In summary, the purposes of the take-off can be identified as (1) to give the jumper-ski system a maximum vertical velocity, (2) to produce a favorable body position at the jump's edge, and (3) to provide an initial turning moment for the forward rotation of the body of the skis immediately after take-off.

To aid in accomplishing these purposes, the ski jumper should perform the take-off with the center of gravity in a forward position. This position is related to the angle of the lower leg. If the center of gravity is not forward prior to the take-off movement, an adjustment in the run position should be made by decreasing the angle of the lower leg.

The ski jumper should generate a large vertical velocity by rapidly extending at the knee and hip joints during the take-off and maintaining the lower leg angle. This large force with the forward position of the center of gravity will generate an initial turning moment to rotate the skier forward after take-off. This turning moment forward allows the jumper to expose the trunk to the air and to generate a lifting force early and to produce a favorable aerodynamic position during the preflight. The position of the trunk should not make an angle of more than 30° with the air flow.

FLIGHT

The goal of the ski jumper during the flight phase is to obtain the most favorable, or aerodynamically efficient, jumper-ski position to maximize flight distance. It has previously been stated that among highly skilled ski jumpers the take-off has the most significant effect on distance jumped. This is true primarily because these jumpers have mastered proper flight techniques and are highly skilled at controlling their ski and body positions. Skiers who are not as skilled can greatly improve performance by mastering proper flight technique.

The flight curve of a ski jumper is determined by the velocity and direction of motion of the jumper at take-off, as well as the acceleration due to gravity and the aerodynamic forces acting on the jumper-ski system. Once the ski jumper is airborne, the forces acting on him or her are gravitational and lift and drag forces. The gravitational force cannot be altered by the jumper and can be considered a constant. Therefore, the only means the jumper has to change the flight path once he or she is airborne is to change the aerodynamic lift and drag forces. The drag force (D) acts in a direction opposite to the direction of motion. The lift force (L) acts perpendicular to the drag force, or direction of motion, and tends to raise the

flight path. The formulae for calculating the lift (L) and drag (D) forces are:

$$D = (SV^2C_D)/2$$

$$L = (SV^2C_L)/2$$

where: S = area exposed to the flow
      V = relative velocity
      C_D = drag coefficient
      C_L = lift coefficient

and ($C_D + C_L$) is dependent on the size of the jumper, including angle of attack of the ski, the jumper's posture, and the equipment worn by the skier. From these equations, it can be seen that as speed (relative velocity) increases, the aerodynamic forces also increase. It also can be seen that for a given velocity, the jumper can vary the lift and drag forces by altering body and ski positions to change the area exposed to air flow as well as the lift and drag coefficients.

It is often stated that for the best flight, a ski jumper should generate large amounts of lift and only small drag forces. However, this is not possible. As lift increases, there is a corresponding increase in drag. This is explained by the increased surface area. As the lifting area increases, the drag area also increases. The most favorable or most efficient flight position is one that generates a large lift:drag ratio. The lift:drag ratio is found by dividing the lift force by the drag force. A high lift:drag ratio for a ski jumper is generally 1.0 or greater, indicating more lift than drag. However, a low lift:drag ratio (e.g., 0.67) indicates a larger drag force than lift force.

Researchers have studied the flight position and have found the optimal jumper-ski orientation for producing maximum distance in stable conditions.[1] This position is defined by four angles: (1) angle of attack (AA); (2) forward lean angle (FL); (3) trunk bend angle (TB); and (4) arm angle (Fig. 34–4).

The angle of attack (AA, Fig. 34–4) is defined as the angle between the ski and the air flow. For jumps between 70 and 90 meters, the optimal angle of attack is between 20 and 30°. As the length of the jump increases from 70 to 90 meters, or as speed increases, the angle of attack decreases. The forward lean angle (FL, Fig. 34–4) is defined as the angle measured between the ski and the extended

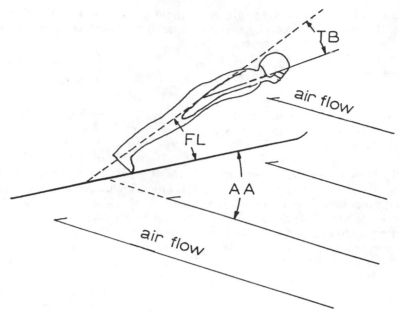

Figure 34–4. Proper flight position as described by (1) the angle of attack (AA), (2) the forward lean angle (FL), (3) the trunk bend angle (TB), and (4) the arm angle.

legs. The optimal value for this angle is 20°. The trunk bend angle (TB) is measured from the extension of the line through the legs to the trunk (see Fig. 34–4). The optimal position yields a trunk bend angle of 22°. This creates a position with the trunk being only 2° from parallel with the skis. The arm angle (not shown in Fig. 34–4) is the angle the arm makes with the trunk. An arm angle of 180° would place the arm directly along the midline of the trunk. The optimal position for the arm is slightly in front of the trunk, producing an arm angle of 165°.

It is possible to further define proper flight position by examining the positioning of the hands and skis. The hands should be held palms down as a natural extension of the arms with the little fingers four inches from the thighs. In this manner, the hands will increase the lifting surface area and therefore the lift force. Research has indicated that the skis should be four to six inches apart, which will result in the legs being fully extended and slightly spread.[1,3]

The optimal jumper-ski positioning for flight as described above has been determined for stable conditions through wind-tunnel tests and mathematical modeling.[1,5] In actual ski jumping, conditions are rarely stable, and the jumper must make modifications

in position to account for this. However, these modifications are only slight, and the optimal position described generally serves as a sound basis for most flight conditions.

After take-off, the jumper must quickly move into the stable flight position. Generally, the proper hip angle is obtained early. The angle between the legs and skis must be reduced from between 70 and 80° at 0.1 seconds after take-off to between 20 and 30° during the first 15 to 20 meters of flight. This is accomplished by utilizing the angular momentum or turning moment created during take-off and by using the aerodynamic forces to cause rotation. If the resultant aerodynamic force is acting below the center of gravity, a forward turning moment will be created and aid in the move into the strong forward-leaning flight position. If the resultant aerodynamic force is acting above the center of gravity, there will be a backward rotating moment, which will slow the move into the flight position.

The location of the resultant aerodynamic force can be altered by varying the flight position. Increasing the hip angle to expose more upper body surface area will tend to raise the location of the resultant aerodynamic forces (called the center of pressure). If the trunk is kept down, less surface area will be exposed above the center of gravity. The result will be a lower position of the center of pressure and an increased rate of forward rotation.

SUMMARY

During the flight, the jumper must move quickly into a stable flight position. The most efficient flight position is described by four angles: (1) angle of attack (the angle between the skis and airflow) should be 20 to 30°; (2) the forward lean angle (measured as the angle between the legs and skis) should be approximately 20°; (3) the trunk bend angle (angle between the extension of a line through the legs and the trunk) optimally should be 22°; and (4) the optimal arm angle (the angle between the trunk and arm) position should be 165°.

The jumper must move into the strong forward leaning position described above by utilizing the turning moment created at take-off and the aerodynamic forces to create ad-ditional turning moments. After flight position is reached, there must be a continued slight forward rotation of the jumper-ski system. However, recent studies indicate that near the end of the flight, the angle of attack should increase, and that forward rotation is not necessary. As the jumper prepares for landing, rotation is stopped, and a backward moment is created by increasing the forward lean and trunk angles and decreasing the arm angle.

REFERENCES

1. Baumann, W: The Biomechanical study of ski jumping, In Scientific Study of Skiiing in Japan. Tokyo, Japan, 1978, pp 70–95.
2. Campbell, KR: A kinematic analysis of the take-off phase in ski jumping. Unpublished master's thesis, University of Illinois, Urbana, IL, 1979.
3. Remizov, LP: Factors affecting the speed of straight descent of a downhill skier. Teorria I. Pratitka Fizicheskoi Kultury 30 (11):23–24, 1970.
4. Strauman, F: Ski jumping and its mechanics. Ski, Schweizer Jarbuch 34–64, 1927.
5. Strauman, F: Jumping style and its evaluation. Sport, Zurich, 1957.

CHAPTER 35

Ski-Jumping Injuries

JAMES R. WRIGHT, JR., M.D.

EDWARD G. HIXSON, M.D.

JAY J. RAND, B.A.

Although Scandinavians have been skiing for several thousand years, organized competitive skiing did not begin until the 1860s in Norway. These early competitions were either ski jumping or combined jumping and cross-country events. During the late 19th century, large numbers of Scandinavians immigrated to northern New England, the northern Midwest, and the Pacific Northwest, bringing ski jumping with them to North America.

Here, ski jumping competitions held during the 1880s in the new Scandinavian communities attracted national media attention and the interest of event promoters such as Barnum and Bailey. Ski-jumping exhibitions and competitions became popular attractions in the early 20th century. Professional jumpers, usually Norwegian, traveled around the country competing for large cash prizes. Promoters constructed temporary, often poorly designed, jumping hills for these spectacles. Many experienced jumpers were injured because they did not know how far they could safely jump and still land on the steep portion of the landing hill. Jumpers outjumping the hill were sometimes injured because of the harder impact of landing in the transition or on the outrun (see Chapters 33, 34, and 36). Poorly groomed landing hills, short outruns, and outrun obstacles also contributed to injuries. Inexperienced jumpers, attracted by money or challenge, were especially susceptible to injuries. Spectators came to perceive ski jumping as a very dangerous sport and ski jumpers as daredevils.

Jumping facilities and jumpers are now strictly regulated to maximize safety. Modern jumping hills (see Chapter 36) are permanent structures consisting of a carefully designed inrun scaffold or inrun contoured from the natural landscape, a landing hill of a designated size and shape, and a long outrun that is free of obstacles. The height of the starting gate at the top of the inrun is set so that most jumpers will land on the steepest portion of the landing hill and so that the best jumpers will land near, but not beyond, the critical point. If jumpers exceed the critical point, the starting gate is lowered to decrease the jumpers' takeoff velocities and the likelihood of injuries.

Ski clubs regulate access to jumping facilities during competition and training. Inexperienced jumpers train on smaller jumping hills under the supervision of coaches and must demonstrate proficiency on smaller jumping hills before advancing to larger hill sizes (see Chapter 36). This strict regulation tends to decrease the frequency of injuries.

Although several authors have suggested that jumping-related injuries are now rare,[2,4] little specific information is available in the medical literature or elsewhere pertaining to types and frequencies of Nordic ski jumping* injuries.[6,10,13] Much of the information in this chapter is from our retrospective study, in which we tabulated the types and frequencies of ski-jumping injuries that occurred at the Intervale Ski Jumping Complex in Lake Placid.[16] Selected preliminary results from an injury survey of active American ski jumpers registered with the United States Ski Association (USSA) are included where appropriate.[17]

INJURY RATES

Injury rates were estimates using data from competitions held at Intervale from

---

*Ski flying (jumping on hills with a normal point of 120 meters) is excluded from this review because detailed injury information is not available. The injury rate for ski flying is probably much higher than that for ski jumping. Nevertheless, there are very few jumpers qualified to ski fly, and there are only six FIS-approved ski-flying hills in the world.

1980 to 1985, excluding the World Cup and Olympic games. Eight injuries occurred during 1881 skier days, giving an injury rate of 4.3 injuries per 1000 skier days. We estimate that approximately 8.5 hard falls occurred per 1000 scored jumps. We were not able to estimate the injury rate during training.[16]

We also analyzed injury data for the eight World Cup competitions held at Intervale. Only one injury was sustained during 864 skier days and 2233 training, practice, or competitive jumps. We estimate that only one hard fall occurred in 902 scored jumps.[16]

Only one injury occurred at the Intervale Ski Jump Complex during the 1980 Winter Olympic games held at Lake Placid or during official training. This was a clavicular fracture sustained by a Swedish skier during his first competition jump.

These injury figures are similar to those reported for recreational Alpine skiing but are higher than those reported for cross-country skiing. Recent studies have reported Alpine skiing injury rates varying from 2.6 to 6 injuries per 1000 skier days;[5,8,12] injury rates for adolescents have been reported to be as high as 9.1 injuries per 1000 skier days.[7] Comparable figures for competitive Alpine skiing are not available, but injury rates are probably much higher than those for recreational Alpine skiing.[9] Cross-country injury rates are less than one per 1000 skier days.[3,4]

Limited injury figures for Nordic ski jumping are available from two Scandinavian studies. Eriksson surveyed all general and orthopedic surgeons in Sweden and reported that 22 ski-jumping injuries occurred in Sweden during the 1973–1974 season, but he was unable to estimate an injury rate.[6] Sandelin and colleagues[10] reported that during the 3 year period from 1976 to 1978, 39 ski-jumping injuries were reported to the insurance company that insures all competitive skiers in Finland. He estimated the annual injury rate for competitive jumping to be 4.7 percent (based on 275 licensed competitive jumpers in Finland). He reported a 1.8 percent annual injury rate for competitive Alpine skiers.

INJURY VICTIMS

The age range of injured jumpers in our retrospective study was 6 to 57 years (mean = 21.7, SD = 11.4). Of the 47 injured skiers,

21 were juniors (jumpers less than 18 years of age), 13, seniors (jumpers between 18 and 27); 8, masters (jumpers greater than 27 years of age); and 5, unclassified (jumpers of unstated age). All but one of the injured jumpers in our study were male.[16]

Webster[13] observed that injuries were rare in jumps under 12 years of age, and our data confirm this observation. Only one jumper injured during the period of our retrospective study was under the age of 12 years. Very young jumpers usually jump on small jumping hills. Lightweight jumpers on small hills cannot attain the high speeds that promote injuries (see Chapter 36).

TYPES AND FREQUENCIES OF INJURIES

Forty-seven jumpers at the Intervale Ski Jump Complex sustained 72 total injuries during the 5-year period covered by our retrospective injury study.[16] Most of these ski-jumping injuries were minor, and none resulted in permanent disability (Table 35–1). The most frequent injuries (26.4 percent) were contusions, usually involving the shoulder, knee, or elbow. Abrasions and mild concussions were also common.

Table 35–2 shows the frequency and distribution of fractures. The majority of these were nondisplaced simple fractures; none required surgical repair. Upper extremity fractures, usually involving the wrist or shoulder, outnumbered lower extremity fractures (see Table 35–2). Similarly, the ratio of upper extremity and lower extremity fractures in our survey population was 2:1.[17] In contrast, lower extremity fractures are more common than upper extremity fractures in Alpine skiers[12]. Unlike Alpine skis, jumping skis do not have metal edges that can dig into the snow and force the lower extremity to external rotation. Furthermore, the cable-binding system used to attach ski jumpers to their skis does not firmly fix the heel. Therefore, external rotation of the leg is less likely to result in fractures. Both of these features protect the ski jumper's leg. Three of the four lower extremity fractures occurring at Intervale involved the ankle. The predominance of ankle fractures is probably due to the design of jumping boots: soft construction with low top. Ankle fractures have become uncommon in Alpine skiers since the development of tall, rigid plastic ski boots.[8,12]

Dislocations accounted for 9.7 percent of injuries sustained by jumpers in our study (see Table 35–1). These included five anterior shoulder dislocations and two acromioclavicular joint separations.

Only 6.9 percent of the injuries were sprains (see Table 35–1), the most common Alpine skiing injury.[5] All sprains involved the medial collateral ligament of the knee joint. None of our survey respondents or

Table 35–1. FREQUENCIES OF VARIOUS TYPES OF SKI-JUMPING INJURIES SUSTAINED AT INTERVALE FROM 1980 TO 1985*

	Number	Percentage of Injured Jumpers	Percentage of Total Injuries
Contusions	19	40.4	26.4
Fractures	11	23.4	15.3
Abrasions	10	22.1	13.9
Concussions	7	14.9	9.7
Dislocations	7	14.9	9.7
Visceral injuries	5	10.6	6.9
Sprains	5	10.6	6.9
Muscular strain	4	8.5	5.6
Lacerations	3	6.4	4.2
Epistaxis	1	2.1	1.3
Total injured jumpers		n = 47	
Total injuries			n = 72

*Reprinted from Wright et al,[17] with permission.

Table 35–2. TYPES OF FRACTURES SUSTAINED SKI JUMPING AT INTERVALE
FROM 1980 TO 1985*

Patient	Hill Size	Type of Fracture
14-year-old male	40 m	distal radius and ulna (incomplete fx)
13-year-old male	70 m	metacarpal of thumb
16-year-old male	70 m	styloid process of radius
46-year-old male	70 m	greater tuberosity humerus (nondisplaced)
14-year-old male	?	clavicle
20-year-old male	?	tip of scapula (nondisplaced)
16-year-old male	70 m	compression fx thoracic vertebra (equivocal, x-ray −, bone scan +)
6-year-old male	15 m	proximal tibia
19-year-old male	70 m	medial malleolus ankle, chip fx (nondisplaced)
21-year-old male	70 m	medial malleolus ankle (periosteal tear only)
30-year-old male	90 m	medial malleolus ankle (nondisplaced)

*Reprinted from Wright et al,[17] with permission.

jumpers injured at Intervale suffered sprains to the ulnar collateral ligament of the metacarpophalangeal joint of the thumb ("skier's thumb"), possibly the most common injury in Alpine and cross-country skiers.[14] This observation further implicates the ski pole in the pathogenesis of skier's thumb.

Ten percent of the injured jumpers at Intervale sustained some sort of visceral injury (see Table 35–1). These included a renal contusion, two pulmonary contusions, and three ruptured spleens. All three patients with ruptured spleens required surgery. Visceral injuries are uncommon in Alpine skiing.[11]

SERIOUS INJURIES AND FATALITIES

A recent study by Webster[13] attempted to determine the frequencies of serious ski-jumping injuries (i.e., those resulting in permanent disability). He was able to determine that at least 12 serious injuries occurred in Norway between 1977 and 1981 by evaluating data from three sources: (1) the insurance company insuring all licensed Norwegian jumpers, (2) Nordic ski clubs, and (3) all Norwegian hospitals. These included three cervical fractures with spinal transections, an intracerebral hematoma/contusion requiring resection of a temporal lobe, two leg amputations, a unilateral blindness, and five lower extremity fractures with subsequent complications. Webster[13] estimated that serious injuries occur in 0.003 percent of ski jumps (based on 2200 registered ski jumpers aver-

aging an estimated 400 jumps each per year). He estimated that the risk of being seriously injured during a 5-year period was approximately 5 percent, but he was not able to estimate the frequency of nondisabling injuries.

No serious or debilitating injuries occurred at the Intervale Ski Jump Complex during the period of our retrospective study.[16] Our study suggests that serious injuries are extremely rare at well-maintained, modern ski-jumping hills like Intervale. Data from Intervale cannot be extrapolated to estimate the overall frequency of serious injuries in the United States because injury rates are affected by variables such as hill maintenance and design (see Chapter 36). These depend largely on the age of the ski jump and the budget of the ski club maintaining the jumping facility. Obviously, our survey of active ski jumpers is biased toward healthy athletes.[17] Serious injuries or fatalities would be missed because these athletes would no longer be able to compete, would not be active members of the USSA, and would not have received questionnaires. The results of our survey cannot be used to estimate the frequencies of serious injuries.

A group of seasoned jumpers, former jumpers, and jumping officials from the USA's Eastern, Central, and Rocky Mountain divisions as well as the far West (a region that no longer has any active jumping facilities) were informally surveyed to estimate the number of serious injuries and fatalities that have occurred at jumps in North America. A list of six jumping fatalities occurring since 1939 was compiled. All occurred on older-style jumps built prior to Federation Internationale de Ski (FIS) standards (see Chapter 36). There have been no Nordic ski-jumping fatalities in the last decade. The fatality rate for Nordic ski jumping, estimated to be roughly 12 fatalities per 100,000 participants annually, appears to be within the range for other "risky" outdoor sports. Cervical fractures appear to be the most frequent fatal ski-jumping injury.[15]

It is more difficult to estimate the number of jumpers paralyzed, because our experts were frequently unable to remember them by name; they were remembered only by the location of the jump and the approximate date. It appears that these incidents are almost as rare as fatalities (see Chapter 36). However, several have resulted in litigation with large settlements for the injured jumpers.

TYPES OF FALLS

Falls can be divided into three types: inrun falls, falls in which the jumper lost control at take-off or while in the air, and outrun falls. Inrun falls occur when a jumper loses balance before he or she reaches the take-off point. Inrun falls are exceedingly rare and are due to uneven snow conditions, usually unexpected spots of new snow in the track, which result in sudden deceleration. These jumpers either fall forward onto the knoll or off the side of the inrun scaffold. All three of the spinal cord transections in Webster's study[13] occurred in this type of fall. He also suggested that this type of fall may be associated with the use of exceesively high heel blocks. Heel blocks, designed to allow the jumper to reach the airfoil position earlier by moving the jumper's center of gravity forward, make the jumper more susceptible to losing balance when encountering small decelerations in the inrun track. Bland[2] reports that concussions and shoulder injuries occur frequently during inrun falls.

Falls resulting from the jumper losing control immediately after take-off (i.e., while in the air) happen when the skier starts the jump too early and is unable to keep the ski tips angled upward to form an airfoil. Bland[2] considers these falls to be the most serious type because the jumper lands on the head and/or shoulder. Some of these falls result in hyperextension of the neck and, if the hyperextension is severe, cervical compression fractures. Fortunately, these serious injuries are exceedingly rare.

Falls on the landing hill and outrun are the most frequent type. Falls on the steep portion of the landing hill tend to be less serious than those described above because the trajectory of the jumper parallels the angle of the landing hill (see Chapter 33 and 34). Therefore, the impact of the fall is minimized, and a fallen jumper merely slides down the slope of the landing hill, dissipating the kinetic energy. If a jumper travels too far in the air (i.e., outjumps the hill) and lands in the transition, the impact upon landing will be great and the probability of a hard fall is increased.

FACTORS AFFECTING INJURY RATES

Various factors affect injury rates. Foremost among these is the weather. Gusting winds are very hazardous (see Chapter 36). A gusting head wind can suddenly lift the ski tips, causing the jumper to pitch forward abruptly. Loss of the gust suddenly lessens the air resistance against the skis and jumper. Consequently, a tip roll can occur, especially if the air pressure gets on top of the skis. A sudden, strong crosswind can pull the lengthy jumping skis to the side and cause the jumper to land perpendicular to the landing hill. Constant head winds and tail winds are not usually dangerous for experienced jumpers but may confuse less experienced jumpers.

The landing hill should be very smooth and firm so that the jumper's skis do not sink or catch an edge. Warm weather or big snowfalls soften the landing hill (see Chapter 36). Furthermore, a fallen jumper's shoulder, arm, or other body part may dig into a soft landing hill and become fixed while the jumper is traveling very fast. These injuries are usually preventable by proper hill grooming (see Chapter 36).

Jumping on plastic during the summer is a very recent development, and, as such, it may be premature to evaluate whether injury rates are different (see Chapter 33). However, our retrospective study suggests that summer jumping has a higher injury rate than winter jumping. The injury rate for competitive ski jumping on plastic was four times higher than the injury rate for competitive jumping on snow.[16] However, this observation is based on relatively few skier days. At this time, few jumping facilities are equipped with plastic and, therefore, few jumpers have very extensive experience on plastic. As plastic jumping becomes more commonplace, the rate of injury will probably decrease. The most frequent summer injuries are contusions and abrasions from falling and sliding on the plastic mats. There is no evidence that the frequency of more serious injuries is increased on plastic-covered jumping hills.

More than 60 percent of the athletes responding to our injury survey believe that summer jumping is more dangerous than winter jumping.[17] They suggested that this is due to the following factors: (1) plastic mats are hard and abrasive, (2) plastic outruns are often too short or narrow, (3) plastic requires more self-confidence, and (4) plastic mats deteriorate, resulting in speed variations. Only about 20 percent of surveyed jumpers believed that winter jumping is more dangerous. These jumpers suggested that plastic was safer because the conditions were constant; whereas snow conditions vary depending on the weather.

PREVENTION OF INJURIES

The frequency of injuries increases when jumping hills are soft or poorly groomed, when winds are strong and variable, and when inexperienced jumpers attempt to jump on larger hills than their skills permit. The relatively low incidence of ski-jumping injuries can be attributed to strict regulation of the jumpers and ski-jumping facilities by the individual ski clubs, the USSA, and the FIS (see Chapter 36). Improvements in the design of jumping hills during the past few decades have probably also contributed to lower injury rates.*

In our survey of active ski jumpers, we asked the athletes for suggestions about how ski-jumping safety could be improved. The most frequent suggestions were (1) improve maintenance of landing hill and outrun surfaces, (2) cancel competitions when conditions are adverse, (3) improve binding design, and (4) establish strict criteria for advancement to larger jump sizes.[17]

As is true of most sports, training should be supervised whenever possible. This serves both to prevent injuries and to facilitate management of injuries when they do occur. In addition, jumpers should be in excellent physical and psychologic condition.[1] Ski jumping requires strength, timing, balance, depth perception, and concentration. Although athletes who are ill may still want to compete, they should be discouraged from jumping.

ACKNOWLEDGMENTS

We are indebted to the Lake Placid Sports Medicine Society for sponsoring our studies and to the Olympic Regional Development Authority of Lake Placid and the United States Ski Association for their cooperation.

We would also like to thank our panel of ski-jumping experts: Hermod Bakke, Dr. Phil Bland, Ed Brisson, Dave Bradley, Nic Cohen, Stan DuRose, Tom Harrington, Don Kinney, Dr. Jack Koenig, Warren Lowry, Bill Mahre, Al Merrill, Gus Raaum, Lloyd Severud, Ralph Symalla, Dr. Frank Trudeau, and Dr. Don West.

Finally, we would like to recognize the recent centennial year of competitive ski jumping in North America. The first competition was held in Red Wing, Minnesota, in 1887.

REFERENCES

1. Allaria, A: Snow skiing (jumping). In Larson, LA (ed): Encyclopedia of Sports Sciences and Medicine. MacMillan, New York, 1971, pp 469–470.

---

*Several improvements on the design of ski-jumping hills have been instituted during the past two decades, and they appear to have made jumping a safer sport. Older, less aerodynamically efficient ski-jumping techniques required that the jumper be projected high into the air and then "free fall" while flying horizontally. The modern jumping style is aerodynamically more efficient. The jumper actually mimics an airfoil and generates lift. Therefore, the modern jumper can fly farther without having to gain as much altitude (i.e., the vertical component of the flight curve relative to the horizontal component has decreased). This has allowed the landing curve to be redesigned. The modern ski-jump landing hill is not as steep, and as a result, the knoll and transition are not as flat. These have increased the margin of safety because the landing hill more closely resembles the flight curve on very long and very short jumps.

2. Bland, PT: Ski jumping injuries. Physician and Sportsmedicine 3:63–66, 1975.
3. Boyle, JJ, Johnson, RJ, Pope, MH, Pierce, JC, and Brady, MM: Cross-country skiing injuries. In Johnson, RJ and Mote, CD (eds): Skiing Trauma and Safety: Fifth International Symposium. American Society for Testing and Materials, Philadelphia, 1985, pp 411–422.
4. Clancy, WG and McConkey, JP: Nordic and alpine skiing. In Schneider, RC, Kennedy, JC, and Plant, ML (eds): Sports Injuries: Mechanisms, Prevention, and Treatment. Williams & Wilkins, Baltimore, 1984, pp 247–270.
5. Ellison, AE: Skiing injuries. Ciba Clinical Symposia 29:1–40, 1977.
6. Eriksson, E: Ski inuries in Sweden: A one year survey. Ortho Clin North Am 7:3–9, 1976.
7. Garrick, JG and Requa, RK: Injury patterns in children and adolescent skiers. Am J Sports Med 7:245–248, 1979.
8. Johnson, RJ, Ettlinger, CF, Campbell, RJ, and Pope, MH: Trends in skiing injuries: Analysis of a 6-year study (1972 to 1978). Am J Sports Med 8:106–113, 1980.
9. Margreiter, R, Raas, E, Lugger, LJ: The risk of injury in expereinced alpine skiers. Ortho Clin North Am 7:51–53, 1976.
10. Sandelin, J, Kiviluoto, O, Santavirta, S: Injuries of competitive skiers in Finland: A three year study. Annales Chirurgiae et Gynaecologiae 69:97–101, 1980.
11. Scharplatz, D, Thurleman, K, and Enderlin, F: Thoracoabdominal trauma in ski accidents. Injury 10:86–91, 1978.
12. Tapper, EM: Ski injuries from 1939 to 1976: The Sun Valley experience. Am J Sports Med 6:114–121, 1978.
13. Webster, K: Serious ski jumping injuries in Norway. Am J Sports Med 13:124–127, 1985.
14. Wright, J: Skier's thumb. Ski Patrol Magazine 2:38–39, 1986.
15. Wright, JR: Nordic ski jumping fatalities in the United States: A 50 year summary. Journal of Trauma 28:848–851, 1988.
16. Wright, JR, Hixson, EG, and Rand, JJ: Injury patterns in Nordic ski jumpers: A retrospective analysis of injuries occurring at the Intervale ski jump complex from 1980 to 1985. Am J Sports Med 14:393–397, 1986.
17. Wright, JR, Hixson, EG, and Rand, JJ: Nordic ski jumping injuries: A survey of active American jumpers. (In preparation.)

CHAPTER 36

Ski Jumping Hills

JEFF HASTINGS, B.S.

DAVID BRADLEY, M.D.

Ski jumping is unique. No other sport packs such excitement, poise, finesse, and occasional glory into so few seconds. The whole intense experience—even on the big hills—lasts only 25 seconds, whereas the controlling instant—the act of launching out to catch the air—must be carried out in a fraction of a second. Then the jumper is alone with his or her destiny.

With jumping, the skier rides an invisible wave of air (Fig. 36–1), a curved medium the skier must foresee and grasp and feel on the body—the chest, the face, and especially the feet.

AERODYNAMICS

The glory of modern ski jumping is in its aerodynamic flight (see Chapter 34). This is the vision all young jumpers hold. Figure 36–2 is a photograph of Mike Holland riding to a new world's record of 189 meters on the Yugoslav ski-flying hill. Note carefully the skis and ankles, the relaxed legs and body, and the face. The aerodynamic benefits of leaning out over the skis are obvious. A jumper who jumps and stands vertically in the air will meet a strong wind resistance and be dropped back down to earth before the flight has begun. A jumper who minimizes wind resistance by jumping forward with the chest down will float and feel the air supporting him or her. The photograph clearly shows that the jumper's position in the air—

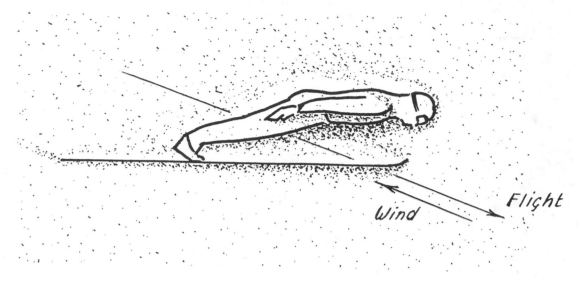

Figure 36–1.

stream approaches that of a proper airfoil, similar to the cross section of a subsonic airplane wing. Air is compressed along the incident surfaces of skis, legs, chest, and head, while a partial vacuum develops along the jumper's back. Both provide lift. Lifting is most clearly seen on large jumps, where higher inrun and air speeds amplify its effect. Occasionally in ski flying, the best jumpers actually fly away from the ground, gaining relative altitude as they glide down the hill. Only by breaking out of their flight position,

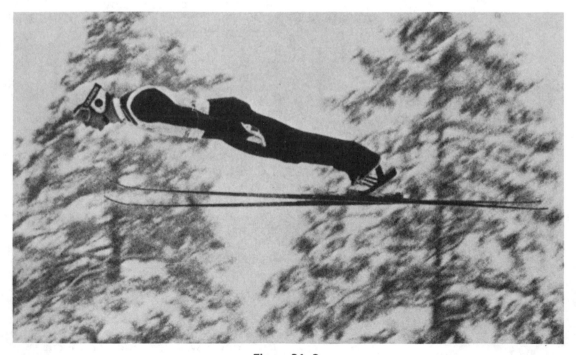

Figure 36–2.

and thereby breaking the airfoil, are these jumpers able to avoid outjumping the landing hill.

INJURIES

Most people consider ski jumping dangerous. Racing down the slope at speeds of 100 km per hour, the jumper must be committed, whether the take-off is good or bad. If the take-off is good, the result will be an act of pure ecstasy. The skier will fly for 5 or 6 seconds and land with two slim planks of wood on an inclined slope, then ride it out standing. With a "perfect" take-off, the transition from snow to air is natural. A good flight position is simply the extension of a good take-off move. If the take-off is bad, the ski jumper will struggle to catch up with the flight, but serious accidents are infrequent.

By and large, serious ski-jumping injuries are similar to those seen among Alpine skiers (see Chapters 35 and 39), but there are no obstructions on a jumping hill. As a result, ski jumpers need not fear that their bodies may be hurled against trees or may go over cliffs. We can recall only three ski-jumping fatalities and two accidents resulting in paraplegia over the past 6 decades. In each case the accident was much more the result of bad hill design, poor snow preparation, or foolish official judgment than it was the skier's error. Even broken bones are rare. This is because there are no obstructions on a jumping hill

and because loose bindings let the skis fly off during a hard fall. Sprained ankles and knees occur almost always as a result of soft or rutted conditions in the dip. Torn ligaments of the knee and dislocations of the shoulder also happen occasionally.

SKI HILLS

The laws of physics being what they are, a skier's flight must follow closely the parabolic curve of falling bodies. Therefore, in the design, the hill engineer has only to compute the take-off speed and then fit a nice parabola of wide smooth snow under the jumper (see Chapter 35, page 329, footnote). Figure 36–3 demonstrates the elements of a jumping hill. Galileo's laws are absolute for small hills, where air pressure is minimal. Whatever may be the forward speed at take-off, the jumper will drop 4 feet in the first half second, 16 feet in 1 second, 64 feet in 2 seconds, and so on.[2]

However, the situation is very different on big hills, where air is moving past the skier at 50 to 80 mph. Here,

distance = parabola of fall, shortened by drag, extended by lift.

On larger hills, drag and lift become huge components. A jumper moving from a 40-meter hill (take-off velocity about 40 mph) to a ski-flying hill (80 mph) will have to deal with four times more wind pressure on the

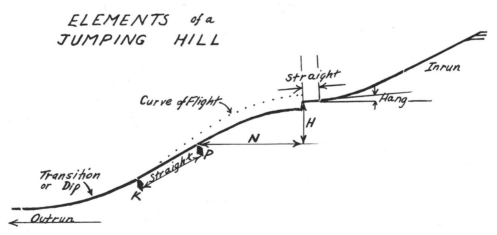

Figure 36–3.

larger hill. Thus, the poor jumper, fighting the air, will land well up on the knoll, but the real flyer may float 200 feet further and seem in danger of coming down in the parking lot.

Fortunately, such serious variables of flight and distance scarcely exist with small hills and beginning jumpers. Here, wind is no problem, and changing snow conditions can be handled in a commonsense way. Parents will worry eternally, of course, but the boys and girls can go ahead and jump.

Small Hills

The speed, the drop, the time in air, and the impact of landing—even on a small hill—are unfamiliar and awesome to the beginning ski jumper. A young jumper's early anxieties are perfectly natural, but if the hill is a good one and the snow is packed hard and smooth, there is really little danger.

Confidence is what young jumpers learn on small hills. Confidence is the sine qua non, the essential mind-set, of good ski jumpers. Confidence comes in stages, in learning little by little, and practicing over and over the basic skills:

- good inrun position
- quickness and timing on the take-off
- jumping off the whole foot
- jumping up and out, over the ski tips
- holding tips up, skis parallel
- floating, poised in air, and preparing for landing
- landing softly and in good balance

In the course of making thousands of jumps on many different hills, the young ski jumper also will learn to analyze what different hills will do to him or her. The young jumper will learn how to deal with wind, how to remain balanced on bumpy air, and how to sustain a confident flight.

Big Hills

By international requirements, big hills (70 and 90 meters) must be designed by a certified hill engineer. A jumping jury and a technical delegate are appointed to oversee safety and to assure fairness at each sanctioned competition. All officials are required to follow Federation Internationale de Ski (FIS) rules regarding permissible snow and wind conditions.

Safety Considerations

Two danger areas in all jumping hills, big or small, are depicted in Figure 36–4. These areas demand the most care in snow preparation and the most expert attention during practice or competition. Especially in these areas, patches of ice, sticky new snow, mushy corn snow, or bumps and ruts can create conditions difficult for skiers to manage. These zones are special because the centrifugal force of a rapid change of direction piles 2 to 3 G on a jumper just when balance means everything. The upper curve comes suddenly when the ski jumper is readying all faculties for the crucial act of flinging himself or herself out on the air. The lower curve comes when the jumper has maximum speed in the most vertical part of the flight, when the jumper must absorb the impact of land-

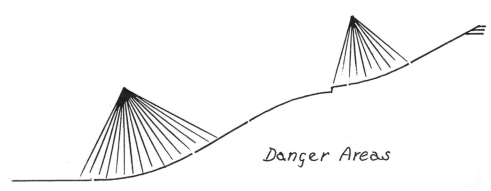

Danger Areas

Figure 36–4.

ing at 80 mph and finish the jump with a flourish of grace and balance.

Three special problems need to be mentioned:

1. *Inrun Speed.* It is possible for a good jumper to jump beyond the K point into the upper part of the transition. This is of no particular harm if that transition is not quick. A sudden change of climatic conditions causing damp snow to begin freezing, or a wrong decision on the part of race officials, can throw a jumper well beyond K into a crash.

Hence all big hills have photoelectric cells placed on the take-off to give officials fair and timely warning as to changes in take-off velocity (Vo). Furthermore, all big hills must have a mechanism for changing the starting point in order to hold take-off speeds to a reasonable optimum.

This is vital, because on big hills it is very hard indeed to predict how far a good jumper will fly. A mere increase of 2 km per hour on the take-off can make a difference of 10 to 12 meters down below. A good jumper might just crank a perfect jump or get the lift of a perfect breeze up the landing hill and ride right over the K point.

Fortunately, small hills do not pose such speed and/or distance problems.

2. *Wind.* Although wind is not a serious problem on small hills, gusty, puffy, or rolling side wind is a frequent complication and sometimes a danger on big hills where a good ski jumper can stay aloft for 5 seconds or more. Occasionally, although rarely, a meet must simply be postponed or canceled because of wind. Therefore, the help of a good meteorologist with local experience is absolutely necessary in conducting a ski-jumping event.

3. *Snow.* If a hill has been left unprepared and soft, it must be compacted and hardened. Small hills can be set up by boot tramping top to bottom, including the outrun. Large hills always require special mechanical rolling and scraping equipment.

When a new storm dumps a half foot of powder on a well-prepared hill, it should be shoveled off. The whole hill should be cleaned, with particular attention paid to the danger areas noted above. If a warm spell or rain followed by freezing has changed the hill to a small glacier, the surface should be scarified, and salt should be mixed with the snow at about 20 pounds for a 40-meter hill in order to get a good skiing surface.

Conversely, if the weather has suddenly turned warm, leaving the take-off and landing like mush, it may be advisable to rake in some form of "snow cement," which can actually freeze snow and keep it hard for a few hours. Some use ammonium chloride or rock salt. Others prefer ammonium nitrate fertilizer, which acts more slowly. Chemicals are tricky, however. Sometimes just the opposite result will occur. On a small hill, one may judiciously experiment with chemicals, but on a big hill, a recognized expert should be called.

ACCIDENTS

In any major competition, and in any big hill jumping, the responsible officials must anticipate accidents. Ski patrol or first-aid people need to have special training in handling injuries to the head and neck. Jaw screws, airways and oxygen, toboggans, blankets, and snowmobiles always should be present. Ambulances, of course, should be in readiness. And in remote locations, a helicopter directed to a good general hospital is often the best way to care for a seriously injured skier.

Finally, jumping helmets are light and strong. Young jumpers should get used to protective helmets right from their first days on small hills. Young jumpers should be outfitted with, and appropriately use, safe clothing, skis, boots, and bindings. Horseplay on the hill should not be tolerated.

CONCLUSION

Figures 36–5, 36–6, and 36–7 represent the best ski-jumping styles of 1900, 1925, and 1948. How far the evolution had to come! In Figure 36–5, we see essentially a small-hill style on a medium-size hill. In Figure 36–6 and Figure 36–7, the jumpers' heels are held down much too tightly by cable bindings adapted from downhill skiing. Therefore, the ski tips cannot ride up and plane on the wind.

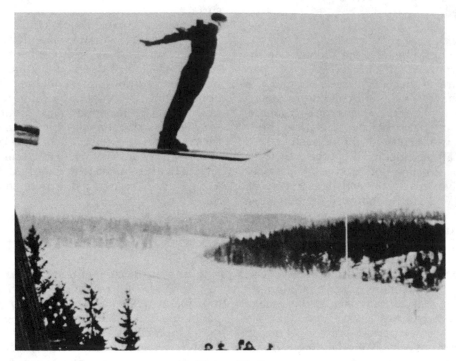

Figure 36—5.

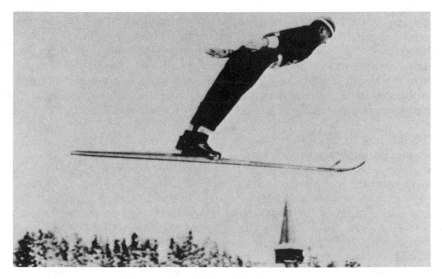

Figure 36—6.

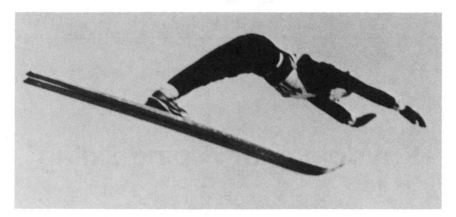

Figure 36–7.

Following World War II, the modern style emerged, and present-day jumpers are flying the length of two football fields. Now look back once more to Mike Holland's jump (Figure 36–2). He is flying almost 600 feet, yet he looks relaxed, loose, happy, even playful, as though he were body surfing on the air. No words could so graphically portray the importance of proper hill design and maintenance, strict adherence to official rules regarding snow and wind conditions, and the prompt availability of first-aid and evacuation equipment to ensuring the safety of ski-jumping athletes.

REFERENCES

1. Bradley, DJ: Ski Jumping, ed 2. R Burt, Hanover, NH, 1964.
2. Bradley, D, Miller, R, and Merrill, A: Expert Skiing. Holt, Rinehart & Winston, New York, 1960.
3. Federation Internationale de Ski: International Ski Competition, Book 3: Joint Regulations for Ski Jumping, Ski Flying, and Nordic Combined Competition. Dühlmann and Company, Bern, Switzerland, 1983.

CHAPTER 37

Physiology of Alpine Skiing

GENE R. HAGERMAN, Ph.D.

The recreational or competitive Alpine skier must adequately prepare for many things. These may include environmental encounters (e.g., altitude, sun, storms, terrain), equipment selection, and physical and mental preparation. To enjoy and/or to compete in this physically demanding sport requires a knowledge of how the body functions and what a skier can do for training preparation. Having the opportunity to be a member of the United States Alpine Ski Team's Sportsmedicine Council for the past eight years has demonstrated to me the importance of complementing physical training with physiology.

PHYSIOLOGIC COMPONENTS

The physiology of Alpine skiing emphasizes general fitness (aerobic, anaerobic, and flexibility); motor fitness (balance, agility, and coordination); and body composition. Each of these physiologic components has specific requirements as part of dry-land training or on-snow preparation.

General Fitness

During Alpine skiing the majority of propulsive force is provided by gravity. In the absence of active work to prevent descent, the skier will come down the hill more or less without effort. Thus, the dominant locomotor problem for the Alpine skier represents the control of motion down the hill. Muscular activity is required to Alpine ski, and this activity is dependent on the breakdown of adenosine triphosphate (ATP), a high-energy chemical bond. Some ATP is available in skeletal muscle cells for immediate use, but a majority of ATP is stored as cellular substrates (carbohydrates and fats) that must undergo a chemical breakdown in the muscle cell prior to producing ATP. There are two metabolic pathways that use ATP for muscle contraction: aerobic and anaerobic. Aerobic metabolism requires the presence of oxygen. During extended periods of skiing at low to moderate intensity, ATP is generally readily available. Substrates for aerobic metabolism are carbohydrates, fats, and a trace of protein. On the other hand, anaerobic metabolism does not use oxygen for the production of ATP but relies on stored carbohydrates (muscle glycogen). Anaerobically, the chemical breakdown of muscle glycogen is known as glycolysis, and lactic acid is an end product of this process. Anaerobic metabolism is very important during short-duration, high-intensity Alpine skiing.

Another integral component of general fitness is flexibility. This can be described as the range of movement at an anatomic joint and its surrounding connective tissue. Without adequate flexibility, energy production in the muscles may not be adequately transferable into useful work.

Muscular Fitness

Leg muscles will contract repeatedly in a dynamic and static manner during skiing. Muscles of the torso need to be developed for total body balance, stabilization, coordination, and pole planting.

Muscular strength or the ability to exert an all-out force for a maximum effort in a muscle or muscle group is the basis for strength training. Because Alpine skiing relies on repeated contractions over a period of time, muscular endurance must also be a part of the training program. As the skier becomes more proficient and needs to turn quicker and respond faster, muscular power becomes an important factor. The skill level of the skier will dictate the aforementioned strength-training modes. Elite competitive skiers should incorporate all three (strength, power, and endurance) in their training programs to accommodate for speed, snow, and

terrain changes. Beginners and intermediates should concentrate on strength and endurance.

World class Alpine ski racers need muscular strength, power, and endurance to perform the slalom, giant slalom, super g, and downhill events. In the World Cup competitions, men ski a slalom course in 50 to 55 seconds, giant slalom in 1:00 to 1:15 minutes, super g in 1:30 to 1:50 minutes, and downhill in 2:00 to 2:30 minutes. Men's courses are slightly longer than women's courses. Muscular fitness can be developed through aerobic and anaerobic training sessions, but more specifically by using strength-training equipment. This equipment should usually be some combination of free weights or specialized machines. In addition, body-weight exercises or stretch-cord exercisers made of surgical tubing can provide excellent means of muscular strength training when the athlete travels. A strength-training regimen should parallel general and motor fitness programs.

While directing the Sports Physiology Laboratory for the United States Olympic Committee at Squaw Valley, California (1977–1980), I had an opportunity to evaluate isokinetic leg strength in the men's and women's US Alpine Ski Team. These elite skiers recorded some of the highest values for leg strength relative to body weight compared with US Olympic athletes.[2]

Motor Fitness

Coordination, the neuromuscular integration or development of a natural or smooth technique, is the result of balance and agility. Physically "weighting and unweighting" on skis is a form of balance which requires correct weight distribution and body harmony. To move quickly with fluid or smooth body motions involves the agility aspect of neuromuscular control. Motor fitness skills are part of the kinesthetic or body positioning sense, an important learning process for Alpine skiing.

Acquiring the motor skills of balance, agility, and coordination at too late an age may affect the elite racer's opportunity of making it to the top. Usually these skills are nurtured during the early years of growing up and demand repeated neuromuscular movements so that the learned skills become part of the brain's computer center. Generally, the world's top ski racers started skiing at a very early age.

Because Alpine skiing involves more than aerobic, anaerobic, and strength training, development of motor skills is important for both elite and recreational skiers. There is debate as to what extent motor skills can be acquired by the older athlete. Obviously, skills learned later in life need to be programmed and repeated for correct neuromuscular control. Thereby, neural positioning and control usually improve with time, so the skier must be patient and motivated for this improvement to take place. Participation in other skill sports and/or exercises may assist the older skier in developing coordination, balance, and agility.

Body Composition

Body composition can be defined as the proportions of the body that are comprised of fat and fat-free tissue (e.g., muscle, bone). Physiologically, most advanced and elite skiers have a lower percentage of body fat than the general population. This does not suggest that the lower the body fat, the better the skier. But it does recommend that each skier will benefit from maintaining a desired body weight that transfers into efficient skiing performance. Body weight can be altered with adequate nutrition and exercise habits (see also Chapters 2 and 4).

Body composition evaluations using skinfold calipers, underwater weighing, and a couple of new "high-tech" systems can estimate the percentage of body fat. Body fat percentages for the general population range from 13 to 18 percent for young men and 22 to 27 percent for young women. Elite male Alpine racers are from 8 to 11 percent fat, and elite women range from 15 to 20 percent fat (see Chapter 6).

PHYSIOLOGIC APPLICATION

Once the physiologic components have been ascertained, the skier can begin to understand functional application.

Flexibility

Stretching or flexibility exercises are usually incorporated during the warm-up before a training session or a day of skiing and again after the session during cool-down. Some skiers will often perform a series of two or three stretches after a chair lift or T-bar ride. A flexibility program assists in preparing the muscles of the body for the skiing activity, thereby preventing muscle and surrounding soft tissue injuries, and alleviating muscle soreness. A flexibility program should emphasize the upper and lower body and use at least three to four exercises for each. The athlete should concentrate on static stretching without any bouncing movements. The stretch should be held for 15 to 30 seconds and repeated a total of three times. Flexibility regimens are important not only for exercise programs but also for rehabilitation of athletic injuries.

Aerobic and Anaerobic

Alpine skiers should combine aerobic and anaerobic metabolism as part of their training tools. The type of terrain, snow conditions, length of run, and skiing ability of the skier will dictate the need for one or the other. Every skier needs some type of aerobic base or foundation. If the skier wishes to complete tighter, faster turns, it is necessary for the anaerobic component of fitness to be included in the training program. Aerobic and anaerobic sessions can be practiced either on snow or during dry land training.

To develop aerobic and anaerobic training concepts, a basic understanding of skeletal muscle is imperative. Skeletal muscles are composed of two fiber types: slow (type I, red) and fast (type II, white) twitch fibers. The properties of each fiber type vary, but generally, aerobic (or endurance) training develops the slow twitch muscle fibers, whereas anaerobic (or sprint) training is more specific to fast twitch fibers. The human body is not capable of changing twitch fiber types slow to fast (or vice versa). Fiber type ratios can cover a broad spectrum in human skeletal muscle, but the elite Alpine skier has approximately equal distribution of fast and slow twitch muscle fibers. The general nonathlete population has similar muscle fiber distribution. This half-and-half ratio is important to the Alpine skier, because downhill, giant slalom, and slalom racing and all levels of recreational skiing require slow twitch muscles for sustaining power and endurance, whereas the fast twitch muscles are used for balance, coordination, dynamic power, and quickness. The Alpine skier can develop these fiber types to their potential through well-organized aerobic and anaerobic training programs.

Aerobic development should involve a minimum of 30 minutes, three to four times per week. The frequency, duration, and intensity of training can be progressively increased as the skier becomes more fit. Intensity or the degree of difficulty per session will vary for each individual. Heart rate monitoring using light finger pressure on the carotid artery or a heart rate watch is ideal for intensity calculation.

After at least 8 weeks of aerobic training, the skier should begin to use one or two high-intensity anaerobic training workouts. These workouts can consist of jog-run intervals, speed hiking, and bike sprints or intervals. When anaerobic training is done, the intensity is higher but still controlled. As the skier works anaerobically, lactic acid (a metabolic end product) is formed. This is the result of insufficient oxygen to the working muscles, so the muscle cells must rely on the incomplete breakdown of stored glycogen for energy. As the training intensifies, lactic acid accumulation escalates. Too much lactate in muscle cells can prevent adequate muscle contraction and lead to fatigue. Lactic acid usually forms in the fast twitch muscle fibers, because slow twitch fibers contain a low anaerobic capacity. A specific problem encountered with Alpine skiing is the intense or forceful contractions of the leg muscles. In many instances the circulation of the blood to the legs is inhibited; this produces an anaerobic environment. During aerobic training it is very important to maintain an intensity that does not extend into the anaerobic zone, because this will result in excessive build-up of lactic acid. On the other hand, anaerobic training with proper rest intervals permits the skier to develop the anaerobic energy system in a methodic, progressive manner. By progressively training the anaerobic system, the skier becomes more able to tolerate increases in lactic acid production.

Nutrition

The primary nutritional fuels for muscular energy are carbohydrates and fats; protein may supply a very small percentage. Carbohydrates are converted into blood glucose and glycogen, a storage form of glucose. Glycogen can be found in skeletal muscles as well as in the liver. Fats are carried in the blood as free fatty acids and stored as triglycerides in skeletal muscle and adipose tissue. A day of Alpine skiing can deplete muscle glycogen stores in both the fast and slow twitch muscle fibers. In fact, skiing injuries at the end of the day may be a direct result of lowered glycogen stores. Fats are not an important fuel for Alpine skiing; however, dryland training sessions of longer duration may call on fat utilization for muscular fuel.

Good nutritional habits are important for elite as well as recreational skiers (see Chapter 4). Well-balanced meals from the four food groups form the basis for good nutrition. If necessary, these may be supplemented with one or two nutritional snacks. An often forgotten dietary need during dryland training and/or Alpine skiing is fluid replacement. This may be particularly important at higher altitudes, because there the amount of insensible water loss is increased (see Chapters 42 and 43). Water is the best form of fluid replacement, but several commercially prepared electrolyte drinks and fruit juices are very good substitutes.

Strength Training

Both recreational and elite Alpine skiers are constantly using muscle groups throughout the body, whether skiing or doing dryland training. To develop these muscles, strength training should be undertaken at least two to three days per week. Three or four exercises should be assigned to the upper body, and two to three to the lower body. Generally, three to four sets of 10 repetitions for each exercise are adequate. A lifting sequence can be performed via the traditional method in which all three sets are completed for one exercise before starting the next exercise. The more popular method is circuit training. The circuit is organized into stations for each exercise, and the athlete completes one set of an exercise before moving to the next station. The United States Alpine Ski Team uses a combination of both methods.

Development of leg strength is very important for Alpine skiing, because this will be the key factor for controlling dynamic and static muscular movements. A strength-training program, unlike aerobic or anaerobic training sessions, can specifically emphasize muscular training. Through strength training there can be hypertrophy of the muscle cells, some increased metabolic capacities, and concomitant gains in muscle tissue mass. Although on-snow skiing will also develop the muscular functions needed to ski all types of terrain and conditions, a strength-training program will assist in preparing those muscles prior to getting on snow (see Chapter 2). When skiing, both the fast and slow twitch muscle fibers are recruited. The advanced skier uses a higher percentage of slow twitch muscle fibers than the beginning skier. This suggests that more highly skilled skiers are performing more efficiently.

Motor Performance

During dry-land or on-snow training, motor skill activities or exercises should complement the remainder of the skier's program. These activities should include eye–hand and eye–foot coordination, visual recognition, balance, and simple-to-complex movement patterns. The following is a list of suggested activities: basketball, diving, ice skating, karate, racquetball, soccer, tennis, volleyball, water skiing, and wind surfing. An outdoor or indoor "homemade" general and motor fitness circuit using body-weight exercises can also assist in motor skill development.

SUMMARY OF TRAINING

The United States Alpine Ski Team trains on a year-round basis (see also Chapter 2). Upon completion of the World Cup circuit at the end of March, the month of April is one of rest and relaxation. Off-season dry-land training begins in May and continues until the middle of August. The middle of August until the first of November constitutes the preseason. The competitive season continues from November until the end of March. These elite skiers will be on snow during the off season and the preseason for a total of 1 to 2 months prior to the first race. Dry-land training sessions are individually organized for the team members and require a few hours each day. When on-snow camps con-

vene during the offseason and preseason, 4 to 6 hours of skiing are followed by 1 to 2 hours of dry-land training. During the competitive season, dry-land sessions are held three times a week for maintenance purposes. During on-snow training, the skiers repeat training runs and receive technical advice. The purpose is to learn how to tolerate and maximize performance sessions leading to race day.

Of course, training for the recreational skier will be different from that for a member of the United States Ski Team. However, recreational skiers should consider a program that at least will prepare them in advance for the first on-snow experience. If the end of November is the target ski date, recreational skiers should begin dry-land training workouts at least 10 to 12 weeks before that date. The major difference between the elite and recreational skiers' programs is the manipulation of the following training variables: (1) frequency, (2) duration, and (3) intensity of training. Workout sessions require time, and the amount of time devoted to training will always be individualized. Each of the physiologic components deserves specific attention in every case, and a variety in training workouts will assist in alleviating boredom.

An example training week for the recreational skier may include a daily 5-minute warm-up and cool-down, aerobic and/or anaerobic training of 30 to 40 minutes three to four days per week, and strength training of 30 minutes three days per week. One should be progressive in the dry-land training schedule; for motivational purposes, a simple training diary may be kept. Without adequate maintenance training (at least 2 to 3 days per week) during the ski season, the physiologic components achieved through dry-land training will not be maintained during the skiing season.

SUMMARY

When the principles of neuromuscular physiology are applied to the demands of Alpine skiing, a rational program emerges that is composed of the following elements: flexibility exercises, aerobic and anaerobic training, strength training, and motor performance training. This work is fueled by proper nutrition and adequate fluid replacement. The elite Alpine skier's required dedication to year-round training should inspire the serious recreational skier to undertake preseason preparation and continue maintenance conditioning throughout the ski season. By so doing, the risk of injury may be diminished, and the fitness gains and joy from skiing will be enhanced.

REFERENCES

1. Fox, EL: Sports Physiology. WB Saunders, Philadelphia, 1985.
2. Hagerman, GR: Unpublished data, 1980.
3. Hagerman, GR, Davis, S, Rozenek, R, and Stone, J: United States Ski Team: A review of physiological parameters. Journal of the United States Ski Coaches Association 3:42–46, 1979.
4. Haymes, EM and Dickinson, AL: Characteristics of elite male and female ski racers. Med Sci Sports Exercise 12:153–158, 1980.
5. Karlsson, J, Eriksson, A, Forsberg, A, Kallberg, L, and Tesch, P: The physiology of alpine skiing. The United States Ski Coaches Association, Park City, UT, 1978.
6. Knuttgen, HG: Physiology of fatigue in winter sports. Contemporary Orthopaedics 2:246–253, 1980.
7. The National Alpine Staff: United States Ski Team Training Manual. United States Ski Team, Park City, UT, 1985.
8. Tesch, P, Larsson, L, Eriksson, A, and Karlsson, J: Muscle glycogen depletion and lactate concentration during downhill skiing. Med Sci Sports 10:85–90, 1978.

CHAPTER 38

Biomechanics of Alpine Skiing

JOHN G. McMURTRY, M.A.

Alpine or downhill skiing is a unique and noninstinctive sport. One of the first major motor experiences of young children is learning to walk, followed by running and later by skill games. A beginning skier will find, however, that typical early childhood motor activities have very little transfer value to skiing. Without exception, champion ski racers started skiing on a regular basis at a young age.

In Alpine skiing, no two consecutive turns or runs down a mountain are ever exactly the same. There is always something new to experience. Perhaps the most difficult aspect of the sport is mastering the many variables that influence technique and biomechanics.

Technique, for example, will vary with terrain. The steeper the slope, the more important it is to control speed by turning and edging. The flatter the slope, the less edge angle is required. Changes in terrain from steep to flat or vice versa require a change in technique and turn radius.

Snow conditions can be as variable as terrain, and technique must be adjusted accordingly. Besides reliable and well-maintained equipment, skiing on hard icy snow should emphasize edging and pressuring of the skis. Soft snow necessitates a more subtle, sensitive touch.

To the variables of terrain and snow must be added weather. Rain, snow, wind, and sun affect skiing conditions. There is tremendous concern about weather conditions during World Cup and Olympic Alpine events. Changing weather can drastically speed up or slow down a race course.

Finally, the equipment and its present condition directly alter the turning and sliding ability of the skier. For competition, the skis must be prepared according to snow, weather, and terrain conditions.

BALANCE AND FORCE IN ALPINE SKIING

In its simplest form, Alpine skiing is sliding downhill on skis and making turns to control speed and avoid obstacles. For the racers who compete in the four Alpine disciplines of downhill, super g, giant slalom, and slalom, turning ability and carrying speed around gates are highly developed skills. The turn can be either short or long in radius and is completed by edging and directing forces to the skis. The technique will vary accordingly, depending on speed, radius of the turn, snow conditions, and terrain changes.

Center of Gravity

The skier is continually striving to maintain balance. The center of gravity is the imaginary point inside or outside the body around which all body parts balance. The location of the center of gravity in a stationary skier is lower because of the added weight of the boots and skis. Roughly, the center of gravity is below the pelvic region between the thighs. By bending the different body parts such as the arms, legs, and trunk, the center of gravity can be moved. Expert skiers move their body parts efficiently in order to maintain proper balance. The arms are specifically used as a balance and counterbalance system.

A lower center of gravity and a wider base of support increase the stability of the skier. This enables the skier to use an independent foot action or pressurizing from one foot to the other. Feet should be hip width apart, with arms and poles in front and to the sides. A pole plant to initiate turns broadens the base of support.

The forces that develop in skiing and influence the technique and balance of skiers are (1) air friction, (2) snow friction, (3) gravity, (4) centrifugal force, (5) centripetal force, and (6) resultant force.

Air Friction

As a skier moves, the air hits the body and creates friction. The faster one skis, the more this can be noticed. In high-speed racing events, particularly the downhill and super g, a good aerodynamic "tuck" position is important to reduce air friction. For the recreational skier, a slight forward lean with the arms in front and to the sides will help prevent being pushed back by the force of the air hitting the body.

Snow Friction

Snow beneath the running surface of the skis creates friction. Fresh soft powder snow creates the most friction because of its sharp crystalline structure and requires more unweighting by the skier to start a turn. Icy and man-made snow have a ball-bearing structure and therefore offer much less friction. The skis accelerate fastest on icy surfaces; so it is possible to unweight too much on hard, slick surfaces and lose contact with the slope throughout the turn. This problem results in skidded turns.

Gravity

The force of gravity pulls the skier down the mountain and is responsible for the increasing velocity. Gravity also pulls the skier into the mountain, which many times results in a fall.

Centrifugal Force

In turning, centrifugal force is created, which pulls the skier to the outside of the turn. Proper technique and strength is needed to keep the skier fixed on a curved path.

Centripetal Force

In order to maintain control, the skier must create an equal and opposite reaction to centrifugal force while completing a turn. This equal and opposite centripetal force is developed by leaning inward, edging, and placing pressure on the skis. Muscle power also plays an important role. Without centripetal force, the skier would travel in a straight line. The higher the skill level, the more efficiently the centripetal force is applied by the skier.

Resultant Force

A skier making a turn must contend with both centrifugal force and gravity. The summation of these forces or the resultant force pushes the ski into a bend, causing it to turn. Ideally, the line of the resultant force should pass from the center of gravity to the inside edge of the outside ski throughout a turn. The outside ski should feel most of this pressure while the inside ski is used for balance and stability.

Alpine skis are designed to turn when the resultant force together with muscular force is correctly applied. The ski is made wider at the tip and tail and narrower at the waist. This curved portion of the ski along the edge and sidewall is called the *side cut*. The ski has a flexible arch called the *camber*. When the resultant force in a turn is directed to the ski, it is bent into a *reverse camber*. This bend in the center of the ski causes a curved path, or arc, when sliding in the snow. The radius of the arc will depend on the speed, edge angle, pressure, and applied muscle power.

TECHNICAL TERMS USED IN ALPINE SKIING

Inside and Outside Ski

The outside ski, which is also referred to as the "downhill" ski, is farthest from the center of the radius of the turn. The inside ski, or uphill ski, is closest to the center of the turn radius.

Inside and Outside Edges

Each ski has an inside edge and an outside edge. The inside edges are directly under the arches of the feet. The outside edges are under the outside of the feet. The inside edge of the outside ski is used primarily for turning. Turns made on the outside edge of the uphill ski are risky because the base of support is so narrow.

Angulation

The skis are placed on edge by an inward lean, or angulation. This is physically performed when two or more body parts bend to form an angle. Angulation is a combination of lateral hip and knee flexion. During high-speed turns, the skis are placed on edge because of an inward lean resulting from the increase in centrifugal force. In slower speed turns, edging is achieved with hip and knee angulation. In extremely short radius turns, knee angulation becomes even more important. Because a reduced edge angle is needed in soft snow, less angulation tends to be used. Hard and icy conditions demand more edging, hence more angulation.

Fall Line

If a ball is rolled down the slope, it will follow the most direct line of descent, because it is pulled by gravity. This is referred to as the fall line. In a turn, the skis intersect this imaginary fall line at a perpendicular angle. When skiing a turn, the fall line is intersected twice: first at the turn's initiation, and then during its completion.

THE FOUR PHASES OF A SKI TURN

The basic athletic skiing position begins with the feet placed a hip width apart. The feet should lie as flat as possible in the boots with equal pressure on both the heel and the ball of the foot. The knees should be flexed well forward to absorb bumps, with the hips directly over the boots. The trunk should be slightly bent at the waist, and the upper back should be semiflexed, or rolled. The arms should be in front of the body and to the sides. This flexed position allows the body to maintain balance while absorbing bumps. From this neutral position the skier is able to react quickly.

Bumps and rolls can then be absorbed by actively contracting the hip flexors to pull the knees up or by passively allowing the bump to push the knees upward. Because the center of gravity moves behind the feet, the hands should be driven forward as a counterweight. After passing the apex or crest of a bump, the skier must extend to keep the skis on the snow and be ready to absorb the next bump (Fig. 38–1).

The ability to carve correct, round turns from the neutral position is a demanding skill. Practicing round turns across the fall

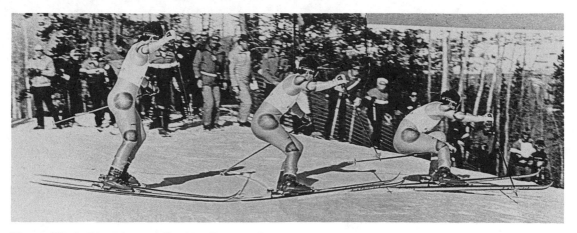

Figure 38–1. Olympic medalist Jure Franco of Yugoslavia absorbs a bump in this sequence photo. The first frame shows him extended, followed by a flexing motion in frames 2 and 3. This keeps the skis on the snow. Notice that in frame 3 the center of gravity is behind the boots, with the arms in front for counterbalance. (Courtesy of Doug Smith, Poudre Publishing Company, La Porte, Colorado 80535.)

line is a good exercise to improve skiing skills, because this exercise allows adequate time to execute each phase of the turn.

Phase One: Preparation

Starting from the neutral position, in phase one the skier transfers weight from the old outside ski of the previous turn to the new outside ski of the upcoming turn (Figs. 38–2, 38–3). This unweighting phase is done either by upward extension or downward flexion of the legs. A third method of unweighting, primarily employed in short radius turns, utilizes the energy or spring built into a ski when it is bent into reverse camber. With release of pressure at the end of a turn, the ski rebounds, springing back to its normal shape. This is referred to as rebound unweighting. Whether to use the unweighting method of upward extension, downward flexion, or rebound depends on the terrain and turn radius. Unweighting is necessary to make a definitive weight transfer from one ski to the other. The ski pole should be planted in front and slightly down the hill during phase one. The pole plant is important for unweighting and for balance. On steep slopes and short radius turns, the pole plant blocks the upper body and hips to allow the legs in phase two to twist or rotate into the turn. Throughout phase one, the upper body faces the direction of the turn and slightly down the hill.

Phase Two: Turn Initation

The turn starts immediately in phase two with pressure on the new outside ski and a lean down the hill or to the inside of the turn (see Fig. 38–2). The centrifugal force and pressure bend the ski into a reverse camber, which starts the turn. The inside lean places the ski on edge. The greater the speed, the more inward inclination and forward pressing of the knees are needed. This increases tip pressure in the snow and aids in turn initiation. Simultaneously, the outside thigh and leg should rotate medially and the inside thigh and leg should rotate laterally. Throughout the turn, the center of gravity will then follow a shorter path than the skis and legs, and the upper body will come to face in a downhill direction.

Phase Three: The Fall Line

During this phase, the speed will increase, because the skis are pointed down the hill (see Fig. 38–2). Gravity and centrifugal forces are at right angles to each other. The edge angle should be increased by angulating at the knees and hips. Because the centrifugal force in short radius turns is not as

PHASES OF THE SKI TURN

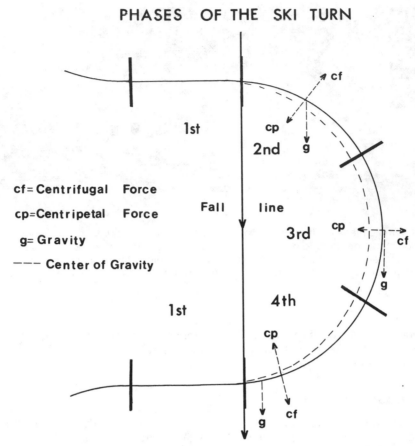

Figure 38–2. The four phases of the turn are shown: Phase 1, preparation; phase 2, initiation; phase 3, the fall line; and phase 4, completion. The center of gravity follows a shorter path as compared with the feet.

great as it is in long radius turns, less inward lean and more knee and hip angulation should be used. Through phases three and four the outside leg continues its medial rotation and adduction, and the inside leg rotates and abducts. Most importantly, the pelvis and upper body should remain blocked to provide the firm resistance for the lower legs to turn against (Fig. 38–4). A very common error for even expert skiers is to allow the hip and shoulders to rotate to the inside of the turn. When this happens, the tails of the skis lose their hold and slide out. In phase three the arms, shoulders, and hips should remain quiet and face downhill.

Phase Four: Turn Completion

Phase four is the most difficult part of the turn and requires the most strength and tech-

nical ability (see Fig. 38–2). Gravity and centrifugal force are pulling together in the same direction down the hill. Angulation and pressure on the skis continue to increase. The hips and shoulders will face the direction of the next turn. Arms should remain in front and to the sides as counterweights for balance. Theoretically, the turn is completed when the skis are perpendicular to the fall line or pointed in the direction of the next turn. At the end of phase four, the centrifugal force, as well as the pressure on the skis, has decreased, and the skier returns to the neutral position. The weight of the body should fall in the middle of the outside ski. To carry speed out of the turn and into the next one, it is important to end the turn by decreasing the angulation with leg extension. To slow down, the skis are simply kept turning up the hill by pressuring and edging them.

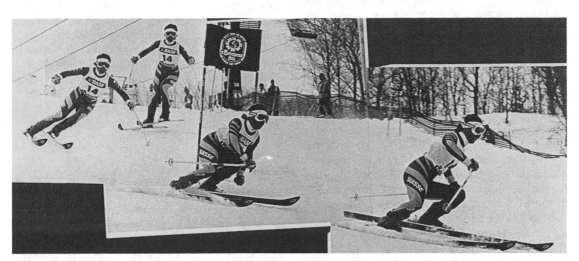

Figure 38–3. 1986 World Cup champion Maria Walliser of Switzerland clearly demonstrates the major phases of the giant slalom turn. Frame 1, unweighting and weight transfer; frame 2, inward inclination places the skis on edge; frame 3, turn completion—note the down motion and the increased angulation in this most demanding phase; frame 4, end of completion phase and beginning of preparation for next turn—notice the bend or reverse camber in the outside ski. (Courtesy of Doug Smith, Poudre Publishing Company, La Porte, Colorado 80535.)

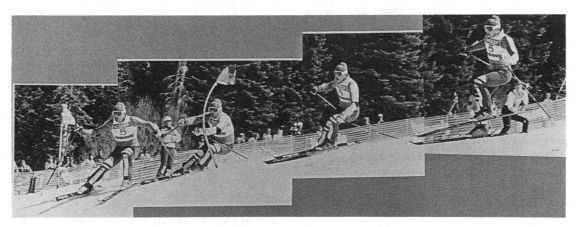

Figure 38–4. This sequence illustrates the dynamic and powerful slalom skiing of two-time World Cup champion Marc Girardelli of Luxemburg. Frames 1, 2, and 3 show Marc skiing from the fall line phase to the completion phase of a slalom turn; upper body and pelvis remain blocked and facing down the hill while the legs rotate into the turn. Notice the down motion from frame 1 to frame 2; this places an eccentric load on the quadriceps of the thighs. By frame 4, the turn is completed as Marc steps onto the new outside ski of the next turn and prepares to make a pole plant. This is the preparation phase of the next turn. (Courtesy of Doug Smith, Poudre Publishing Company, La Porte, Colorado 80535.)

MUSCLE GROUPS

One of the unique aspects of Alpine skiing is that many of the movements are resisting and moderating the force of gravity and centrifugal force. For this reason, extensor muscle groups are used both eccentrically and concentrically. The quadriceps muscles in the upper thigh are most important.

The internal and external rotators in the hip and thigh assist in rotating the femur and tibia against the pelvis in the turns. The hip flexors and extensors are important muscle groups for unweighting, skating, and absorbing terrain. Lateral stepping movements, angulation, and holding the skis together in a turn or straight running position requires use of the adductors and abductors of the thighs.

Muscles of the lower leg are used extensively in skiing for fine edge control and for shifting the body weight forward and backward. While the foot and ankle are immobilized in a stiff plastic boot, a considerable amount of muscle activity occurs both isometrically and isotonically. The anterior tibialis and gastrocnemius are used when pressing the knees forward and backward in phases two and four of the turn. For fine edge control and pressure distribution on the inside edges of the outside ski, the peroneal groups are used. Therefore, lower leg strength and muscle endurance are important in Alpine skiing.

Muscles in the midsection and upper body are also called on by the Alpine skier for dynamic use. Flexion, extension, and rotation of the trunk as well as stabilization occur in generating muscle force for turning and absorbing terrain. Stabilization of the pelvis, particularly in short radius turns, is important to provide the resistance against which considerable twisting forces occur in the legs. The erector spinae, internal and external obliques, and the rectus abdominis play an active role in these movements.

An important technique is the pole plant, which is useful on steep, demanding terrain and short radius turns. In these maneuvers, much of the skier's weight is supported for an instant by the arm and shoulder joints.

Pushing with the ski poles is also used to generate speed. In competition, races may be won or lost in the starting gate. The forearm flexors are used to grip the pole; and the triceps, latissimus dorsi, and deltoids assist in extending and planting the pole at the start.

Because of the importance of muscle strength, power, and endurance in Alpine skiing, the United States Alpine Ski Team has developed an extensive off-season and in-season strength-training program for its athletes.

CONCLUSION

A keen understanding of the biomechanics employed by the greatest Alpine ski racers is mandatory for developing competitive skiers and to sharpen their personal techniques. Working to integrate these techniques into the skills of recreational skiers will provide greater satisfaction in participation and appreciation for the physical demands of the sport.

Proper execution of biomechanically correct Alpine skiing technique requires muscle strength, power, and endurance, which cannot be gained just by occasional skiing sessions. For the serious skier, year-round training is in order (see Chapter 2). And the dedicated recreational skier should begin dry-land training several weeks or months before winter and continue an intelligent conditioning regimen throughout the skiing season.

BIBLIOGRAPHY

Atkins, JW and Hagerman, GR: Alpine skiing. National Strength and Conditioning Association Journal 5:6–8, 1984.

Howe, JG: Skiing Mechanics. Poudre Press, Laporte, CO, 1983.

Joubert, G: Skiing an Art . . . a Technique. Poudre Press, Laporte, CO, 1978.

The National Alpine Staff: United States Ski Team Training Manual. United States Ski Team, Park City, UT, 1985.

Wells, KF: Kinesiology: The Scientific Basis of Human Motion. WB Saunders, Philadelphia, 1971.

CHAPTER 39

Alpine Skiing Injuries

ROBERT J. JOHNSON, M.D.

STEPHEN J. INCAVO, M.D.

Alpine skiing enthusiasts and physicians and other health professionals are increasingly aware of the injuries sustained from downhill skiing. This chapter outlines the basic biomechanical principles of skiing injuries as well as the epidemiology and trends of Alpine ski injuries. The more common ski injuries are discussed, including their mechanisms, diagnosis, and treatment.

To understand the biomechanical basis of ski injuries, one must consider that the ski becomes an extension of human anatomy by the coupled skier-boot-binding-ski system. Because this is a relatively rigid system, the ski can act as a lever, thereby imparting high loads to the lower extremity. In the early days of skiing, boots were both low and flexible, and the result of the ski acting as a lever was often a spiral fracture of the fibula within the ankle joint.[10] As boots became higher and stiffer, ankle injuries decreased, but tibial fractures increased in frequency.[8] With improvements in the design of the release binding, tibial fractures subsequently declined. In recent years, an alarming increase in the number of anterior cruciate ligament (ACL) sprains has been observed and seems to be associated with today's higher and stiffer boots along with the inability of present bindings to protect the knee.[4]

During the 1970s, the overall injury rate appeared to be declining.[7,8] However, injuries that involve twisting the leg (spiral tibial fractures and ankle sprains) were declining at

351

the highest rate. Bending injuries (transverse tibial fracture and boot-top contusions) are now only modestly declining. Improved binding function and settings are related to these changes through the years. Unfortunately, the improvements in injury rates observed in the 1970s do not appear to be continuing into this decade.[8,15]

SKI BINDINGS

The objective of the ideal ski binding is to release the foot and leg within the boot from the ski when loads approach the threshold of injury to the lower extremity. Also, the binding should ignore those forces and moments that are not dangerous to the leg but are generated when the skier maneuvers to control the skis.

Ski binding retention settings are based on biomechanical studies of tibial strength in torsion and bending.[10] Therefore, with improvements in design, one would expect decreases in tibial fracture rates, and in fact these have been observed. Unfortunately, not enough is yet known about the mechanical characteristics of the knee during skiing to provide for binding design that can reliably protect the knee.

There are two general classifications for bindings based on release capabilities: two-mode (Fig. 39–1) and multimode (Fig. 39–2). Two-mode release bindings release in outward and inward twist at the toe and forward lean at the heel. Most ski bindings on the market today fall into this category. These bindings do not sense loads that require release in backward lean, twist at the heel, or lateral roll and shear from the top of the ski. Fortunately, most falls in skiing result in loads that release two-mode release bindings. Multimode release bindings release in one or more additional directions; however, the more modes of release chosen, the more difficult it is to construct a binding that avoids inadvertent releases. We believe these bindings should be used by beginner skiers who fall frequently and by persons who have previously sustained knee ligament injuries, because theoretically they should prevent knee injuries better than conventional two-mode bindings.

There are many other factors involved in binding performance. Common sense dictates, and clinical studies have shown, that proper binding maintenance is associated with fewer injuries.[5,9] Release settings are very important. In all skier groups tested, the release settings were too high.[7-9] An antifriction device (a pad with a low friction surface placed beneath the toe of the boot) is used with most modern bindings. Antifriction devices have two functions. First, they function as a fulcrum for the forward release mechanism. Second, they prevent friction in twists during combined forward lean and twisting falls. If a high coefficient of friction is present, the likelihood of binding-related injuries increases. From a safety standpoint, the binding is the most important piece of ski equipment because it is the link between the lever (ski) and the foot and leg. The ski binding's function depends not only on design principles but also on its proper mounting, adjustment, and maintenance.

The number of skiers in the United States has increased at least 40-fold over the last 30 years. Current estimates reveal that as many as 8 to 10 million people now ski in this country, and 200,000 to 600,000 skiing injuries are incurred each year.[14] Skiing injuries probably exceed 1 million per year worldwide. The injury rate in Alpine skiing is about 2.5 to 3.5 per thousand skier days.[7,8,15] Nationwide, this appears to be a decreased incidence from the 1940s, 1950s, and 1960s, when rates were nearly eight per thousand skier days.[6,11] In a study at Sugarbush North, Vermont, a small decline from nearly 5.0 to 3.3 injuries per thousand skier days was observed over the nine seasons from 1972 through 1981. However, wider fluctuations

RELEASE CAPABILITY

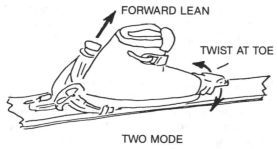

Figure 39–1. Two-mode release capability releases in twist at the toe and forward lean at the heel. Most ski bindings are in this category. (From Eriksson and Johnson,[3] with permission.)

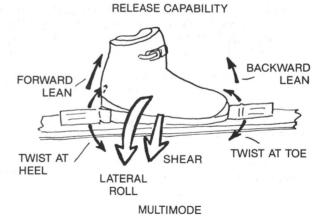

Figure 39–2. Multimode release capability releases in additional directions, including backward lean at the toe, twist at the heel, and shear and lateral roll. (From Eriksson and Johnson,[3] with permission.)

were observed within specific types of injuries. Twist-related lower leg injuries dropped from 17 percent in year one to 5 percent in year nine. In contrast to this, bending injuries declined from 12 to 10 percent of all injuries. The dramatic decline in the rate of twist-related injuries can be explained in terms of an overall improvement in the ability of the toepieces of bindings to release in twist. However, the modest improvement in rates of bending injuries suggests that the function of the bindings to release in response to bending loads at the boot top (i.e., forward lean at the heel) has been only minimally improved. Because a significant number of these injuries probably result from backward bending, a plea for a release mechanism in that direction is implied.

The vast majority of ski injuries in the past involved the lower extremity, but as boot design and binding function have improved to protect the lower extremity, the relative incidence of upper body injuries has increased.[7,8,15] Nonetheless, the incidence of upper body injuries relative to the population at risk has changed little through the years.[2,8,15]

RISK FACTORS

Certain risk factors have been identified in skiing injuries.[1,8] In general, beginner skiers sustain more injuries than experienced skiers. Female skiers are more likely to sustain lower extremity injuries than their male counterparts. However, expert skiers who sustained serious knee injuries showed no male or female predominance. Also,

younger, smaller, and lighter skiers are more likely to injure themselves.

There is a difference in the type of skier who sustains a mild medial collateral ligament (MCL) sprain of the knee and the skier who sustains a more serious MCL or ACL sprain. The mild injury is most likely to occur to a young inexperienced female skier; whereas skiers sustaining more serious injuries are no different from the general skiing population.[8,10]

Weather conditions play a role in the observed injury rates. When edging conditions are poor, such as on ice or extremely hard packed snow, upper extremity and trunk injuries are more common.[7] Lower extremity injuries are more frequent when good edging conditions exist.

CLASSIFICATION OF INJURIES

Before specific skiing injuries are discussed, a few basic concepts must be defined. A fracture is a break in the continuity of the cortex of the bone. When the overlying soft tissues and skin are intact, it is a closed fracture. When the overlying tissues and skin have been lacerated, it is an open fracture. Open fractures usually result from high-energy injuries and are much more serious. Open fractures are associated with a great potential for infection and delayed healing and require immediate operative treatment. Fortunately, most fractures from skiing injuries are closed factures resulting from relatively low-energy injuries.

When a ligament is damaged or disrupted, it is defined as a sprain. Ligamentous injuries should be graded, because treatment varies depending on the degree of disruption. The American Medical Association guidelines for grading ligamentous injuries[13] are

Grade I: Pain, mild disability, microscopic damage to collagen fibers, no clinical instability

Grade II: Pain, moderate disability, stretching of ligament produces mild to moderate clinical instability

Grade III: Pain, severe long-term disability, complete disruption of ligament produces marked clinical instability

KNEE SPRAINS

Knee ligament injuries are the most commonly reported injuries in skiing (Table 39–1) and have accounted for 20 to 25 percent of all injuries since the 1940s.[8] In spite of the steady overall incidence of knee sprains, there have been dramatic changes in the rates of specific injuries. We reported a significant decline in mild MCL sprains between 1972 and 1978.[7] However, at that time no change in the rates of complete ligament tears was perceived. About 1980 we ob- served an increase in the relative severity of knee ligament sprains. For instance, during the 1976–1977 ski season we treated 73 knee sprains at Sugarbush, Vermont. Of that group, 13 (18 percent) had sustained complete tears of one or more of the major ligaments. During the 1985–1986 season, we evaluated 205 knee sprains. Of these, 116 (57 percent) had a total disruption. Before 1980, the most common severe sprains involved primarily the medial collateral ligament, but since that time the major problem has become tears of the anterior cruciate ligament.[4] The increase in incidence of anterior cruciate sprains is the only major injury that has significantly worsened in the past 15 years. This information suggests that changes in modern equipment, which have proven to be so effective in preventing injuries of the tibia and ankle, may inadvertently result in this disastrous trend in knee ligament injuries. Our evaluation of video tapes of ski competitors sustaining acute anterior cruciate ligament injuries tends to confirm these findings. It appears that a combination of high, stiff boots with a built-in forward lean angle, bindings that are unable to release upward at the toe, and a backward

Table 39–1. SUGARBUSH NORTH, VT, 3690 INJURIES 1972–1973 TO 1981–1982

	Percent of Total Injuries	Number
Knee sprains	21.4	788
Thumb MCP-UCL sprains	10.6	391
Lower extremity contusions	8.4	311
Sutured lacerations	7.4	272
Ankle sprains	5.1	187
Shoulder contusions with AC separations	4.7	172
Tibia fractures	4.5	165
Knee contusions	3.3	123
Arm and hand contusions	3.0	112
Shoulder dislocations	2.7	98
Ankle fractures	2.1	77
Abdomen, chest, flank contusions	2.0	75
Possible meniscal tears	1.8	65
Concussions	1.6	60
Metacarpal fracture	1.6	60
Back sprain or contusion	1.6	58
Skull or face contusion	1.4	52
Patellar pain or chondromalacia	1.4	51
Thumb, finger, phalanx fracture	1.3	48
Gastrocnemius strain	1.1	42

fall—or even loss of balance backward not resulting in a fall—may be contributing to the problem that we now face. It is distressing that over 95 percent of bindings currently manufactured do not have upward toe release capability.

Injuries to the ACL can occur from a variety of mechanisms. An external rotation-valgus force may disrupt the ACL after the MCL has been disrupted, and internal rotation of the knee with or without hyperextension can result in disruption of the ACL. Moreover, there now appears to be a boot-induced ACL injury that occurs when an airborne skier wearing high, stiff boots lands with the weight on the back of the ski and with the knee in extension. The boot pushes the tibia forward on the femur, thereby injuring the ACL. Also, we believe that ACL injuries may be caused by a third mechanism, in which a skier falling backward drives all the weight onto one leg that is flexed at the knee. The inside edge of the back of the ski catches and forces the ski to rotate internally, thereby rupturing the ACL. These mechanisms were postulated from watching slow-motion video tapes of accidents in which skiers had torn their ACL.

An ACL sprain is often accompanied by a loud snapping sensation from within the joint and severe but brief discomfort. Occasionally, a skier will be able to ski for several more runs after such an injury before realizing that something significant has occurred. Mild to moderate swelling develops within a few hours of the injury and is associated with stiffness and mild to moderate discomfort. In a few days, the knee may seem to have recovered, only to give way when the patient attempts to increase the level of activity.

Posterior cruciate ligament (PCL) injuries are very uncommon. They are usually the result of a posteriorly directed blow to the tibial tubercle when the knee is flexed.

Medial collateral ligament injuries most commonly result from sudden external rotation of the leg with a valgus (inward) directed force at the knee joint. These usually result when a skier catches an inside edge, which forces the ski tip outward while the skier continues to fall forward. Sequentially, this will injure the superficial MCL, then the capsular (deep) MCL, and finally the ACL.

Lateral collateral ligament (LCL) injuries are only about 10 percent as common as

MCL injuries and usually occur with forced internal rotation of the leg from catching an outside edge.

Knee ligament ruptures may or may not be accompanied by severe pain, but localized tenderness and swelling along the ligament is almost always present. Knee ligament sprain must be identified by the examination of a relaxed lower extremity. Stress tests must be done by a skilled examiner, for even complete tears of the ACL are often difficult to perceive. X-ray images should be obtained during a complete examination to rule out tibial plateau fractures or bony avulsions. Occasionally the muscles crossing the knee cannot be adequately relaxed for a good examination of the joint. If there is any question as to the extent of injury, an examination under anesthesia or even arthroscopy may be necessary to establish the diagnosis. Arthroscopy also has a role in distinguishing between acute and chronic ACL tears.

To establish the diagnosis of a ligament sprain, it is essential to test the uninjured knee first to establish a basis for comparison. Varus-valgus stress testing is done to assess the degree of disruption of the collateral ligaments (MCL, LCL). This is most often done with the knee in 20° of flexion. In the past, only the anterior drawer test was used to establish the diagnosis of a torn ACL; however, the accuracy of this test is often very poor. The more accurate Lachman test (Fig. 39–3) is now used by most examiners and is performed with the knee in 20° of flexion.

The treatment of the torn ACL is controversial. Many well-qualified orthopedists believe that proper muscle rehabilitation, bracing, and modification of sports activities are adequate for the average individual. However, many orthopedists specializing in sports medicine feel that the best treatment for young, vigorous athletes is surgical. If surgical repair is not made within two weeks, the ACL function can be reestablished only by surgical reconstruction of the ligament. Our preference for ACL repair, in the appropriate patient, is to routinely augment the ACL repair with a fascia lata graft or hamstring tendon graft. If less than one half of the ligament can be approximated, we prefer to perform a primary reconstruction with a patellar tendon graft. Primary ACL reconstruction, utilizing arthroscopic techniques,

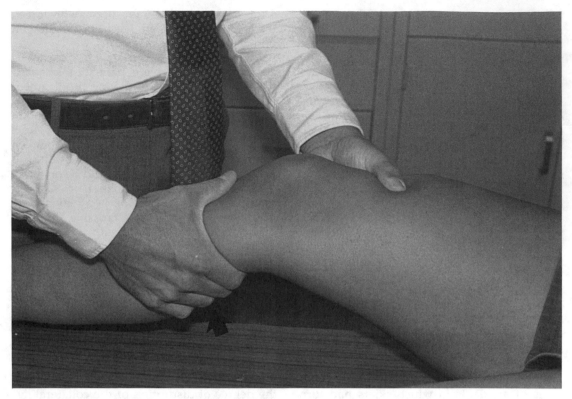

Figure 39–3. The Lachman test. To examine the right knee, the examiner stabilizes the femur with the left hand and applies an anterior movement to the posterior aspect of the proximal tibia with the right hand. An intact ACL has a solid end point with this maneuver. The knee is held in about 20° of flexion.

is gaining acceptance among orthopedic surgeons,

Treatment is generally nonoperative for isolated MCL tears of all grades. Grade I injuries require minimal protection and rehabilitation, and the subject can resume skiing usually at 2 weeks. Grade II and III injuries should be immobilized with immediate institution of isometric quadriceps exercises. Range of motion exercises are begun when comfort allows (1 to 2 weeks). At 2 to 3 weeks, when range of motion and complete comfort allows, running without cutting or turning is started and weight lifting is advanced. When cutting and turning can be done painlessly, usually after 4 to 8 weeks, the patient can return to skiing if the quadriceps and hamstrings are equal in strength to those of the normal side.

OTHER KNEE INJURIES

Knee lacerations and contusions constitute 13 percent of knee injuries in skiers and are generally minor. Contusions must be carefully evaluated to avoid missing more serious ligamentous injuries. An isolated contusion is a rare cause of hemarthrosis.

Meniscal injuries may accompany severe knee injuries, but isolated meniscal injuries constitute only 7 percent of all knee injuries. Initial treatment of meniscal injuries is immobilization, nonsteroidal anti-inflammatory drugs, and an exercise program when the patient is comfortable. The only exception to this management is a displaced bucket-handle tear in which the knee is locked or cannot be fully extended. This should be treated with traction and then arthroscopy. If possible, meniscal repair is the treatment of choice for symptomatic meniscal injuries, but often a portion of the meniscus must be removed arthroscopically.

Patellofemoral injuries result from an external rotation mechanism in which the medial retinaculum is torn and the patella subluxates or even dislocates laterally. These injuries are not rare and often are accompanied by intense hemarthrosis. The differentiation from MCL injuries is often difficult. Occasionally, an avulsion fracture of the patellar may be seen on an axial patellar x-ray examination. Patellar pain syndromes, including chondromalacia, due to patellofemoral mechanism malalignment are often associated with vigorous skiing, although no specific injury has occurred. Conservative care—including decreased skiing activity, short arc quadriceps exercises of 20° to full extension, nonsteroidal anti-inflammatory drugs, and patellar alignment braces—may be beneficial in treating these troublesome conditions.

THUMB INJURIES

Thumb injuries, particularly damage to the ulnar collateral ligament (UCL) of the thumb metacarpal phalangeal (MCP) joint ("skier's thumb"), are probably underreported by 75 percent.[2] Thumb injuries account for 40 percent of all upper extremity injuries, the majority (85 percent) being skier's thumb. This means that skier's thumb is probably the most common ski injury today.

Tears of the ulnar collateral ligament of the thumb MCP joint, although seeming rather innocuous, may lead to permanent instability. If these injuries are not promptly recognized and surgically repaired, they can result in an inability to grasp and pinch between the thumb and index finger. The injury results from forced abduction and hyperextension of the thumb, which is often driven into the snow during a forward fall (Fig. 39–4).[2] The ski pole has been implicated in the production of these injuries by directing the skier's thumb into the snow when the skier does not or cannot release the pole from the hand. Occasionally, the ski pole itself acts as a lever to increase force on the ligament.

Our studies revealed no decrease in incidence of these thumb injuries when using molded plastic grips, which do not allow the pole to leave the skier's hand when the grip is released.[2] However, this injury is less frequent if the handle is gripped outside the straps so that the pole can be discarded during a fall.

The diagnosis of skier's thumb is confirmed by tenderness and swelling over the ulnar aspect of the MCP joint. X-ray images should be examined for bony avulsion from the proximal phalanx, which occurs in ap-

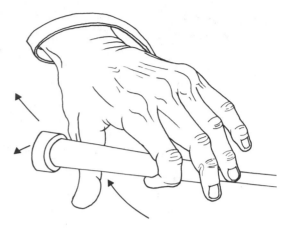

Figure 39–4. Skier's hand still grasping the pole as the hand is placed onto the snow surface. The tip of the thumb is directed into the snow and thus can be driven into abduction and extension.

proximately 20 percent of the cases. We do not routinely obtain stress views with these x-ray studies; instead, we perform arthrography when even mild instability is observed. In this manner, the danger of increasing the severity of the injury by applying a stress is avoided. Arthrography determines whether or not a surgical lesion exists.[12] Grade I injuries are treated with immobilization until pain resolves. Grade II injuries are treated with 4 to 5 weeks by cast immobilization, followed by strengthening exercises. Grade III ligamentous avulsions may require surgical repair.

TIBIAL FRACTURES

The rate of tibial fractures has declined in recent years. Our data indicate that over a 9-year period they decreased from 7 to 3 percent of all injuries.[8] In the past, spiral fractures of the tibia were the most common, but in recent years nonspiral, bending fractures have become most prevalent.[7]

The diagnosis of tibial fracture is often obvious with pain, swelling, and deformity being present. Occasionally, however, a nondisplaced fracture can be confirmed only by x-ray examination. Because tibial fractures are low-energy injuries and have a high likelihood of healing, the overwhelming majority are treated with casting after fracture reduction, and usually limited weight bearing is allowed. Some short oblique or transverse tibial fractures near the boot top can be difficult to treat in a cast, and because of this, many physicians recommend internal fixation.

SHOULDER INJURIES

Acromioclavicular (AC) joint separations combined with shoulder contusions make up about 5 percent of all skiing injuries (see Table 39–1).[7,8] The mechanism of AC separation most often involves a direct blow to the shoulder driving the acromion down with respect to the clavicle. The diagnosis is made by observing tenderness directly at the AC joint. In a severe injury, the clavicle is elevated or depressed with respect to the acromion.

Treatment of AC joint injuries is somewhat controversial, but most orthopedic surgeons agree that the majority of AC injuries may be treated adequately with conservative measures, the most important being resting the injured shoulder. This represents a major change from the feelings of 10 years ago, when a greater number of surgeons felt surgical repair was most efficacious.

Anterior dislocation of the glenohumeral joint accounts for about 3 percent of all injuries (see Table 39–1). The mechanism is commonly a fall on an outstretched arm. The arm abducts and externally rotates. This forces the humeral head anteriorly and inferiorly out of the joint. Examination reveals a tender shoulder that the patient refuses to move. Fullness corresponding to the dislocated humeral head is present anteriorly. The neurovascular status in the rest of the extremity should be checked, as it is occasionally compromised with this injury. Treatment of glenohumeral joint dislocation consists of immediate reduction followed by immobilization for 3 weeks. After this, gentle range of motion exercises should be instituted and followed later by extensive strengthening of the internal rotators of the shoulder.

CONCLUSIONS

Alpine skiing, although both challenging and enjoyable, all too frequently results in an unexpected injury. This is true for experts as well as for beginners. Although progress has been made in decreasing skiing injuries, there are still too many. Presently, reducing the number of serious knee injuries is the main challenge for the ski industry.

REFERENCES

1. Campbell, RJ, Ettlinger, CH, Pope, MH, and Johnson, RJ: High risk injury groups in downhill skiing. In Ski Trauma and Skiing Safety III. Technischer Uberwachungs, Verein Bayern, Munich, 1982, pp 126–134.
2. Carr, D, Johnson, RJ, Pope, MH: Upper extremity injuries in skiing. Am J Sports Med 9:378–383, 1981.
3. Eriksson, E and Johnson, RJ: The etiology of downhill ski injuries. In Hutton, RS and Miller, DI (eds): Exercise and Sports Sciences Reviews, Vol 8. Franklin Institute Press, Philadelphia, 1981, pp 1–17.
4. Ettlinger, CF: Why all the knee injuries? Skiing 48(7):70–78, 1986.
5. Ettlinger, CF and Johnson, RJ: The state of the art in preventing equipment related Alpine Ski injuries. Clin Sports Med 1:199–207, 1982.
6. Haddon, W, Ellison, AE, and Carroll, RE: Skiing injuries. Epidemiologic study. Public Health Reports 77:1–11, 1962.
7. Johnson, RJ, Campbell, RJ, Ettlinger, CF, and Pope, MH: Trends in skiing injuries. Analysis of a six year study (1972–1978). Am J Sports Med 8:106–113, 1980.
8. Johnson, RJ and Ettlinger, CF: Alpine injuries. Changes through the years. Clin Sports Med 1:181–197, 1982.
9. Johnson, RJ, Pope, MH, and Ettlinger, C: Ski injuries and equipment function. J Sports Med 2:299–307, 1974.
10. Johnson, RJ, Pope, MH, Weisman, G, White, BF, and Ettlinger, CF: Knee injury in skiing. A multifaceted approach. Am J Sports Med 7:321–327, 1979.
11. Moritz, JR: Ski injuries. Am J Surg 98:493–505, 1959.
12. Mogan, JV and Davis, PH: Upper extremity injuries in skiing. Clin Sports Med 1:295–308, 1982.
13. Rachum, A: Standard nomenclature of athletic injuries, pp. 99–100. Prepared by the subcommittee on classification of sports injuries and the Committee on Medical Aspects of Sports. American Medical Association, Chicago, 1968.
14. Shealy, JE: Death in downhill skiing. In Johnson, RJ and Mote, CD Jr (eds): Skiing Trauma and Safety: 5th International Symposium. American Society for Testing and Materials, Philadelphia, 1985, pp 342–357.
15. Young, LR and Crane, HD: Thumbs up: The changing pattern of ski injuries. In Johnson, RJ and Mote, CD Jr (eds): Ski Trauma and Safety: 5th International Symposium. American Society for Testing and Materials, Philadelphia, 1985.

Hillside Evacuation

DAVID H. MOORE, M.S.

When we picture winter sports we imagine superbly trained, thoroughly conditioned athletes performing flawlessly, and in most cases that is exactly what happens. But when it does not happen, we must have an equally highly trained and competent medical team prepared to meet all emergencies.

Inasmuch as the National Ski Patrol provides this sort of coverage for local, national, World Cup, and Olympic events, certain elements are common to all rescue work regardless of venue. To this end, National Ski Patrol members are required to have training in advanced first aid, emergency care, and cardiopulmonary resuscitation. This training must be updated each year with a first-aid refresher course and an 8-hour "on the hill" practicum.

Standard equipment used for rescue operations at ski jump, cross-country, and downhill events varies somewhat but falls into the same general categories.

At the ski jump, a Stokes' litter is used to carry the injured party. At ski-jump venues the distances are short from where injuries occur to the waiting ambulance. A Stokes' litter affords great speed and is then easy to fit into an ambulance. Each litter is equipped with an orthopedic "scoop" stretcher. This combination affords absolute rigidity for immobilizing the injured jumper.

At downhill and cross-country events a toboggan-type sled is used to evacuate the injured person. The cross-country sled has smooth runners on the bottom, thills at the front, and a drop-chain brake. The rescuer skis between the thills, pulling the sled behind. The downhill sled is slightly different in that it has stabilizing fins underneath to prevent it from slipping to either side as well as a drop chain on the front to be used as a brake.

To immobilize the accident victim, both of these sleds carry backboards, quick splints, hare traction splints, airplane splints, and a cervical collar. Blankets are carried on both sleds, and the cross-country rescue sled carries a sleeping bag as well.

In addition to this equipment, each rescuer is expected to carry the following items in a pack: airway, triangular bandages, large dressing, Ace or Kling bandage, assorted bandage compresses, assorted butterfly bandages, adhesive tape or perforated athletic tape, Steri-strip bandages, sterile compresses (e.g., $2'' \times 2''$, $4'' \times 4''$) roller bandages, soap, moist towelettes, scissors, single-edge razor blades, tweezers, clamps, seam ripper, and a sheet of plastic or Saran wrap.

Any of these materials may be used by the rescuer during a normal day of competition; however, the higher the level of competition, the less likely it seems that an accident will occur.

OPERATING PROCEDURES

Let us now consider a well-defined operating procedure for hillside evacuation. In discussing the removal of an injured party from the course we will use the ski jump as the main example and compare the differences encountered with Alpine and cross-country skiing.

The protocol for the ski jump and each of the other events was developed with maximum concern for treatment of the injured party. The Intervale Olympic Ski Jump protocol, which follows, is an example of a plan for a specific event: the XIII Olympic Winter Games in Lake Placid, 1980.

Ski Jump Patrol—XIII Olympic Winter Games Operating Procedure

1. Hill stations
   a. Top of hill: sled under jump lip (lip team)
      – 3 patrollers near markers' stairway in full view of inrun;

   – 1 patroller moving through VIP lounge (rotate this job);
   – 4 patrollers will be wearing crampons;
   b. Station 1: Base medical facility-side of jump on the lower part of transition. The team on this station is the designated cardiac team.
   c. Station 2: Base of other side of jump on the flat (hot-spot team);
   d. All patrollers on station will watch either the lip of the jump or the tower for early detection.
2. Accident procedure
   a. Team nearest the approximate stopping site moves there immediately.
   b. Team leader takes charge (if for some reason leader is not with the team, he or she must have appointed a new leader).
   c. If the fall starts before or at the lip of the jump, take a litter to the site.
   d. If the fall occurs after touch down on skis, send one patroller to the site.
3. Examination on course
   a. Breathing
   b. Easily detected bleeding
   c. Cervical injury
   d. Lumbar injury
   e. Remainder of spine
   f. Other extremities (quick palpation)
4. Removal from course—no spinal injury, conscious, and breathing
   a. Move into rescue litter immediately.
   b. Move off course to ambulance or medical facility.
5. Removal from course—spinal injury or life-threatening injury present
   a. Use orthopedic stretcher.
   b. Use Velcro strap on orthopedic stretcher to immobilize head.
   c. Move off course immediately.
   d. Physician on team will direct triage from there.
   e. Physician may wish to take charge earlier with life-threatening injury; team leaders defer to physician.
6. Team replacement
   a. Spare team will fill in immediately for team working on injured skier.
   b. Second accident may leave only one team on the hill (top team can be called down).
   c. Second accident may indicate jump

problems. Jumpmaster may already have stopped competition; if not, alert first-aid chief to discuss the problem with him or her.

7. An alert patrol is most effective—no idle chatter or horseplay while on station.

EQUIPMENT AND SPECIAL TRAINING

In all rescue work, the critical issue is stabilizing the injured party, preparing for transportation, and then transporting. Time is often of the essence. Jumping competitions stop while an injured athlete is on the course; the injured jumper is treated at the site of the accident unless he is able to walk off the course without aggravating the injuries. Injured cross-country and Alpine skiers must be removed immediately, however, because other competitors will be already on the course. The first-aid staff in these events must therefore learn to increase their speed without losing any skill.

Because actual treatment of the injured ski racer begins only after the removal from the immediate course, the most effective methods for removal in the least amount of time should be employed. For this purpose the quick splint (Fig. 40–1) is particularly useful. The quick splint is totally self-contained. It should have no missing ties. It can be applied within seconds. Also, it affords excellent support with maximum patient comfort. The quick splint is easily made from two 9½ × 36 inch pieces of ⅜-inch plywood, two 2 × 7 × 35 inch pieces of foam-rubber vinyl material for hinges, and 9 feet of ⅛-inch nylon line. Slots are made along the edge of the plywood where the board is wider than the foam, to permit lacing the splint shut. This type of splint may be used for both upper or lower extremities and reduces splinting time to a minimum (see Fig. 40–1).

The airplane splint is used for supporting extremities at joints where an angle is required (Fig. 40–2). This splint is foam padded and has ties attached for efficient use. The angle can be adjusted as necessary. The airplane splint can be made from ⅜-inch plywood. Two pieces of 4 × 12 inch, one piece of 3¼ × 8½ inch and one piece of 3¼ × 10 inch boards are used. These are attached

with three 3 × ¾ inch hinges and padded with 1 inch foam. A bolt with a wing nut is used to fix the angle of the splint.

The orthopedic scoop stretcher has Velcro straps attached for immobilizing the head, and side straps to complete the immobilization (Fig. 40–3). All these straps should be held separately in position by rubber bands for immediate use.

The Rockford plastic litter also has straps that should be held in position by rubber bands for immediate use (Fig. 40–4).

Blankets and Warmth

Blankets carried in the litter or sled may be used for padding and support and for keeping the victim warm during transport. Alpine and cross-country rescue sleds have fabric covers attached to the sled to protect the injured person on the way off the course and down the hill. Cross-country rescue sleds are pulled by snow machines to speed return of the injured skier to the aid station or ambulance, so blankets should be used to provide cover and to maintain warmth.

The use of special equipment requires extra training for each particular item. This may consist of a complete educational program to develop the necessary skills. Patrollers who participated in the 1980 Olympics Winter Games at Lake Placid were required to have emergency medical training and received specialized training for the use of oxygen and medical antishock trousers (MAST) (Fig. 40–5) (see Chapter 21).

EVACUATION METHODS

We will now consider some of the more common problems encountered with winter sports injuries.

Quick Splint of Extremities

A suspected fracture of the arm or leg can in most cases be quickly and effectively immobilized with a quick splint. The exception to this is the case of two broken legs. Two separate splints can be utilized for this immobilization; but if only one quick splint is

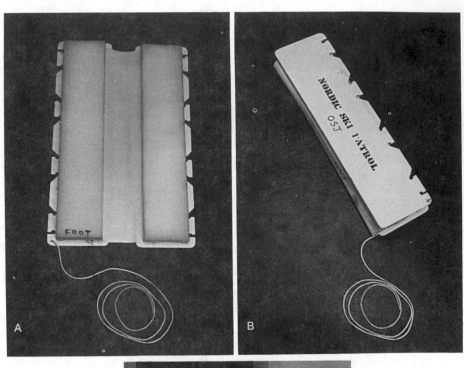

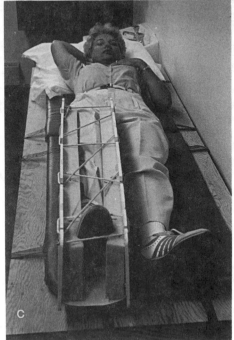

Figure 40–1. Quick splint: (A) open, (B) shut, and (C) in use.

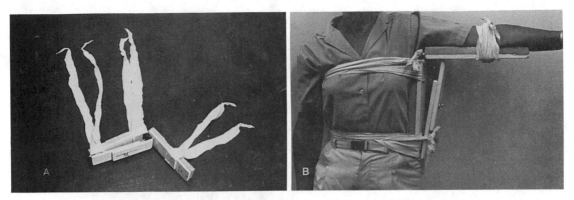

Figure 40–2. Airplane splint: (A) with ties extended, (B) in use.

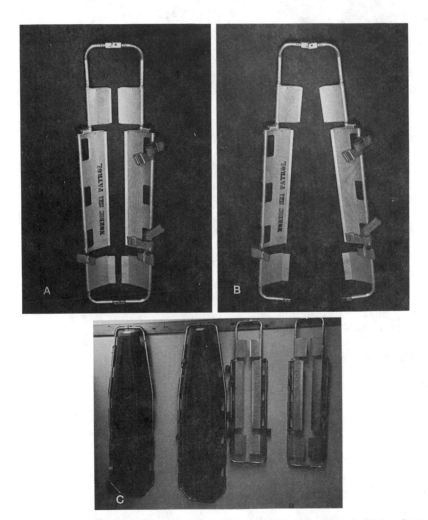

Figure 40–3. Orthopedic stretcher. (A) Note Velcro headband and straps held in place with rubber bands. (B) Orthopedic stretcher open. (C) Orthopedic stretchers and Rockford litters hanging in place on first-aid room wall.

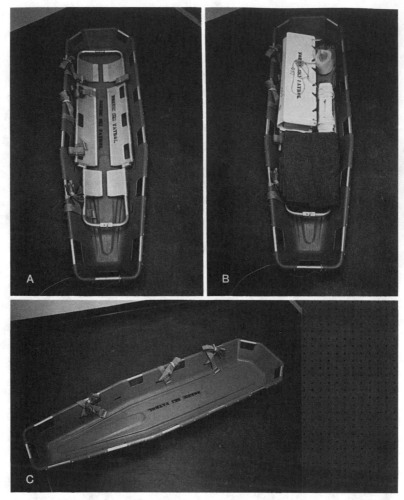

Figure 40–4. (A) Rockford litter with orthopedic stretcher. (B) Rockford litter with stretcher splints, cervical collar, and so forth. (C) Rockford litter with straps held in place with rubber bands.

available, it may be used to immobilize what appears to be the more severely fractured extremity, and then the other fractured leg may be attached along the outside of the quick splint. The victim may then be placed on the litter or sled and removed from the course.

Back and Neck Injuries

Suspected cervical spine and back injuries require extreme care in immobilizing the injured party on an orthopedic scoop stretcher or backboard. A cervical collar should be immediately available and used when cervical injuries are suspected. The scoop stretcher has a release mechanism at each end. This permits one half of the stretcher to be disconnected from the other at the center. The halves of the scoop stretcher are constructed with the thinnest part of the support along the center of the long axis. The scoop then does what its nickname implies when the two pieces are slid under the victim and reconnected. This permits loading the injured party with a minimum of movement and discomfort. The Velcro head and body straps should be held in place with rubber bands to keep them out of the way while the victim is loaded. The scoop stretcher fits well into a Rockford litter, and when it is strapped in place a rigid and protective carrier is formed

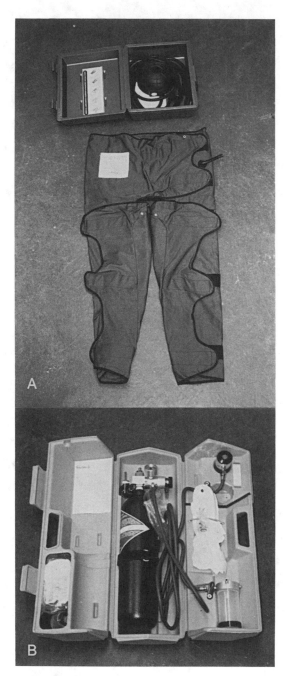

Figure 40–5. (A) MAST pants. (B) Oxygen and equipment for use.

and safest method for transporting an injured skier over steep, rugged terrain, where movement from a rescue sled may be transferred to the injured party.

Specific Injuries

Some of the injuries common to winter events require special splints.

The fractured femur may require the use of a traction type of splint. The hare traction splint is applied quickly and has an easily utilized windlass to apply traction and to prevent the bone ends from overriding. The injured party is then loaded onto a litter or sled and carried or skied off the hill.

The airplane-type splint is used for any application to the upper extremity that requires an angle, such as a dislocated shoulder in which the arm should remain at a right angle to the body. Certain knee injuries may require keeping the leg bent at an angle while transporting, and the airline splint is very effective for this particular use. The splint is placed under the extremity and adjusted to the correct angle. Then the ties are attached and can be quickly tied. When the first-aid station is close at hand, as is usually the case at the ski jump, and the injury is an upper extremity injury, the injured skier often can be walked to the aid room or ambulance with an airplane splint in place. On the other hand, at Alpine or cross-country events where many meters of terrain must be traversed, the victim should sit up in the rescue sled with a patroller riding in the sled to provide support.

CONCLUSION

Excellent training and a high level of skill, a carefully constructed operating plan, and equipment appropriate for the particular sport are all necessary for effective and efficient evacuation of injured winter athletes. Moreover, the rescuers themselves must be in excellent physical condition to enable them to perform their skills under extreme conditions of weather, terrain, and stress. Alpine rescue sled handling skills require training and regular practice on the steepest and most difficult trails. Cross-country rescuers must be able to ski long distances rapidly to attend to an injured person and then move

for removing the injured party. The same technique is utilized at Alpine and cross-country events to load the injured skier with a scoop stretcher onto backboards or rescue sleds. The backboard is the most effective the rescue sled for some distance to an intersecting road to meet the power snow sled. At the ski jump, some rescues have taken place on the steepest part of the outrun, where it was necessary to use crampons for traction and belaying methods to move the litter down the remainder of the slope.

Such skills, plans, equipment, and conditioning are necessary not only to conduct the successful evacuation of an injured winter sportsman safely but also to avoid having a rescuer become a victim—an event that could turn a simple rescue into a complex, time-consuming operation or even a tragedy.

CHAPTER 41

Medical Aspects of Bobsled and Luge

EDWARD G. HIXSON, M.D.

MURRAY JOSEPH CASEY, M.D.

Sledding and sled racing, originally with animal skins stretched between wooden runners, probably date to ancient times. During the late 1800s, the toboggan first made its appearance in Switzerland and began to evolve into the modern bobsled. The first official luge race on wooden sleds was recorded in 1883 at Davos, also in Switzerland.

The sport of bobsledding was introduced to Olympic competition in 1924. Since that time, bobsledding has been a part of every winter Olympics, except for the Squaw Valley Games of 1960, because there was no bobsled course in Squaw Valley. Presently, there are only two bobsled runs in North America. These are at the sites of the 1932 and 1980 winter Olympics—Lake Placid, New York—and the site of the 1988 Olympic Winter Games, Calgary, Alberta. Modern bobsled runs are well-designed iced tracks, which are often refrigerated to maintain consistent conditions. The Mount van Hoevenberg bobsled run near Lake Placid is 5,160.96 feet (1,557 meters) long with a 485.44-foot (146.5-meter) vertical drop. There are 15 turns along the course.

Olympic luge competition officially commenced in 1964 and has been held in every winter games since then. In North America, there are only two internationally sanctioned luge runs. These are also at Lake Placid and Calgary. The Mount van Hoevenberg track measures 3,326 feet (1076.73 meters), and it, too, is refrigerated.

Olympic bobsled competitions are presently restricted to male athletes, who participate in two-man and four-man events. The first man of a bobsled team is the driver, who is responsible for managing the steering mechanism; the second or last man of the four-man team is the brakeman, who works the braking mechanism to bring the sled to a halt at the end of each run. Bobsled races are begun with the teams pushing their sleds in a running start to develop the momentum for their course downhill. Two-man bobsleds with their riders must weigh no more than 858 lb, and four-man sleds weigh no more than 1387 lb. In world class competition, speeds of around 100 mph are reached.

Both men's and women's Olympic luge competitions are held. Men compete in both singles and doubles events, but only singles events are held in Olympic women's luge competitions. The length of the men's singles course at Mount van Hoevenberg is 3281 feet (1000 meters) and that of the men's doubles and women's singles is 2429 feet (740.5 meters). The vertical drop is 306 feet (93.3 meters), with 14 curves in the men's singles course and 11 curves in the women's singles and men's doubles courses. The racers begin on their sleds in a seated position, and then with a strong fling of their upper extremities propel themselves down the course lying feet first with their backs on the sled. A luge has no steering or breaking device, and approaching turns are accommodated by subtle shifts in weight and by pressure of the inner legs against the anterior upturned curves of the sled's runners, affording remarkable control of these surprisingly flexible sleds. The weight of the sleds may not exceed 48.4 lb (22 kg) for singles and 55 lb (25 kg) for doubles. In some international competitions, speeds of 80 mph are reached. Olympic competition involves four runs for the lowest aggregate times. At the Mount van Hoevenberg track, known for its technical demands, luge speeds of around 70 mph are attained.

The Mount van Hoevenberg bobsled and luge bahns are maintained and operated by the Olympic Regional Development Authority, which hosts world class competitions each year. Both tracks are active training facilities as well. All significant injuries occurring at the Mount van Hoevenberg sledding courses have been recorded since 1979.

ACCIDENTS

Bobsled and luge share the common potential for serious injuries due to the high speeds that are attained during competition.

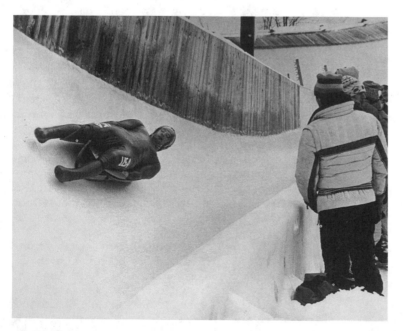

Figure 41–1. Luge negotiating curve can reach forces up to 4 G and speeds of 70 to 80 mph. Spills can be dangerous, so expert design and meticulous care of the track are essential to minimize accidents and to afford the safest possible conditions for training and competition. (Courtesy of the United States Luge Association.)

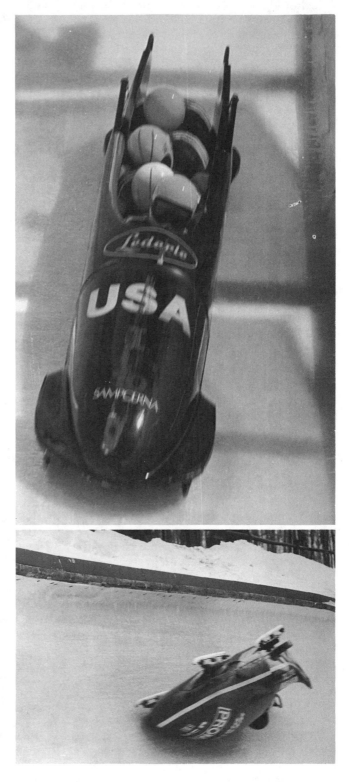

Figure 41–2. At speeds around 100 mph, bobsledders crouch below the cowling of the sled to maintain their aerodynamic streamline *(top)* and to protect themselves from impact with the sides of the track and in case of accidental rolls *(bottom)*. (Deborah L. Wight, courtesy of the United States Bobsled & Skeleton Federation.)

However, modern bahns are constructed so that should a spill occur, the competitors and sled remain in the track held by the banking of the turns and the retaining lips constructed along the top of the track (Fig. 41–1). When spills do occur, this construction usually allows the athletes to slide to a safe stop. In the event of an accident, bobsled competitors try to remain in their sleds beneath the protective cowling (Fig. 41–2, *top*). These quarter-ton sleds can be a hazard in themselves as they career uncontrolled down the course (Fig. 41–2, *bottom*). In luge accidents, the smaller, lighter sleds usually precede the unseated athlete down the course, so impacts with the sled are much less likely and less dangerous in this sport. When luge collisions occur, they are usually with the retaining lip of the track.

BOBSLED AND LUGE INJURIES

Injuries at Mount van Hoevenberg, 1980 Winter Olympic Games

During the 1980 pre-Olympic trials, 85 accidents occurred at the Mount van Hoevenberg bobsled and luge runs.[4] Eight required hospitalization, but none required major surgery. Three fractures were encountered. During the 1980 Olympic Winter Games, 81 bobsled and 22 luge athletes were seen by Lake Placid Olympic Organizing Committee physicians. There were no serious bobsled accidents during the course of these events. Two luge accidents resulted in significant injuries. One athlete sustained a leg contusion that required emergency fasciotomy, and another suffered a cerebral concussion after which there was complete recovery.

Injuries at Mount van Hoevenberg, 1983 to 1985

In a study of bobsled and luge accidents at Mount van Hoevenberg during the 1983–1984 and 1984–1985 winter seasons, a total of 84 bobsled injuries and 94 luge injuries were reported for 6,465 bobsled slides and 24,754 luge slides.[2] This gave an incidence of 13 injuries per 1000 bobsled slides and 3.8 injuries per 1000 luge slides (Table 41–1). To gain an idea of relative injury rates, these incidences may be compared with the rates of injury occurring at the Lake Placid Alpine

Table 41–1. BOBSLED AND LUGE INJURIES, MT. van HOEVENBERG OLYMPIC REGIONAL DEVELOPMENT AUTHORITY

	Injuries/Number of Slides	
	1983–1984	**1984–1985**
Bobsled	30/1,657	54/3,808
Luge	30/10,635	64/14,119

Data taken from Dick et al.[2]

skiing site on White Face Mountain, where during the 1983 to 1985 winter seasons there were 3.6 injuries per 1000 skier days.[2] If we assume that a slider takes five runs daily, there would be 71 bobsled and 23 luge accidents per 1000 sled days. So the sliding sports appear to be relatively more dangerous than Alpine skiing.

The types of sledding injuries occurring during the 1983–1984 and 1984–1985 winter seasons at Mount van Hoevenberg were primarily contusions (53 percent), but these injuries were often very severe, with a significant amount of bleeding into the soft tissues. Lacerations were the next most common injury (24 percent), and fractures occurred in 12 percent. Although a displaced coccygeal fracture during a bobsled accident resulted in a rectal laceration during 1986–1987, most of the fractures I saw[6] from Mount van Hoevenberg were nondisplaced. Twenty-eight percent of the injuries occurring at the Mount van Hoevenberg sledding sites between 1983 and 1986 required ambulance evacuation. However, only 2 percent of these injuries were ultimately classified as serious by the Abbreviated Injury Scale (AIS),[1] and 14 percent were moderate. Fifteen percent required hospital admission, and 57 percent required only emergency room treatment and release.

Critical Injuries and Fatalities

Although there have been no deaths, life-threatening injuries, or permanent disabilities resulting from accidents at Mount van Hoevenberg since 1976,[7] several critical injuries and fatalities are reported worldwide from sledding accidents each year. Two fatalities occurred from luge accidents during the 1985–1986 seasons.[7] One of these was reported by the German Democratic Republic and the other was from the Soviet Union. Both luge-related fatalities followed head injuries. And a cervical vertebral fracture, which occurred during bobsled competition in Innsbruck during 1985–1986 resulted in the death of a Soviet sledder.[5] Most of the fatalities from both sports have resulted from injuries to the head and neck.

In the United States sledding programs, there have been no fatalities or life-threatening injuries since before the 1980 Olympics. Much of the safety success of the United States bobsled and luge programs has been due to their insistence that no runs may be taken by their athletes at facilities under their supervision unless a responsible coach, an emergency medical technician, and an ambulance are present.

HEADACHES IN SLEDDING ATHLETES

Perhaps more perplexing to the sledding athlete than the ever present danger of serious injuries from accidents are the frequent

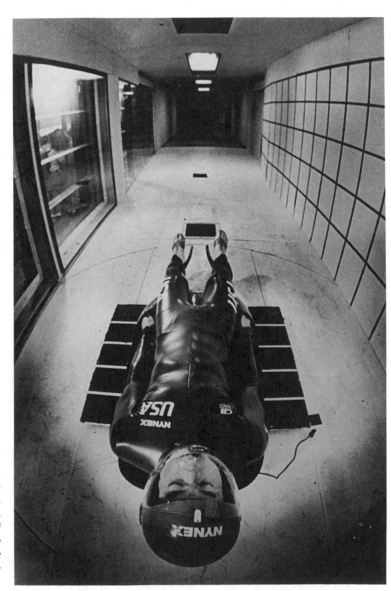

Figure 41–3. The luger is exposed to the potential of very severe injury in case of an accident. There is considerable current attention to the design of highly aerodynamic protective equipment. (Courtesy of the United States Luge Association.)

headaches that are associated with these sports. Nearly every competitor in the sliding sports suffers from this malady, which may persist for less than an hour to several days following a run (see Chapter 20). In bobsledding, sore necks and headaches almost invariably affect each team member seated behind the driver, and often the driver is affected, too.[5] Although the exact mechanism for these headaches is as yet uncertain, it is pointed out that bobsled and luge riders are subjected to the constant jarring of their sleds as they speed along the curving courses, reaching gravity force of nearly 4 G. The physical and mental exertion involved in sliding may be reflected in the release of high levels of enzymes usually associated with isometric muscle tension, emotional stress, and tissue damage.[3] Some relief from the headaches that accompany luge racing has been reported by athletes fitted with orthodontic mouthpieces, which were designed to compensate for malocclusions (mandibular orthopedic repositioning appliances), on the presumption that misaligned condyles in the temporomandibular joint (TMJ) may be contributing to the occurrence and severity of these headaches.[8] Some experimentation is also underway to determine the effectiveness of cervical stabilization in preventing headaches in sliding athletes.[9]

CONCLUSION

While North American bobsledding training and competition are quite confined to the Lake Placid and now newly developed Calgary sites, training courses for luge athletes have been developed in Marquette and Muskegon, Michigan, and Fairbanks, Alaska. As a result, the luge is rapidly gaining popularity, and with this popularity comes the prospect of injuries to novice sledders. In addition, skeleton sledding is gathering notice. Competitions with this singles, head-first sled were held during the Olympic Winter Games at St. Moritz in 1928 and 1948. The USA skeleton successes in the two St. Moritz events cannot have escaped the attention of budding young American sledders. Now with greater access to training sites and

the development of refrigerated courses throughout the world, there has been a movement for Olympic recognition of skeleton sledding.

National and international associations and federations of bobsled, skeleton, and luge have worked steadfastly to assure the safety of their athletes. With increasing participation in these sports, the sledding federations and associations are conscious of their responsibilities to protect and develop the young aspirant. The presence of emergency medical technicians and the availability of ambulance personnel are required at even the earliest level of sanctioned competition. Teams of physicians, emergency medical technicians, and evacuation personnel are developed for all higher levels of competition. Great stress has been placed on the development of protective clothing, padding, and helmets (Fig. 41–3). Expert maintenance of sanctioned bahns, which includes careful inspection of the profile and shape of the ice cover, is overseen by the sledding federations and associations to assure the safety of all competitions held under their purview.

REFERENCES

1. Abbreviated Injury Scale (AIS): American Association for Automotive Medicine, rev ed, 1980.
2. Dick, B, Hornet, J, and Pazienza, J: Sports injuries at Lake Placid: 1983–1985, a descriptive study. Department of Family Practice, Albany Medical College, Albany, NY, 1986.
3. Haralambie, G, Cerny, FJ, and Huber, G: Serum enzyme levels after bobsled racing. J Sports Med 54–56, 1976.
4. Hart, GG: Final report, frequency of visits by ICD-9 diagnostic code. Medical Report of the XIII Winter Olympic Games. Lake Placid Olympic Organizing Committee Medical Services, Lake Placid, NY, 1980.
5. Heim, D, Executive Director, United States Bobsled and Skeleton Federation: Personal communication, Lake Placid, NY, 1987.
6. Hixon, EG: Unpublished observations, 1989.
7. Hughes, B, Resource Development Director, United States Luge Association: Personal communication, Lake Placid, NY, 1987.
8. Kaufman, A and Kaufman, RS: Use of the MDRA to reduce headaches on members of the U.S. Olympic Luge Team. Basal Facts 5:129–133, 1983.
9. Mullally, WJ, Department of Medicine, Section of Neurology Medical Center at Princeton: Personal communication, 1989.

PART VI

Climbing, Trekking, and Winter Camping

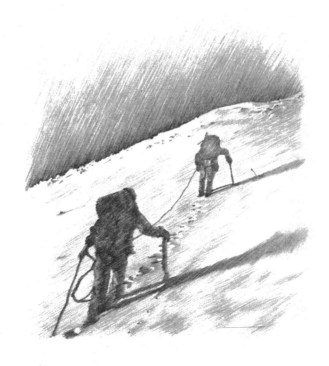

CHAPTER 42

Physiology of Mountaineering

JAMES D. ANHOLM, M.D.

In 1978, Reinhold Messner and Peter Habeler successfully climbed the 29,108-foot peak of Mount Everest without supplemental oxygen. Until then, many respiratory physiologists felt that such a feat was impossible. Inasmuch as the alveolar partial pressure of oxygen (Po_2) of only 35 torr would cause unconsciousness within seconds, and death soon thereafter in an unclimatized person, how, then, was this remarkable feat accomplished? What adjustments does the body make to allow survival, and even small amounts of work to be done, under such adverse conditions?

At high altitudes, hypoxia is certainly the most important factor affecting one's performance; however, cold and isolation, as well as the frequent bad weather, usually accentuate the difficulties. Nevertheless, some 15 million people live at elevations over 10,000 feet, and in the Andes, there are permanent residents living between 16,000 and 17,000 feet (see also Chapter 44). Most of these populations have had many months or even generations of time to adjust to the hypoxia at altitude. Mountaineers, however, have only a few weeks to accomplish the physiologic changes required. In the process of acclimatizing, the climber faces a significant risk of developing altitude illness.

Although the percentage of oxygen in the air remains constant at all altitudes, barometric pressure at 18,000 feet is only about one half of the normal sea-level value of 760 millimeters of mercury. Thus, after taking into account the 47 millimeters mercury of water vapor pressure in the body, the inspired PO_2 at 18,000 feet is approximately 70 millimeters of mercury; whereas on the summit of Mount Everest, with a barometric pressure of 253 torr, the inspired PO_2 is only 43. Actual samples of his own expired breath were taken by Christopher Pizzo, a physician climber on John West's 1981 expedition, as he stood on the summit of Mt. Everest. These showed an alveolar PO_2 of 35 torr and a calculated arterial PO_2 of less than 30.

One of the most important responses the body makes to hypoxia is hyperventilation. In fact, nearly a fourfold increase in ventilation occurs during an ascent to 29,000 feet. This hyperventilation reduces the partial pressure of carbon dioxide (PCO_2) in arterial blood from 40 millimeters mercury at sea level to around 10 millimeters mercury at 29,000 feet. Another important change occurring along with this is an increase in hemoglobin and hematocrit in the blood. In addition, there are shifts in the oxygen dissociation curve, which may result in better unloading of oxygen to the tissues at moderate altitudes and improved loading of oxygen onto hemoglobin in the lungs at much higher altitudes. These and other adjustments will be considered in more detail later.

Climbers going to altitudes over 10,000 feet may suffer from a number of forms of altitude illness. Thousands of other trekkers or skiers who go rapidly from sea level to 8000 or 9000 feet are at risk of developing altitude illness. In this chapter, we will deal with the three main types of altitude illness: acute mountain sickness, high-altitude pulmonary edema, and high-altitude cerebral edema. In addition, we will touch briefly on high-altitude retinal hemorrhage before going on to describe acclimatization in more detail. Finally, we will discuss who should not go to high altitudes.

ACUTE MOUNTAIN SICKNESS

Acute mountain sickness, as well as the other forms of altitude illness, occurs when the body is unable to adapt fast enough to the increase in altitude. Following rapid ascent to 8000 feet or above, many people experience headache within a few hours after arrival. In addition, nausea (sometimes vomiting), shortness of breath, and disturbed sleep frequently occur. Fatigue, anorexia, and dizziness also commonly occur.

Edward Fitzgerald wrote of his experiences in the Andes, "I got up, and tried once more to go on, but I was only able to advance one or two steps at a time, and then I had to stop, panting for breath, my struggles alternating with violent fits of nausea. At times I would fall down, and each time had greater difficulty rising: black specks swam across my sight; I was like one walking in a dream so dizzy and sick that the whole mountain seemed whirling around me."[7] This vivid account of acute mountain sickness was written long before much was known of the pathophysiology. Others experience similar symptoms but to a lesser degree, and in fact, one of the most notable features of acute mountain sickness is the variability from one person to another. The reasons for this individual variability are not completely understood at this time.

An important factor in determining the severity of acute mountain sickness is the rate of ascent and the altitude reached.[6] The length of stay and the severity of the exertion to get to the altitude also appear to be important contributing factors. Although no hard rules can be made, probably most people can go from sea level to 9000 or 10,000 feet without too much difficulty. Above 10,000 feet, further ascents of 1,000 feet per day are usually tolerated. Above 16,000 or 18,000 feet, however, each climber will have to find his or her own safe rate of ascent.

The incidence of acute mountain sickness (AMS) is variable depending on how fast one climbs. Hackett[4] recently reported an incidence of approximately 50 percent in climbers on Mount McKinley, and an even higher percentage has been reported on Mount Rainier.[9] At ski resorts between 8000 and 9500 feet, the incidence of AMS is probably about 25 percent.[4]

The mechanisms responsible for AMS are still not completely known. Hypoxia is the most important cause of AMS and results in many changes, especially problems with water and sodium balance, leading to edema formation in the hands, feet, lungs, and brain. The headache may be caused by the hyperventilation but may also result from a minor degree of cerebral edema. However, AMS certainly is different from the severe problems seen in overt high-altitude cerebral edema. Nevertheless, the different types of altitude illness are not separate diseases but are closely related to one another and often occur together.

Treatment

Acute mountain sickness by itself is not dangerous unless the symptoms are ignored and it progresses to high-altitude pulmonary or cerebral edema. Generally, a few days of rest at altitude results in complete recovery, and descent is not usually needed. If symptoms are severe or manifestations of pulmonary or cerebral edema develop, then descent to lower altitude is essential. Oxygen, if available, can be helpful, but it is less important than descent. Most other medications have not been studied adequately at altitude to allow definitive statements. Some have found aspirin helpful for the headache. Prochlorperazine (Compazine) appears effective for the nausea and vomiting. Sleeping medications should not be used, because they tend to depress ventilation and may make the hypoxia during sleep worse. Furosemide (Lasix) probably should not be used because of its potential for causing hypovolemia in subjects who often are already dehydrated.

Acetazolamide (Diamox), a carbonic anhydrase inhibitor, has been used successfully for the treatment as well as the prevention of AMS.[3,9] Its mechanism of action in AMS is not known, but it has been shown in several well-controlled studies to be effective in eliminating or decreasing the symptoms of AMS. Diamox is also effective in reducing the periodic breathing during sleep at altitude, and this results in a higher arterial oxygen saturation.

Prevention

The most important and effective means of preventing AMS as well as the other types of altitude illness is gradual ascent. Other probably important factors are maintaining adequate hydration and a high-carbohydrate diet (see Chapter 43). A pure carbohydrate diet may lower the altitude effects by as much as 2000 feet. We, and others, have shown that a balanced diet with 70 to 80 percent of the calories from carbohydrates does reduce the symptoms of AMS.[1] Acetazolamide in a dose of 250 mg two to three times daily beginning the day prior to ascent and continued for the first two days at altitude has been well established as an effective prophylactic medication. Dexamethasone also appears to be effective, but data are limited at present, and possible side effects make dexamethasone less attractive at present.

HIGH-ALTITUDE PULMONARY EDEMA

Twenty-four to 36 hours after arrival to altitude, a few persons for unknown reasons develop an accumulation of fluid in the lungs. Originally thought to be a "cardiac" form of altitude illness, high-altitude pulmonary edema (HAPE) is now known to be a noncardiogenic pulmonary edema caused by increased permeability of the pulmonary capillaries.[13] HAPE typically strikes young, fit, active climbers or skiers at altitudes of 9000 feet or higher. The following is a typical case history.

Case History ————————————

JA, a 25-year-old man and two companions drove from sea level to approximately 7800 feet in the Sierra Nevada mountains of California, then hiked to 9000 feet, where they spent their first night. The next day they hiked and skied to 11,000 feet. The day after that, they continued to 12,400 feet, where they dug a snow cave and spent the night. That night JA developed a slight cough but otherwise was asymptomatic. The next morning (about 60 hours after leaving sea level) they set off ice climbing. Initially all went well, except that JA noted considerable fatigue and shortness of breath and was unable to keep up with his climbing partners. In the early afternoon they abandoned the climb and began the descent. By this time JA was extremely fatigued but had only a slight headache. His cough increased, and shortly after starting down he began coughing thin straw-colored fluid from his chest. He was able to descend slowly, and after midnight, some 12 hours or more after starting the descent, the party arrived at their car. After driving to 4000 feet, JA felt markedly improved but exhausted. A chest x-ray examination was obtained after arriv-

ing home some 18 hours after descent (Fig. 42–1). A second x-ray examination was made 3 days later (Fig. 42–2).

HAPE may occur on the first exposure to high altitude, but often the subject has previously been to the same or higher altitudes. The incidence of HAPE is not known, but it is probably less than 2 percent. Some 20 percent or more of persons probably develop subclinical pulmonary edema, then recover completely, often never realizing they had mild HAPE.[5] The symptoms of fatigue and shortness of breath are common at altitude, but when they get out of proportion to the others in the climbing party, HAPE should be suspected, especially if a cough or cerebral symptoms are also present. The cough frequently becomes productive and may at times produce pink, frothy sputum.

The cause of HAPE is not known, and the pathogenesis is unclear. Subjects who get HAPE appear to have accentuated hypoxic pulmonary vasoconstriction compared with normal subjects. This pulmonary hypertension is probably not evenly distributed throughout the lungs, and some areas become overperfused with blood; the edema develops in these areas. Recent studies have

clearly shown that the edema fluid is high in protein.[13] Thus, HAPE is a type of pulmonary edema due to increased capillary permeability and is similar in some aspects to the adult respiratory distress syndrome (ARDS).

Treatment of HAPE depends on the situation, but the most important response is immediate descent to lower altitude. HAPE has been treated successfully in the hospital environment by bedrest and supplemental oxygen, but this is rarely available on an expedition. The sooner the diagnosis of HAPE is made, the more effective the treatment; in early cases, a descent of only 500 to 1000 feet may provide substantial, even lifesaving, relief.

Drugs for treating HAPE have not been studied sufficiently to be recommended. Furosemide (Lasix) may be useful, but hypovolemia may change a walking patient into a litter evacuation case. Digoxin and other cardiac drugs have not been shown to be beneficial. Morphine sulfate may improve oxygenation but must be used carefully because it is a respiratory depressant. Clearly, the best treatment once HAPE is present is immediate descent. Delay for even a few hours because of darkness or inclement weather may be fatal.

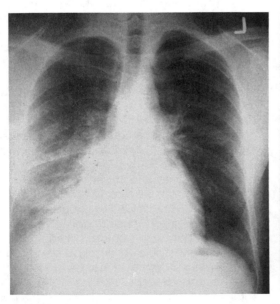 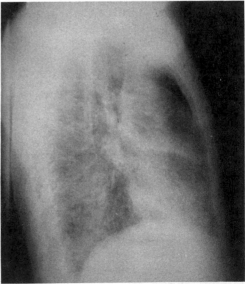

Figure 42–1. Posterior-anterior *(left)* and lateral *(right)* chest roentgenograms taken 18 hours after descent to near sea level, showing edema involving the right lung.

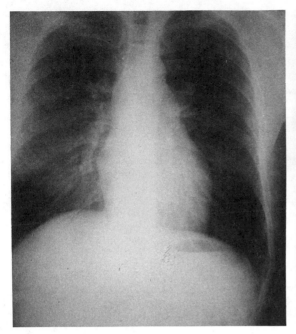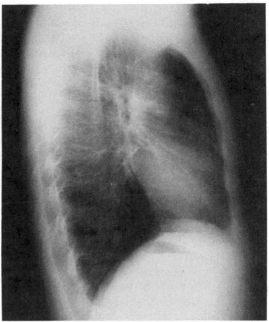

Figure 42–2. Chest roentgenograms taken 3 days after those in Figure 42–1, showing nearly complete clearing of the right lung fields.

HIGH-ALTITUDE CEREBRAL EDEMA

The third and even more dangerous form of altitude illness is high-altitude cerebral edema (HACE). Fortunately it is less common than AMS and HAPE. The signs and symptoms of HACE are similar to those of severe acute mountain sickness, and there undoubtedly is overlap between these forms of altitude sickness. Subjects may have severe headache and changes in consciousness. The subject with HACE, though, often shows progressive neurologic dysfunction; hallucinations and gait ataxia are common. In general, there is loss of judgment.

The precise pathophysiologic events that take place are not known. Intracranial pressure is increased, as is cerebral blood flow, but the mechanism for edema formation is unclear.

Whatever the mechanism, the treatment of HACE is immediate and rapid descent. Improvement may be dramatic after only a few thousand feet of descent but typically occurs more slowly than with HAPE. Although controlled trials are lacking, diuretics (Lasix) and dexamethasone have been used and probably are reasonable as long as descent is not delayed. Oxygen, if available, is useful, but descent is the only truly effective therapy.

HIGH-ALTITUDE RETINAL HEMORRHAGE

High-altitude retinal hemorrhages occur in about one half of persons going to 17,000 feet or above.[10] In most cases the hemorrhages are not noticeable to the subject unless the macula, or central vision area, is involved. Asymptomatic retinal hemorrhages by themselves are not considered an indication for descent.

OTHER ALTITUDE PROBLEMS ENCOUNTERED BY MOUNTAINEERS

Changes in the blood coagulation system, in addition to periods of forced inactivity from inclement weather, contribute to a higher than expected incidence of venous thrombosis and pulmonary embolism (see Chapter 44). The possible role of platelet aggregation and other coagulation abnormalities in the pathogenesis of HAPE has not been defined at this time.

Sleep at high altitude is frequently disturbed, and breathing often is irregular. The breathing pattern consists of a series of waxing and waning breaths followed by a short pause (so-called Cheyne-Stokes respiration). This periodic breathing with apnea is not harmful itself but may contribute to the sleep disruption and to arterial oxygen desaturation. Additionally, during sleep there is a decrease in ventilation. This may be insignificant at sea level, but at altitude decreased pulmonary ventilation can result in significant desaturation of the arterial blood oxygen. Acetazolamide (Diamox) has been used successfully in preventing marked arterial blood oxygen desaturation during sleep.[14]

In a recent decompression chamber study called Operation Everest II, rapid eye movement sleep was significantly depressed, and prolonged periods of wakefulness occurred during the night. Arterial oxygen saturation during sleep decreased with increasing altitudes, and at 25,000 feet some subjects spent the entire night with saturations below 50 percent. These disturbances in sleep and blood oxygen saturation undoubtedly contribute to daytime symptoms of altitude illness.[2]

ACCLIMATIZATION

Many persons going to altitude develop some type of altitude illness, especially if the ascent is rapid. Under the same circumstances, many others have few, if any, symptoms. The physiologic changes that allow one to function at altitude have been called acclimatization. Some of the changes seen with acclimatization were mentioned earlier, but a more complete explanation is needed.

Acclimatization has been called a "series of integrated changes which tend to restore the oxygen pressure in the tissues toward normal sea level values."[8] Some of the changes occur immediately or soon after ascent to altitude, whereas other changes take much longer. Table 42–1 lists a number of the important physiologic changes that take place. Some of these changes will now be discussed.

On ascent to altitude, increased minute ventilation at rest occurs. This causes an increase in the arterial P_{O_2} but also a decrease in P_{CO_2}. The fall in P_{CO_2} makes the blood

Table 42–1. RESPONSES TO HYPOXIA

Early Responses to Hypoxia
Increased ventilation
Increase in cardiac output
Increased hemoglobin
Shift to right of oxygen-hemoglobin dissociation curve
Increase in blood pH
Changes in distribution of blood flow
Increased myoglobin

Later Responses to Hypoxia
Changes in glucose consumption and hormone levels
Changes in cellular metabolic pathways
Increased number of mitochondria
Increased hemoglobin formation
Change back to normal distribution of blood flow
Restoration of acid balance
Changes in neurotransmitters

more alkaline and, along with the lower P_{CO_2}, partially suppresses further increments in ventilation. This alkalosis stimulates the kidneys to excrete bicarbonate, which in turn helps restore the acid-base balance to normal.

In addition to the changes in acid-base balance due to hyperventilation, there is an increase in the enzyme 2,3 diphosphoglycerate (2,3 DPG) within the red blood cells. The higher 2,3 DPG causes the oxygen-dissociation curve to shift to the right, allowing improved extraction of the oxygen at the tissue level. At very high altitudes, the loading of oxygen onto the red cells in the lungs is a more important limiting factor in oxygen transport than is the unloading of oxygen in the peripheral tissues. Consequently, shifting of the oxygen dissociation curve to the left due to the respiratory alkalosis results in improvement in the maximal oxygen consumption.[16]

Soon after arrival at altitude, the circulating hemoglobin is transiently increased. This improves the oxygen-carrying capacity of the blood. Gradually over weeks to months at altitude, though, there is increased formation of new red blood cells.

The resting cardiac output following ascent is elevated compared with the sea level cardiac output due to the hypoxia. Maximal working capacity, however, is decreased even after complete acclimatization has occurred. In general there is an approximately 3 percent decrease in maximal oxygen uptake for each thousand feet of elevation. The precise mechanisms of the decrease in maximal working capacity are beyond the scope of this paper. In fact, considerable debate still exists as to what really limits exercise at altitude. Recent evidence, though, suggests that the heart is not the primary cause of decreased exercise capacity.

Ultimately, changes in mitochondria and cellular enzymes are what bring about the most important aspects of acclimatization. Unfortunately, very little is known about these changes, except that the number of mitochondria in the cells is increased in acclimatized subjects.

Inasmuch as the majority of climbers who have attempted peaks over 25,000 feet have been unable to make the summit, it is reasonable to wonder whether successful high-altitude climbers were unique physiologically. Men climbed to within 1000 vertical feet of the summit of Mount Everest as early as 1924, but it was not until 1978 that the summit was attained without the use of supplemental oxygen. Extrapolation of the fall in maximal oxygen consumption with increasing altitude suggests that on the summit of Mount Everest, maximal oxygen consumption is very low. This information was used by some to claim that Mount Everest could not be climbed without oxygen. Although we now know this to be false, at 29,000 feet there is very little reserve left. Recently a study was published that evaluated six elite high-altitude mountaineers.[11] These were all climbers who had been over 27,000 feet on at least one of the four highest peaks in the world without supplemental oxygen. Interestingly, these climbers did not have unusual lung function or maximal oxygen consumption at sea level. There were no differences that could account for their remarkable tolerance of severe hypoxia. Undoubtedly, some important factors unmeasured in this study are responsible.

WHO SHOULD NOT GO TO HIGH ALTITUDES

Because the whole process of altitude illness and acclimatization is complex and in-

dividual variability great, no hard rules can be given. Nevertheless, a few general guidelines may be helpful. Children and infants tend to have more problems at high altitude than young adults. At the other end of the spectrum, the elderly may be at increased risk because of other underlying medical problems, such as heart or lung diseases. Therefore, in these individuals, special care must be taken if going above 10,000 feet is considered. Patients who are symptomatic at sea level from heart, lung disease, and sleep apnea should probably not go high. On the other hand, those with diabetes mellitus, hypertension, or gastrointestinal diseases that are well controlled do not need to fear ascent to altitude.[12] Those who have previously gone to altitude and have gotten sick may be at an increased risk of altitude illness on reascent; however, many have been able to successfully climb to high altitude after having recovered from high-altitude pulmonary or cerebral edema. Advising them not to climb does not seem justified at this time.

REFERENCES

1. Anholm, JD, Anderson, CL, Peters, JA, and Estes-Bruff, V: Effects of diet on acute mountain sickness at 3780 meters altitude (abstr). Med Sci Sports Exercise 14:121, 1982.
2. Anholm, JD, Powles, ACP, Houston, CS, Sutton, JR, Tyler, D, and Bonnet, MH: Arterial oxygen saturation and sleep cycles at high altitude—Operation Everest II (Abstract). Fed Proc 46:1092, 1987.
3. Hackett, PH: Mountain Sickness. American Alpine Club, New York, 1980.
4. Hackett, PH: Acute mountain sickness. Seminars in Respiratory Medicine 5:132–140, 1983.
5. Hackett, PH and Rennie, D: Rales, peripheral edema, retinal hemorrhage and acute mountain sickness. Am J Med 67:214–218, 1979.
6. Hackett, PH, Rennie, D, and Levine, HD: The incidence, importance and prophylaxis of acute mountain sickness. Lancet 2:1149–1154, 1976.
7. Houston, CS: Going Higher: The Story of Man and Altitude, ed 3. Little, Brown & Co, Boston, 1987.
8. Houston, CS and Riley, RL: Respiratory and circulatory changes during acclimatization to high altitude. Am J Physiol 149:565–588, 1947.
9. Larson, EB, Roach, RC, Schoene, RB, and Hornbein, TF: Acute mountain sickness and acetazolamide: Clinical efficacy and effect on ventilation. JAMA 248:328–332, 1982.
10. McFadden, DM, Houston, CS, Sutton, JR, Powles, ACP, Gray, G, and Roberts, RS: High altitude retinopathy. JAMA 245:581–586, 1981.
11. Oelez, O, Howald, H, dePrampero, PE: Physiological profile of world-class high altitude climbers. J Appl Physiol 60:1734–1742, 1986.

12. Rennie, D and Wilson, R: Who should not go high. In Sutton, JR, Jones, NL, and Houston, CS (eds): Hypoxia: Man at Altitude. Thieme-Stratton, New York, 1982, pp 186–190.

13. Schoene, RB: Pulmonary edema at high altitude: Review, pathophysiology, and update. Clin Chest Med 6:491–507, 1985.

14. Sutton, JR, Houston, CS, Mansell, AL, McFadden, MD, Hackett, PH, Rigg, JRA, and Powles, ACP: Effect of acetazolamide on hypoxemia during sleeep at high altitude. N Engl J Med 301:1329–1331, 1979.

15. West, JB, Hackett, PH, Monet, KH, Milledge, JS, Peters, RM, Pizzo, CJ, and Winslow, RM: Pulmonary gas exchange on the summit of Mount Everest. J Appl Physiol 55:678–687, 1983.

16. West, JB and Wagner, PD: Predicted gas exchange on the summit of Mount Everest. Resp Physiol 42:1–16, 1980.

CHAPTER 43

Nutrition for High Altitudes and Mountain Sports

JULIE ANN LICKTEIG, M.S., R.D.

Many visitors to altitudes above 2400 meters (8000 feet) are unaware of the discomforts and risks of altitude illness or fail to appreciate how these can be prevented. Some 15 percent of all persons visiting resorts at 2400 to 2500 meters will experience unpleasant symptoms due to altitude, and about 0.5 percent may die. The most common symptoms at these altitudes are headache, weakness, anorexia or even nausea, sleep disturbance, and shortness of breath. Most visitors recover in 2 or 3 days, but during their malaise they may miss some of the recreation they sought. It has been estimated that simple altitude illness causes a loss of 50 to 75 million dollars a year to Colorado resort owners.[13]

Each year some 61.5 million persons go camping, and 19 million engage in skiing, many at altitudes above 2500 meters. Although the numbers can only be estimated, many thousands of mountain climbers and trekkers go much higher, where the unwary are far more often victims of the heights. The incidence of altitude sickness and the death rate increase as the altitude increases. Of those who go too rapidly to 4500 meters (15,000 feet), almost half will be ill. Avoidance of mountain sickness depends on three simple rules: (1) eat and drink appropriately, (2) take time to go up, (3) and heed what your body tells you. Unfortunately, too many people ignore these rules, feeling "it can't happen to me." This chapter will address the first rule: eat and drink appropriately. A scientific approach to diet can be a significant factor in avoiding mountain sickness.

Altitude illnesses are due to a reversible failure of the body's handling of salt and water, which results in the accumulation of fluid within and around the cells. Acclimatization is an integrated series of adaptive changes that enables the body to stay well at great altitudes. Gradual ascent is necessary to allow the body to physiologically adapt to high altitude (see Chapters 42 and 45). A low-salt diet and high fluid intake are essential for the excretion of ample urine to carry off bicarbonate, a fundamental process in physiologic acclimatization.

Most of the dietary research regarding adaptation to altitude and its low atmospheric pressures has been done during medically oriented mountain expeditions and through controlled studies carried out in hypobaric chambers. My personal observations gained through walking, talking, and working with skiers, climbers, and trekkers have provided insights into a pattern of selecting, eating, and absorbing certain foods that may be beneficial to those who will be engaged in sports at high elevations.

HISTORICAL BACKGROUND

An excellent review of the history and physiology of altitude illness by Houston,[14] an experienced high-altitude mountaineer, quotes a prominent physician, Conrad Meyer-Ahrens, who wrote in 1854: "The principal symptoms of altitude illness . . . are discomfort, distaste for food . . . intense thirst . . . nausea and vomiting." Although Meyer-Ahrens suggested that lack of oxygen was the cause of these symptoms, this was not established until the end of the nineteenth century.

All bodily functions are dependent on oxygen and compete for scarce oxygen molecules in the rarified atmosphere of high altitude. Digestion, absorption, and the metabolism of ingested food is essential to energy production. The more efficiently oxygen can be used in these functions, the less likely problems at altitude will be. Among early writers, Boycott and Haldane[4] suggested using a carbohydrate diet and continuing to eat between meals during expeditions at low atmospheric pressures. Boothby,

Lovelace, and Benson[3] estimated a 300- to 600-meter (1000- to 2000-foot) gain in altitude tolerance through eating high-carbohydrate meals. Eckman and colleagues[9] confirmed this, using psychomotor and psychologic tests after high-carbohydrate meals.

Carbohydrate and Oxygen

It is generally accepted that whatever foods are eaten, the carbohydrates are "burned" first, initially giving a favorably high respiratory quotient (RQ), which subsequently decreases as the metabolism turns to fats and proteins. Therefore, frequent small feedings of high-carbohydrate foods should be beneficial to sports persons at high altitudes. Theoretically, a pure carbohydrate diet allows more efficient use of oxygen by burning one molecule to form one molecule of carbon dioxide, making an RQ of 1.0; whereas a mixed diet containing protein and fat as well as carbohydrate will yield a lower RQ.[12,14] Athletes in training are often encouraged to increase carbohydrate intake to 55 percent of their diets, using primarily complex carbohydrates as a source. For those working at higher altitudes, particularly climbers, the percentage of carbohydrate in the diet should be increased even more. The original work by physiologist Griffith Pugh[20] on the British Cho Oyo expedition in 1952 served as a prelude to the successful climb of Everest in 1953. Carbohydrate usage during that expedition ranged from 66 to 75 percent of the consumed calories. This may be compared with the current ordinary American diet, which consists of 46 percent carbohydrate, 42 percent fat, and 12 percent protein. Total caloric intakes on the Cho Oyo expedition were 3220 kcal to 4370 kcal per day. A most important observation made by Pugh[20] was that acclimatization improved by taking large amounts of fluid—more than four to five liters per day.

Prior to the successful Everest expedition of 1953, the food preferences of members were collected and incorporated into food planning. General improvement in weight maintenance during this climb was attributed to carefully planned acclimatization and to dietary patterns. Table 43–1 contains the overall figures for three Himalayan expeditions. This shows an 80 percent car-

Table 43–1. HIGH ALTITUDE DAILY DIETARY INTAKE

Expedition	Protein	Fat	Carbohydrate	Total Kcal	Fluid (Liters)
	(Percent of Diet)				
Cho Oyo 1952*					
5758 m–7818 m[a]	5	20	75	3960	2–3
Everest 1953*					
5454 m[b]	9	45	46	3786	2–3
6212 m–6424 m[a]	8	43	49	3869	2–3
6667 m +[c]	6	15	80	3208	2–3
Everest 1981†					
6300 m[b]	15	34	51*[d]	2224	—

[a]Climbing
[b]Base camp
[c]Assault on peak
[d]Mean daily intake during 3-day studies; highest carbohydrate consumption reached 63%.
*Cho Oyo 1952 and Everest 1953 figures adapted from Pugh.[20]
†Everest 1981 figures adapted from Boyer and Blume.[5]

bohydrate intake for the Everest assault. According to expedition leader Sir Edmund Hillary, he and Tensing Norgay spent most of the night before reaching the summit making tea at a 8454-meter (27,900-feet) camp. To each cup they added milk and three to four dessert spoons heaped with sugar.[20] Their solid food included sardines and wheat biscuits.

Additional research by Chinn and Hannon,[6] Consolazio and colleagues,[8] and Hansen and associates[12] further supported high carbohydrate consumption for improving performance at high altitudes. Consolazio and colleagues[8] found that carbohydrate diets as high as 68 percent were associated with "less nausea, less severe headache, less shortness of breath," and climbers "were more energetic, lively and happy." The 1981 American Research Expedition to Everest (AMREE) estimated dietary intake at 6300 meters (20,790 feet) to be 2224 kcal per day, of which approximately 63 percent was carbohydrate.[5] During the 1981 AMREE, Caucasian expedition members lost a great deal of weight, estimated to be more than 50 percent fat. The Sherpa porters, however, who were exposed to similar altitude and work but ate a largely cereal diet, lost little or no weight. Similar findings have occurred with virtually every Himalayan expedition.[24] Moreover, during Everest II, six men taken slowly over 45 days to an equivalent of 8787 meters (29,000 feet) in a decompression

chamber also lost a great deal of weight despite comfortable living conditions and ample, appetizing meals of their own selection.[22] Currently available evidence suggests that the low atmospheric pressures of high altitude result in malabsorption of food from the digestive tract.

ACCLIMATIZATION

Four factors are important in acclimatization to high altitude: (1) speed of ascent, (2) altitude reached, (3) intensity of work done, and (4) amount and nature of food and liquid consumed. Length of stay at altitude is important in determining the degree to which acclimatization is achieved. Individual characteristics are also important, but for reasons not well understood, an individual may be well on one occasion but become ill during a similar expedition at another time.

The rate of ascent should be tailored to the individual, but most people can go to 1500 meters (5000 feet) in a few hours, and then take one day for each additional 600 meters (2000 feet) ascent without developing symptoms. But many people who choose to stay overnight at 1500 meters and go to 2100 to 2400 meters (7000 to 8000 feet) the next day can expect slight symptoms. Above 3600 meters (12,000 feet) individuals must listen to their bodies and choose a rate of climb accordingly.

Persons flying in jet aircrafts from sea level

to resorts at high altitudes are taken within the first half hour of flight to cabin pressures equivalent to 2100 to 2300 meters (7000 to 7500 feet). For this reason it is recommended that individuals—particularly athletes, trainers, and coaches—going above 2500 m (8500 feet) should increase their carbohydrate consumption the day before departure. Fluid intake should be increased throughout the journey and during the stay at these moderately high altitudes. Alcohol intake should be minimized, because at high altitudes one drink can have the same central nervous system effects as two at lower levels. Furthermore, alcohol consumption tends to dehydrate the body.

Acclimatization begins with arrival at high altitude but takes days or weeks to mature. This depends on many factors, only some of which are controllable. Moderate exertion enhances acclimatization, but extreme effort slows the process. Because of increased ventilatory rate and consequent loss of body water in the rare dry mountain air, much more fluid is necessary. Consumption of four or five liters of fluid a day is not too much. To minimize abnormal fluid retention, a slight decrease in customary salt intake is desirable.

Transition Diet

To minimize nausea and headaches at high altitudes, the diet should be modified from sea level. Lighter foods should be used, and the percentage of carbohydrate and fluids should be significantly increased. Being in shape nutritionally before arrival at high altitudes will not alone prevent mountain sickness, but these measures can lessen symptoms during the usual 3 days of transition time. During the transition period, appetites and, therefore, total consumption may be diminished by as much as 40 to 60 percent.[7,11,19] Light, satisfying foods include soups, crackers, gelatin, turkey, chicken, fish, eggs, canned fruits, breads, cereals, skim milk, sherbet, mashed potatoes, rice, noodles, vanilla wafers, and plain cookies. Baked or broiled foods are preferred to frying because frying increases the total dietary fat. Usually the nauseated traveler will shun fried or fatty foods. As mentioned previously, fluid consumption should be increased. This is done with frequent intake of small amounts of teas or other mild liquids. Alcoholic beverages should be minimized if they are used at all. Spicy and exotic foods should be avoided, thereby lessening the possibility of dyspepsia, flatulence, diarrhea, and other digestive complaints. Sample adjustment menus for two altitude and activity levels are given in Tables 43–2 and 43–3.

Staying at Altitude

Fluids

Rapid breathing is a normal response to high altitude. This increases loss of water from the lungs because dry mountain air is humidified as it enters the nasopharynx and bronchopulmonary tree, and then this water is lost with exhalation. Adequate fluid intake is needed to avoid subtle dehydration. Enough fluids should be taken to produce copious amounts of clear urine. Cool plain water is the fluid of choice, especially during early acclimatization. Concentrated fluids can cause nausea at any altitude and if not retained, may defeat the purpose.[16] Sugared drinks in a concentration of 5 to 7.5 g sugar per 100 ml water (about 1 to 1½ tsp per ½ cup) are suggested at sea level; at altitude, 2.5 g sugar per 100 ml water (about ½ tsp per ½ cup) may be a starting point and increased accordingly. Soda and salty beverages should be decreased so that fluid is not abnormally retained. Of current interest are glucose polymer drinks, which provide another source of calories and fluid and are evenly absorbed.[18] This is especially true when high concentrations (e.g., 20 to 25 percent solutions) are needed for appropriate glycogen replacement following heavy expenditures of energy. Normal meals usually contain the essential nutrients, including electrolytes, which tend to remain in balance at altitude according to Consolazio and colleagues.[7]

Foods

Diets composed of 55 to 65 percent carbohydrate, 20 percent fat, and 15 percent protein taken in small frequent feedings are easy to digest and provide a steady stream of energy. An overloaded stomach takes a long time to feel "good" because absorption

Table 43–2. ALTITUDE ADJUSTMENT MENUS: CASUAL TRAVELER/RESTAURANT CHOICES—MODERATE ALTITUDE*

Meal	Fluids—Ad Lib	Snack Foods
Breakfast		
125 ml (½ C) orange juice	250 m (1 C) tea	½ banana
15 g (¾ C) corn flakes	5 g (1 tsp) sugar	
10 g (2 tsp) sugar	500 ml (2 C) water	
250 ml (1 C) skim milk		
1 slice toast		
5 g (1 tsp) marg		
5 g (1 tsp) jelly		
Lunch		
125 ml (½ C) chicken noodle soup	500 ml (2 C) lemonade	1 med apple
6 crackers	250 ml (1 C) water	
113 g (½ C) cottage cheese		
120 g (½ C) gelatin salad		
120 g (½ C) peach halves		
Dinner		
90 g (3 oz) broiled fish	250 ml (1 C) tea	
120 g (½ C) parslied potatoes	5 g (1 tsp) sugar	
90 g (½ C) mixed vegetables	500 ml (2 C) water	
96 g (½ C) sherbet		

Resume normal patterns after 36 to 48 hours.

General Hints
Minimum exercise
No alcohol; increase other fluids
2 to 3 liters of water; drink frequently
Eat foods with higher fluid content
Increase carbohydrates; complex carbohydrates preferred
Eat light meals; smaller amounts
Avoid fried foods
Easy Activity, 1500 Calories
75% carbohydrate
12% fat
13% protein
2½ liters fluid

*From data in Lickteig.[16]

tends to be delayed at altitude and is less totally efficient.[5,6] For the same reason, time is needed between feeding and training. Because the lungs and the digestive tract compete for oxygen, exercising at any intensity immediately after eating should be avoided. Due to expansion of gases under decreasing atmospheric pressure, there is more flatulence at altitude; therefore, low-gas-forming foods should be chosen. Supplements of vitamins and minerals may be required for long stays at high altitude. Athletes involved in very intensive training or competition, such as ultramarathoners, and women in borderline iron balance due to menstrual losses are susceptible to anemia and therefore low oxygen-carrying capacity. Such individuals should have their hemoglobin levels checked before going to high altitude. When iron deficiencies are demonstrated, the cause should be sought and corrected (see Chapters 6 and 13).

Calories

At 3600 meters (12,000 feet), 20 percent of sea-level work capacity is lost; by 5500 meters (18,000 feet) this loss increases to 50 percent.[14] Even after full acclimatization, sea-level work capacity is not restored, so caloric intake must be adjusted accordingly. The

Table 43–3. ALTITUDE ADJUSTMENT MENUS: AGGRESSIVE
SPORTSPERSON/FREEZE-DRIED CHOICES—HIGH ALTITUDE*

Meal	Fluids—Ad Lib	Snack Foods
Breakfast		
120 g (½ C) applesauce	500 ml (2 C)	8 fig cookies
1 pkg oatmeal/10 g (2 tsp)	milk cocoa	
sugar	250 ml (1 C) tea	
250 ml (1 C) skim milk	5 g (1 tsp) sugar	
1 sl bread	500 ml (2 C) water	
5 g (1 tsp) margarine		
5 g (1 tsp) jelly		
Lunch		
1 granola bar	500 ml (2 C) lemonade	50 g (½ C) dried fruit
100 g (1 C) banana chips	250 ml (1 C) water	
73 g (½ C) raisins	250 ml (1 C) tea	
	5 g (1 tsp) sugar	
	250 ml (1 C) eggnog	
Dinner		
250 ml (1 C) vegetable soup	375 ml (1½ C) hot-	hard candies
200 g (1 C) macaroni and cheese	spiced cider mix	
1 pita bread	500 ml (2 C) hot	
125 g (½ C) fruit cocktail	flavored gelatin	
	500 ml (2 C) water	

Gradually increase calories as activity increases.

General Hints
Plan one-pot meals that cook in 15 minutes
3 to 5 liters of water per day; drink frequently
It takes 15 to 20 minutes to melt snow to water
It takes 10 to 15 minutes to boil water
Drastic increase of carbohydrate intake
Moderate Climbing, 3500 Calories
4.4 kg (2 lb) dry food per person
75% carbohydrate
15% fat
10% protein
4 liters fluid
Heavy Climbing, 5000 Calories
5 kg (2¼ lb) dry food per person
5 liters of fluid

*From data in Lickteig.[16]

---

total calories needed include amounts sufficient to cover the basal metabolic rate (BMR), exercise, dietary thermogenesis (DT) of protein, plus additional caloric needs for loss of efficiency of metabolism and effort at the higher elevations and loss from extenuating circumstances such as low wind chill (see Chapter 18).[5,25]

Dietary records of a British-American party that spent 4 months at 5800 meters (19,000 feet) in 1961 during the Silver Hut research studies showed intakes of 3000 to 3200 kcal per day despite decreased appetites.[21] Although usually not much strenuous work was done, weight losses of 9.45 to 1.36 kg per week occurred.[21] Decreased absorption and fat intolerance were suspected during that project, and this was confirmed by the AMREE in 1981.[5]

A significant observation for climbers from the Silver Hut studies was that training at 3600 to 4500 meters (12,000 to 15,000 feet) for an 8000-meter (26,400-foot) climb allowed better weight and muscle maintenance; above that elevation, the overall physical deterioration far outweighed any acclimatization advantage. During the 1981 AMREE, it was found that up to 5400 meters (17,820 feet), 70 percent of weight loss related to depletion of body fat, and catabolism of muscle protein occurred even with high-carbohydrate, protein-sparing diets.[5] "On Top Everest '89" will focus on nutritional studies, specifically caloric input and energy expenditure. When deterioration exceeds the process of adaptation, periodic returns to a lower altitude are necessary to recuperate nutritionally.

SPECIFIC SPORTS

Several sports that characteristically take place at higher elevations deserve special mention regarding their nutritional demands.

Ski Touring

Cross-country skiing, ski touring, and snowshoeing put great demands on the body, especially the larger muscle groups. If these activities are continued for many hours, energy demands range from 50 to 100 kcal per kilometer, dependent on technical ability, sex, weight, age, temperature, and wind speed. Female marathon skiers require between 2800 and 4000 kcal per day while training, and the male skiers require 4100 to 5300 kcal.[23] Small amounts of carbohydrate-rich foods eaten at frequent intervals assure the athlete a consistent supply of energy. (For endurance ski racing, see the carbohydrate-loading menu patterns listed in Tables 4–2 and 4–3 in Chapter 4.) Ski tourers require nutrient-dense, lightweight foods that take up water easily and require minimal cooking. Depending on the altitude, 55 to 75 percent of the calories may be selected from the carbohydrate family.

Adequate fluid intake is absolutely essential for cross-country skiers. When practicing or racing in a dry cold mountain atmosphere, 125 ml (½ cup) of water or 5 to 7.5 percent sugared drinks should be taken every 15 minutes. Beverages containing alcohol should be avoided because they cause peripheral vasodilation and thus heat loss, and they may create problems with judgment and coordination. Too much cold blood returned to the body core sets the stage for hypothermia. Eating snow requires consider-

able energy to melt the crystals internally, which leads to shivering, with more heat and energy loss. Four to 6 cups of snow are needed for 1 cup of water; melting this over a fire or stove can be a slow and tedious task for a fatigued body at altitude. Cool liquids—14 to 32°C (40 to 50°F)—are absorbed more rapidly than warm. To maintain water supplies, ski tourers should carry an insulated canteen or even a stove, matches, fuel, and pots for melting snow on longer expeditions.

Alpine Skiing

An Alpine skier uses aggressive spurts of energy in contrast to the long steady progress of the cross-country skier. A recreational Alpine skier weighing 57 kg (125 lb) requires 480 kcal per hour, whereas a recreational skier weighing 93 kg (205 lb) requires 789 kcal per hour. Alpine racers may spend long cold hours studying a course or waiting at the starting gate. To contend with the cold, wind, sleet, and snow, a high-carbohydrate breakfast totalling 300 to 500 kcal is essential. If meals are to be delayed, portable sources of calories may be carried in the skier's pack or pocket (Table 43–4).

Eriksson and colleagues[10] have reported higher incidences of injuries during afternoons of the first two days of skiing. They also showed that experienced skiers used more glycogen than beginners, and glycogen gradually diminishes in the thigh during the day. By attentive inclusion of adequate carbohydrate intake in their diets, the skier's glycogen values returned to normal. These researchers suggested eating carbohydrate-

Table 43–4. HANDY POCKET FOODS IN THE FOUR FOOD GROUPS

Milk products	Cheese wedges, string cheese, yogurt
Meats	Beef sticks, peanut butter sandwiches, nuts, hard-boiled eggs
Fruits and vegetables	Dried apricots, apples, banana chips, raisins, fruit leather, date bars, fig- or fruit-filled cookies
Grains	Granola, bread sticks, crackers, popcorn, bagels, bran muffins, soft pretzels

rich meals containing spaghetti, breads, pancakes, and so forth in the evening before skiing to allow 8 to 12 hours for glycogen restoration.

Trekking

During most trekking expeditions the use of animals and porters provides increased weight-carrying capacity for fresh and canned foods and a portable kitchen. Therefore, appetites are more likely to be stimulated by foods that resemble a familiar diet than by the freeze-dried foods that are so essential in ski touring, backpacking, and climbing. However, the selection of foods during trekking in foreign lands is often dependent on native patterns of cooking.

A typical trek to Nepal might provide the following menu for breakfast: tea, apple juice, eggs, and shortbread wafers; for lunch: tea, eggs, chapattis, boiled potatoes, and lemonade; for snack time: tea and butter cookies; for dinner: vegetable soup, noodles, cabbage, carrots, ground beef, gelatin, and tea. In a 2326-kilocalorie diet, protein would make up 12 percent; carbohydrate, 66 percent; and fat, 22 percent of this particular menu. Two and a half liters of fluid would complete the daily intake. Foods are prepared by the trekking staff, which allows more rest time before walking is resumed. This aids the digestion and breathing processes during the period immediately after eating.

A typical pattern of food and liquid consumption during a 20-day Everest trek is shown in Table 43–5. This is compared with the average food intakes of a party of 16 climbers on Mount Kilimanjaro (see Table 43–5). The Mount Kilimanjaro party generally consumed native foods at meals, and these were supplemented by self-selected snacks. Considerable individual differences, attributable to individual preferences and energy outputs, were demonstrated by members of the Mount Kilimanjaro party at various altitudes (Table 43–6).

Winter Camping and Climbing

Quick Alpine ascents require nutrient-dense, ready-to-eat foods. Tents, stoves, clothes, and food are lightened or omitted in preference to climbing quickly and efficiently, with little room for error. Many winter expeditions have failed or ended in tragedy due to inadequate fluids or inappropriate food. There is little room for error in winter climbing at high altitudes or in winter camping when extreme weather may occur.

For expeditions to major peaks, food supplies are specifically selected for the approach march, the base camp, sometimes an advanced base camp, and the climb. For campers and climbers, the following steps are suggested:

1. Survey participants for acceptable and unacceptable foods. Omit the unacceptable items.
2. Taste test the foods under conditions in which they will be eaten. If all food has the possibility of freezing at given altitudes, try the food frozen.
3. Organize menus around the number of man days when fresh or local food can still be purchased and the days when the expeditioners will be out of reach of such supplies. There is a preponderance of anecdotal notes in the climbing literature that state that traditional and fresh food items are preferred over freeze-dried counterparts. This approach has the advantages of both an open commissary and a set menu.
4. Purchase selections.

Table 43–5. DIETARY INTAKE USING NATIVE FOODS

Expedition	Protein	Fat	Carbohydrate	Total Kcal	Fluid in Liters
	(Percent of Diet)				
Mount Kilimanjaro*	16	28	56	1488	2.3
Everest Trek†	12	28	60	1342	2.0

*1982, 5 days, 16 people from Lickteig.[15]
†1985, 20 days, 1 person, from Lickteig.[17]

Table 43–6. MOUNT KILIMANJARO—5 DAY INTAKE RANGES
BY ALTITUDE*

Expedition	Protein	Fat	Carbohydrate	Total Kcal	Fluid in Liters
	(Percent of Diet)				
1364 m–2727 m	8–21	25–39	46–65	1098–2853	1.2–4.7
2727 m–3787 m	12–14	12–37	39–62	1340–2335	1.0–4.0
3787 m–4697 m	7–16	9–32	54–82	807–2142	1.2–4.5
4697 m–5855 m 5855 m–3787 m	6–26	8–44	30–92	683–1474	0.5–3.0
3787 m–1364 m	13–29	22–49	30–60	727–2281	1.5–5.0

*8 men, 8 women; native food for meals, self-selected snacks; data taken from Lickteig.[15]

5. Repackage items into one meal per bag with simple preparation instructions.

To facilitate menu writing along the Basic Four guidelines (see Chapter 4) with high-altitude percentages of nutrients in mind, the following suggestions are made. Both grocery store and backpack store items are listed; freeze-dried items are specifically indended for higher elevations. Note that meat proteins also have a fat component, and carbohydrate foods, such as cereals, also have proteins. Because casseroles have all three—protein, fat, and carbohydrate—they may be classified in more than one nutrient group.

Protein

Grocery store. Fresh eggs; cheese; dried milk; dried meats such as chipped beef, ham, jerky, and meat sticks; nuts; peanuts; soy products; bacon chips; peanut M & M's; legumes; tuna; chicken; shrimp; canned meats; instant breakfasts; eggnog mix; cereals.

Backpack store. Powdered cheese; freeze-dried eggs; omelettes; cottage cheese; cheese spreads; casseroles; diced ham, beef, and chicken; freeze-dried shrimp; peanut butter; instant cereals.

Fats

Grocery store. Sauce and gravy mixes, bacon chips, coconut, liquid margarine, oils, soft margarine, butter, cheesecake, chocolate bars, nuts, seeds, eggs, eggnog mix.

Backpack store. Bacon bars, meat bars, pre-fried canned bacon, protein foods with a fat component: meats, cheese, eggs, nuts, seeds, milk products.

Carbohydrates

Grocery store. Cocoa, syrups, jelly, honey, soup mixes, instant soups, noodles,* instant rice,* macaroni,* dehydrated potatoes,* granola,* candy bars, dried fruit*—such as raisins, apples, apricots, prunes, figs, and banana chips—whole-grain breads,* crackers,* bagels,* biscuits,* cornbread,* gelatins,* puddings,* cider mix, fruit drinks, lemonade, iced tea with sugar, instant breakfasts, eggnog mix, fruit leather, popcorn,* whole-grain cereals,* pancakes,* cookies*—especially fig, apple, and blueberry bars—breakfast bars, fruit tarts,* gumdrops, and hard candy.

Backpack store. Dehydrated jelly, syrup, freeze-dried casseroles, specialized fruit bars, freeze-dried fruits, banana chips, ice cream, fruit crystals, tomato crystals.

SUMMARY AND CONCLUSION

Appendices to the climbing literature often include complete lists of foods, menus, fuel, equipment, and so forth. For example, Bonington[2] has chronicled the idiosyncracies of the Annapurna climb as well as Everest.

From these dietary recommendations, published research, and my own observations during numerous high-altitude treks and climbs, the following conclusions may be drawn: (1) The reaction to altitude is affected by several factors, including diet, digestion, metabolism, and hydration. (2) Lack of appetite will reduce food intake during acute and chronic exposure to altitude.

---

*Complex carbohydrate

(3) High fluid intake is a major physiologic need that must be satisfied during the entire stay at altitude. (4) A good altitude diet should increase carbohydrate content to 55 to 65 percent or higher at the expense of fat while maintaining protein intake during the extended time of stay. (5) Fat and carbohydrate are not well absorbed over 6300 meters, and at these altitudes, muscle catabolism probably occurs, at least in most Caucasians. (6) Above 6060 meters, physical deterioration outstrips acclimatization and exceeds the limits of nutritional replacement. (7) Over long periods of time, familiar, fresh, and canned foods have greater acceptance than their freeze-dried counterparts. (8) The weights of specific food items will often determine the altitudes and the points at which they are used during particular expeditions.

ACKNOWLEDGMENT

I gratefully acknowledge the review of the manuscript and comments by Charles S. Houston, M.D., of Burlington, Vermont.

REFERENCES

1. American Alliance for Health, Physical Education, Recreation and Dance: Nutrition for Sports Success. National Association for Sport and Physical Education, Reston, VA, 1984.
2. Bonington, C: Annapurna South Face. Penguin Books, Middlesex, England, 1971.
3. Boothby, WA, Lovelace, WR II, and Benson, OO: High altitude and its effect on the human body. Journal of Aeronautic Science 7:461–468, 1940.
4. Boycott, AE and Haldane, JS: The effects of low atmospheric pressures on respiration. J Physiol 37:354–377, 1908.
5. Boyer, SJ and Blume, FD: Weight loss and changes in body composition at high altitude. J Appl Physiol 57:1580–1588, 1984.
6. Chinn, KSK and Hannon, JP: Efficiency of food utilization at high altitude. Federation Proceedings 28:944–947, 1969.
7. Consolazio, CF, Johnson, HL, Krzywicki, HJ, and Daws, TA: Metabolic aspects of acute altitude exposure (4300 meters) in adequately nourished humans. American Journal of Clinical Nutrition 25:23–29, 1972.
8. Consolazio, CF, Matoush, LO, Johnson, HL, Krzywicki, HJ, Daws, TA, and Isaac, GJ: Effects of high-carbohydrate diets on performance and clinical symptomatology after rapid ascent to high altitude. Federation Proceedings 28:937–943, 1969.
9. Eckman, M, Barach, B, Fox, CA, Rumsey, CC, and Barach, AL: Effect of diet on altitude tolerance. Aviation Medicine 16:328–340, 1945.
10. Eriksson, E, Nygaard, E, and Saltin, B: Physiological demands in downhill skiing. The Physician and Sports Medicine 5:29–34, 1977.
11. Hannon, JP, Klain, GJ, Sudman, DM, and Sullivan, FJ: Nutritional aspects of high-altitude exposure in women. American Journal of Clinical Nutrition 29:604–613,1976.
12. Hansen, JE, Hartley, LH, and Hogan, RP: Arterial oxygen increase by high-carbohydrate diet at altitude. J Appl Psychol 33:441–445, 1972.
13. Houston, CS: Incidences of acute mountain sickness: A study of winter visitors to six Colorado ski resorts. The American Alpine Journal 27:162–165, 1985.
14. Houston, CS: Going Higher: The Story of Man and Altitude, ed 3. Little, Brown & Co., Boston, 1987.
15. Lickteig, JA: Computerized dietary analysis of sixteen climbers on Mount Kilimanjaro (computer program). Michael Lucas, Computer Science Division, Cardinal Stritch College, Milwaukee, 1984.
16. Lickteig, JA: Dietary adjustments to altitude. Sports-Nutrition News 3:1–4, 1985.
17. Lickteig, JA: Dietary analysis of Everest Trek. Unpublished data, 1986.
18. Marcus, JB (ed): Sports Nutrition: A Guide For the Professional Working With Active People. Sports and Cardiovascular Nutritionists of the American Dietetic Association, Chicago, 1986, pp 56–60.
19. McArdle, WD, Katch, FI, and Katch, VL: Exercise Physiology, Energy, Nutrition and Human Performance, ed 2. Lea & Febiger, Philadelphia, 1986.
20. Pugh, LGC: Himalayan rations with special reference to the 1953 expedition to Mount Everest. Proceedings of Nutrition Society 13:60–69, 1954.
21. Pugh, LGCE: Physiological and medical aspects of the Himalayan scientific and mountaineering expedition, 1960–61. Br Med J 2:621–627, 1962.
22. Rose, M, Houston, CS, and Fulco, C: Operation Everest II: Effects of a Simulated Ascent to 29,000 Feet on Nutrition and Body Composition. US Army Research Institute of Environmental Medicine, Natick, MA, May 1987.
23. Ulrich, D: Cross-country concerns. Sports-Nutrition News 1:1–3, 1982.
24. West, JB: Everest: The Testing Place. McGraw-Hill, New York, 1985, p 12.
25. West, JB: Human physiology at extreme altitudes on Mount Everest. Science 223:784–788, 1984.

CHAPTER 44

Medical Aspects
of Mountaineering

EDWARD G. HIXSON, M.D.

Mountaineering is an individual sport with informality a prime attraction. Its goals are personal and hard to define. The sport is protean and difficult to adapt to empirical analysis. This chapter will first discuss the sport itself, then the mountain environment, and finally the medical problems encountered in mountaineering.

MOUNTAINEERING

The sport of mountaineering is becoming quite popular. High altitude is reached by more than 5000 people yearly in the Nepal Himalaya.[5] The American Alpine Club (1979) has estimated that there are more than 100,000 active climbers in the United States. Although the Grand Teton National Park records more than 8000 climbs annually,[9] most climbs in North America are done by small groups and are unrecorded. Because of this, injury and illness rates cannot be accurately determined, and much of the knowledge of medical problems involved in mountaineering is based on anecdotal information. Moreover, the available data are often obtained and collected under extreme conditions. Although undocumented, it is my impression that mountaineering is among the most dangerous of all sports. The obvious potential for injury and illness is combined with the hazards of the mountain, where environmental and logistical problems usually accentuate the effects of illness and injury in a remote area.

Mountaineering is constantly changing. During the golden age of mountaineering (1850 to 1875), when small groups of several rope teams were usual, the emphasis was on the conquest of the summits of the European Alps. Individual skill, prowess, and climbing technique were foremost. During the 20th century, the highest peaks of the Himalaya were attempted. The initial attempts on Himalayan summits were by large expeditions. A major Himalayan expedition was on the order of a military campaign. Climbers were supported by Sherpa porters who brought in their supplies. Prior to the summit attempt, a series of camps would be established and supplied. A summit team could then move from camp to camp on the ascent while others supplied their food and equipment along an established route. The supply pyramid consisted of many porters and support climbers at the base camps supplying the summit climbers at the highest camp. Successive attempts could be made on the summit as long as supplies, weather, and the strength of the party were maintained. No summit can indefinitely withstand this expedition style of attack. All 14 of the Himalayan peaks higher than 8000 meters were thereby climbed. However, the climbing world is returning to simpler ways. Climbing "by fair means" is now emerging.

Rock walls previously climbed only with direct aids (e.g., e'triers, holts, pitons) are now climbed "free" and "clean" without the use of such apparatus in a fraction of the time formerly required. Formerly, Himalayan expeditions were preoccupied with developing more sophisticated oxygen apparatus; but since ascent of Everest without oxygen by Reinhold Messner and Peter Habelar in 1978, the use of supplemental oxygen has declined. Now all of the 8000-meter peaks have been climbed also "without oxygen." Solo climbing has been recently popularized. The tedious "expedition style" ascent has been replaced by "Alpine style" ascent. An Alpine ascent is short and rapid, with all of the equipment being taken by the climbers themselves, who make successive camps or bivouacs en route to the summit. Even the giants of the Himalaya have succumbed to solo assaults. Although the return to Alpine style climbing is intellectually and emotionally appealing, in the Himalaya, when there is little available within the resources of the

team itself to cope with a major illness, the potential dangers are greatly increased.

The hazards of mountaineering are considered in two categories: objective and subjective. Objective hazards are those over which the climber has no control, for example, avalanche, rock fall, lightning, storms, and altitude itself. Subjective hazards are those that may be controlled by the climber. Examples are problems related to route finding, technique, experience, skill, fitness, and group dynamics. The climber should have maximum awareness of objective hazards through a combination of knowledge and experience. He or she must have maximum control of subjective elements. Despite the conscientiousness of experienced climbers, the danger is always present.

Between 1921 and 1979, 77 climbers in 17 successful expeditions reached the 29,028-foot summit of Mount Everest during the 43 attempts on the mountain.[10] In this period, 44 deaths occurred.

ENVIRONMENT

In discussing illness and injury in mountaineering, several elements of the mountain environment deserve particular attention: altitude, cold, radiation, and geography.

Altitude

Altitude is the most important aspect of the mountain environment. Houston[6] has classified mountain altitudes as ordinary, 6000 to 7000 feet (2000 meters); moderate, 7,000 to 12,000 feet (3600 meters); high altitude, 12,000 to 18,000 feet; and very high altitude, above 18,000 feet (5500 meters). It is important to note that rapid ascent to very high altitude may be fatal. This was first shown in 1875 when during the ascent of the balloon Zenith to above 25,000 feet, only one of its three occupants survived. Messner and Habelar's 1978 ascent of Mount Everest (29,028 feet) without supplemental oxygen was previously thought to be impossible without mortality or extreme morbidity. Attainment of such altitudes is possible only through the process of acclimatization to the hypoxic environment.

Acclimatization to the hypoxic mountain environment is usually obtained by residing at high altitude (above 3000 meters) for 3 to

4 weeks. If one attempts to acclimatize at very high altitude, above 5000 meters, the body will deteriorate at a greater rate than the benefits of acclimatization can occur. Rates of acclimatization are considered in the logistic plans of Himalaya climbs. If one ascends slowly and limits strenuous activity during ascent to 1000 feet of ascent per day above 10,000 feet at less than 75 percent of maximum perceived effort, acclimatization is maximized and altitude illness can be avoided.

The ability of man to utilize oxygen decreases with altitude ($\dot{V}O_{2max}$ decreases 3 percent per 1000 feet above 5000 feet). At the summit of Mount Everest, where the barometric pressure is 253 torr, man without oxygen is near death.[1] Dr. Chris Pizzo obtained an aveolar air sample on the summit of Mount Everest in 1981. From this sample, estimated arterial blood would have a PO_2 of 30 torr, and a PCO_2 of 6 torr.[11] Oxygen saturation could be as low as 10 percent, making life itself barely maintainable. A more complete discussion of altitude physiology can be found in Chapter 42.

Cold

The mountains are cold. As altitude increases, ambient temperature decreases at a rate of 10°C (50°F) for every 150-meter increase in altitude.[1] Mountaineers must be concerned also with wind chill. Wind chill tables relate the combined effect of cold and wind on living tissue. These hazards are discussed in Chapter 18. Subzero temperatures at night may progress to balmy tropical temperatures during the day within a few hours after sunrise. In the shadows and after sunset, the oppressive cold returns. At high altitudes, the humidity of air is decreased, so the hyperventilating climber loses a great deal of water by evaporation from the lungs. Cold air and desiccation of the mucous membranes result in a constant sore throat and dry cough.

Radiation

Climbers are well aware of the warmth from solar radiation reflected by snow. At the rarefied atmosphere of high altitude, the intensity of solar radiation is great because there is little filtration by the intervening at-

mosphere. The ultraviolet segment of solar radiation reflected by snow is increased at altitude, and severe sunburn and "snow blindness" will occur to unprotected skin and eyes within hours (see Chapter 17).

Geography

The geography in which high-altitude mountaineering takes place and the related social and economic conditions of these foreign lands are extremely important when considering the availability of food, supplies, and medical facilities and the illnesses to which the expedition may be exposed (see Chapters 43 and 45). Himalaya means "abode of snow"; here the flora and fauna of high altitude are significant by their absence. Above 5000 meters there is very little to sustain life. No human habitation has ever persisted above 5500 meters (see Chapter 42). With minimal bacterial and viral life at these altitudes, the mountaineer with a cough and shortness of breath is more likely to have high-altitude pulmonary edema than pneumonia. Above the base camps, the waterborne bacterial and parasitic infestations common to the economically undeveloped Third World do not occur. When hepatitis and gastrointestinal illnesses are seen, they were probably brought up from below (see Chapters 16 and 45).

MEDICAL PROBLEMS

Trauma

Trauma is the major cause of morbidity and mortality in mountaineering. Estimates of injury rates can be obtained only from locations where climbing has been regulated over a 10-year period. During the 1970s, 71,655 climbers were registered at Grand Teton National Park. One hundred and forty-four accidents occurred, injuring 158 people. Thirty of these injuries were fatal. This is an injury rate of 2 per 1000 climbers.[9] Subjective errors accounted for the majority of the injuries in this study. Comparative injury rates of 3.4 to 10 per 1000 skier days are seen in Alpine skiing, and 1.5 to 2 per 1000 skier days in cross-country skiing are reported.[2] The prevention of mountaineering accidents is mainly a problem of education and experience. Properly used equipment seldom fails.

Because as mountaineering accidents often occur in remote areas, an injured climber's companions are the most readily available help. All mountaineers should be trained in first aid and be as knowledgeable in technical extrication as they are in technical climbing. In remote areas of the Third World, expedition parties will have to depend upon their own resources for the initial care of ill and injured members. Mountain rescue teams complete with the capabilities of helicopter evacuation, which are available to many climbing areas in North America and Europe, are usually not available in the rest of the world. Therefore, every expedition should include individuals trained in "advanced life support level" first aid and capable of sophisticated rescue and evacuation.

Altitude Illness

The syndromes of altitude illness are acute mountain sickness (AMS), high-altitude pulmonary edema (HAPE), high-altitude cerebral edema (HACE), high-altitude retinal hemorrhage (HARE), chronic mountain sickness or Monge's disease (CMS), and high-altitude cachexia (HAC). Hypoxia is the etiologic factor of altitude sickness. It is most often seen in those who climb too high too fast. The universally accepted treatment is descent and oxygen, the former being most important. Altitude illness is possible for those who go even to moderate altitudes.

Acute mountain sickness is a mild self-limited illness seen in trekkers, skiers, or other outdoor enthusiasts who ascend too rapidly to elevations above 10,000 feet. At 14,000 feet in the Andes, 52.5 percent of climbers were noted to have symptoms of AMS.[7] Mountaineers often will avoid AMS because the logistics of approaching the peak require load carrying and therefore slow ascent. I noted lack of AMS symptoms among climbers on the 1983 Everest expedition, because 2 to 3 weeks were required to get personnel and equipment to base camp at 17,000 feet.[4] However, trekking groups, which ascended to base camps in less than 10 days, almost universally developed members with AMS symptoms, and several "dropouts" usually occurred.[4]

HACE and HAPE are a worry for the inexperienced and unacclimatized trekkers at moderate altitudes and of major concern for elite climbers at very high altitudes. At very high elevations, acclimatization is not preventative. The only effective measure is immediate descent when early symptoms develop.

For HAPE, climbers should descend when there is persistent cough and dyspnea in excess of what is usual at that altitude, particularly when the climber's condition is "slipping" and decreased performance is noticed. To avoid the serious complications of HAPE (see Chapter 42), descent should occur well before the development of rales and pink, frothy sputum.

With HACE, descent should occur when headache increases and with the first signs of ataxia or lethargy. If subtle signs are acted upon with early descent, catastrophe often can be prevented.

High-altitude retinal hemorrhage is common in mountaineers, occurring in 56 percent at 5360 meters. These hemorrhages can be seen easily with the ophthalmoscope. They are usually benign and resolve spontaneously with no residua. In themselves, asymptomatic retinal hemorrhages do not indicate the need for descent, although an occasional hemorrhage will involve the macula and leave a permanent scotoma. The importance of HARE is that one may consider the retina as a window to the brain. Although it may be hypothesized that HARE might herald the onset of cerebral problems, no clinical correlation with HACE has yet been demonstrated. This relationship needs further evaluation.[8]

Chronic mountain sickness results from long-term residence at moderate to high altitudes and is generally not a problem for mountaineers.

High-altitude cachexia affects virtually all who go above 17,000 feet for more than a few days. No permanent human habitation has ever persisted above this elevation, and very high altitude is considered by some as "the death zone." Here the rate of deterioration of the body exceeds the benefits of acclimatization from the hypoxic stimulus. The HAC syndrome is similar to starvation; associated with weight loss is the loss of strength and mental vigor. Climbers on a 2- to 3-month expedition to the Himalaya may lose 25 percent or more of their body weight.

The old climbing philosophy of "bulking up" prior to an expedition is erroneous. Leaner individuals lose less muscle mass than obese climbers. Because roughly half of altitude weight loss is fat and half is muscle, excess fat does not protect against muscle loss.

Diet and Fluid

High-altitude cachexia may be minimized or eliminated for a short period of time[4] with a high-carbohydrate diet, as emphasized in Chapter 43. A high-carbohydrate diet "lowers the summit by 2000 feet." The hypoxic environment makes carbohydrates very appropriate. More oxygen is required to burn fat and protein. In addition, protein is dehydrating, because more water is required for its metabolism. A particular problem for climbing expeditions is the large amounts of fluid and calories that are required at high altitudes, where each climber may need 5 liters of water and 6000 kcal daily.[3] Equally important in maintaining body reserves is rest. Rest days should follow hard climbing days. This should be considered in planning logistics of the ascent. Forty-eight or more hours on a high-carbohydrate diet may be required to replace the depletion of muscle glycogen of a hard day's climb.

Thromboembolic Disorders

Thromboembolic disorders are another significant problem faced by climbers at high altitudes (see Chapter 42). The hematologic response to altitude is increased erythropoiesis. Dehydration, due to hyperventilation and the difficulty of getting adequate fluid from melting ice and snow, aggravates the hemoconcentration of the increased red blood cell mass. Hemoglobin concentrations are commonly above 20 g per liter, with hematocrits above 55 to 60 percent. These changes take 3 to 6 weeks to develop. Theoretically, a hematocrit of 57 percent is optimum for its oxygen-carrying capacity.[6] However, this level of hemoconcentration may lead to thromboembolic problems, such as phlebitis, pulmonary emboli, and cerebral thromboses and emboli. Treatment of these disorders is difficult, and they are best avoided. Some have recommended phlebotomy when hematocrits exceed 60 percent. I

believe that the key to avoiding thromboembolic disorders lies in limiting exposure above 17,000 feet and avoiding dehydration—both factors seem to be common denominators in the development of these problems.

Hypothermia and Frostbite

Hypothermia and frostbite are major medical problems to the mountaineer. Altitude hypoxia severely aggravates frostbite and contributes to hypothermia. This topic is well described by Dr. Murray Hamlet in Chapter 18. From a practical standpoint, several points deserve emphasis. Oxygen use contributes to the sensation of warmth and is of great benefit in avoiding and treating both hypothermia and frostbite. The climber "without oxygen" at very high altitude is especially at risk for cold injury. When frostbite does occur, climbers should descend on frozen feet with their boots on. Controlled thawing should be done only after the individual has descended to the point that evacuation can be achieved without further walking. In itself, walking on hard frozen feet harms them very little if at all. However, thawed feet create quite a different case, and walking on thawed feet greatly accentuates the tissue damage of frostbite.

CONCLUSION

In many areas of the world the entire responsibility of prevention, extrication, and evacuation—as well as initial primary care of illness and injuries—will rest on the climbers themselves. In addition to understanding and appreciating the sport and techniques of climbing, it is the responsibility of the climbers and the responsibility of the expeditionary physician to be knowledgeable and adept in handling the most common problems that may befall their party in the often hostile environment of the high mountains.

REFERENCES

1. Heath, D and Williams, DR: Man at High Altitude: The Pathophysiology of Acclimatization and Adaptation, ed 2. Churchill Livingstone, London, 1981.
2. Hixson, EG: The Physician and Sportsmedicine Guide to Cross-Country Skiing. McGraw Hill, New York, 1980.
3. Hixson, EG: Unpublished observations. Shaklee

Clinical Symposium on High Altitude Nutrition, San Francisco, 1981.

4. Hixson, EG: Unpublished observations, 1983.
5. Houston, CS: Altitude illness. Emergency Medicine Clinics of North America 2:503–512, 1984.
6. Houston, CS: Going Higher: The Story of Man at Altitude, ed 3. Little, Brown & Co, Boston, 1987.
7. Hultgren, HN and Markovena, EA: High altitude pulmonary edema epidemiologic observations in Peru. Chest 74:372–376, 1978.
8. McFadden, DM, Houston, CS, and Sutton, JD: High altitude retinopathy. JAMA 245:581–586, 1981.
9. Schussman, LC and Lutz, LJ: Mountaineering and rock climbing accidents. The Physician and Sportsmedicine 10:52–61, 1982.
10. Unsworth, W: Everest, A Mountaineering History, Appendix 4–5. Houghton-Milton, Boston, 1981.
11. West, JP and Hahiri, S: Barometric pressures of extreme altitudes on Mount Everest: Physiologic significance. J Appl Physiol 54:1166–1194, 1984.

CHAPTER 45

Medical Aspects of Trekking and Winter Camping

WALTER R. HAMPTON, M.D.

Today, an increasing number of persons are participating in "adventure travel" experiences and may consider these vital for their physical and spiritual health. Adventure travel implies the undertaking of a trip to remote areas far from conventional means of transport and support services. Participants should be in good physical health, be fit, and have the ability to cope with the unexpected.

TREKKING

A trek is an organized, long-distance hike, usually lasting from 10 to 30 days. The trekking group is largely self-sufficient. Support services, usually provided by a trekking or travel company, include food, tentage, and/or other forms of lodging. Equipment and personal gear are carried by porters or pack animals, so that in most expeditions, the trekker needs only to carry a day pack containing the personal items that may be required for that day's activities.

A typical trekking day in the Kingdom of Nepal begins with a wake-up from the Sherpa guide at about 6:00 A.M. with "washee water" for personal use and a steaming mug of "bed tea." Gear is quickly stowed, and a substantial breakast is served. As the Sherpas and porters break camp and pack, the group moves out for the day's hike. The pace can be leisurely, but for many it is also strenuous, because many feet of altitude are gained and lost in a single day. A lunch stop of about 2 hours at midday allows a chance to rest and to enjoy magnificent scenery. After lunch, another 3 or 4 hours of walking ends by about 4:00 P.M. at a camp site set up ahead by the guides. Afternoon tea is provided as well as more "washee water" to enable the hikers to freshen up. Dinner is usually served by 6:00 P.M. and is followed by early retirement in the comfort of a spacious two-person tent. The food, packed in by the group and prepared by Sherpa cooks, is largely vegetarian in nature (see Chapter 43).[2]

Though trekking is generally healthful, it is not without its hazards. Most trekking agencies attempt to guide their clients as to the degree of difficulty by a grading system. For example, trips may be graded on the basis of *A* through *E* and rated with the subscripts of (1) easy, (2) moderate, and (3) strenuous. *A* trips leave hiking as an option and may include simple walking tours or jeep safaris. Trips rated *B* involve some required physical activity with a degree of difficulty ranging from 1 (easy) to 3 (strenuous). *C* trips generally denote that some of the hiking takes place at high altitude. *D* trips generally require some basic mountaineering skills. Trips rated *E* usually require advanced mountaineering skills for which a reputable trekking agency will require a résumé of experience before accepting one on such a venture.

Pretrek Evaluation

The physician is frequently called upon to certify that a client is fit to participate in a proposed trek. Although the examination usually will be performed on an apparently healthy, even robust, individual, it is important for the examiner to assess the patient's physical condition in relation to the demands of the proposed trek. The chief purpose of the preparticipation examination is to reveal problems that might be present that could preclude participation in a trip or require attention before departure. For instance, the finding of an asymptomatic inguinal hernia might require elective surgical repair prior to the venture rather than risking an emergency in a remote setting. A history of anaphylactic reactions to insect stings would prompt the physician to equip the patient with instructions in self-administration of adrenaline.

Certain medical conditions, such as primary pulmonary hypertension, congenital absence of the right pulmonary artery, chronic obstructive pulmonary disease, arteriosclerotic heart disease with angina, and/or congestive heart failure, should preclude the patient from going to high altitude.

It is important for the physician to document and initiate records of ongoing medical problems that may require advance planning and medication schedules. Consideration should be given to the problems of medical evacuation from remote areas. Search and rescue capability is limited at best in undeveloped countries and when available, guarantee of payment is often required before that transport will be provided.

There are several agencies that are able to provide information and/or insurance and the availability of medical resources in foreign countries. The International Association for Medical Assistance to Travelers (736 Center Street, Lewiston, New York, 14092) provides a worldwide directory of English-speaking doctors who have agreed to standardize fees. International information on malaria, immunizations, and weather is also available from the association. These services are free, but donations are appreciated. NEAR Services (1900 North Mac Arthur Boulevard, Oklahoma City, Oklahoma 73127) is one of many organizations that provide medical and other insurance coverage for international and domestic travelers.

It is important for the physician to recognize the significance of the trip grading system. The distinction between *B* and *C* trips is usually that of high altitude. It is possible that a trip rated B_3 may be more strenuous than a C_2 or C_3 trip because of differences in support services or terrain despite the altitude.

Prior to any trek, a physical conditioning program should be instituted. Although conditioning does not influence the ability of one to adjust to altitude (see Chapter 42), being physically fit does help one in meeting the demands of hiking 6 to 12 miles a day. Running, hiking with a heavy pack, cycling, and other forms of aerobic exercise are recommended. A standard prescription of 30 minutes of exercise achieving a target pulse rate of 60 to 80 percent of the predicted maximum pulse rate, three times weekly, should begin at least 2 months before departure.

Immunoprophylaxis

It is important for trekkers to be provided with necessary immunizations and recomendations for prevention of infectious disease before they depart (see Chapters 15 and 16). Useful references are *Health Information for International Travel,* published annually by the United States Department of Health and Human Services as a supplement to their weekly publication, *Morbidity & Mortality Weekly Report* (MMWR). A subscription to the MMWR provides the physician with updated information regarding patterns of disease throughout the world. Another useful publication is the *Guide for Adult Immunization,* published by the American College of Physicians.

Hepatitis

Trekkers in developing countries, especially those in tropical areas, are at risk of exposure to hepatitis. Hepatitis immune globulin given on departure in a single intramuscular dose of 0.02 ml/kg body weight provides partial protection against hepatitis A for the short term (i.e., up to 3 months). It is recommended that those who are at risk for longer periods should have larger doses of immune globulin, up to 0.05 ml/kg every 4 to 6 months.

Although the risk to the international traveler of contracting hepatitis B (HBV) is generally low, it may be significant under certain circumstances. These include travel to countries in which the prevalence of HBV carriers is high in the resident population, especially if there is likely to be intimate exposure and/or contact with blood and secretions of infected persons. If such an exposure is anticipated, the use of HBV vaccine is recommended.[10] The vaccine is considered safe, and the initial concern that the vaccination carries infectious acquired immunodeficiency syndrome (AIDS) virus (HIV) has been discounted.[6]

Cholera

Cholera is prevalent in Africa and Asia, where there are periodic localized outbreaks, but this disease is a relatively small risk to travelers. The best prevention is scrupulous avoidance of fecally contaminated food and water (see Chapter 16). Cholera vaccine is generally not recommended unless required by a specific country as a condition of entry.[1] The vaccine is given in two 0.5-ml intramuscular doses spaced 1 month apart. This provides about 50 percent protection for as long as 3 to 6 months. Despite these limitations, I feel more comfortable taking cholera vaccine when venturing to undeveloped African or Asian countries.

Meningitis

Meningitis vaccine is not routinely recommended for international travel. However, occasional epidemics in specific areas may necessitate its use in selected circumstances. For instance, the apparent outbreak of meningitis in Nepal has resulted in the recommendation that travelers to that kingdom should receive a single dose of bivalent A-C meningitis vaccine.

Yellow Fever

Yellow Fever, transmitted by the *Aedes aegypti* mosquito, occurs only in part of Africa and South America. Vaccination with yellow fever vaccine is required for travel to countries requiring an International Certificate of Vaccination and can be obtained in the United States at designated Yellow Fever Vaccination Centers. The location of the nearest Yellow Fever Vaccination Center may be obtained from local and state health departments.

Diphtheria/Tetanus

Diphtheria and tetanus remain serious health problems on a global scale. Booster doses of tetanus/diphtheria vaccine are recommended for all persons every 8 to 10 years, regardless of their travel status.

Polio

Though no longer a problem in this country, poliomyelitis continues to be endemic in many undeveloped countries. Fully immunized persons should be given one dose of polio vaccine before traveling to such areas, and previously unvaccinated persons should complete a primary series. For adults, the use of inactivated polio vaccine is preferred over oral polio vaccine because of the slightly increased risk of vaccine-induced paralysis with use of the live vaccine.

Malaria Prophylaxis

Malaria is probably the most common serious infectious disease in the world today. It is transmitted by the Anopheles mosquito. Chloroquine phosphate (Aralen), 300 mg base (500 mg salt) orally, once weekly, started 1 to 2 weeks prior to travel and continued for 6 weeks after return provides effective prophylaxis against *Plasmodium vivax* and chloroquine-sensitive *Plasmodium falciparum.* Fansidar (pyrimethamine-sulfadoxine) has been used to protect against chloroquine-resistant *Plasmodium falciparum.* However, incidence of severe, sometimes fatal mucocutaneous reactions and of severe liver disease in some who have taken Fansidar has prompted the Centers for Disease Control to revise the recommendations for the prophylactic use of this drug.[4] Now travelers who expect only short-term exposure of less than 3 weeks to resistant malaria forms should carry with them three Fansidar tablets to be taken at once if fever develops and there is no access to medical help. In all instances, it is important to emphasize the importance of protection from mosquitos such as insect repellant, sleep netting, and long-sleeve clothing.

Rabies

During trekking expeditions, local animals should be avoided, as rabies is prevalent in many economically developing countries. Rabies vaccine developed in human diploid cell lines has been shown to elicit effective neutralizing antibody response against the virus. Postexposure vaccination has been the recommended approach for persons at low risk of rabies exposure in the United States.[9] However, pre-exposure immunization with human diploid cell rabies vaccine may offer protection to those who are at risk for inapparent exposure or delays in postexposure treatment. For many years human diploid cell rabies vaccine has been used without significant untoward effects for pre-exposure vaccination of United States Peace Corps volunteers assigned to endemic areas.[5] In view of the remoteness from medical facili-

ties of many trails in underdeveloped countries, pre-exposure vaccination should be considered for all trekkers going to rabies-endemic areas. It is vitally important to point out, however, that pre-exposure vaccination has not been proven to be completely protective; so any trekker in a rabies-endemic area who suffers an animal bite, whether or not he or she has been pre-immunized, should be managed by thorough cleansing of the wound and immediate evacuation to the nearest facility to begin the recommended procedure of prophylactic vaccination and administration of rabies immune globulin.[9] A final caveat is that recent observations and vaccination research have called into question the effectiveness of human diploid cell rabies vaccination of persons receiving chloroquine doses for malaria prophylaxis.[12] The final resolution of this dilemma has yet to unfold.

Common Problems

The majority of medical problems arising in the course of trekking are minor in nature but may cause concern because of their occurrence in unfamiliar, remote locations. Good foot care is essential (see Chapter 17). The trekker is advised to have well-broken-in hiking boots. The feet should be kept dry and the socks frequently changed in order to prevent blisters. Muscle aches and strains are common during the first few days out and may be managed by rest, stretching, warm soaks, and aspirin. Small wounds can be treated in the conventional manner. It is probably best not to attempt primary closure of larger lacerations in the field, but rather, they should be cleansed as well as possible and then kept covered with a dry, sterile dressing. Sunburn and actinic burns to the eyes are more common at high altitude, because of increased exposure to ultraviolet radiation and reflection from ice and snow (see Chapter 17). The tendency to sunburn may be enhanced in those who use doxycycline as prophylaxis against traveler's diarrhea. Protective sunscreens and appropriate sunglasses should be used. Persons requiring prescription eyeglasses should carry a spare pair, and because the care of contact lenses may be difficult in trekking situations, the user should also have a back-up pair of prescription eyeglasses.

Traveler's Diarrhea

Diarrhea is probably the most common affliction that the trekker may encounter (see Chapter 16). Although the disease is generally not serious, it is at best inconvenient and in some instances may cause significant dehydration. Prevention is the best measure. Uncooked fruits and vegetables and suspect water sources must be avoided. The trekker is advised to purify his or her own water supply by the method to be described below.

Although routine antibiotic prophylaxis against traveler's diarrhea is sometimes discouraged, I continue to prefer the use of chemoprophylaxis, because the occurrence of diarrhea could impair the trekker's ability to move the usual 6 to 12 miles a day with the group in remote terrain. If the illness does occur, recommended treatment schedules include (1) limiting the diet to clear liquids, (2) avoiding antimotility agents until absolutely necessary, and (3) using an effective antimicrobial agent. One trimethoprim sulfa double-strength tablet daily or one 100 mg of doxycycline daily should suffice. Neither of these medications should be continued for more than 3 weeks, and the user should be aware of the possible untoward side effects, including photosensitivity, skin rashes, and vaginal infections.[3]

Water Purification

For those venturing to remote and underdeveloped areas to engage in mountaineering or wilderness activities, the safety of the drinking water is of critical concern. Consideration should even be given to disinfecting water obtained from the "pristine and pure" streams of New England and the Adirondacks, where in recent years, some rural communities have had outbreaks of giardiasis apparently caused by contamination of their water sources by animal vectors (see Chapter 16).

Several methods of water purification are available. Boiling water in a wilderness situation is time consuming, and the efficacy of water coming to a boil at lower temperatures at high altitude is questionable. Chlorine products have enjoyed wide popularity, but they are not really suitable to wilderness situations because of their impaired efficacy due to temperature, pH changes, and particulate matter.

I favor using saturated aqueous iodine solution as described by Kahn and Visscher.[11] We have used this method on several expeditions to the Himalayas and found it convenient and effective. The method is as follows: Four to 6 g of resublimed iodine crystals are placed in a 1-ounce (30-ml) clear glass bottle with a Bakelite top from which the metal liner has been removed. The bottle is filled with water and shaken vigorously, producing a tea-colored solution as the crystals resettle on the bottom. At a temperature of 20°C (68°F) an iodine concentration of 9 mg per liter will be reached. To disinfect one liter of water, 12.5 ml of this solution is carefully poured into a poly-bottle containing 1 liter of the water to be purified. When decanting the prepared iodine solution, care should be taken not to allow the crystals to flow out, though there is no health risk from accidentally ingesting a few crystals. Metal containers should not be used, because a toxic reaction may take place between the iodine solution and metal. After about 1 half hour, the disinfected canteen will have an iodine concentration that has destroyed bacteria, viruses, parasites, and parasitic cysts. Longer contact times are required at cold temperatures and to eradiate giardial cysts. Water should be added to the stock iodine solution to bring the volume back up to 30 ml. This amount of iodine can handle about 500 liters of water. As long as crystals are visible at the bottom of the bottle, they are sufficient for use.

Cold Injuries and High Altitude

The medical problems of high altitude, hypothermia, and frostbite are covered in more detail elsewhere in this volume (see Chapters 17, 18, 42, and 44). Hypothermia, defined as a core body temperature of less than 35°C (95°F) occurs when factors contributing to heat loss exceed the physiologic mechanisms of heat production. Conduction, convection, radiation, evaporation, and respiration are the principal sources of heat loss. These are influenced by both intrinsic and extrinsic factors. Metabolic processes of heat production as well as exercise capability and shivering can be impaired by disease processes and nutritional status. The pathophysiologic consequences of hypothermia involve the cardiovascular, respiratory, and neuromuscular systems and are associated with metabolic and respiratory acidosis. Manifestations of altitude sickness can further complicate associated hypothermia.

The trekker at moderately high altitudes (3000 meters/10,000 feet) may be prone to various manifestations of acute mountain sickness (AMS), high-altitude pulmonary edema (HAPE), and high-altitude cerebral edema (HACE) (see Chapters 42 and 44). These several forms of altitude sickness vary in their onset and mode of presentation, depending upon the rate and method of mountain ascent, the altitude reached, and the presence or absence of dehydration and hypothermia.

The symptoms of each syndrome of altitude sickness overlap, but they include headache, insomnia, mental aberrations, loss of coordination, weakness, anorexia, nausea, vomiting, and respiratory difficulties. At high altitude, a proportionally greater amount of heat is lost from the lungs during the process of warming and humidifying cold dry air. Although the exact pathophysiology of altitude illness is unknown, it is postulated that the hypoxia common to all forms of mountain sickness interferes with the cellular adenosine triphosphate (ATP)—the oxygen-dependent "sodium pump."[8] Intracellular sodium retention and osmotic swelling occur, and symptoms develop depending upon the location and degree of swelling of the cells involved.

The only definitive treatment of mountain sickness is immediate descent to a lower altitude. However, it may be prevented by an ascent slow enough to achieve adequate acclimatization. The degree of physical fitness is no protection against altitude sickness. Acetazolamide (Diamox) taken before going to altitude may prevent some of the symptoms of acute mountain sickness without impairing the subsequent physiologic adjustment to high altitude, but its routine use is not recommended.[7]

Trip Physician and Medical Kit

The physician on a trek should be flexible and have the ability to improvise. He or she should have a good sense of humor and the ability to cope with the unexpected. A medical kit suitable for trekking can be packaged in a variety of ways. A large fishing tackle box with tiered trays and a large bottom bay has been found to be useful. Larger items, such as stethoscope, blood pressure cuff, otoscope, ophthalmoscope, and bandages, are stored in the lower bay. Other supplies and medications are displayed for easy access in the upper tiers. The basic list of medications includes aspirin, a codeine-containing analgesic, and a selection of antibiotics and antispasmodics. Indispensable is a copy of *Medicine for Mountaineering*, edited by James A. Wilkerson, M.D.,[13] which is currently in its third edition.

Posttrek

Most persons return from their trekking experience relaxed, healthy, and fit. A patient presenting to a physician with an unexplained illness following a trek or an adventure travel experience should be questioned closely about the exposures encountered along the way. Conditions that should be considered may include hepatitis, malaria, and parasitic disorders such as giardiasis.

WINTER CAMPING

The appeal of winter camping lies in the beauty of the winter wilderness and the freedom from crowds, summer insects, heat, and humidity. To these are added the risk and challenge of activities in a harsh, cold environment, which make winter camping a true adventure experience.

The winter camping group should make provision for proper nutrition and maintenance of hydration (see Chapter 43). Shelter and sleeping bags should be selected to meet and exceed the anticipated temperature extremes. The winter camper should be fully aware of the hazards involved in this sport and should be prepared to anticipate and prevent frostbite and hypothermia (see Chapter 18).

Hypothermia can occur insidiously, when the body loses heat at a rate beyond that which it can produce. Exposure to wind and wetness, fatigue, and inadequate protection can predispose to its onset. A sensation of feeling cold and the onset of shivering may be the first and only indications of hypothermia. These symptoms may be accompanied or rapidly followed by a subtle lapse of judgment (e.g., dropping a hat or glove and failing to retrieve it, or an inappropriate expression of bravado or despair). Uncontrollable shivering, accompanied by further intellectual impairment may then occur. As hypothermia progresses, shivering will cease and the hypothermic person will lapse into unconsciousness. At this point the victim is at severe risk of death unless appropriate intervention occurs (see Chapter 18).

Frostbite is the actual freezing of cellular tissues, accompanied by the shifting of blood flow to vital tissues (see Chapter 18). Exposed areas, including the ears, nose, cheeks, fingers, and toes, are usually involved. Unless frostbite is recognized early, serious damage and loss of tissue can occur. To prevent frostbite, one should make sure that footwear is not too tight. Too many layers of socks can impair the circulation and result in frostbite of the feet. Spraying the feet with an ultradry deodorant daily for 3 to 5 days prior to an outing will effectively eliminate foot perspiration, and dry feet are warm feet (see Chapter 17). When camping and hiking in the cold, the outdoorsperson should always be able to feel the toes. If the toes cannot be felt, the boots should be removed and the toes inspected. Mittens are generally more effective than gloves in keeping hands warm. Finally, wearing pierced earrings in the cold is to be avoided. The metal posts predispose to frostbite of the ear lobes.

The secret of staying warm and safe in cold winter activities is to stay dry! For this, knowledge and proper use of clothing is essential. Polypropylene underwear should be worn as a base. This allows moisture (perspiration) to be passed from the skin to the next layers of clothing, which should be wool or pile garments that can be easily opened and/or shed as the situation dictates. Because physical activity generates body heat, time should be taken to "layer down," so that none of the clothing becomes wet. It is always a good idea to carry some extra dry gear, such as a sweater, gloves, socks, and a hat. The outer garment should be made of a windproof, waterproof shell material such as Gortex. A hat is important, as 50 percent of the body's heat can be lost from the scalp. Hence, the mountaineer's dictum "When your feet are cold, put on your hat!"

Finally, a stalled car on a cold winter's night can ruin the whole next day and cause one to put off thoughts of pleasant days spent among snow-clad trees in the mountains. For those who engage in winter wilderness activities, I would just like to suggest keeping the following items in the automobile trunk: (1) a sleeping bag rated to 0°F (− 17.8°C), (2) a milk crate containing (a) jumper cables, (b) starting fluid, (c) tire inflator, (d) road flares, (e) rain gear, (f) hat, gloves, sweater, waterproof boots, wind shell, and space blanket, (g) headlamp-type flashlight, which allows use of the hands while providing light, (h) windproof/waterproof matches and candles, (i) candy bars or granola bars and a couple of cans of soup, and (j) some loose change just in case there is a phone booth handy!

CONCLUSION

Mountain trekking, winter camping, hiking, and snowshoeing are rapidly becoming among the most popular participatory winter sports. The beauty and thrill of these activities can provide a sense of high adventure and many evenings of lingering impressions for years to come. But to avoid and rectify bad situations that could lead to serious untoward results and even the tragedy of permanent illness, injury, or death, participants, group leaders, physicians, and other health care providers involved in these activities should be aware of their inherent risks and be prepared to prevent and deal with them.

REFERENCES

1. Auerbach, PS: Travelers diarrhea. Wilderness Medicine Conference. University of California, San Diego School of Medicine, Showmass, CO, 1987.
2. Bezrcuhka, SA: A Guide to Trekking in Nepal, ed 5. Sahayaha Press, Kathmandu, 1985.
3. CDC Health Information for the International Traveler: Public Health Service, United States Department of Health and Human Services, Publication No. (CDC) 85-8280, Atlanta, 1985.
4. Centers for Disease Control: Revised recommendations for preventing malaria in travelers to areas with chloroquine-resistant *Plasmodium falciparum*. MMWR 34:185–190, 1985.
5. Fishbein, DB, Viral and Rickettsian Zoonosis Branch, Centers for Disease Control: Personal communication, Atlanta, 1987.
6. Francis, DP, Feorino, PM, McDougal, S, Warfield, D, Getchell, J, Cabradilla, C, Tony, M, Miller, WJ, Schultz, LD, Bailey, FJ, McAleer, WJ, Scolnick, EM, and Ellis, RW: The safety of hepatitis B vaccine: Inactivation of the AIDS virus during routine vaccine manufacture. JAMA 256:869–872, 1986.

7. Hackett, PH and Rennie, D: Acute mountain sickness. Sem Respir Med 5:132–140, 1983.

8. Houston, CS: Going Higher: The Story of Man and Altitude, ed 3. Little, Brown & Co, Boston, 1987, pp 181–185.

9. Immunization Practices Advisory Committee: Rabies prevention—United States, 1984. MMWR 33:393–402, 407–408, 1984.

10. Immunization Practices Advisory Committee: Update on hepatitis B prevention. MMWR 36:353–366, 1987.

11. Kahn, FH and Visscher, BR: Water disinfection in the wilderness. Western Journal of Medicine 122:450–453, 1975.

12. Pappaianou, M, Fishbein, DB, Dreesen, DW, Schwartz, IR, Campbell, GH, Sumner, JW, Patchen, LC, and Brown, WJ: Antibody response to pre-exposure human-diploid cell rabies vaccine given concurrently with chloroquine. N Engl J Med 314:280–284, 1986.

13. Wilkerson, JA: Medicine for Mountaineering, ed 3. The Mountaineers, Seattle, 1985.

Index

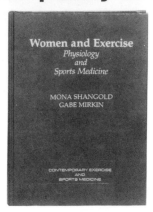

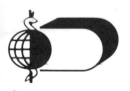

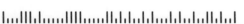